Applied
Laboratory Medicine

with contributions by

Naif Z. Abraham, Jr.
Kenneth B. Ain
Ted L. Anderson
Dean A. Arvan
David N. Bailey
William F. Balistreri
Drora Berkowitz
Robert V. Blanke
Donald C. Bondy
William Z. Borer
Emmanuel L. Bravo
Nausherwan K. Burki
Robert M. Carey
Michael L. Cibull
Rex B. Conn
Marcel E. Conrad
Avram M. Cooperman
Gibbons G. Cornwell, III
Carol M. Cottril
Susan Cox
William Eugene Davis
Paul D. DePriest
David G. Elliott
Z. Myron Falchuk
Jerome M. Feldman
Susan A. Fuhrman
Holly Gallion
Joseph M. Gertner
Fred Gorstein
George F. Gray, Jr.
Philip R. Greipp
Gordon P. Guthrie
A. Ralph Henderson
Steven L. Hoover
Douglas W. Huestis
Zilla Huma
Eric L. Hume

John C. Hunsaker, III
C. Darrell Jennings
Jamshed F. Kanga
Dennis G. Karounos
Michael J. Kelner
John A. Koepke
Paul A. Luce
Patricia L. Mann
Ewa Marciniak
Richard A. Mc Pherson
William E. Neeley
Douglas A. Nelson
Kevin R. Nelson
Robert C. Noble
William N. O'Connor
Anjana Lal Pettigrew
Jonathan E. Plehn
William H. Porter
Deborah E. Powell
Elizabeth L. Pruden
Larry E. Puls
Dennis Ross
Albert I. Rubenstone
H. William Schnaper
Douglas J. Schneider
Margie A. Scott
Steven I. Shedlofsky
Denise F. Shuey
Mikel D. Smith
Phyllis W. Speiser
John C. Spinosa
Lisa A. Sprague
Evan A. Stein
Michael W. Stelling
J. R. van Nagell, Jr.
Nelson B. Watts
Ronald J. Whitley

Applied

Laboratory
Medicine

Editor:

NORBERT W. TIETZ
Professor, Department of Pathology and Laboratory Medicine
Director, Division of Clinical Chemistry
University of Kentucky Medical Center
Lexington, Kentucky

Associate Editors:

REX B. CONN
Director, Clinical Laboratories, Thomas Jefferson University Hospital
Professor and Vice-Chairman, Department of Pathology
Thomas Jefferson University
Philadelphia, Pennsylvania

ELIZABETH L. PRUDEN
Clinical Chemist, Diagnostic Pathology, Schumpert Medical Center
Associate Professor, Graduate School, Louisiana State University
Shreveport, Louisiana

W.B. SAUNDERS COMPANY
Harcourt Brace Jovanovich, Inc.
Philadelphia   London   Toronto   Montreal   Sydney   Tokyo

W. B. SAUNDERS COMPANY
Harcourt Brace Jovanovich, Inc.

The Curtis Center
Independence Square West
Philadelphia, Pennsylvania 19106

Library of Congress Cataloging-in-Publication Data

Applied laboratory medicine / editor, Norbert W. Tietz; associate editors, Rex B. Conn, Elizabeth L Pruden.

p. cm.

ISBN 0–7216–6474–1

1. Diagnosis, Laboratory.   I. Tietz, Norbert W.
   II. Conn, Rex B.   III. Pruden, Elizabeth L.

[DNLM: 1. Diagnosis, Laboratory. QY 4 A652]

RB37.A715 1992

616′.07′56—dc20

DNLM/DLC

for Library of Congress   92-13381

Editor: Joan T. Meyer
Cover Designer: Joan Wendt
Production Manager: Peter Faber
Manuscript Editor: RoseMarie Klimowicz
Indexer: Angela Holt

Applied Laboratory Medicine   ISBN 0–7216–6474–1

Copyright © 1992 by W. B. Saunders Company

All rights reserved. No part of this publication may be reproduced or transmitted in any form or by any means, electronic or mechanical, including photocopy, recording, or any information storage and retrieval system, without permission in writing from the publisher.

Printed in Mexico.

Last digit is the print number: 9   8   7   6   5   4   3   2   1

In thankfulness dedicated to

MY WIFE GERTRUD

and to my children

MARGARET ANN, KURT RICHARD,

ANNETTE MARIE *and* MICHAEL GERHARD

and to

JUDY *and* JON

Acknowledgments

I would like to express my thanks to all contributors who submitted so willingly to the editorial process and adhered to a relatively tight production schedule. Their understanding and cooperation made this book possible.

My special thanks goes to the associate editors, Rex B. Conn, M.D., and Elizabeth L. Pruden, Ph.D., and to the various reviewers who gave me significant support in the editing process and who made many valuable contributions.

Ms. Patricia L. Mann, B.A., was responsible for the layout and typesetting, as well as general editorial assistance. Ms. Norma Stewart supported our efforts by typing manuscripts, and Ms. Denise F. Shuey, B.H.S., gave us general support. Their contributions are greatly appreciated and have made it a pleasure to work on this book project.

The effort and cooperation of the staff of W. B. Saunders Company, especially of Joan Meyer, Medical Editor, are gratefully acknowledged.

Norbert W. Tietz
Editor

Contributors and Reviewers

Naif Z. Abraham, Jr., M.D., Ph.D.
Hematopathology Fellow, Department of Pathology, SUNY Health Science Center, Syracuse, NY
Case 46, A Woman with Fatigue and Pallor (Pernicious Anemia)

Kenneth B. Ain, M.D.
Assistant Professor of Medicine, Division of Endocrinology and Metabolism, Department of Medicine, University of Kentucky Medical Center; Veterans Administration Medical Center, Lexington, KY
Case 23, Anterior Neck Mass (Graves' Disease); Case 24, The Fatigued Attorney (Hashimoto's Thyroiditis); Case 25, The Reluctant Chef (Medullary Thyroid Carcinoma)

Ted L. Anderson, Ph.D.
Shapiro Scholar, Department of Pathology, Vanderbilt University Medical School, Nashville, TN
Case 28, Woman with Irregular Menses, Hirsutism, and Depression (Adenoma of the Pituitary with Cushing's Disease)

Dean A. Arvan, M.D.
Professor, Department of Pathology and Laboratory Medicine, University of Rochester; Director, Clinical Laboratories, Strong Memorial Hospital, Rochester, NY
Case 63, Child with Lethargy and Coma (Reye's Syndrome)

David N. Bailey, M.D.
Professor and Chairman, Department of Pathology, University of California at San Diego; Director of Clinical Laboratories, UCSD Medical Center, San Diego, CA
Invited Reviewer

William F. Balistreri, M.D.
Professor of Pediatrics and Medicine, Dorothy M. M. Kersten Professor of Pediatrics, Department of Pediatrics, University of Cincinnati College of Medicine; Director, Division of Pediatric Gastroenterology and Nutrition, Children's Hospital Medical Center, Cincinnati, OH
Case 21, Persistent Jaundice in Infant (Extrahepatic Biliary Atresia)

Drora Berkowitz, M.D.
Fellow, Division of Pediatric Gastroenterology and Nutrition, Children's Hospital Medical Center, Cincinnati, OH
Case 21, Persistent Jaundice in Infant (Extrahepatic Biliary Atresia)

Robert V. Blanke, Ph.D.
Professor, Department of Pathology; Affiliate Professor, Department of Pharmacology and Toxicology, Medical College of Virginia, Virginia Commonwealth University; Consultant Toxicologist, Richmond, VA
Case 60, High Anion-Gap Acidosis with High Osmolal Gap (Ethylene Glycol Poisoning); Case 61, An Anemic Child from an Upper Middle-Class Family (Lead Poisoning)

Donald C. Bondy, M.D.
Professor, Department of Medicine, University of Western Ontario; Chief, Department of Gastroenterology, University Hospital, London, Ontario, Canada
Case 20, Woman with Chronic Diarrhea and Weight Loss (Diarrhea)

William Z. Borer, M.D.
Director of Clinical Chemistry and Toxicology, Department of Pathology and Cell Biology, Thomas Jefferson University Hospital, Philadelphia, PA
Introduction: Selection and Use of Laboratory Tests

Emmanuel L. Bravo, M.D.
Head, Department of Heart and Hypertension, Research Institute; Staff, Cleveland Clinic Foundation, Cleveland, OH
Case 31, Weakness, Weight Loss, and Hypotension (Chronic Adrenal Insufficiency)

Nausherwan K. Burki, M.D.
Professor, Department of Medicine, University of Kentucky College of Medicine; Chief, Division of Pulmonary and Critical Care Medicine, University of Kentucky Medical Center; Staff, Veterans Administration Medical Center; Staff, Humana Hospital, Lexington, KY
Case 4, Shortness of Breath with Productive Cough (Chronic Obstructive Pulmonary Disease)

Robert M. Carey, M.D.
Dean and James Carroll Flippin Professor of Medical Science, University of Virginia School of Medicine, Charlottesville, VA
Case 27, Sudden Onset of Polyuria and Polydipsia (Hypothalamic Cushing's Syndrome)

Michael L. Cibull, M.D.
Associate Professor, Department of Pathology and Laboratory Medicine, University of Kentucky Medical Center; Director, Surgical Pathology, University of Kentucky Medical Center, Lexington, KY
Case 32, Boy with Thick Lips (MEN 3)

Rex B. Conn, M.D.
Professor and Vice-Chairman, Department of Pathology, Jefferson Medical College of Thomas Jefferson University; Director, Clinical Laboratories, Thomas Jefferson University Hospital, Philadelphia, PA
Case 9, A 35-Year-Old Man with Fulminant Liver Failure (Hepatitis D); Case 10, A Nurse with Metastatic Cancer (Hepatocellular Carcinoma)
Associate Editor

Marcel E. Conrad, M.D.
Professor of Medicine and Pathology, University of South Alabama; Director, USA Cancer Center; Director, Division of Hematology and Oncology, University of South Alabama Medical Center, Mobile, AL
Case 47, Pneumona, Leukopenia, and Ecchymoses (Acute Promyelocytic Leukemia)

Avram M. Cooperman, M.D.
Professor of Surgery, New York Medical College, Valhalla, NY; Director of Surgery, St. Clare's Hospital, New York, NY
Case 14, Patient with Abdominal Pain (Cholelithiasis)

Gibbons G. Cornwell, III, M.D.
Professor of Medicine and Pathology, Director of Clinical Cancer Research Program, Norris Cotton Cancer Center, Dartmouth-Hitchcock Medical Center; Staff Hematologist, Staff Clinical Pathologist, Mary Hitchcock Memorial Hospital, Hanover, NH
Case 65, Heart Failure in a Middle-Aged Woman (Primary Amyloidosis)

Carol M. Cottrill, M.D.
Professor of Pediatrics (Cardiology), University of Kentucky College of Medicine; Medical Director, Pediatric Intensive Care Unit; Director, Pediatric Cardiac Catheterization Laboratory, University of Kentucky Medical Center, Lexington, KY
Case 1, Child with Heart Murmur and Cyanosis (Congenital Heart Disease); Case 22, A Three-Week-Old Infant with Vomiting (Pyloric Stenosis)

Susan Cox, M.D.
Associate Professor of Maternal-Fetal Medicine, Department of Obstetrics and Gynecology, University of Kentucky College of Medicine; Director, Maternal-Fetal Medicine, University of Kentucky Medical Center, Lexington, KY
Case 38, Pregnancy Complicated by Abdominal Pain (Pregnancy with Sickle Cell Crisis)

William Eugene Davis, M.D.
Clinical Assistant Professor of Medicine, Department of Internal Medicine, Tulane University Medical Center; Staff Clinician, Department of Internal Medicine, Section of Rheumatology, Ochsner Clinic and Foundation Hospital, New Orleans, LA
Case 66, A Man with Fever and Acute Polyarthritis (Gout)

Paul D. DePriest, M.D.
Assistant Professor, Department of Obstetrics and Gynecology, Division of GYN Oncology, University of Kentucky College of Medicine, Lexington, KY
Case 42, Woman with Abdominal Distention (Ovarian Cancer)

David G. Elliott, M.D.
Resident Physician, Department of Pathology, University of Kentucky College of Medicine, Lexington, KY
Case 30, Middle-Aged Man with Weakness and Weight Gain (Lung Tumor with Cushing's Syndrome)

Z. Myron Falchuk, M.D.
Associate Professor, Department of Medicine, Harvard Medical School; Physician, Medical Service, New England Deaconess Hospital, Boston, MA
Case 19, Recurrent Diarrhea (Gluten-sensitive Enteropathy)

Jerome M. Feldman, M.D.
Associate Professor, Department of Medicine, Duke University Medical School; Attending Physician, Duke University Hospital; Chief, Endocrinology and Metabolism Section, Durham Veterans Administration Hospital, Durham, NC
Case 37, Woman with Facial Flushing (Carcinoid Syndrome)

Susan A. Fuhrman, M.D.
Assistant Professor, Department of Laboratory Medicine and Pathology; Director of Pathology Education; Director of Critical Care, Chemistry Laboratory, University of Minnesota Hospital and Clinics, Minneapolis, MN
Case 33, A Woman with Psychosis and Hypercalcemia (Primary Hyperparathyroidism); Case 68, Child with Nausea and Vomiting Eight Days Post-Craniotomy (SIADH)
Invited Reviewer

Holly Gallion, M.D.
Associate Professor, Department of Obstetrics and Gynecology, University of Kentucky College of Medicine, Lexington, KY
Case 39, Woman with Amenorrhea (Gestational Trophoblastic Neoplasia)

Joseph M. Gertner, M.B., M.R.C.P.
Professor, Department of Pediatrics, Cornell University Medical College; Attending Pediatrician, New York Hospital-Cornell Medical Center, New York, NY
Case 70, Gait Disturbance after Extensive Bowel Resection (Rickets)

Fred Gorstein, M.D.
Chairman and Professor, Department of Pathology, Vanderbilt University Medical Center; Pathologist-in-Chief, Vanderbilt University Hospital, Nashville, TN
Invited Reviewer

George F. Gray, Jr., M.D.
Professor, Department of Pathology, Vanderbilt University Medical Center; Director of Surgical Pathology, Vanderbilt University Medical Center, Nashville, TN
Case 17, Woman with Jaundice (Carcinoma of the Ampulla of Vater)

Philip R. Greipp, M.D.
Professor of Medicine, Division of Hematology and Internal Medicine; Cell Kinetics Laboratory, Department of Laboratory Medicine and Pathology, Mayo Clinic, Rochester, MN
Case 50, Patient with Pleuritic Pain and Hypergammaglobulinemia (Multiple Myeloma)

Gordon P. Guthrie, M.D.
Professor, Department of Medicine, University of Kentucky College of Medicine; Director, Division of Endocrinology and Metabolism, University of Kentucky Medical Center, Lexington, KY
Case 35, Episodic Hypertension (Pheochromocytoma)

A. Ralph Henderson, M.B., Ch.B., Ph.D.
Professor, Department of Biochemistry, University of Western Ontario; Chief, Department of Clinical Biochemistry, University Hospital, London, Ontario, Canada
Case 16, Severe Epigastric Pain (Acute Pancreatitis); Case 36, Diarrhea and Gastrointestinal Hemorrhage (Zollinger-Ellison Syndrome); Case 64, Low Back Pain (Prostatic Carcinoma)

Steven L. Hoover, M.D.
Clinical Neurophysiology Fellow, Department of Neurology, University of Kentucky College of Medicine, Lexington, KY
Case 52, Acute Hemiparesis (Multiple Sclerosis)

Douglas W. Huestis, M.D.
Professor, Department of Pathology; Chief, Transfusion Medicine, University of Arizona College of Medicine, Tucson, AZ
Case 40, A Healthy Multiparous Woman Whose Babies Became Jaundiced (Rh Hemolytic Disease of the Newborn)

Zilla Huma, M.B., M.R.C.P.
Research Fellow, Department of Pediatric Endocrinology, Cornell University Medical College; Clinical Fellow, New York Hospital, New York, NY
Case 70, Gait Disturbance after Extensive Bowel Resection (Rickets)

Eric L. Hume, M.D.
Assistant Professor, Department of Orthopedic Surgery, Jefferson Medical College; Director of Bone Center; Director of Trauma, Thomas Jefferson University Hospital, Philadelphia, PA
Case 69, An Elderly Woman with Bilateral Hip Pain (Osteoporosis)

John C. Hunsaker, III, J.D., M.D.
Associate Professor, Department of Pathology and Laboratory Medicine; Director, Forensic Pathology, University of Kentucky College of Medicine; Associate Chief Medical Examiner, Kentucky Justice Cabinet, Lexington, KY
Case 67, Sudden Death of a Cocaine Addict in Police Custody (Accidental Death due to Cocaine)

C. Darrell Jennings, M.D.
Associate Professor, Department of Pathology and Laboratory Medicine; Director of Immunopathology, University of Kentucky College of Medicine; Associate Director of Clinical Laboratories, University of Kentucky Medical Center, Lexington, KY
Case 5, Oliguria with Metabolic Acidosis after Renal Transplantation (Renal Tubular Acidosis after Renal Transplantation); Case 6, Man with Hypertension and Fever (Acute Tubular Necrosis); Case 7, Glomerulonephritis, Uremia, Pulmonary Infiltration, and Hemoptysis (Acute Glomerulonephritis and Uremic Syndrome)

Jamshed F. Kanga, M.D.
Associate Professor, Department of Pediatrics, University of Kentucky College of Medicine; Chief, Division of Pulmonology, University of Kentucky Medical Center, Lexington, KY
Case 3, Child with Recurrent Pneumonia, Anemia, and Failure to Thrive (Cystic Fibrosis)

Dennis G. Karounos, M.D.
Assistant Professor, Division of Endocrinology and Metabolism, Department of Medicine, University of Kentucky College of Medicine, Lexington, KY
Case 18, Abdominal Pain and Polyuria (Diabetes Mellitus)

Michael J. Kelner, M.D.
Associate Professor, Department of Pathology, School of Medicine, University of California at San Diego; Associate Director, Clinical Chemistry and Toxicology, Division of Laboratory Medicine, UCSD Medical Center, San Diego, CA
Invited Reviewer

John A. Koepke, M.D.
Professor, Department of Pathology; Associate Professor, Division of Hematology/Oncology, Department of Medicine, Duke University School of Medicine; Medical Director, Clinical Hematology Laboratory, Duke University Medical Center, Durham, NC
Case 44, Woman with Anemia and Hypertension (Chronic Anemia); Case 45, Child with Pneumonia (Sickle Cell Disease)

Paul A. Luce, B.S.
Medical Student, Vanderbilt University School of Medicine, Nashville, TN
Case 17, Woman with Jaundice (Carcinoma of the Ampulla of Vater)

Patricia L. Mann, B.A.
Data Coordinator, Department of Pathology and Laboratory Medicine, University of Kentucky College of Medicine, Lexington, KY
Editorial Assistant and Compositor

Ewa Marciniak, M.D.

Professor, Department of Medicine, University of Kentucky College of Medicine; Director, Coagulation Laboratory, University of Kentucky Medical Center, Lexington, KY
Case 57, Woman with Malaise and Bleeding (Disseminated Intravascular Coagulopathy); Case 58, A Young Girl with Deep Vein Thrombosis and Abnormal Coagulation Tests (Systemic Lupus Erythematosus with Lupus Anticoagulant); Case 59, Medical Student with Mild Bleeding Disorder (Hemophilia)

Richard A. Mc Pherson, M.D.

Clinical Professor, Department of Pathology, University of California at San Diego; Director, Scripps Immunology Reference Laboratory, The Scripps Institute; Head, Laboratory Medicine, Department of Pathology, Scripps Clinic and Research Foundation, San Diego, CA
Case 49, A Case of Impotence and Progressive Fatigue (Hairy-Cell Leukemia)
Invited Reviewer

William E. Neeley, M.D.

Associate Professor, Department of Laboratory Medicine, Yale School of Medicine, New Haven; Chief, Laboratory Services, Department of Veterans Affairs Medical Center, West Haven, CT
Invited Reviewer

Douglas A. Nelson, M.D.

Professor, Department of Pathology, State University of New York Health Science Center at Syracuse; Attending Pathologist and Director of Hematology Section, Division of Clinical Pathology, University Hospital, SUNY-Health Science Center at Syracuse, Syracuse, NY
Case 46, A Woman with Fatigue and Pallor (Pernicious Anemia); Case 48, A Man with Splenomegaly (Chronic Myelogenous Leukemia)

Kevin R. Nelson, M.D.

Associate Professor, Department of Neurology, University of Kentucky College of Medicine; Director, Neuromuscular Program; Director, Electromyography/Nerve Conduction Study Laboratory, University of Kentucky Medical Center, Lexington, KY
Case 52, Acute Hemiparesis (Multiple Sclerosis)

Robert C. Noble, M.D.

Professor, Department of Medicine, University of Kentucky College of Medicine, Lexington, KY
Case 71, Persistent Cough and Dyspnea (Acquired Immune Deficiency Syndrome)

William N. O'Connor, M.D.

Director of Residency Training Program and Associate Professor, Department of Pathology and Laboratory Medicine, University of Kentucky College of Medicine; Director, Autopsy Service, University of Kentucky Medical Center, Lexington, KY
Case 1, Child with Heart Murmur and Cyanosis (Congenital Heart Disease); Case 2, Woman with Angina Pectoris (Myocardial Infarction)

Anjana Lal Pettigrew, M.D.

Assistant Professor, Departments of Pathology, Pediatrics, and Obstetrics and Gynecology, University of Kentucky College of Medicine; Director, Cytogenetics Laboratory, University of Kentucky Medical Center, Lexington, KY
Case 51, Pregnancy with Elevated Maternal Serum α-Fetoprotein (Neural Tube Defect)

Jonathan E. Plehn, M.D.

Associate Professor, Department of Medicine, Dartmouth Medical School; Director, Cardiac Ultrasound Laboratory, Dartmouth-Hitchcock Medical Center, Hanover, NH
Case 65, Heart Failure in a Middle-Aged Woman (Primary Amyloidosis)

William H. Porter, Ph.D.

Professor, Department of Pathology and Laboratory Medicine, University of Kentucky College of Medicine; Associate Director, Clinical Chemistry Laboratory, University of Kentucky Medical Center, Lexington, KY
Case 34, A Child with Osteopenia and Retarded Growth (Renal Osteodystrophy); Case 62, Suicide Attempt by Drug Overdose (Acetaminophen Intoxication)
Invited Reviewer

Deborah E. Powell, M.D.
Professor and Chairman, Department of Pathology and Laboratory Medicine, University of Kentucky College of Medicine, Lexington, KY
Case 41, Woman with a Family History of Breast Cancer (Breast Tumor); Case 43, Polydipsia, Polyuria, and a Perisellar Mass (Dysgerminoma)

Elizabeth L. Pruden, Ph.D.
Associate Professor, Graduate School, Louisiana State University; Consultant and Clinical Chemist, Diagnostic Pathology, Schumpert Medical Center, Shreveport, LA
Associate Editor

Larry E. Puls, M.D.
Fellow, Department of Obstetrics and Gynecology, University of Kentucky College of Medicine, Lexington, KY
Invited Reviewer

Dennis Ross, M.D., Ph.D.
Adjunct Professor, Department of Pathology, University of North Carolina-Chapel Hill; Pathologist, Forsyth Memorial Hospital, Winston-Salem, NC
Invited Reviewer

Albert I. Rubenstone, M.D.
Professor, Department of Pathology, Chicago Medical School; Chairman, Department of Pathology, Mount Sinai Hospital Medical Center, Chicago, IL
Case 13, Middle-Aged Alcoholic with Jaundice and Ascites (Cirrhosis)

H. William Schnaper, M.D.
Associate Professor, Department of Pediatrics, George Washington University; Department of Nephrology, Children's National Medical Center, Washington, DC
Case 8, Young Woman with Edema and Decreased Urine Output (Nephrotic Syndrome)

Douglas J. Schneider, M.D.
Resident Physician, Departments of Pediatrics and Internal Medicine, University of Kentucky College of Medicine, Lexington, KY
Case 22, A Three-Week-Old Infant with Vomiting (Pyloric Stenosis)

Margie A. Scott, M.D.
Pathology Housestaff, Department of Pathology, Vanderbilt University School of Medicine, Nashville, TN
Case 29, Intermittent Right Flank Pain (Adrenal Cortical Neoplasm)

Steven I. Shedlofsky, M.D.
Associate Professor, Department of Medicine and Graduate Center for Toxicology, University of Kentucky College of Medicine; Staff Gastroenterologist, Veterans Administration Hospital and University of Kentucky Medical Center, Lexington, KY
Case 11, Adult Male with New Onset Ascites (Genetic Hemochromatosis); Case 12, Adolescent Female with Tremor, Depression, and Hepatitis (Wilson's Disease); Case 13, Middle-Aged Alcoholic with Jaundice and Ascites (Cirrhosis); Case 15, Young Woman with Recurrent Abdominal Pain (Acute Intermittent Porphyria)
Invited Reviewer

Denise F. Shuey, B.H.S., M.T.(ASCP)
Research Assistant, Department of Pathology and Laboratory Medicine, University of Kentucky Medical Center, Lexington, KY
General Support

Mikel D. Smith, M.D.
Associate Professor of Medicine/Cardiology, Division of Cardiology; Associate Professor, Department of Medicine, University of Kentucky College of Medicine; Director of CV Training Program; Associate Director of Echocardiography Laboratory, University of Kentucky Medical Center, Lexington, KY
Case 2, Woman with Angina Pectoris (Myocardial Infarction)

Phyllis W. Speiser, M.D.
Associate Professor, Department of Pediatrics, Cornell University Medical College; Associate Program Director, Children's Clinical Research Center, New York, NY
Case 26, Child with Rapid Growth and Precocious Sexual Maturation (Congenital Adrenal Hyperplasia)

John C. Spinosa, M.D.
Fellow in Hematopathology, Department of Pathology, Scripps Clinic, The Scripps Research Institute, San Diego, CA
Case 49, A Case of Impotence and Progressive Fatigue (Hairy-Cell Leukemia)

Lisa A. Sprague, M.D.
Resident Physician, Department of Obstetrics and Gynecology, University of Kentucky College of Medicine, Lexington, KY
Case 38, Pregnancy Complicated by Abdominal Pain (Pregnancy with Sickle Cell Crisis)

Evan A. Stein, M.D., Ph.D.
Clinical Professor, Department of Pathology and Laboratory Medicine; Director, The Christ Hospital Cardiovascular Research Center; President, Medical Research Laboratories, Cincinnati, OH
Case 53, Young Man with Chest Pain (Familial Hypercholesterolemia); Case 54, Middle-Aged Woman with Recurrent Abdominal Pain (Familial Hypertriglyceridemia)

Michael W. Stelling, M.D.
Associate Professor, Department of Pediatrics, University of Kentucky College of Medicine; Pediatric Endocrinologist, University of Kentucky Medical Center, Lexington, KY
Invited Reviewer

Norbert W. Tietz, Ph.D.
Professor, Department of Pathology and Laboratory Medicine, University of Kentucky College of Medicine; Director of Clinical Chemistry, University of Kentucky Medical Center; Consultant, Veterans Administration Hospital, Lexington, KY
Editor

J. R. van Nagell, Jr., M.D.
Professor and Director, Division of GYN Oncology, Department of Obstetrics and Gynecology; American Cancer Society Professor of Clinical Oncology, University of Kentucky College of Medicine, Lexington, KY
Invited Reviewer

Nelson B. Watts, M.D.
Associate Professor of Medicine, Division of Endocrinology and Metabolism, Emory University School of Medicine, Atlanta, GA
Invited Reviewer

Ronald J. Whitley, Ph.D.
Associate Professor, Department of Pathology and Laboratory Medicine, University of Kentucky College of Medicine; Assistant Director, Clinical Chemistry Laboratory, University of Kentucky Medical Center, Lexington, KY
Case 32, Boy with Thick Lips (MEN 3); Case 55, Child with Recurrent Vomiting (Ornithine Transcarbamylase Deficiency); Case 56, Hyperactive Boy with Infantile Speech (Phenylketonuria)
Invited Reviewer

Preface

Over the last few decades there has been an information explosion in the field of Laboratory Medicine. This development has been triggered not only by the ever-growing increase in diagnostic knowledge and skills, but also by the impressive technological advances in diagnostic equipment and analytical techniques. These developments call for educational material that discusses the clinical aspects of diseases in the context of readily acquired diagnostic data. Only the synthesis of clinical, laboratory, and other diagnostic data can lead to an efficient and accurate diagnostic process and the subsequent treatment.

APPLIED LABORATORY MEDICINE provides teaching material geared predominantly toward the second-year medical student; however, this material should also be helpful for training of residents and even for continuing education of practicing physicians. The case studies provide a proper clinical setting for a thorough discussion of history, clinical evaluation, laboratory and other diagnostic data, differential diagnosis, definition of the disease, and principle of treatment. Material on microbiology, except for one case study on AIDS, is not included in this book, since this topic is generally taught in medical school in a course separate from that in Pathology or Laboratory Medicine.

Approaches for teaching Laboratory Medicine are undergoing revolutionary changes. "Problem-based learning" is rapidly supplementing traditional didactic teaching and in some schools has fully replaced the older teaching approaches. APPLIED LABORATORY MEDICINE is designed to support various teaching modes in the following ways:

>The material can be used for *programs that solely engage in problem-based learning*, since it provides an appropriate clinical setting characteristic for a given disease; it supplies the appropriate description of the diagnostic process; and it provides other background information essential for the medical student and, indeed, for the practicing physician.

>*Programs that supplement didactic teaching with problem-based learning* can use the text not only for the functions explained above but for supplementary reading for the didactic component of the teaching program.

>*Programs that engage in didactic teaching only*, particularly those heavily weighted toward anatomical pathology, will find the information most helpful to reinforce and supplement lecture material presented for Laboratory Medicine.

>*Graduates in medicine and practicing physicians* will find the information helpful to update their knowledge, since the material contains the latest diagnostic information and is supplemented with the most recent pertinent literature citations.

Contributors, the editorial staff, and invited reviewers have tried to present the material in a fashion that will live up to the requirements of modern teaching approaches. This process, however, is evolutionary and therefore subject to continuous change. We would appreciate receiving from teachers and students alike comments that will help us to streamline further the teaching approach and make future editions of this text most useful to our readership.

Norbert W. Tietz
Rex B. Conn
Elizabeth L. Pruden

Abbreviations

AAA	aromatic amino acids	anti-EBV	Epstein-Barr virus antibody
AAT	α_1-antitrypsin	anti-GBM	glomerular basement membrane antibodies
Ab	antibody		
(aB)	arterial blood	anti-HAV	hepatitis A virus antibody
ABO	one of 4 blood groups	anti-HBc	hepatitis B core antibody
ACHE	acetylcholinesterase	anti-HBe	hepatitis B e antibody
ACTH	adrenocorticotropic hormone; corticotropin	anti-HBs	hepatitis B surface antibody
		anti-HCV	hepatitis C virus antibody
ADH	antidiuretic hormone; vasopressin	anti-HDV	hepatitis D virus antibody
AFP	α-fetoprotein	anti-HIV	human immunodeficiency virus antibody
AHA	American Heart Association	anti-HSV1	*Herpes simplex* virus 1 antibody
AIDS	acquired immune deficiency syndrome	anti-HSV2	*Herpes simplex* virus 2 antibody
		anti-Rh$_O$(D)	antibody to Rh D antigen
AIP	acute intermittent porphyria	APL	acute promyelocytic leukemia
ALA	δ-aminolevulinic acid	Apo B100	apolipoprotein B100
ALA-D	δ-aminolevulinic acid dehydratase	Apo E	apolipoprotein E
ALD	alcoholic liver disease	ASO	antistreptolysin O
all-TRA	all-*trans* retinoic acid	AST	aspartate aminotransferase
ALP	alkaline phosphatase	ATN	acute tubular necrosis
ALT	alanine aminotransferase	(B)	whole blood
AMI	acute myocardial infarction	BAL	British anti-Lewisite
AML	acute myelogenous leukemia	BAO	basal acid output
AMP	adenosine monophosphate	BAS	bile acid sequestrant
ANA	antinuclear antibody	BCAA	branched-chain amino acids
anti-DNA	antibody to deoxyribonucleic acid	BH$_4$	tetrahydrobiopterin

b.i.d.	twice daily (*bis in die*)	CO_2	carbon dioxide
BPH	benign prostatic hyperplasia	COD	cause of death
BPM	beats per minute	COPD	chronic obstructive pulmonary disease
°C	degree Celsius	COPRO-O	coproporphyrinogen oxidase
C3	complement factor 3	CPPD	calcium pyrophosphate dihydrate
C4	complement factor 4	CRF	corticotropin-releasing factor
CA 125	cancer antigen 125	CRH	corticotropin-releasing hormone
CAH	congenital adrenal hyperplasia	Cr_S	serum creatinine
CALLA	common acute lymphoblastic leukemia-associated or CD10 antigen	Cr_U	urinary creatinine
$CaNa_2EDTA$	calcium disodium edetate	CSA	cyclosporine A
CAT	computed axial tomography	CSF	cerebrospinal fluid
Ca_U	urinary calcium	CT	calcitonin
CBC	complete blood count	CT	see CAT
2-CDA	2-chlorodeoxyadenosine	CYP21	gene detected in 21-hydroxylase deficiency
CDCA	chenodeoxycholic acid	d	day
CEA	carcinoembryonic antigen	DALA	δ-aminolevulinic acid
CEP	congenital erythropoietic porphyria	DCF	deoxycoformycin
CESD	cholesteryl ester storage disease	DDAVP	1-desamino-8-D-arginine vasopressin
CF	cystic fibrosis	DHPR	dihydropteridine reductase
CFTR	cystic fibrosis transmembrane regulatory protein	DI	diabetes insipidus
cGy	centigray	DIC	disseminated intravascular coagulopathy
CHF	congestive heart failure	D_LCO	carbon monoxide diffusing capacity
CK	creatine kinase	DKA	diabetic ketoacidosis
CK-BB	creatine kinase isoenzyme 1	DM	diabetes mellitus
CK-MB	creatine kinase isoenzyme 2	DNA	deoxyribonucleic acid
CML	chronic myelogenous leukemia	DVT	deep vein thrombosis
CMV	cytomegalovirus	ECG	electrocardiogram
CNS	central nervous system		

ECHO	enteric cytopathogenic human orphan (virus)	GC	gas chromatography
EGD	esophagogastroduodenoscopy	GFR	glomerular filtration rate
EGFR	epidermal growth factor receptors	GGT	γ-glutamyltransferase
		GH	genetic hemochromatosis
ELISA	enzyme-linked immunosorbent assay	GI	gastrointestinal
		Gla protein	osteocalcin
EMG	electromyography	G-6-PD	glucose-6-phosphate dehydrogenase
EPP	erythrocytic protoporphyria		
ER	estrogen receptors	GSE	gluten-sensitive enteropathy
ERCP	endoscopic retrograde cholangiopancreatography	GTN	gestational trophoblastic neoplasm
Ercs	erythrocytes	GTP-CH	guanosine triphosphate cyclohydrolase
ESR	erythrocyte sedimentation rate		
EtOH	ethanol	h	hour(s)
(F)	feces	HAV	hepatitis A virus
FA	fluorescent antibody	Hb	hemoglobin
FAB	French-American-British	Hb A	hemoglobin A
FDA	Food and Drug Administration	Hb A$_1$	subspecies of hemoglobin A
FDP	fibrin degradation products	Hb A$_2$	subspecies of hemoglobin A
FEP	free erythrocyte protoporphyrin	Hb C	hemoglobin C
FEV$_1$	forced expired volume in one second	Hb D	hemoglobin D
		Hb F	hemoglobin F; fetal hemoglobin
FH	familial hypercholesterolemia	Hb S	hemoglobin S
FHTG	familial hypertriglyceridemia	Hb SS	hemoglobin SS; sickle cell disease
FI O$_2$	fraction of inspired oxygen		
FNA	fine-needle aspiration	HBcAg	hepatitis B core antigen
FRC	functional residual capacity	HBeAg	hepatitis B virus e antigen
FSH	follicle-stimulating hormone; follitropin	HBsAg	hepatitis B surface antigen
		HBV	hepatitis B virus
FTI	free thyroxine index	HCC	hepatocellular carcinoma
FVC	forced vital capacity	hCG	human chorionic gonadotropin
GABA	γ-aminobutyric acid	β-hCG	human chorionic gonadotropin, β-subunit

HCL	hairy-cell leukemia	IL-2	interleukin-2
HCP	hereditary coproporphyria	IM	intramuscular
HCV	hepatitis C virus	IMP	inosine monophosphate
HD	hemodialysis	IRMA	immunoradiometric assay
HDL	high-density lipoprotein	IQ	intelligence quotient
HDV	hepatitis D virus (delta agent)	IU	international unit
HEV	hepatitis E virus	IV	intravenous
5-HIAA	5-hydroxyindoleacetic acid	IVC	inferior vena cava
HIV	human immunodeficiency virus	IVP	intavenous pyelogram
HLA	human leukocyte antigen	kg	kilogram
HMG-CoA	3-hydroxy-3-methylglutaryl-CoA reductase	17-KS	17-ketosteroids
hpf	high power field	LA	left atrium
hPL	human placental lactogen	LAD	left anterior descending
HPLC	high-performance liquid chromatography	LDH	lactate dehydrogenase
		LDL	low-density lipoprotein
HPRT	hypoxanthine guanine phosphoribosyltransferase	Leu	leucine
5-HT	5-hydroxytryptamine	LH	luteinizing hormone; lutropin
5-HTP	5-hydroxytryptophan	LH-RH	luteinizing hormone-releasing hormone
HUS	hemolytic uremic syndrome	LMP	last menstrual period
123I	123-radiolabeled iodine	Lp(a)	lipoprotein little A antigen
^{131}I	131-radiolabeled iodine	LPL	lipoprotein lipase
^{131}I-MIBG	131-radiolabeled iodine-m-iodobenzylguanidine	L/S	lecithin/sphingomyelin ratio
		LV	left ventricle
IDL	intermediate-density lipoprotein	M1	acute myeloblastic leukemia without maturation
IF	intrinsic factor	M2	acute myeloblastic leukemia with maturation
IgA	immunoglobulin A		
IgD	immunoglobulin D	M3	acute promyelocytic leukemia
IgE	immunoglobulin E	M4	myelomonocytic leukemia
IgG	immunoglobulin G	M5	monocytic leukemia
IgM	immunoglobulin M	M6	erythroleukemia

M7	acute megakaryocytic leukemia	NIDDM	noninsulin-dependent diabetes mellitus; diabetes mellitus II
MBP	myelin basic protein	nm	nanometers
MCH	mean corpuscular hemoglobin	NMR	nuclear magnetic resonance
MCHC	mean corpuscular hemoglobin concentration	NSAID	nonsteroidal anti-inflammatory drug
MCNS	minimal change nephrotic syndrome	5'-NT	5'-nucleotidase
MCT	medium-chain triglycerides	NTD	neural tube defect
MCV	mean cell volume	OCB	oligoclonal bands
MEN	multiple endocrine neoplasia	O.D.	oculus dexter; right eye
MHC	major histocompatibility complex	O.S.	oculus sinister; left eye
MIBG	m-iodobenzylguanidine	17-OHCS	17-hydroxycorticosteroids
min	minute(s)	$1,25(OH)_2D$	1,25-dihydroxyvitamin D
MM	normal α_1-antitrypsin phenotype	21-OHD	21-hydroxylase deficiency
MOD	manner of death	25(OH)D	25-hydroxyvitamin D
MoM	multiples of median value as defined by maternal age, weight, race, diabetic status, and weeks of gestation	OTC	ornithine transcarbamylase
		(P)	plasma
MPGN	membranoproliferative glomerulonephritis	PA	pernicious anemia
		PA	pulmonary artery
MRI	magnetic resonance imaging	PABA	p-aminobenzoic acid
MS	multiple sclerosis	PAH	phenylalanine hydroxylase
MTC	medullary thyroid carcinoma	PAO	peak acid output
NA	nicotinic acid	Pap	Papanicolaou test
NAC	N-acetyl-L-cysteine	PAS	periodic acid-Schiff
NAD	nicotinamide adenine dinucleotide	PBG	porphobilinogen
		PB-T_4	protein-bound thyroxine
NADH	nicotinamide adenine dinucleotide, reduced	pCO$_2$	carbon dioxide, partial pressure
NCEP	National Cholesterol Education Program	PCT	porphyria cutanea tarda
		PCW	pulmonary capillary wedge
NH$_3$	ammonia	PCWP	pulmonary capillary wedge pressure
NH$_4^+$	ammonium ion		

PDA	patent ductus arteriosus; abnormal communication between the great arteries	RFLP	restriction fragment length polymorphism
PG	phosphatidylglycerol	Rh	Rh group of erythrocyte antigens
pH	hydrogen ion concentration	RhIg	Rh immune globulin
Ph^1	Philadelphia chromosome	r-HuEPO	recombinant human erythropoietin
PICU	pediatric intensive care unit	RI	reductase inhibitors
PKU	phenylketonuria	RNA	ribonucleic acid
(Plt)	platelets	ROC	receiver-operating characteristic
pO_2	oxygen, partial pressure	RPGN	rapidly progressive glomerulonephritis
POMC	pro-opiomelanocortin	RPR	rapid plasmin reagin test
ppb	parts per billion	RSV	respiratory syncytial virus
PR	progesterone receptors	RTA	renal tubular acidosis
PRA	plasma renin activity	RV	right ventricle
PRPP	5-phosphoribosyl-1-pyrophosphate	RV	residual volume
PSA	prostate-specific antigen	s	second(s)
PSE	portosystemic encephalopathy	(S)	serum
PT	prothrombin time	SC	hemoglobin S + hemoglobin C (hemoglobinopathy)
PTC	percutaneous transhepatic cholangiography	SD	hemoglobin S + hemoglobin D (hemoglobinopathy
PTH	parathyroid hormone; parathormone	SD	standard deviation
PTHrP	parathyroid hormone-related peptide	SGA	small for gestational age
6-PTS	6-pyruvoyl tetrahydropterin synthase	SID	syndrome of inappropriate diuresis
PTT	partial thromboplastin time	SIADH	syndrome of inappropriate antidiuretic hormone secretion
PVR	pulmonary vascular resistance	sIL-2R	serum-soluble interleukin-2 receptor
q.i.d.	four times a day (*quater in die*)	SLE	systemic lupus erythematosus
RA	right atrium	SLVL	splenic lymphoma with circulating villous lymphocytes
RAR-α	retinoic acid receptor		
RDS	respiratory distress syndrome	STS	serological test for syphilis

SVC	superior vena cava
(Sw)	sweat
$t_{1/2}$	terminal half-life
T_3	triiodothyronine
T_4	thyroxine; tetraiodothyronine
TBG	thyroxine-binding globulin
^{99m}Tc	radionuclide-labeled technetium
TdT	terminal deoxynucleotidyl transferase
THBR	thyroid hormone-binding ratio
TIBC	total iron-binding capacity
TLC	thin layer chromatography
TLC	total lung capacity
TORCH	*TO*xoplasmosis, *R*ubella, *Cy*tomegalovirus, and *H*erpes simplex (virus titers)
t-PA	tissue-type plasminogen activator
TPN	total parenteral nutrition
TRAP	tartrate-resistant acid phosphatase
TRH	thyrotropin-releasing hormone
TRL	triglyceride-rich lipoprotein
TSH	thyroid-stimulating hormone; thyrotropin
TT	thrombin time
TTP	thrombotic thrombocytopenic purpura
TTP-HUS	thrombotic thrombocytopenic purpura-hemolytic uremic syndrome
TVS	transvaginal sonography
(U)	urine
UDCA	ursodeoxycholic acid
uE_3	estriol, unconjugated
u-PA	urokinase-type plasminogen activator
URI	upper respiratory infection
Val	valine
VDRL	Venereal Disease Research Laboratory
VLDL	very low-density lipoprotein
VMA	vanillylmandelic acid
VP	variegate porphyria
VP-16	etoposide
VSD	ventricular septal defect; abnormal communication between the ventricles
ZPP	zinc protoporphyrin

Table of Contents

Introduction: Selection and Use of Laboratory Tests 1
     by William Z. Borer, M.D.

CARDIAC AND CARDIOVASCULAR DISEASES

Case 1. Child with Heart Murmur and Cyanosis 7
     (Congenital Heart Disease)
     by William N. O'Connor, M.D., and Carol M. Cottrill, M.D.

Case 2. Woman with Angina Pectoris 11
     (Myocardial Infarction)
     by William N. O'Connor, M.D., and Mikel D. Smith M.D.;
     William H. Porter, Ph.D., Reviewer

PULMONARY DISEASES

Case 3. Child with Recurrent Pneumonia, Anemia, and Failure to Thrive 15
     (Cystic Fibrosis)
     by Jamshed F. Kanga, M.D.

Case 4. Shortness of Breath with Productive Cough 21
     (Chronic Obstructive Pulmonary Disease)
     by Nausherwan K. Burki, M.D.; David N. Bailey, M.D., Reviewer

RENAL DISEASES

Case 5. Oliguria with Metabolic Acidosis after Renal Transplantation 27
     (Renal Tubular Acidosis after Renal Transplantation)
     by C. Darrell Jennings, M.D.; William H. Porter, Ph.D., and
     Richard A. Mc Pherson, M.D., Reviewers

Case 6. Man with Hypertension and Fever 33
     (Acute Tubular Necrosis)
     by C. Darrell Jennings, M.D.; David N. Bailey, M.D., Reviewer

Case 7. Glomerulonephritis, Uremia, Pulmonary Infiltration, and Hemoptysis .. 39
     (Acute Glomerulonephritis and Uremic Syndrome)
     by C. Darrell Jennings, M.D.; Richard A. Mc Pherson, M.D., Reviewer

Case 8.   **Young Woman with Edema and Decreased Urine Output** 45
          (Nephrotic Syndrome)
          by H. William Schnaper, M.D.; David N. Bailey, M.D., Reviewer

DISEASES OF THE LIVER AND BILIARY TRACT

Case 9.   **A 35-Year-Old Man with Fulminant Liver Failure** 53
          (Hepatitis D)
          by Rex B. Conn, M.D.; Steven I. Shedlofsky, M.D., Reviewer

Case 10.   **A Nurse with Metastatic Cancer** 61
          (Hepatocellular Carcinoma)
          by Rex B. Conn, M.D.; Steven I. Shedlofsky, M.D., Reviewer

Case 11.   **Adult Male with New Onset Ascites** 65
          (Genetic Hemochromatosis)
          by Steven I. Shedlofsky, M.D.

Case 12.   **Adolescent Female with Tremor, Depression, and Hepatitis** 71
          (Wilson's Disease)
          by Steven I. Shedlofsky, M.D.

Case 13.   **Middle-Aged Alcoholic with Jaundice and Ascites** 77
          (Cirrhosis)
          by Albert I. Rubenstone, M.D., and Steven I. Shedlofsky, M.D.

Case 14.   **Patient with Abdominal Pain** 85
          (Cholelithiasis)
          by Avram M. Cooperman, M.D.; Susan A. Fuhrman, M.D., Reviewer

Case 15.   **Young Woman with Recurrent Abdominal Pain** 89
          (Acute Intermittent Porphyria)
          by Steven I. Shedlofsky, M.D.

PANCREATIC AND GASTROINTESTINAL DISEASES

Case 16.   **Severe Epigastric Pain** 99
          (Acute Pancreatitis)
          by A. Ralph Henderson, M.B., Ch.B., Ph.D.; Steven I. Shedlofsky, M.D., Reviewer

Case 17.   **Woman with Jaundice** 107
          (Carcinoma of the Ampulla of Vater)
          by Paul A. Luce, B.S., and George F. Gray, Jr., M.D.;
          Fred Gorstein, M.D., Reviewer

Case 18.   **Abdominal Pain and Polyuria** 111
          (Diabetes Mellitus)
          by Dennis G. Karounos, M.D.; Susan A. Fuhrman, M.D., Reviewer

Case 19. Recurrent Diarrhea 119
(Gluten-sensitive Enteropathy)
by Z. Myron Falchuk, M.D.; David N. Bailey, M.D., Reviewer

Case 20. Woman with Chronic Diarrhea and Weight Loss 123
(Diarrhea)
by Donald C. Bondy, M.D.

Case 21. Persistent Jaundice in Infant 127
(Extrahepatic Biliary Atresia)
by Drora Berkowitz, M.D., and William F. Balistreri, M.D.

Case 22. A Three-Week-Old Infant with Vomiting 133
(Pyloric Stenosis)
by Douglas J. Schneider, M.D., and Carol M. Cottrill, M.D.

THYROID DISEASES

Case 23. Anterior Neck Mass 137
(Graves' Disease)
by Kenneth B. Ain, M.D.; Nelson B. Watts, M.D., Reviewer

Case 24. The Fatigued Attorney 141
(Hashimoto's Thyroiditis)
by Kenneth B. Ain, M.D.

Case 25. The Reluctant Chef 145
(Medullary Thyroid Carcinoma)
by Kenneth B. Ain, M.D.

ADRENOCORTICAL DISEASES

Case 26. Child with Rapid Growth and Precocious Sexual Maturation 149
(Congenital Adrenal Hyperplasia)
by Phyllis W. Speiser, M.D.

Case 27. Sudden Onset of Polyuria and Polydipsia 155
(Hypothalamic Cushing's Syndrome)
by Robert M. Carey, M.D.; Michael J. Kelner, M.D., Reviewer

Case 28. Woman with Irregular Menses, Hirsutism, and Depression 161
(Adenoma of the Pituitary with Cushing's Disease)
by Ted L. Anderson, Ph.D.; Fred Gorstein, M.D., Reviewer

Case 29. Intermittent Right Flank Pain 167
(Adrenal Cortical Neoplasm)
by Margie A. Scott, M.D.; Fred Gorstein, M.D., Reviewer

Case 30. Middle-Aged Man with Weakness and Weight Gain 171
(Lung Tumor with Cushing's Syndrome)
by David G. Elliott, M.D.

Case 31. Weakness, Weight Loss, and Hypotension 177
(Chronic Adrenal Insufficiency)
by Emmanuel L. Bravo, M.D.; Michael J. Kelner, M.D., Reviewer

MISCELLANEOUS ENDOCRINE DISEASES

Case 32. Boy with Thick Lips 183
(Multiple Endocrine Neoplasia [MEN 3])
by Michael L. Cibull, M.D., and Ronald J. Whitley, Ph.D.;
Michael J. Kelner, M.D., Reviewer

Case 33. A Woman with Psychosis and Hypercalcemia 189
(Primary Hyperparathyroidism)
by Susan A. Fuhrman, M.D.; Ronald J. Whitley, Ph.D., Reviewer

Case 34. A Child with Osteopenia and Retarded Growth 195
(Renal Osteodystrophy)
by William H. Porter, M.D.; Richard A. Mc Pherson, M.D., Reviewer

Case 35. Episodic Hypertension 201
(Pheochromocytoma)
by Gordon P. Guthrie, Jr., M.D.

Case 36. Diarrhea and Gastrointestinal Hemorrhage 207
(Zollinger-Ellison Syndrome)
by A. Ralph Henderson, M.B., Ch.B., Ph.D.

Case 37. Woman with Facial Flushing 213
(Carcinoid Syndrome)
by Jerome M. Feldman, M.D.

GYNECOLOGICAL AND OBSTETRICAL DISEASES

Case 38. Pregnancy Complicated by Abdominal Pain 219
(Pregnancy with Sickle Cell Crisis)
by Lisa A. Sprague, M.D., and Susan Cox, M.D.

Case 39. Woman with Amenorrhea 225
(Gestational Trophoblastic Neoplasia)
by Holly Gallion, M.D.; Larry E. Puls, M.D., Reviewer

Case 40. A Healthy Multiparous Woman whose Babies Became Jaundiced ... 229
(Rh Hemolytic Disease of the Newborn)
by Douglas W. Huestis, M.D.

Case 41. Woman with a Family History of Breast Cancer 235
(Breast Tumor)
by Deborah E. Powell, M.D.

Case 42. Woman with Abdominal Distention 239
(Ovarian Cancer)
by Paul D. DePriest, M.D.; J. R. van Nagell, Jr., M.D., Reviewer

Case 43. Polydipsia, Polyuria, and a Perisellar Mass 245
(Dysgerminoma)
by Deborah E. Powell, M.D.

HEMATOLOGICAL DISEASES

Case 44. Woman with Anemia and Hypertension 249
(Chronic Anemia)
by John A. Koepke, M.D.; Richard A. Mc Pherson, M.D., Reviewer

Case 45. Child with Pneumonia 253
(Sickle Cell Disease)
by John A. Koepke, M.D.; Richard A. Mc Pherson, M.D., Reviewer

Case 46. A Woman with Fatigue and Pallor 257
(Pernicious Anemia)
by Naif Z. Abraham, Jr., M.D., Ph.D., and Douglas A. Nelson, M.D.;
Susan A. Fuhrman, M.D., Reviewer

Case 47. Pneumonia, Leukopenia, and Ecchymoses 265
(Acute Promyelocytic Leukemia)
by Marcel E. Conrad, M.D.; Susan A. Fuhrman, M.D., Reviewer

Case 48. A Man with Splenomegaly 269
(Chronic Myelogenous Leukemia)
by Douglas A. Nelson, M.D.; Richard A. Mc Pherson, M.D., Reviewer

Case 49. A Case of Impotence and Progressive Fatigue 275
(Hairy-Cell Leukemia)
by John C. Spinosa, M.D., and Richard A. Mc Pherson, M.D.;
Dennis Ross, M.D., Reviewer

Case 50. Patient with Pleuritic Pain and Hypergammaglobulinemia 281
(Multiple Myeloma)
by Philip R. Greipp, M.D.; David N. Bailey, M.D., Reviewer

CENTRAL NERVOUS SYSTEM DISORDERS

Case 51. Pregnancy with Elevated Maternal Serum α-Fetoprotein 285
(Neural Tube Defect)
by Anjana Lal Pettigrew, M.D.

Case 52. Acute Hemiparesis 291
(Multiple Sclerosis)
by Kevin R. Nelson, M.D., and Steven L. Hoover, M.D.

LIPID DISORDERS

Case 53. Young Man with Chest Pain 297
(Familial Hypercholesterolemia)
by Evan A. Stein, M.D., Ph.D.

Case 54. Middle-Aged Woman with Recurrent Abdominal Pain 303
(Familial Hypertriglyceridemia)
by Evan A. Stein, M.D., Ph.D.

CONGENITAL DISEASES

Case 55. Child with Recurrent Vomiting 309
(Ornithine Transcarbamylase [OTC] Deficiency)
by Ronald J. Whitley, Ph.D.; Michael W. Stelling, M.D., Reviewer

Case 56. Hyperactive Boy with Infantile Speech 315
(Phenylketonuria [PKU])
by Ronald J. Whitley, Ph.D.

COAGULOPATHIES

Case 57. Woman with Malaise and Bleeding 321
(Disseminated Intravascular Coagulopathy [DIC])
by Ewa Marciniak, M.D.

**Case 58. A Young Girl with Deep Vein Thrombosis and Abnormal
Coagulation Tests** 325
(Systemic Lupus Erythematosus with Lupus Anticoagulant)
by Ewa Marciniak, M.D.

Case 59. Medical Student with Mild Bleeding Disorder 331
(Hemophilia)
by Ewa Marciniak, M.D.; Richard A. Mc Pherson, M.D., Reviewer

TOXICOLOGICAL CONDITIONS

Case 60. High Anion-Gap Acidosis with High Osmolal Gap 335
(Ethylene Glycol Poisoning)
by Robert V. Blanke, Ph.D.

Case 61. An Anemic Child from an Upper Middle-Class Family 341
(Lead Poisoning)
by Robert V. Blanke, Ph.D.

Case 62. Suicide Attempt by Drug Overdose 347
(Acetaminophen Intoxication)
by William H. Porter, Ph.D.

MISCELLANEOUS DISORDERS

Case 63. Child with Lethargy and Coma 353
(Reye's Syndrome)
by Dean A. Arvan, M.D.; William E. Neeley, M.D., Reviewer

Case 64. Low Back Pain 359
(Prostatic Carcinoma)
by A. Ralph Henderson, M.B., Ch.B., Ph.D.

Case 65. Heart Failure in a Middle-Aged Woman 365
(Primary [AL] Amyloidosis)
by Jonathan E. Plehn, M.D., and Gibbons G. Cornwell, III, M.D.

Case 66. A Man with Fever and Acute Polyarthritis 371
(Gout)
by William Eugene Davis, M.D.

Case 67. Sudden Death of a Cocaine Addict in Police Custody 377
(Accidental Death due to Cocaine)
by John C. Hunsaker, III, J.D., M.D.

Case 68. Child with Nausea and Vomiting Eight Days Post-Craniotomy 385
(SIADH)
by Susan A. Fuhrman, M.D.; Ronald J. Whitley, Ph.D., Reviewer

Case 69. An Elderly Woman with Bilateral Hip Pain 391
(Osteoporosis)
by Eric L. Hume, M.D.; William H. Porter, Ph.D., Reviewer

Case 70. Gait Disturbance after Extensive Bowel Resection 397
(Rickets)
by Zilla Huma, M.B., M.R.C.P., and Joseph M. Gertner, M.B., M.R.C.P.

INFECTIOUS DISEASES

Case 71. Persistent Cough and Dyspnea 403
(Acquired Immune Deficiency Syndrome [AIDS])
by Robert C. Noble, M.D.

INDEX 407

Introduction

SELECTION AND USE OF LABORATORY TESTS

William Z. Borer, Contributor

Appropriate use of laboratory tests in the management of disease processes is one of the most important aspects of medical decision-making. Skillful use of the wide array of laboratory and imaging studies available to the practicing physician begins in the formative years of medical school and is further refined throughout the postgraduate years. The ultimate goal, however, lies beyond the analytical and synthetic logic leading to a clinical diagnosis and plan of management. The ultimate goal is the relief of patient suffering and the prolongation of well-being. Only 50 to 60 of the hundreds of readily available laboratory tests account for 70% of the results generated by the modern hospital clinical laboratory. The implication is that "common diseases" are investigated using "common tests." When taken in the context of the clinical situation, the results of these tests provide discrete bits of data to be added to those already derived from the medical history and physical examination. Many correct clinical decisions are made in the absence of any laboratory data. Others require the results of one or more selected laboratory tests to arrive at the next step in the decision-making process. It is uncommon for a single laboratory test to make a diagnosis. However, a small number of well-chosen laboratory tests may be very useful to confirm a clinical suspicion or to rule out one or more of the candidates in the differential diagnosis.

Choosing Laboratory Tests

The appropriate selection of laboratory tests is the result of an incremental decision-making process. That is, the physician orders tests to answer questions regarding a disease process so that another series of medical decisions may be made. Several commonly asked questions may be answered, at least in part, by laboratory testing.

1. Is the diagnosis correct? Properly selected laboratory tests may corroborate or refute a working diagnosis. For example, a hemoglobin concentration or hematocrit may be ordered on a patient who complains of fatigue and shortness of breath and who appears unusually pale. A low value may confirm the diagnosis of anemia.

2. What is the etiology of the disease? Following the diagnosis of anemia in the patient described above, the physician may order a serum iron assay or vitamin B_{12} and folate assays to help determine the cause of the anemia.

3. How severe is the disease? The severity of anemia may be ascertained from the hemoglobin concentration. The patient with a hemoglobin concentration below 12 g/dL (7.45 mmol/L) is technically defined as anemic; however, anemia may not be obvious to the physician until the hemoglobin concentration falls below 9 g/dL (5.59 mmol/L). Severe anemia (hemoglobin <6 g/dL; <3.72 mmol/L) usually results in symptoms of dyspnea and extreme fatigue.

4. Has the patient's condition improved or deteriorated? Laboratory testing is also useful in following the course of a disease or the success of a therapeutic regimen. The anemia detected above may have been found to be caused by inadequate iron intake in an otherwise healthy young woman whose diet was strictly vegetarian. Treatment with oral iron sulfate would be started, and the success of this treatment could be documented by an increased hemoglobin concentration a few weeks later. Therapeutic drug monitoring is another example of the use of laboratory testing in clinical follow-up. Patients receiving drugs such as theophylline, phenytoin, or digoxin often need to have the serum drug concentration measured so that the optimal therapeutic concentration may be maintained.

5. *Is the patient at risk for disease or is there a disease not clinically apparent (subclinical)?* Many of the tests performed in an outpatient setting are directed toward wellness screening. Examples of these kinds of tests are the serum cholesterol assay to detect patients at risk for coronary heart disease and the Papanicolaou (Pap) test for early detection of cancer of the uterine cervix.

Interpreting Test Results

After the clinical questions have been formulated and the appropriate tests ordered, the results must be interpreted in the context of the clinical situation. This process usually begins with the comparison of a quantitative value (test result) with the reference interval for that test. Reference intervals (reference ranges) are established by performing tests on a population of healthy individuals in order to determine the distribution of test results that may be expected in the absence of disease. These distributions — when gaussian — are characterized by the mean and the standard deviation.* The reference interval is defined as the mean of the distribution plus or minus two standard deviations and includes about 95% of the population tested. By this definition the probability is that 1 out of 20 (about 5%) single test results will fall outside the reference interval. If 14 tests are ordered on a healthy subject, the probability is about 50% that at least one result will fall outside of the reference interval. Appropriately derived reference intervals should account for important population variables that include age, gender, race, geographics, social economics, diet, and life style.

A second distribution may be compiled to represent individuals with a given disease (see Figure 1). This distribution is characterized by a mean and standard deviation different from that of the healthy population. Theoretically the two distributions should provide a method by which the individual with disease may be differentiated from the individual without disease. Unfortunately, complete separation between the two populations is nearly always impossible. The area of overlap in the example (see Figure 1) is described by points A through C. This area of overlap may also be statistically defined. The terms sensitivity and specificity measure the diagnostic performance of a laboratory test. The values for these two parameters depend upon the selection of the referent value as well as the degree of separation between the two populations. The *sensitivity* of a test estimates the frequency of a positive test in the presence of a specific disease, whereas the *specificity* of a test measures the frequency of a negative test in the absence of the same disease. These frequencies are commonly expressed as percentages. The ideal laboratory test would be 100% sensitive and 100% specific. Under these circumstances the test result would always distinguish between health and disease. Regrettably such perfection only exists in hypothetical cases.

Real clinical situations usually require a compromise between sensitivity and specificity (as sensitivity increases, specificity decreases, and conversely). If the referent value (cutoff point) is adjusted to provide 100% sensitivity (point A in Figure 1), the specificity will be markedly reduced as healthy individuals are misclassified into the population with disease (false positive results). Conversely, if the specificity is fixed at 100% (cutoff at point C in

---

* In the case of a nongaussian distribution of reference values, the mean ± 2 SD cannot be used to determine the reference interval. Instead, a frequent approach is the calculation of the central 95th percentile after elimination of any possible outliers.

Figure 1), the sensitivity will diminish as a large number of individuals with the disease are misclassified as healthy (false negative results). Point B represents the referent value that provides the best discrimination between the healthy and diseased populations and that provides the best compromise between sensitivity and specificity in most, but not all, clinical situations. When a simple, inexpensive test is being used to screen a population for disease, it may be desirable to adjust the referent value to provide greater sensitivity (closer to point A), so that more subjects with the disease will be detected. This means that a second, more specific test must be used to identify the healthy individuals (false positives) who were misclassified by the screening test and to confirm the presence of the disease in subjects with true positive test results.

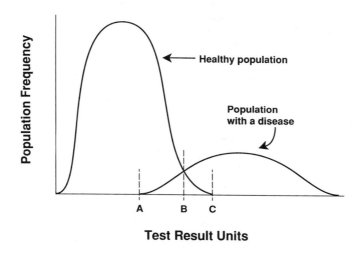

Figure 1. Assignment of referent value based upon test results in healthy and diseased populations (see text for explanation).

In addition to sensitivity and specificity, *predictive value* is another indicator of test performance. The predictive value of a positive test result is the ratio of the number of true positive results to the total number of positive results (true positives plus false positives); the ratio is expressed as a percentage. When the *prevalence* (the frequency of a disease in the population at a given time) of a disease is low, the predictive value of the test deteriorates. This phenomenon is important because the sensitivity and specificity of the test are not affected by disease prevalence and may be misleading if they are used as the sole indicators of the diagnostic performance of the laboratory test. Any test will have a higher predictive value when applied to a population with a high prevalence of the disease for which it is testing than when it is applied to a population with a low prevalence of that disease. As an example, consider a test with a sensitivity of 99% and a specificity of 98%. At a disease prevalence of 10% (i.e., 10,000 in 100,000), the predictive value of a positive result is 85%. However, if the prevalence were only 0.64% (i.e., 640 in 100,000), the predictive value of a positive result would decrease to 25%. This means that for every true positive detected, three false positives would also occur. If the test described in this example were used to screen for HIV infection (a low prevalence disease), which of us would wish to be mistakenly classified as positive?

Using Groups of Tests

Some laboratory tests are commonly ordered in combinations called panels or profiles. Historically, the individual tests in these profiles were combined by the laboratory to reflect physician ordering patterns or the menu of an automated multichannel instrument. Two decades of debate as to the clinical utility of profiles have not resolved the issue of appropriate use as an approach to comprehensive screening for occult disease vs. inappropriate use as a shotgun approach to diagnosis. Inappropriate use of laboratory testing has developed special importance in the current climate of cost control of health care. The problems with panels and profiles lie not so much with the concept as with the test mix included in various forms of profiles. The American College of Physicians has issued guidelines decrying use of general biochemical profiles for routine screening of asymptomatic adults. On the other hand, a comprehensive profile may have valid application for establishing a baseline of biochemical parameters in a sick or well patient. Subsequent testing with well-defined, focused panels or specific single tests, when symptoms appear or abate at a later time, may disclose significant biochemical changes not otherwise apparent and lead to a more rapid diagnosis or therapeutic response.

The guidelines of the American College of Physicians suggest that serum tests for cholesterol, glucose, and renal function (creatinine and urea nitrogen) may be useful in wellness screening. Others suggest that this profile is too limited and would add screening tests for detection of iron deficiency and iron overload and evaluation of thyroid function. For example, early detection and treatment of the hyperthyroid condition experienced by President Bush would quite likely have prevented the related heart condition (atrial fibrillation) from developing. This, however, is anecdotal and does not speak to the vexing clinical problem of whether, how extensively, and how often screening tests on asymptomatic adults should be performed.

The value of *serial testing* has been alluded to in a previous section. Clinical situations exist in which repeated testing of one or two analytes in serum provides much more diagnostic information than does a single result. This testing approach is particularly applicable to the diagnosis of acute myocardial infarction (AMI). Typically, when the patient is seen in the emergency room with acute chest pain, the activities of the enzymes creatine kinase (CK) and lactate dehydrogenase (LDH) in serum are not yet increased. Myocardial release of these enzymes is usually detectable within hours, and CK activity in serum reaches a peak 12 to 24 hours following AMI. Three or four consecutive measurements of serum CK (or CK-MB isoenzyme) that show a rise and fall ("peaking") of the enzyme over 24 to 36 hours strongly support the diagnosis of AMI.

Serial measurements of CK-MB are almost three times more sensitive than is a single measurement in the detection of early AMI. By contrast, LDH activity peaks between three and six days after an AMI and is usually not needed to support the diagnosis, unless the onset of chest pain occurred more than 24 hours prior to admission.

Optimizing the Use of Laboratory Tests

Experience has shown that physicians who take the time to learn about both the benefits and limitations of laboratory tests are those who use the laboratory most productively and cost effectively. A few simple guidelines may be emphasized:

1.   Carefully select tests to answer questions about a specific clinical situation.

2.   Be certain that orders are clear and that the patient is correctly identified.

3. Obtain the appropriate specimen and see that it is correctly labeled and promptly transported to the laboratory.

4. Review the results of all tests in a timely manner and take appropriate action.

5. Integrate laboratory findings with other clinical data from the medical history, physical examination, and imaging studies.

6. Investigate any puzzling or unexpected laboratory result as thoroughly as you would a puzzling or unexpected physical finding or imaging abnormality.

Additional Reading

Friedman, R.B., and Young, D.S.: Effects of Disease on Clinical Laboratory Tests. Washington, AACC Press, 1989.

Jacobs, D.S., Kasten, B.D., Jr., DeMott, W.R., et al.: Laboratory Test Handbook, 2nd ed. Baltimore, Williams and Wilkins, 1990.

Kassirer, J.P., and Kopelman, R.I.: Learning Clinical Reasoning. Baltimore, Williams and Wilkins, 1991.

Sox, H.R., Jr., Ed.: Common Diagnostic Tests: Use and Interpretation, 2nd ed. Philadelphia, American College of Physicians, 1990.

Speicher, C.E.: The Right Test: A Physician's Guide to Laboratory Medicine. Philadelphia, W.B. Saunders Co., 1990.

Wallach, J.: Interpretation of Diagnostic Tests: A Synopsis of Laboratory Medicine, 5th ed. Boston, Little, Brown and Co., 1992.

CHILD WITH HEART MURMUR AND CYANOSIS

William N. O'Connor, Contributor
Carol M. Cottrill, Contributor

A seven-year-old white male was referred to the University Hospital for evaluation of a heart murmur that had been present all of his life. He had been a 3 lb 9 oz (1978 g) premature infant who had tachypnea and oxygen dependency in the early neonatal period as well as difficulty feeding and a high caloric requirement. He was discharged from the hospital at four months of age. During the rest of his childhood, he had been a sickly child, always thin, who failed to thrive and was unable to tolerate infection. He had, in fact, several hospitalizations for pneumonia, respiratory viruses, and fevers. He had been cyanotic since age five and was placed on digitalis therapy by the referring physician. He had age-appropriate performance at school but tired easily.

On physical examination, the patient was thin and weighed 33 lb (15 kg). The mucous membranes were cyanotic, with mild clubbing of the fingers and toes. His blood pressure was 105/65 mm Hg. On cardiac examination, there was a very active right ventricle and a left ventricular heave. A prominent click was noted in the pulmonary area. The second heart sound was very loud and was followed by an early diastolic blow of pulmonary insufficiency. A soft, systolic ejection murmur was maximal at the lower left sternal border. The lungs were clear. The abdominal examination was unremarkable. The peripheral pulses were full and equal.

The following laboratory results were reported:

Analyte	Value, conventional units	Reference range, conventional units	Value, SI units	Reference range, SI units
Sodium (S)	139 mmol/L	138-145	Same	
Potassium (S)	4.6 mmol/L	4.1-5.3	Same	
Chloride (S)	108 mmol/L	98-108	Same	
CO_2, total (S)	22 mmol/L	20-28	Same	
Urea nitrogen (S)	7.0 mg/dL	5-18	2.5 mmol urea/L	1.8-6.4
Creatinine (S)	0.3 mg/dL	0.2-0.4	27 µmol/L	18-35
Glucose (S)	96 mg/dL	60-100	5.3 mmol/L	3.3-5.6
Protein, total (S)	5.6 g/dL	6.2-8.0	56 g/L	62-80
Albumin (S)	3.0 g/dL	3.8-5.4	30 g/L	38-54
Urate (S)	5.9 mg/dL	2.0-5.5	350 µmol/L	119-327
Cholesterol (S)	86 mg/dL	120-200	2.22 mmol/L	3.10-5.17
Bilirubin, total (S)	0.3 mg/dL	0.2-1.0	5 µmol/L	3-17
pH (aB)	7.44	7.35-7.45	Same	
pCO_2 (aB)	38 mm Hg	35-45	5.1 kPa	4.7-6.0
pO_2 (aB)	50 mm Hg	83-108	6.7 kPa	11.1-14.4
Oxygen saturation (aB)	85 %	95-98	0.85	0.95-0.98
Hemoglobin (B)	17.0 g/dL	11-16	10.55 mmol/L	6.83-9.93
Hematocrit (B)	48 %	31-43	0.48	0.31-0.43
Erythrocyte count (B)	$6.4 \times 10^6/\mu L$	3.8-5.5	$6.4 \times 10^{12}/L$	3.8-5.5

A chest X-ray examination showed mild cardiac enlargement and increased pulmonary vascularity without evidence of frank pruning (rapid tapering of the pulmonary vessels). The main pulmonary artery was quite large. An electrocardiogram was notable for right axis deviation, right ventricular hypertrophy, and right atrial enlargement.

At cardiac catheterization, the patient was found to have a large muscular ventricular septal defect (VSD) and a patent ductus arteriosus (PDA). Pulmonary artery pressure was 100/60 mm Hg, with a mean of 76 mm Hg. Aortic pressure was 100/60 mm Hg, with a mean of 80 mm Hg. Oxygen saturations were as follows:

Superior vena cava (SVC)	59%	(70 ± 5)
Right atrium (RA)	59%	(68 ± 5)
Right ventricle (RV)	65%	(66 ± 5)
Pulmonary artery (PA)	65%	(64 ± 5)
Pulmonary capillary (wedge) (PCW)	96%	(95-100)
Left atrium (LA)	96%	(95-100)
Left ventricle (LV)	80%	(95-100)
Aorta	80%	(95-100)

The significance of decreased venous saturation in the superior vena cava and right atrium is that either oxygen consumption at the periphery is excessive or blood with decreased oxygen saturation is being delivered to the periphery. In this case, the aortic saturation of only 80% with normal oxygen extraction would yield a superior vena caval oxygen saturation lower than normal. The significance of an increase in oxygen saturation between the right atrium (59%) and the right ventricle (65%) indicates oxygenated blood from the left side is mixing with the systemic venous blood. This is usually termed a left-to-right shunt. The pulmonary capillary wedge oxygenation and the left atrial oxygenation were normal. This suggested that the patient had a normal ability to oxygenate blood in the lungs and therefore had normally oxygenated pulmonary venous blood. The fact that oxygen saturation decreases from 96% in the left atrium to 80% in the left ventricle suggests that right-to-left shunting is occurring at the ventricular level.

Since oxygen is a potent pulmonary vasodilator, 100% oxygen was administered by mask during cardiac catheterization while sampling catheters were present in the aorta and the pulmonary artery. Pulmonary vascular resistance is measured by calculating the drop in pressure across the pulmonary vascular bed (the left atrial pressure subtracted from the mean pulmonary artery pressure) and dividing that by the pulmonary flow. Similarly, systemic vascular resistance is calculated by subtracting the right atrial mean pressure from the mean aortic pressure and dividing that by the systemic flow (cardiac output). In this child, systemic and pulmonary vascular resistances were equal in room air. However, after the administration of 100% oxygen, the patient's pulmonary vascular resistance decreased to 12 Wood units while the systemic resistance remained at 15 Wood units. This indicated that the pulmonary vascular resistance was poorly responsive to a vasodilator and greater than two-thirds the level of systemic vascular resistance. When pulmonary vascular resistance is elevated to two-thirds of systemic resistance and shunt reversal occurs, the so-called Eisenmenger physiology is present.

Cineangiography with injection of contrast material into the left ventricle documented a large ventricular septal defect. Both great vessels were noted to originate from the right ventricle, the so-called double-outlet right ventricle. In addition, a patent ductus arteriosus was seen. Because the patient was deemed inoperable because of irreversible pulmonary vascular disease, he was referred to another medical center for evaluation for combined heart and lung transplantation.

Discussion

The combination of clinical and laboratory findings and catheterization data explain the presence of congenital heart disease with central cyanosis (Eisenmenger physiology). Prolonged left-to-right shunt with pulmonary vascular volume and pressure overload had led to advanced pulmonary hypertensive vascular disease and ultimately the reversal of left-to-right shunting.

Normal Perinatal Pulmonary Vascular Dynamics. All healthy fetuses and newborns have equal pressures in the systemic (left) and venous (right) ventricles and in their respective great arteries prenatally and at birth. Soon after birth, pulmonary vascular resistance (PVR) falls dramatically, and pulmonary flow increases. The ductus arteriosus closes, and further decrease in pulmonary vascular resistance occurs, soon thereafter reaching normal adult levels.

Congenital Cardiac Shunt-Related Pulmonary Vascular Dynamics. When abnormal communication exists between the right and left ventricles, equalization of pressures is present soon after birth. The pressure in the pulmonary circulation is, therefore, of systemic level. In order to produce effective cardiac output, the left side of the heart must generate enough pressure to maintain adequate systemic arterial perfusion in the face of the normal resistance of the systemic vascular bed with the systemic vascular tone. Hence, with abnormal communication between the ventricles (VSD) or great arteries (PDA), for example, a gradient exists. Because pulmonary vascular resistance is lower than systemic vascular resistance, blood flows from left to right (from high to low pressure side) and results in pressure and volume overload at the right side of the heart and overcirculation of the lungs. This circulatory overload produces prominent pulmonary vascular markings on the chest film. With circulatory overload, the lung is heavier than normal and causes an affected infant to work harder to suck and feed. In addition, tachypnea interferes with feeding ability, and failure to thrive ensues. The abnormal hemodynamic state in the lung predisposes the infant to repeated episodes of pulmonary infection. High pressure and high volume perfusion of the lungs sometimes result in the development of initially reversible and later irreversible morphological vascular changes.

The data gathered at cardiac catheterization in these individuals can help to distinguish the elevated but labile pulmonary artery pressures associated with reversible pulmonary vascular resistance from the more serious elevated but fixed pressures associated with irreversible pulmonary vascular resistance. This can be done by comparing the level of resistance in both the pulmonary and systemic circuits. Pulmonary vascular resistance that is two-thirds or more the level of the systemic resistance is considered a contraindication to surgery for the congenital heart defect. If repaired at this stage, the right side of the heart fails postoperatively as it is unable to overcome the high resistance in the lung, and an opening for decompression no longer exists. The right-sided heart failure of untreated Eisenmenger physiology may ultimately require combined heart and lung transplantation. It is remarkable that this patient remained acyanotic until five years of age.

Complications of Cyanotic Congenital Heart Disease

With reversal of the shunt and right-to-left movement of blood from the desaturated venous (right) ventricle to the arterial (left) ventricle, cyanosis develops, and the patient exhibits hypoxemia in the systemic circuit. The body's adaptation to this process consists of erythropoietin secretion from the kidneys and bone marrow stimulation. This response results in erythroid hyperplasia and an elevated erythrocyte count and hematocrit. If hypoxemia continues, the hematocrit may rise to dangerous levels, as high as 80%. The increased blood viscosity predisposes to sludging, with risk of cerebral venous thrombosis and ischemic necrosis with stroke. The erythrocyte cell survival is also abnormally low.

Increased erythrocyte turnover and breakdown predisposes to secondary hyperuricemia and gout. Also, when venous blood bypasses the "filter" that exists in the pulmonary capillary vasculature, there is increased risk of systemic sepsis. The ischemically injured brain is at risk for seeding by bacteria from the venous circulation, and brain abscess is an important complication. Cerebral necrosis may also be due to a paradoxical embolus across the intracardiac shunt. This allows thrombi, which develop in the deep veins of the lower extremities or pelvis, to circulate through the inferior vena cava and right atrium to the right ventricle and thence into the left ventricle or aorta across the abnormal communication.

The development of finger clubbing in chronic hypoxemic states is readily recognized, but this physical finding is not limited to congenital heart disease. It is found in a variety of conditions such as chronic lung diseases, malabsorption, and other states. The mechanism for clubbing is unclear. When clubbing is limited to the toes, one must consider Eisenmenger physiology complicating isolated patent ductus arteriosus. The liver is hypoxic, and synthesis of proteins suffers. Therefore, the prothrombin time (PT) is sometimes prolonged, and in older female patients there may be a menorrhagia.

Additional Reading

Harris, P., and Keith, D.: The Human Pulmonary Circulation: Its Form and Function in Health and Disease, 3rd ed. New York, Churchill Livingstone Inc., 1986.

Perloff, J.: The Clinical Recognition of Congenital Heart Disease. Philadelphia, W.B. Saunders Co., 1987.

WOMAN WITH ANGINA PECTORIS

William N. O'Connor, Contributor
Mikel D. Smith, Contributor
William H. Porter, Reviewer

A 63-year-old white female was admitted to a community hospital with severe, intractable chest pain. She had been well until five months previously, when she noted the onset of angina pectoris. Initially pain occurred infrequently on climbing stairs. The episodes of angina increased in intensity and frequency over several weeks and led to the development of two days of intractable, severe chest pain. This severe chest pain was present at rest; it was substernal, radiating to the left neck, face, arms and shoulder, and was associated with nausea and diaphoresis. An electrocardiogram (ECG) showed inferior lead (II, III, aVF) ST segment elevation with anterior ST segment depression. Administration of sublingual nitro-glycerin produced transient relief of the pain. The suspected clinical diagnosis was acute myocardial infarction in the inferior wall.

The patient had a past history of chronic obstructive pulmonary disease (COPD), goiter, and arthritis. Her mother died from myocardial infarction at the age of 70, and her father died of lung cancer. She had smoked three packs of cigarettes per day for 44 years (132 pack-years = packs smoked per day × years smoked).

Physical examination showed mild obesity, a regular heart rate of 110 BPM, a blood pressure of 130/95 mm Hg, and a respiratory rate of 12/min. Chest was clear to auscultation, and the abdominal examination was unremarkable. The peripheral pulses were full and equal. The following laboratory results were reported:

Analyte	Value, conventional units	Reference range, conventional units	Value, SI units	Reference range, SI units
Day 1, 0500 h:				
CK (S)	462 U/L	21-215	7.70 µkat/L	0.35-3.58
CK-MB (S)	58 ng/mL	0-5	58 µg/L	0-5
CK-MB, % (S)	12 %	<5	0.12	<0.05
LDH, total (S)	231 U/L	100-190	3.85 µkat/L	1.67-3.17
LDH-1	24 %	18-31	0.24	0.18-0.31
LDH-2	41 %	36-47	0.41	0.36-0.47
AST (S)	Within normal imits			
Day 1, 1000 h:				
CK (S)	557 U/L	21-215	9.29 µkat/L	0.35-3.58
Day 1, 2130 h:				
CK (S)	665 U/L	21-215	11.09 µkat/L	0.35-3.58
Day 2, 1500 h:				
CK (S)	1965 U/L	21-215	32.76 µkat/L	0.35-3.58

Analyte	Value, conventional units	Reference range, conventional units	Value, SI units	Reference range, SI units
Day 2, 1500 h (cont.):				
LDH, total (S)	310 U/L	100-190	5.17 µkat/L	1.67-3.17
LDH-1	45 %	18-31	0.45	0.18-0.31
LDH-2	37 %	36-47	0.37	0.36-0.47
Leukocyte count (B)	14.5 x 10³/µL; 75% polymorpho-nuclear leukocytes	4.8-10.8	14.5 x 10⁹/L	4.8-10.8

Her cardiologist recommended administration of streptokinase (a thrombolytic agent); in addition, treatment with β-blockers, nitroglycerin, and calcium channel blockers was initiated along with aspirin. At noon on day 5, after a pain-free interval of three days' duration, the patient experienced a recurrence of pain involving the left lower chest. She was then transferred from the community hospital to the University Hospital. The pain was constant and exacerbated by deep breathing and left lateral decubitus positioning; it radiated to the left arm and was accompanied by nausea. Findings on admission to the University Hospital included a heart rate of 85/min, a Grade II/VI systolic murmur at the left lower sternal border, and a pericardial friction rub. Abdominal examination revealed mild tenderness in the right epigastrium. Bibasilar rales were present on auscultation of lungs, and a chest X-ray examination showed prominent vascular markings and Kerley B lines. ECG on admission showed ST elevation in leads II, III, and aVF, with ST depression in leads V1 and V2. Q waves were present in leads II, III, and aVF. An echocardiogram revealed left ventricular dilation, dyskinesia of the inferobasal left ventricle, and mild mitral regurgitation. The patient was placed on bed rest in the Coronary Care Unit; nitroglycerin was administered intra-venously, and oxygen was given by nasal cannula. Three hours later, the patient deteriorated rapidly. A Swan-Ganz catheter was placed, and the recorded data showed evidence of low cardiac output and elevation and equalization of right and left heart diastolic pressures.

The following laboratory data were obtained on day 5 at 1700 h:

Analyte	Value, conventional units	Reference range, conventional units	Value, SI units	Reference range, SI units
Urea nitrogen (S)	72 mg/dL	8-21	25.7 mmol urea/L	2.9-7.5
Creatinine (S)	2.4 mg/dL	0.7-1.2	212 µmol/L	62-106
Urea nitrogen/creatinine ratio (calculated)	30:1	12:1-20:1	121.2:1 (urea:creatinine mole ratio)	48.5:1-80.8:1
LDH, total (S)	290 U/L	100-190	4.83 µkat/L	1.67-3.17
LDH-5 isoenzyme	22 %	3-14	0.22	0.03-0.14
ALT (S)	95 U/L	10-40	1.58 µkat/L	0.17-0.67

Very shortly thereafter, the patient suddenly collapsed, and electromechanical dissoci-ation was noted. She was intubated, and bilateral breath sounds were heard. Bilateral chest tubes were placed to rule out tension pneumothorax. During cardiopulmonary resuscitation, a small amount of unclotted blood from the pericardial space was observed during a pericardiocentesis. However, resuscitative efforts were unsuccessful.

Discussion

Typical angina pectoris is defined as chest pain of cardiac ischemic origin that is relieved by rest or sublingual vasodilators. Stable angina usually occurs in a context of fixed calcified and fibrotic stenoses of one or more epicardial coronary arteries. These conditions imply that with increased circulatory demand, the pumping requirements of the heart are increased in the face of a fixed blood supply. Unstable angina, as in this patient, is characterized by rapid progression of severity as an indication of evolving stenosis of the coronary artery tree, secondary to complicated atherosclerosis. Perfusion of the coronary arteries occurs during diastole and is limited when the cross-sectional area of an individual epicardial artery is reduced by >75%. Therefore, with the increased demand of exercise in the presence of a fixed coronary blood supply, transient buildup of metabolites in the ischemic region of the myocardium triggers pain pathways, resulting in the referred pain of cardiac origin onto the corresponding chest wall, arm, or jaw dermatomes. When an increasing intensity of angina pectoris occurs, it implies evolving occlusion of the atherosclerotic vessel by atheromatous intraplaque hemorrhage, thrombosis, or vascular spasm. Fissuring of the fibrous cap of the plaque is the most likely mechanism underlying the complications that lead to accelerated occlusion of the affected atherosclerotic coronary artery.[1]

The onset of intractable chest pain lasting two days in this patient is highly suggestive of an abrupt occlusion of a coronary artery. This assumption was confirmed by the elevated total CK and percentage CK-MB at the time of admission. ECG and echocardiogram findings suggested involvement of the right coronary artery, which normally supplies the posterior basal and septal region of the left ventricle. Involvement probably resulted from athero-thrombotic occlusion of the affected coronary artery. The dependent region of the myocardium then underwent the infarction, and this irreversible injury to the myocardium correlates with the pattern and distribution of changes on the surface ECG. The changes evolved to include deep Q waves reflecting transmural injury and the associated presence of inferior wall dyskinesis on the echocardiogram. Involvement of the posterior/medial papillary muscle resulted in mitral valve insufficiency with elevation of left atrial pressure; the mitral valve insufficiency accounted for the systolic murmur. This murmur, however, could also be due to poor left ventricular wall motion and dilation of the mitral valve ring with mitral insufficiency. "Expansion" due to thinning of the infarct zone as opposed to reinfarction would also contribute to poor left ventricular function and low cardiac output. The net effect of left-sided failure was a rise in pulmonary capillary wedge pressure (PCWP) noted with the Swan-Ganz catheter. The wedged peripheral pulmonary artery open-ended catheter measures precapillary pressure, which is a direct reflection of left atrial pressure.

The serial enzyme studies in serum documented release of constituents of necrotic heart muscle specifically with an early elevation of the MB isoenzyme fraction of CK. The CK-MB level on day 1 in this patient expressed as 12% was obtained by an electrophoretic determination; the quantitation of CK-MB in ng/mL was done by immunochemical measurement.

Elevation of LDH occurred later (day 2) and showed the characteristic "flipped" ratio of LDH isoenzymes 1 and 2. In normal individuals, the ratio of LDH-1/LDH-2 in the serum is less than one. Myocardium contains more LDH-1 than LDH-2, and following myocardial infarction, this pattern is reflected in the serum. The finding of an LDH-1 less than LDH-2 on admission and the peaking of CK on day 2 also indicate that the infarction occurred no longer than a few hours prior to admission to the community hospital and not at the onset of the period of intense chest pain. The elevated leukocyte count after admission reflected the inflammatory response to acute tissue injury (in this case, heart muscle) and not an infection.

The patient received a thrombolytic agent. These preparations, streptokinase and tissue plasminogen activator (t-PA), are generally administered within the first four to six hours after onset of chest pain suspected to be due to acute myocardial infarction. The thrombolytic agent must be given early to lyse the thrombus and to avert irreversible occlusion of the affected coronary artery. After this time frame, the thrombus begins to organize to permanently occlude the coronary lumen. Despite obtaining symptomatic relief from a variety of medications, the patient's chest pain recurred. On transfer to the University Hospital, the presence of auscultatory findings in the lung and changes in the chest film suggested developing left-sided cardiac failure with fluid accumulation in alveoli. The pericardial friction rub was evidence of post-myocardial infarction pericarditis. The pericarditis reflected the presence of the transmural infarct with irritation of the parietal pericardial surface and development of a transient fibrinous inflammatory exudate. The right upper quadrant tenderness (of the liver) and elevation of the ALT and LDH-5 isoenzyme fraction indicated passive congestion with hepatocyte hypoxic injury. Centrizonal liver injury occurs as a result of right cardiac decompensation. Development of congestive heart failure affects hepatic lobular circulation by passive hepatic venous hypertension and predisposes the liver cells around the central vein of the lobule (which have a high oxygen requirement) to injury. In this patient, low cardiac output contributed to underperfusion of the hepatic arterial circuit and the portal venous circuit.

Elevation of the serum urea nitrogen and creatinine in this patient is consistent with prerenal azotemia. The urea nitrogen/creatinine ratio of 30:1 reflects underperfusion of renal tissue rather than intrinsic renal disease. Marked prolonged hypotension following a myocardial infarction may also lead to acute tubular necrosis.

The cause of death in this case was left ventricular wall rupture resulting in escape of blood into the closed pericardial space (pericardial tamponade). The tamponade effectively impedes the systemic and pulmonary venous return to the heart because blood under tension within the pericardial space collapses these thin-walled structures. Rupture of the heart is a recognized complication that most often develops about four days or more following an acute myocardial infarction. The timing reflects maximal softening of the transmural area of necrotic muscle, which also becomes thinned (so-called infarct expansion). Other structures that may rupture include the interventricular septum or papillary muscles.

Reference

1.   Davies, M.J., and Thomas, A.C.: Plaque fissuring — The cause of acute myocardial infarction, sudden ischemic death and crescendo angina. Br. Heart J., *53:* 363-373, 1985.

Additional Reading

Tietz, N.W., Ed.: Textbook of Clinical Chemistry. Philadelphia, W.B. Saunders Co., 1986.

CHILD WITH RECURRENT PNEUMONIA, ANEMIA, AND FAILURE TO THRIVE

Jamshed F. Kanga, Contributor

A two-month-old white male was admitted to the hospital for the second time with pneumonia and respiratory distress. Two weeks prior to this admission he had been seen in the Emergency Department for wheezing, and on chest X-ray examination he was found to have pneumonia. He was hospitalized for 48 hours and was sent home on oral antibiotics. A week after discharge he again presented with respiratory distress, prompting the current admission. His past history included a systolic murmur heard soon after birth and believed to be secondary to aortic stenosis.

On admission, the patient was pale and in moderate distress. The respiratory rate was increased to 35/min, and there was marked tachycardia. He had subcostal and intercostal retractions, and bilateral wheezes were noted. A harsh III/IV systolic ejection murmur was heard along the left lower sternal border. Examination of the abdomen and central nervous system was normal. His body weight of 10 lb (4.5 kg) was only 26 oz (0.75 kg) over birth weight. A chest X-ray examination showed marked hyperinflation with infiltrates in the right middle and right lower lobes.

The following laboratory tests were done on admission:

Analyte	Value, conventional units	Reference range, conventional units	Value, SI units	Reference range, SI units
Leukocyte count (B)	$9.1 \times 10^3/\mu L$	5.0-19.5	$9.1 \times 10^9/L$	5.0-19.5
Erythrocyte count (B)	$2.45 \times 10^6/\mu L$	3.8-5.5	$2.45 \times 10^{12}/L$	3.8-5.5
Hemoglobin (B)	8.1 g/dL	10-15	5.03 mmol/L	6.21-9.31
Hematocrit (B)	24 %	30-40	0.24	0.30-0.40
MCV (B)	95 fL	80-94	Same	
MCH (B)	33 pg	27-31	Same	
MCHC (BErcs)	33.7 g Hb/dL	33-37	21 mmol Hb/L	20-23
Platelet count (B)	$390 \times 10^3/\mu L$	150-450	$390 \times 10^9/L$	150-450
Differential count (B)				
Segmented neutrophils	37 %	41-71	0.37	0.41-0.71
Band neutrophils	3 %	5-10	0.03	0.05-0.10
Lymphocytes	50 %	24-44	0.50	0.24-0.44
Monocytes	8 %	3-7	0.08	0.03-0.07
Eosinophils	2 %	1-3	0.02	0.01-0.03
Reticulocyte count (B)	2.2 %	0.5-3.0	0.022	0.005-0.030
Urinalysis (U)	Within normal limits			
Electrolytes (S)	Within normal limits			
Protein, total (S)	6.1 g/dL	6.2-8.0	61 g/L	62-80
Albumin (S)	3.4 g/dL	3.8-5.4	34 g/L	38-54
Urate (S)	4.1 mg/dL	2.0-5.5	244 µmol/L	119-327
Cholesterol (S)	60 mg/dL	70-175	1.55 mmol/L	1.81-4.53
Liver function tests (S)	Within normal limits			
Folate (S)	>20 ng/mL	1.5-9.0	>45 nmol/L	3-20

Analyte	Value, conventional units	Reference range, conventional units	Value, SI units	Reference range, SI units
Vitamin B$_{12}$ (S)	1393 pg/mL	160-1300	1028 pmol/L	118-959
Ferritin (S)	269 ng/mL	50-200	269 µg/L	50-200
Chlamydiazyme	Negative	Negative		
Chlamydia culture	Negative	Negative		
Respiratory syncytial virus (RSV) direct fluorescent antibodies	Negative	Negative		
RSV culture	Negative	Negative		
Viral respiratory battery (includes influenza, parainfluenza, and adenovirus)	Negative	Negative		
Pertussis fluorescent antibodies	Negative	Negative		
Sputum culture	*Streptococcus pneumoniae, Corynebacterium* species	Negative		

The laboratory tests showed a normochromic anemia, hypoalbuminemia, and hypocholesterolemia. The leukocyte count was normal with a slight lymphocytosis, thus suggesting a viral illness. Cultures and fluorescent antibodies (FA) for viruses, *Chlamydia*, and pertussis were negative. The sputum culture results probably represented bacterial colonization secondary to antibiotic therapy.

The infant's respiratory problems and failure to thrive were initially thought to be secondary to his heart lesion and an intercurrent viral illness. His anemia, hypoalbuminemia, and poor weight gain were attributed to recurrent illness and poor feeding. During the hospitalization, the nurses reported that the patient's bowel movements were poorly formed and greasy and had a pungent odor. These findings led to the suspicion of cystic fibrosis (CF), and a sweat chloride test was performed and revealed the following:

Sweat chloride   82 mmol/L (0-50)
Amount of sweat collected was 0.5958 g.

A repeat sweat test the following day confirmed the previous data (chloride: 86.3 mmol/L; 0.3623 g sweat collected). After the diagnosis of cystic fibrosis was confirmed, the infant was started on a special predigested formula with oral supplementation of pancreatic enzymes, iron, and fat-soluble vitamins, and he began to gain weight. For his pulmonary disease he was treated with erythromycin and nebulized albuterol, and percussion as well as postural drainage was done three times/day. His parents were instructed on the care of infants with cystic fibrosis, and the patient was discharged home eight days later. He has not required subsequent hospitalizations, and his growth is now along the normal growth curve.

Definition of the Disease

Cystic fibrosis affects all the exocrine glands in the body. Secretions from sweat, salivary, and lacrimal glands have abnormal electrolyte content. Secretions of bronchial mucus glands, pancreatic acini, intestinal glands, intrahepatic bile ducts, and the gallbladder have increased viscosity, which causes obstruction. These effects are now believed to be secondary to an abnormality of cystic fibrosis transmembrane regulatory (CFTR) protein, as an expression of the gene defect. The protein defect interferes with chloride ion transfer across cell membranes, thus causing dehydration of the secretions and increased viscosity and electrolyte content.

Incidence and Genetics. Cystic fibrosis (CF) is the most common lethal genetic disease in the Caucasian population, with an incidence of 1 in 2000 live births. It is an autosomal recessive disease with heterozygote frequency of 1:20 in the Caucasian race. The heterozygote frequency and the incidence of the disease is much lower in Afro-Americans (heterozygote: 1:17,000; disease incidence: 1:70,000). The CF gene is extremely rare in Orientals. Heterozygotes or carriers for the CF gene are normal. In 1985 the CF gene was localized to the long arm of chromosome 7, and in 1989 the CF gene was identified.[1,2,3,6] The most frequent mutation, known as ΔF508, is found in approximately 70% of subjects. Over 60 other mutations have now been described and account for the remaining 30%. The different mutations are believed to be responsible for the varying presentations and severity of the disease.[5] Carrier detection and prenatal diagnosis of CF by testing for the CF gene is now available for families that have a child with CF.[4]

Diagnosis

The diagnosis of CF is confirmed by measuring the chloride concentration in sweat. Although sodium and potassium concentrations in sweat are also increased, chloride values are more consistent and better separate normals from CF patients. The standard sweat test (Gibson-Cooke pilocarpine iontophoresis) is considered valid only if >50 mg of sweat are collected. Sweat chloride values greater than 60 mmol/L on two separate days are required to make the diagnosis.[7] Ninety-eight percent of affected individuals have sweat chloride values of >60 mmol/L, and in the remaining 2% of patients the chloride value is in the borderline range (between 40 and 60 mmol/L). Sweat chloride values may also be elevated in untreated adrenal insufficiency, nephrogenic diabetes insipidus, Type I glycogen storage disease, mucopolysaccharidosis, ectodermal dysplasia, and other rare conditions. However, in no other disease is the elevated chloride value as consistent as in CF. False positives are also obtained if the collected sweat was allowed to partially evaporate. False negative results are usually seen when the standardized test is not used and when affected infants with edema and hypoproteinemia are tested. In these cases the test should be repeated using the Gibson-Cooke method after the edema and hypoproteinemia have resolved. To ensure accurate results, it is also important that the patient be afebrile and well hydrated when tested.

Serum immunoreactive trypsin levels are elevated in infants with CF and rapidly decline to subnormal levels within a few months after birth. Measurement of trypsin levels as part of the routine newborn screening tests for congenital disorders is now available in some institutions. In infants with elevated trypsin levels, a sweat chloride test is done to confirm the diagnosis. Newborn screening for CF is presently not done since there is no evidence that early diagnosis of the asymptomatic patient offers any advantage and there would be grave psychological consequences for the child and family.

A sweat test should be performed in any child or young adult with chronic respiratory problems such as cough, bronchitis, recurrent pneumonia, and sinusitis. Gastrointestinal problems, e.g., malabsorption, failure to thrive, meconium ileus, pancreatitis, and cirrhosis, may also be manifestations of CF. All siblings of CF patients should be tested, although in only 10% of newly diagnosed patients is there a family history of CF. A positive sweat test along with chronic respiratory illness, gastrointestinal symptoms, or family history meets the criteria for establishing the diagnosis.

Clinical Features

Approximately 10% of infants with CF present at birth with intestinal obstruction secondary to thick, tenacious meconium (meconium ileus). About 75% of patients are diagnosed within the first two years of life, the majority presenting with chronic respiratory symptoms and failure to thrive. About 1% of patients newly diagnosed each year are adults. The respiratory manifestations of the disease include recurrent bronchitis, pneumonia, and sinusitis. Recurrent lung infection leads to bronchiectasis and pulmonary fibrosis, eventually to cor pulmonale and death. Ninety-five percent of the morbidity and mortality in CF is secondary to lung disease.

Malabsorption secondary to pancreatic duct obstruction is present in 85% of CF patients. The severity of gastrointestinal symptoms is variable, and patients without overt malabsorption tend to have less severe lung disease and survive longer. The severity of the disease does not correlate with the degree of elevation of the sweat electrolytes. Most patients with CF have elevated serum liver enzymes, possibly secondary to partial obstruction and sluggishness of bile flow due to increased viscosity of the bile; 10% of them develop biliary cirrhosis. Cholecystitis and gallstones are frequent complications. Diabetes secondary to destruction of the pancreatic islet cells occurs with increasing age, and 15% of adult patients develop insulin-dependent diabetes. The etiology of anemia occasionally seen in infants with CF is multifactorial since it involves low serum protein, vitamin E deficiency, and chronic infection. Iron deficiency secondary to poor nutritional intake or absorption is uncommon.

Dehydration and heat stroke due to excessive loss of electrolytes via the sweat glands may be a problem in infants and young children during the summer. Most men with CF are sterile because of atrophy and obstruction of the vas deferens, epididymis, and seminal vesicles. Women with CF have decreased fertility secondary to thick cervical mucus acting as a barrier to sperm movement. Nevertheless, many women with CF have borne children.

Treatment

The treatment for children and young adults with CF is palliative. For the pulmonary disease, removal of the thick bronchial mucus is of cardinal importance. The removal is achieved by percussion and postural drainage of the chest. Treatment with bronchodilators and antibiotics also helps to decrease bronchial obstruction and infection and to retard progression of lung destruction. With advancing disease the sputum of patients with CF is colonized with mucoid *Pseudomonas aeruginosa*, which is found most frequently in patients with this disease. The mucoid coating of the organism makes it more resistant to antibiotic treatment, and once colonization of the respiratory tract occurs, the organism is seldom eradicated. Oxygen therapy to relieve hypoxemia and delay development of cor pulmonale is required with advancing disease.

Pancreatic deficiency is treated by giving pancreatic enzymes orally with meals. Most patients with CF require a high calorie, high protein diet to compensate for malabsorption, chronic infection, and the increased effort expended in breathing. Supplementation with fat-soluble vitamins — A, D, E, and K — is also necessary. Many patients receive nutritional supplements in addition to their meals to provide the extra calories, vitamins, and protein.

Heart-lung transplantation has been successfully performed in patients with end-stage lung disease. The transplanted lung does not develop the classic changes of CF. In patients with hepatic failure secondary to cirrhosis, liver transplantation has been carried out.

When CF was first described as a separate disease entity in the 1930's, the life expectancy of patients was less than five years. Today, with better understanding of the pathophysiological mechanism of the disease, the median survival is about 25 years. It is hoped that the discovery of the CF gene and the elucidation of the role of CFTR protein have promise for a cure of this disease in the future.

References

1. Kerem, B., Rommens, J., Buchanan, J., et al.: Identification of the cystic fibrosis gene: Genetic analysis. Science, *245:* 1073-1080, 1989.

2. Rommens, J., Iannuzzi, M.C., Kerem, B.S., et al.: Identification of the cystic fibrosis gene: Chromosome walking and jumping. Science, *245:* 1059-1065, 1989.

3. Riordan, J.R., Rommens, J., Kerem, B.S., et al.: Identification of the cystic fibrosis gene: Cloning and characterization of complementary DNA. Science, *245:* 1066-1073, 1989.

4. Lemna, W., Feldman, G., Kerem, B., et al.: Mutation analysis for heterozygote detection and the prenatal diagnosis of cystic fibrosis. N. Engl. J. Med., *322:* 291-296, 1990.

5. Campbell, P., Phillips, J., Krishnamani, M., et al.: Cystic fibrosis: Relationship between clinical status and F508 detection. J. Pediatr., *118:* 239-241, 1991.

6. Scambler, P.J.: The cystic fibrosis gene. Arch. Dis. Child., *64:* 1647-1648, 1989.

7. The Cystic Fibrosis Foundation guidelines for patient services, evaluation, and monitoring in cystic fibrosis centers. Am. J. Dis. Child., *144:* 1311-1312, 1990.

Additional Reading

Lloyd-Still, J.D., Ed.: Textbook of Cystic Fibrosis. Boston, John Wright PSG Inc., 1983.

Maclusky, I.B., Canny, G.J., and Levison, H.: Cystic fibrosis: An update. Pediatr. Rev. Commun., *1:* 343-389, 1987.

Taussig, L.M., Ed.: Cystic Fibrosis. New York, Thieme-Stratton Inc., 1984.

SHORTNESS OF BREATH WITH PRODUCTIVE COUGH

Nausherwan K. Burki, Contributor
David N. Bailey, Reviewer

A 61-year-old man was admitted to the hospital for treatment of increasing shortness of breath, cough, and sputum production. The patient had neither a family history of pulmonary disease nor a known contact with anyone with tuberculosis. He started smoking cigarettes at the age of 17 and since then had smoked one pack per day. He had been drinking about 1-2 cans of beer a week.

He gave a history of having developed a noticeable cough during the past 10-15 years. This cough had been present daily and had been productive of small amounts of sputum (approximately one tablespoon per day). Sputum production had occurred mainly in the morning. It was usually white but at times had been yellowish green. The patient also gave a history of shortness of breath on exertion that he first noticed about 5-7 years ago. This shortness of breath had steadily progressed until, in the month before admission, he was unable to walk one block or to go up one flight of stairs without pausing to catch his breath.

His current illness started about three days prior to admission when he developed increased frequency or intensity of coughing spells and increased production of sputum that became greenish yellow. He was febrile; his shortness of breath had increased; and he had developed some swelling of his feet and ankles that was particularly noticeable in the evening.

The patient's general health had otherwise been fair, and he had no history of allergies. He gave no history of eczema or childhood asthma. He had been hospitalized four times during the last five years with acute exacerbations of shortness of breath, cough, and increased sputum production. On each occasion, he was treated and discharged from the hospital after about one week; the last admission was approximately four months ago. His current medications consisted of the bronchodilators theophylline and metaproterenol inhaler as well as hydrochlorothiazide tablets.

On physical examination, the patient was alert, cooperative, and short of breath at rest; he had some central cyanosis but showed no pallor, jaundice, or lymphadenopathy. The oral temperature was 100.4 °F (38 °C).

The pulse rate was 110 BPM and regular. The blood pressure in the left arm with the patient in the supine position was 120/76 mm Hg. Jugular venous pressure was elevated to the angle of the jaw, with normal pulsations. The first heart sound was normal, whereas the second heart sound and pulmonic component were accentuated; no murmurs or rubs were heard.

The patient was short of breath at rest and was coughing. The respiratory rate was 20/min, and the patient was using accessory muscles. Percussion noted hyperresonance over both lung fields. Auscultation revealed reduced breath sounds over bases with expiratory rhonchi over both bases. The abdomen was scaphoid, soft; no palpable mass was observed, nor was tenderness elicited. His extremities showed peripheral cyanosis and bilateral 1+ ankle edema. There was no finger clubbing.

The chest X-ray examination showed low, flat diaphragms and a narrow heart. The right diaphragm dome level was below the sixth rib interspace anteriorly; this finding is a strong indication of airways obstruction. Hyperlucent lung fields, i.e., areas of lung parenchyma with decreased density, were observed; these findings were suggestive of emphysema.

The electrocardiogram (ECG) was consistent with a diagnosis of cor pulmonale. The tall (>2.5 mV) P waves suggested right atrial hypertrophy. Right axis deviation suggested right ventricular hypertrophy.

Results of laboratory tests were as follows:

Analyte	Value, conventional units	Reference range, conventional units	Value, SI units	Reference range, SI units
Sodium (S)	138 mmol/L	136-145	Same	
Potassium (S)	3.2 mmol/L	3.8-5.1	Same	
Chloride (S)	100 mmol/L	98-108	Same	
Bicarbonate (S)	44 mmol/L	23-31	Same	
Urea nitrogen (S)	10 mg/dL	8-21	3.6 mmol urea/L	2.9-7.5
Creatinine (S)	0.8 mg/dL	0.8-1.4	71 µmol/L	71-124
FI O_2, 21%				
pO_2 (aB)	46 mm Hg	83-108	6.1 kPa	11.1-14.4
pCO_2 (aB)	56 mm Hg	35-45	7.5 kPa	4.7-6.0
pH (aB)	7.27	7.35-7.45	Same	
FI O_2, 24%				
pO_2 (aB)	50 mm Hg	83-108	6.7 kPa	11.1-14.4
pCO_2 (aB)	62 mm Hg	35-45	8.3 kPa	4.7-6.0
pH (aB)	7.26	7.35-7.45	Same	
After 6 h of FI O_2, 24%				
pO_2 (aB)	52 mm Hg	83-108	6.9 kPa	11.1-14.4
pCO_2 (aB)	54 mm Hg	35-45	7.2 kPa	4.7-6.0
pH (aB)	7.30	7.35-7.45	Same	
Hemoglobin (B)	17.1 g/dL	14-18	10.61 mmol/L	8.69-11.17
Hematocrit (B)	54 %	40-54	0.54	0.40-0.54
Leukocyte count (B)	15.3 x 10^3/µL	4.8-10.8	15.3 x 10^9/L	4.8-10.8
Differential count (B)				
Band forms	14 %	5-10	0.14	0.05-0.10
Polymorphonuclear neutrophils	64 %	41-71	0.64	0.41-0.71
Lymphocytes	17 %	24-44	0.17	0.24-0.44
Monocytes	3 %	3-7	0.03	0.03-0.07
Eosinophils	2 %	1-3	0.02	0.01-0.03

Pulmonary Function Tests

	Actual	% Predicted
Total lung capacity (TLC)	7.20 L	132%
Residual volume (RV)	3.90 L	173%
Functional residual capacity (FRC)	5.20 L	182%
Forced vital capacity (FVC)	3.30 L	76%
Forced expired volume in 1 s (FEV_1)	1.12 L	23%
FEV_1/FVC ratio	34%	>75%
Carbon monoxide diffusing capacity (D_LCO)	17 mL/min/mm Hg	65%

Discussion

An elevated hematocrit suggested polycythemia that was likely caused by the chronic hypoxemia. The total leukocyte count was increased, with a "left shift" (increased band forms and polymorphonuclear neutrophils) suggesting a pulmonary infection.

Decreased serum potassium was probably related to the use of the diuretic drug hydrochlorothiazide.

The sputum revealed many gram-negative coccobacilli, suggesting that the patient had a bronchitis caused by *Haemophilus influenzae*. In patients with chronic bronchitis and emphysema, *Haemophilus influenzae* is the most common infecting organism that causes acute exacerbations. This interpretation was supported by the fact that the patient had an elevated leukocyte count.

Pulmonary function tests and a reduced FEV_1/FVC ratio were evidence of severe airway obstruction. The total lung capacity (TLC) was increased above the normal range, indicating that there was a significant amount of emphysema. Diagnosis of emphysema was further supported by the reduced carbon monoxide diffusing capacity (D_LCO).

Increased airway resistance leads to non-uniform distribution of ventilation in the lungs (since the increase in airway resistance in different lung segments is non-uniform). Because there is also loss of the alveolocapillary bed in emphysema, gas exchange is affected and hypoxemia occurs. As chronic bronchitis and emphysema progress in the patient, alveolar hypoventilation occurs. The reason for this is not clearly understood but is believed to be a combination of the increased mechanical abnormalities hindering ventilation, an alteration in ventilatory pattern, and a reduction in central respiratory drive.

Chronic bronchitis and emphysema may cause cor pulmonale by several mechanisms: hypoxemia is a strong stimulus to pulmonary vasoconstriction; similarly hypercapnia, by increasing H^+ concentration (i.e., by decreasing pH), is also a strong stimulus for pulmonary vasoconstriction. The combination of hypoxemia and hypercapnia thus increases pulmonary vascular resistance and raises pulmonary artery pressure. In addition, emphysema causes destruction of the pulmonary vascular bed, thus reducing the effective capacitance of the system. Finally, prolonged vasoconstriction causes structural alterations in pulmonary arteriolar smooth muscle and narrowing of the arteries. The resulting increase in pulmonary artery pressure increases the afterload on the right ventricle and leads to right ventricular hypertrophy and failure.

The arterial pO_2 and pCO_2 on room air (FI O_2, 21%) indicated severe hypoxemia and alveolar hypoventilation. Elevated pCO_2 and reduced pH suggested that the cause was an acute exacerbation of chronic hypercapnia. When the patient was placed on 24% oxygen, the pO_2 rose but so did the pCO_2, and there was a slight decrease in the pH. This change was presumably due to a reduction in the hypoxic drive, secondary to the rise in pO_2, and resulted in the further reduction in alveolar ventilation, causing the rise in pCO_2. After six hours on 24% oxygen, the patient's pO_2 was not significantly changed, but the pCO_2 decreased — a change that indicated improved alveolar ventilation.

The patient's shortness of breath and cough gradually improved, and after two days, he was afebrile with arterial blood gases on FI O_2, 24%, as follows: pO_2, 56 mm Hg (7.5 kPa); pCO_2, 48 mm Hg (6.4 kPa); and pH, 7.36. His ankle swelling had disappeared.

The patient was readmitted to the hospital six months later with another acute exacerbation but, unfortunately, did not survive this episode.

Comments

Chronic bronchitis usually results from chronic cigarette smoke exposure. The mucous glands of the airway enlarge and increase in number; the mucous membranes become inflamed from prolonged irritation. These processes are first noted in the small (<2 mm diameter) airways but ultimately affect the entire bronchial tree. Thus, narrowed airways increase resistance to airflow.

Emphysema is defined as dilation and destruction of the gas-exchanging portions of the lung. This effect again is most commonly a result of cigarette smoking. The destruction of lung tissue causes a loss of elastic recoil (an increase in lung compliance), which then hinders expiration and causes narrowing of the airways and increased airway resistance.

Cough is one of the cardinal symptoms of disease of the pulmonary airways (the bronchi); it is due to stimulation of the irritant receptors in the airways. Therefore, any condition resulting in inflammation of the airways is likely to cause cough.

Sputum production implies increased secretions in the airways or alveoli. Alveolar inflammation, e.g., pneumonia, causes increased secretions in the alveoli with bronchial inflammation in the airways. Since this patient had a history of chronic cough and sputum production over a period of 10-15 years, it is likely that he had chronic bronchitis at presentation. Indeed, chronic bronchitis is defined as present when a patient has a history of cough for the previous two years with daily sputum production for at least three months in each year. Another possibility to be considered is bronchiectasis; however, the quantity of sputum is usually much greater (a cupful per day or more) in bronchiectasis, and other symptoms and signs are present.

The presence of expiratory rhonchi confirms the airway narrowing. Hyperresonance to percussion and decreased breath sounds are suggestive of the presence of *emphysema*. The 44-pack-year history (= packs smoked per day × years smoked) of cigarette smoking is very significant, since smoking is the major cause of chronic bronchitis as well as of emphysema. Note that there is no history of exposure to dusts or fumes.

Dyspnea or shortness of breath, present in a large variety of pulmonary disorders, is one of the most common symptoms of cardiopulmonary disease. In most cases, dyspnea is first noted on exertion; if dyspnea progresses, the patient may become short of breath on lying down (orthopnea). In very severe cases, dyspnea is present even at rest. The mechanism of production of this symptom is unknown; for further discussion, please see review.[1]

Edema, the swelling of the feet and ankles, indicates salt and water retention. This situation may occur with heart, renal, or liver failure; other causes include severe hypo-albuminemia or secondary hyperaldosteronism or both. In the present case, the elevated jugulovenous pressure indicates right-sided heart failure, and the accentuated pulmonic component of the second heart sound indicates pulmonary hypertension. Since there is no clinical evidence of left-sided heart failure, the right-sided heart failure must be attributed to pulmonary hypertension secondary to lung disease, i.e., *cor pulmonale*. This condition is associated with hypertrophy of the right ventricle. The presence of central cyanosis is suggestive of hypoxemia.

Reference

1.   Burki, N.K.: Dyspnea. Lung, *165:* 269-277, 1987.

Additional Reading

American Thoracic Society: Standards for the diagnosis and care of patients with chronic obstructive pulmonary disease (COPD) and asthma. Am. Rev. Respir. Dis., *136:* 225-244, 1987.

Burki, N.K., and Krumpelman, J.L.: Correlation of pulmonary function with the chest roentgenogram in chronic airway obstruction. Am. Rev. Respir. Dis., *121:* 217-223, 1980.

Fletcher, C., and Peto, R.: The natural history of chronic airflow obstruction. Br. Med. J., *1:* 1645-1648, 1977.

Thompson, A.B., Daughton, D., Robbins, R.A., et al.: Intraluminal airway inflammation in chronic bronchitis: Characterization and correlation with clinical parameters. Am. Rev. Respir. Dis., *140:* 1526-1537, 1989.

OLIGURIA WITH METABOLIC ACIDOSIS AFTER RENAL TRANSPLANTATION

C. Darrell Jennings, Contributor
William H. Porter, Reviewer
Richard A. Mc Pherson, Reviewer

A 37-year-old white male with end-stage renal disease and on chronic hemodialysis presented 10 days after receiving a two A-locus, one B-locus, no DR locus match for a three of six HLA antigen matched kidney transplant (see *HLA Matching*). The kidney functioned within the first 48 hours with good urine output and a rapid decline of serum creatinine to 1.5 mg/dL (133 µmol/L) and urea nitrogen to 23 mg/dL (8.2 mmol urea/L). The patient had been placed on cyclosporine prophylactically because of the relatively poor match.

The patient presented 10 days post transplant with complaints of pain and tenderness over the site of the graft, fever, and reduced urine output. The following laboratory values were obtained:

Analyte	Value, conventional units	Reference range, conventional units	Value, SI units	Reference range, SI units
Urea nitrogen (S)	72 mg/dL	7-18	25.7 mmol urea/L	2.5-6.4
Creatinine (S)	7.0 mg/dL	0.8-1.4	619 µmol/L	71-124
Urea nitrogen /creatinine ratio	10.3:1	12-20:1	41.6:1 (urea:creatinine mole ratio)	48.5-80.8:1
Sodium (S)	142 mmol/L	136-145	Same	
Potassium (S)	5.9 mmol/L	3.8-5.1	Same	
Chloride (S)	99 mmol/L	98-108	Same	
CO_2, total (S)	13 mmol/L	23-29	Same	
Phosphorus (S)	9.5 mg/dL	2.7-4.5	3.07 mmol/L	0.87-1.45
Urate (S)	14.0 mg/dL	4.5-8.0	833 µmol/L	268-476
Calcium, total (S)	8.0 mg/dL	8.4-10.2	2.00 mmol/L	2.10-2.55
Cyclosporine, trough (B)	50 ng/mL	Therap.: 100-200	42 nmol/L	83-166
Creatinine clearance(S,U)	18 mL/min	90-130	0.17 mL/s per m^2	0.87-1.25
pH (aB)	7.28	7.35-7.45	Same	
pCO_2 (aB)	29 mm Hg	35-48	3.9 kPa	4.7-6.4
pO_2 (aB)	98 mm Hg	83-108	13.1 kPa	11.1-14.4
Urinalysis (U)	pH, 5.0; glucose, 1 +; leukocytes, 3-5/hpf			

Because of the low cyclosporine trough level, it was felt that cyclosporine toxicity was not likely the cause of the acute renal dysfunction. The urea nitrogen /creatinine ratio did not suggest pre-renal causes. Consequently, a renal biopsy was obtained and showed diffuse lymphocytic infiltration of the interstitium. There was interstitial edema and some loss of tubules. Renal vessels were patent, and there was no acute intimal injury. The patient's cyclosporine dose was increased, and he was given high-dosage steroids and the immunosuppressant anti-OKT3, a murine monoclonal antibody to CD3 that is a T-cell marker protein on the surfaces of human lymphocytes. This treatment resulted in an improvement in his overall state. The steroids were then rapidly tapered, and the anti-OKT3 course was completed. Several days later the patient presented for a routine follow-up and complained of feeling weak, tired, and somewhat nauseated, but his urine output was normal. Laboratory results obtained at this visit were as follows:

Analyte	Value, conventional units	Reference range, conventional units	Value, SI units	Reference range, SI units
Urea nitrogen (S)	19 mg/dL	7-18	6.8 mmol urea/L	2.5-6.4
Creatinine (S)	1.6 mg/dL	0.8-1.4	141 µmol/L	71-124
Creatinine clearance (S,U)	82 mL/min	90-130	0.79 mL/s per m^2	0.87-1.25
Sodium (S)	139 mmol/L	136-145	Same	
Potassium (S)	4.0 mmol/L	3.8-5.1	Same	
Chloride (S)	112 mmol/L	98-108	Same	
CO_2, total (S)	15 mmol/L	23-29	Same	
pH (aB)	7.31	7.35-7.45	Same	
pCO_2 (aB)	31 mm Hg	35-48	4.1 kPa	4.7-6.4
Urinalysis (U)	pH, 5.0; glucose, 2 +; leukocytes, 1-2/hpf			

Because of the persistent acidosis, the patient was given bicarbonate orally. After 48 hours, repeat laboratory studies revealed the following:

Analyte	Value, conventional units	Reference range, conventional units	Value, SI units	Reference range, SI units
Sodium (S)	141 mmol/L	136-145	Same	
Potassium (S)	3.1 mmol/L	3.8-5.1	Same	
Chloride (S)	112 mmol/L	98-108	Same	
Bicarbonate (aB)	17 mmol/L	18-23	Same	
pH (aB)	7.33	7.35-7.45	Same	
pCO_2 (aB)	33 mm Hg	35-48	4.4 kPa	4.7-6.4
Urinalysis (U)	pH, 7.0; glucose, 2 +; leukocytes, 1-2/hpf			
β_2-Microglobulin (U)	Increased			

The persistent acidosis was felt to be a manifestation of tubulointerstitial disease secondary to acute renal allograft rejection. Despite further therapy, allograft rejection continued, and creatinine clearance further declined. After 10 months, the patient returned for chronic hemodialysis.

Discussion

HLA Matching.[1] All immunocompetent individuals, except identical twins, reject tissues from other human beings. The vigor of the rejection is related to the immune competence of the recipient (host) and the immunogenicity of the graft (donor tissue). The less similar the donor and recipient, the greater the immunogenicity of the graft. The dominant system in immune recognition is the HLA (human leukocyte antigen) system, which consists of several closely linked loci on the short arm of chromosome six. Three loci — the A, B, and DR — are evaluated in clinical transplantation. The degree of the match is expressed as number of matching antigens out of a possible six; the patient in this case was matched for three out of six. Many investigators feel that matching for the B-DR loci is more important than matching for A locus, at least in first transplants. This may be because B-DR matching better predicts matching for the entire D region of the HLA complex than does either locus alone. The D region is very important because it codes for the Class II histocompatibility proteins that are critical in the regulation of T-helper cells, which are themselves the regulators of much of the acquired immune response. Unfortunately, allografts even with six of six matches still may be rejected, albeit less vigorously. Thus, all recipients except identical twins are treated with immunosuppressive agents.

Cyclosporine Effects and Toxicity.[1,3] One of the most important immunosuppressive agents is cyclosporine (CSA). It is such a powerful immunosuppressant that some investigators feel that, with its use, a kidney can be successfully transplanted to even poorly matched recipients. A major international study by Opelz,[2] however, still shows a beneficial effect of matching even when cyclosporine is given. Use of cyclosporine to suppress renal allograft rejection also exposes the patient to the drug's toxicities. Acute cyclosporine toxicity results from increased renal vascular resistance with resulting decreased blood flow and glomerular filtration rate (GFR) and is associated with little morphological change. Thus, development of oliguric dysfunction may be the result of allograft rejection due to insufficient drug levels or the result of drug toxicity. The problem is compounded by the fact that in cyclosporine-treated patients, the classic signs of rejection (graft tenderness and fever) may be suppressed. The clinical and anatomical pathology laboratories can be useful in resolving this question by performing drug level assays and renal biopsy.

Cyclosporine blocks induction of interleukin-2 (IL-2) mRNA in T cells and thus inhibits the cascade leading to T-cell activation and proliferation. Since cyclosporine can cause renal toxicity and dysfunction, monitoring trough levels in blood is very important. The choice of sample and methodology for measurement of cyclosporine levels is somewhat controversial. Whole blood is the preferred specimen, since the drug diffuses variably into red cells in a temperature- and hematocrit-dependent fashion. Measurement may be done by either immunoassay or high-performance liquid chromatography (HPLC). HPLC can distinguish active parent drug from metabolites, but it is time-consuming and requires a relatively large specimen. Immunoassays are faster and use less specimen, but they do not consistently distinguish parent drug from metabolites. The therapeutic range depends on the particular assay utilized. A typical therapeutic range for use in renal transplantation patients, as determined by HPLC using whole blood, is 100-200 ng/mL (83-166 nmol/L). Thus the patient in this case was actually below the therapeutic range and was unlikely to have had drug toxicity.

Allograft Rejection.[3] The biopsy in this case suggested that the renal allograft was being rejected. A rejection that occurs several days post transplant with a predominantly cellular type of immune response is termed acute rejection. Hyperacute rejection occurs within minutes to hours and involves predominantly the humoral arm of the immune response. This occurs in patients with preformed antibody to antigens expressed in the graft, particularly those on endothelial cells. Hyperacute rejections have been virtually eliminated by the laboratory performance of a crossmatch of the recipient's sera against lymphocytes from the donor.

The laboratory findings of acute renal allograft rejection are the same as those of acute renal failure and thus do not distinguish among rejection, acute tubular necrosis, and drug toxicity. Consequently, renal biopsy and a favorable response to antirejection therapy may be the best indicators of rejection. Renal biopsy is associated with significant morbidity. As an alternative, fine-needle aspiration cytology has been tried with some success. Attempts to monitor immunological events by measurement of activation antigens and lymphocyte subsets by flow cytometry have generally been disappointing.

The patient in this case had classic findings of renal allograft rejection with azotemia, oliguria, fever, and graft tenderness. Glomerular filtration was markedly reduced, and the histological picture was compatible with acute rejection. Secondary changes of hyperkalemia and metabolic acidosis were also present.

Uremic Acidosis.[4] Metabolic acidosis of renal failure develops when the kidney is unable to excrete the endogenously generated acid load of approximately 1 mEq/kg body weight per day. The metabolic acidosis that develops in the presence of diffuse renal disease associated with significant reduction of GFR is sometimes referred to as uremic acidosis. It is important to distinguish this entity from the more specific deficit of renal urine acidification in renal tubular acidosis (RTA) that is associated with well-preserved GFR and other renal functions. Because of the accumulation of organic acids, the acidosis of renal failure is usually a normochloremic acidosis with increased anion gap. RTA is typically a hyperchloremic non-anion gap acidosis. However, some studies have suggested that as many as 30% of patients with renal failure may have some component of hyperchloremic acidosis. In addition, potassium retention and hyperkalemia are common in renal failure, whereas some forms of proximal and distal RTA are characterized by potassium loss and hypokalemia.

The vast majority of patients with GFR <20 mL/min will have some degree of acidosis as manifested by a reduction in plasma bicarbonate. In general, the more severe the reduction of GFR, the lower the plasma bicarbonate concentration will be. The basic defect is a failure of tubular function resulting in a net acid excretion that is less than the daily endogenous production. If glomerular function is relatively less compromised than tubular function, the filtration and excretion of organic anions occurs, and a non-anion gap acidosis is the result. If glomerular and tubular function are proportionately reduced, as might be expected in the diffuse injury of advanced renal failure, the organic anions are retained in proportion to the deficit in hydrogen ion excretion, resulting in an increased anion-gap acidosis. In many cases the acidosis will be a mixed-anion gap and non-anion gap acidosis. Additional electrolyte findings in uremia include hyperkalemia, hyperphosphatemia, and hypocalcemia. Generally, in chronic renal failure there is reasonable preservation of distal tubular hydrogen ion excretion so that acidification of the urine occurs appropriately. The major deficit in chronic renal failure is a reduction in ammonium formation and excretion, which is considerably greater than the reduction in titratable acid excretion. The reduction in ammonium excretion appears to be a direct result of the loss of functioning nephron mass.

Renal Tubular Acidosis (RTA).[5-7] After resolution of this patient's episode of graft rejection, much of his renal function returned to near-normal values. In addition, other electrolytes returned to normal except for chloride, which remained moderately elevated. This picture was not compatible with renal failure, and thus the persisting metabolic acidosis would not be expected to be due to renal failure. Furthermore, this is a hyperchloremic metabolic acidosis, which is not the typical form of acidosis seen in renal failure. Certainly, a nonrenal cause of hyperchloremic acidosis could be considered.

Many of the conditions that give rise to hyperchloremic metabolic acidosis can be viewed as secondary to either loss of bicarbonate in urine or stool or the addition of hydrochloric acid or hydrochloric acid-generating compounds. A detailed discussion of the differential of extrarenal causes is not included here but is available.[5] Renal causes include proximal and distal RTA, aldosterone deficiency, hyperkalemia, defective ammoniagenesis, and renal insufficiency. This patient did not have the electrolyte pattern of either aldosterone deficiency or hyperkalemia and did not at this point have renal insufficiency. Patients with distal RTA have an inability to acidify urine in the distal tubule. There is some controversy as to whether this deficit is secondary to back leak of secreted H^+ or inability to secrete H^+. The patient in this case had a urine pH of 5.0, demonstrating the ability to acidify the urine. A significant clue to the underlying problem was obtained when the patient was placed on bicarbonate therapy. In response to bicarbonate therapy, the plasma bicarbonate increased only minimally, and the urine became alkaline despite the preserved ability of the distal tubules to acidify. This must have been due to proximal tubular wasting of bicarbonate and thus represented the proximal form of RTA.

Healthy individuals excrete very little bicarbonate in their urine. Patients with proximal RTA have a reduced renal threshold for bicarbonate, typically between 15 and 20 mmol/L. When plasma bicarbonate is below the renal threshold, urine pH may be appropriately acidic because of preserved distal tubular mechanisms. However, once plasma bicarbonate levels increase, bicarbonate wasting occurs and eventually overwhelms the acid-excreting capacity of the distal nephron, and alkaline urine is produced (pH >6.0). Most of these patients have significant bicarbonate wasting with fractional excretion* >15%; occasional patients may have more moderate wasting with fractional excretion* between 3% and 15%.[7] Many patients have, as did this patient, additional evidence of proximal renal tubular dysfunction such as glucosuria, amino aciduria, and β_2-microglobulinuria. These findings all reflect disordered proximal tubular transport. In addition, because of reduced proximal sodium and bicarbonate resorption, there is increased distal delivery of sodium, which exchanges with potassium and leads to urinary potassium wasting and hypokalemia. Further bicarbonate administration may aggravate the hypokalemia.

Proximal RTA as a pure defect in bicarbonate transport is usually seen only in children. Much more often the defect is a component of a generalized defect in proximal tubular transport with wasting of glucose, phosphate, urate, amino acids, and others (i.e., Fanconi syndrome). Thus, hypophosphatemia and hypouricemia are frequent laboratory findings. The hypokalemia may result in muscle weakness or cramps, paresthesias, polyuria, and thirst. One of the most common symptoms of RTA in children is failure to thrive, presumably secondary to the chronic acidosis. The causes of proximal RTA are numerous but are nicely summarized by Batlle.[6]

In this particular case, proximal RTA was part of a generalized defect in proximal tubular transport brought about by tubulointerstitial injury secondary to renal allograft rejection. The proximal renal tubule is normally very rich in Class II major histocompatibility antigens,

---

* Fractional excretion of a compound is the renal clearance of that compound expressed as a percentage of creatinine clearance or of some other measure of GFR. Clearance is calculated as concentration of analyte in urine divided by its concentration in serum and multiplied by the urine flow rate in mL/min. For example,

$$\text{Creatinine clearance, mL/min} = \frac{\text{Creatinine (U), mg/dL}}{\text{Creatinine (S), mg/dL}} \times \text{Flow rate (U), mL/min}$$

For example , fractional clearance of bicarbonate is determined from assay of bicarbonate and creatinine on the same urine and serum specimens. The value is calculated as the bicarbonate clearance divided by the creatinine clearance in an equation simplified by the cancellation of units and flow rate, thus:

$$\text{Fractional clearance (bicarbonate), \%} = \frac{\text{Creatinine (S), mg/dL} \times \text{Bicarbonate (U), mmol/L}}{\text{Creatinine (U), mg/dL} \times \text{Bicarbonate (S), mmol/L}} \times 100$$

Since bicarbonate is normally almost completely reabsorbed, fractional excretion is <3%. Patients with proximal RTA, however, have significant bicarbonate wasting; thus, fractional excretion is typically >15%.

possibly because of their role in oligopeptide transport, and is thus a vulnerable target for immune attack in patients receiving incompatible renal allografts.

References

1. Strom, T.B., and Carpenter, C.B.: Immunobiology of kidney transplantation. *In:* The Kidney, 4th ed. B.M. Brenner and F.C. Rector, Jr., Eds. Philadelphia, W.B. Saunders Co., 1991.

2. Opelz, G.: The benefits of exchanging donor kidneys among transplant centers. N. Engl. J. Med., *318:* 1289, 1988.

3. Ramos, E.L., Tilney, N.L., and Ravenscraft, M.D.: Clinical aspects of renal transplantation. *In:* The Kidney, 4th ed. B.M. Brenner and F.C. Rector, Jr., Eds. Philadelphia, W.B. Saunders Co., 1991.

4. Madiss, N.E., and Kraut, J.A.: Uremic acidosis. *In:* The Regulation of Acid-Base Balance. D.W. Seldin and G. Giebisch, Eds. New York, Raven Press, 1989.

5. Batlle, D.C.: Hyperchloremic metabolic acidosis. *In:* The Regulation of Acid-Base Balance. D.W. Seldin and G. Giebisch, Eds. New York, Raven Press, 1989.

6. Batlle, D.C.: Renal tubular acidosis. *In:* The Regulation of Acid-Base Balance. D.W. Seldin and G. Giebisch, Eds. New York, Raven Press, 1989.

7. Tietz, N.W., Ed.: Textbook of Clinical Chemistry. Philadelphia, W.B. Saunders Co., 1986.

Additional Reading

Batlle, D.: Renal tubular acidosis. *In:* Symposium on Acid-Base Disorders. Med. Clin. North Am., *67:* 859-878, 1983.

Rock, R.C., Walker, W.G., and Jennings, C.D.: Nitrogen metabolites and renal function. *In:* Textbook of Clinical Chemistry. N.W. Tietz, Ed. Philadelphia, W.B. Saunders Co., 1986.

MAN WITH HYPERTENSION AND FEVER

C. Darrell Jennings, Contributor
David N. Bailey, Reviewer

A 75-year-old man with longstanding hypertension developed a fever and upper respiratory illness two weeks prior to admission. The fever ranged between 103 and 104 °F (39.4-40.0 °C); there were no localized pulmonary findings or productive cough. This illness did not respond to a cephalosporin (Keflex), and thus amantadine was begun one week prior to admission. Four days prior to admission the patient's family stopped all medications, including his antihypertensive drugs, because they felt he was having a reaction to the medicine.

At 3:00 a.m. the morning of admission, the patient awoke with severe dyspnea without chest pain. Upon arrival at the community hospital emergency room, a chest film revealed pulmonary edema. Vital signs were pulse, 140 BPM; temperature, 103 °F (39.4 °C); and blood pressure, 210/110 mm Hg. The patient was treated with intravenous furosemide and intravenous nitroglycerin. The blood pressure decreased somewhat and then fell precipitously to a systolic pressure of 50 mm Hg. Dopamine, bicarbonate, and normal saline were started and returned the systolic pressure to the 100-110 mm Hg range. Laboratory values obtained at the community hospital were as follows:

Analyte	Value, conventional units	Reference range, conventional units	Value, SI units	Reference range, SI units
Sodium (S)	138 mmol/L	136-145	Same	
Potassium (S)	4.2 mmol/L	3.8-5.1	Same	
Chloride (S)	101 mmol/L	98-108	Same	
CO_2, total (S)	32 mmol/L	23-31	Same	
Urea nitrogen (S)	9 mg/dL	8-21	3.2 mmol urea/L	2.9-7.5
Creatinine (S)	1.7 mg/dL	0.8-1.4	150 µmol/L	71-124
Urea nitrogen/creatinine ratio	5:1	12-20:1	20.2:1 (urea:creatinine mole ratio)	48.5-80.8:1
Bilirubin, total (S)	0.9 mg/dL	0.2-1.1	15 µmol/L	3-19
ALT (S)	92 U/L	13-40	1.53 µkat/L	0.22-0.67
AST (S)	107 U/L	19-48	1.78 µkat/L	0.32-0.80
CK (S)	479 U/L	38-174	7.98 µkat/L	0.63-2.90
LDH (S)	433 U/L	110-210	7.2 µkat/L	1.83-3.50
ALP (S)	91 U/L	56-119	1.5 µkat/L	0.9-1.98
Hemoglobin (B)	14 g/dL	14-18	8.69 mmol/L	8.69-11.17
Hematocrit (B)	42 %	40-54	0.42	0.40-0.54
Platelet count (B)	$85 \times 10^3/\mu L$	150-450	$85 \times 10^9/L$	150-450

The patient was transferred by air ambulance to the University Medical Center, a tertiary care hospital. Physical examination suggested pulmonary consolidation, and a chest X-ray examination confirmed right upper lobe pneumonia. No focal neurological deficits were found.   A test for hemosiderin in urine was requested in view of the decrease in hemoglobin and hematocrit compared with values obtained at the community hospital; in the absence of frank hemorrhage, the admitting physician considered the possibility of a hemolytic process.

Three hours after admission and stabilization, the following laboratory results were obtained:

Analyte	Value, conventional units	Reference range, conventional units	Value, SI units	Reference range, SI units
Urea nitrogen (S)	12 mg/dL	8-21	4.3 mmol urea/L	2.9-7.5
Creatinine (S)	1.4 mg/dL	0.8-1.4	124 μmol/L	71-124
Urea nitrogen/creatinine ratio	9:1	12-20:1	36.4:1 (urea:creatinine mole ratio)	48.5-80.8:1
Sodium (S)	136 mmol/L	136-145	Same	
Potassium (S)	3.3 mmol/L	3.8-5.1	Same	
pH (aB)	7.43	7.35-7.45	Same	
pCO_2 (aB)	39 mm Hg	35-48	5.2 kPa	4.7-6.4
pO_2 (aB) (on 30% FI O_2)	116 mm Hg	83-108	15.5 kPa	11.1-14.4
Hemoglobin (B)	13.1 g/dL	14-18	8.13 mmol/L	8.69-11.17
Hematocrit (B)	39 %	40-54	0.39	0.40-0.54
Urinalysis (U)	Within normal limits; negative for hemo-siderin			

The evening of admission, about eight hours later, the following additional laboratory data were obtained:

Analyte	Value, conventional units	Reference range, conventional units	Value, SI units	Reference range, SI units
Hemoglobin (B)	12.9 g/dL	14-18	8.01 mmol/L	8.69-11.17
Hematocrit (B)	38 %	40-54	0.38	0.40-0.54
Platelet count (B)	$67 \times 10^3/\mu L$	150-450	$67 \times 10^9/L$	150-450
Prothrombin time (P)	12.2 s (control: 11.8 s)	11.5-13.5	Same	
Partial thromboplastin time (P)	28.6 s (control: 28.8 s)	23.1-33.3	Same	
Protein, total (S)	5.5 g/dL	6.2-7.8	55 g/L	62-78
Albumin (S)	2.8 g/dL	3.4-4.8	28 g/L	34-48
Amylase (S)	111 U/L	21-150	1.85 μkat/L	0.35-2.50

These data appeared to rule out pancreatitis or a coagulation disorder. Although hemoglobin and hematocrit appeared to have stabilized, thrombocytopenia persisted, and hemolytic anemia remained a possibility. By the second day, however, the patient had virtually no urine output. The following table shows his laboratory results for days 2 and 3:

Analyte	Second day, a.m.	Second day, p.m.	Third day, a.m.
Urea nitrogen (S)	22 mg/dL (7.9 mmol urea/L)	35 mg/dL (12.5 mmol urea/L)	42 mg/dL (15.0 mmol urea/L)
Creatinine (S)	2.1 mg/dL (186 μmol/L)	3.6 mg/dL (318 μmol/L)	4.4 mg/dL (389 μmol/L)
Hemoglobin (B)	11.6 g/dL (7.20 mmol/L)	10.5 g/dL (6.52 mmol/L)	10.6 g/dL (6.58 mmol/L)
Hematocrit (B)	34 % (0.34)	31 % (0.31)	31 % (0.31)

Analyte	Second day, a.m.	Second day, p.m.	Third day, a.m.
Platelet count (B)	54 x 10³/µL (54 x 10⁹/L)	51 x 10³/µL (51 x 10⁹/L)	51 x 10³/µL (51 x 10⁹/L)
Magnesium (S)	1.6 mg/dL (0.66 mmol/L)		
Peripheral blood smear	Unremarkable		Unremarkable
Coagulation studies		Within normal limits	
Urinalysis (U)		Within normal limits	Leukocytes, 1-5/hpf; erythrocytes, 5-10/hpf; renal tubular epithelial cells, 1-5/hpf
Reticulocyte count, corrected (B)			1.8 %
Sodium (U)			44 mmol/L
Osmolality (U)			258 mOsm/kg (258 mmol/kg)

Rapid rise in serum levels of urea nitrogen and creatinine and developing stability of hemoglobin, hematocrit, and thrombocyte values, together with barely elevated reticulocyte count, turned attention away from the hematological findings and focused it on acute renal failure.

Other physicians and the clinical pathologist were called into consultation. The first consultant raised the question of thrombotic thrombocytopenic purpura–hemolytic uremic syndrome (TTP-HUS) and the possibility of plasma exchange. A second consultant thought that acute renal failure secondary to acute tubular necrosis (ATN) was more likely and that anemia and thrombocytopenia were probably due to marrow suppression secondary to the infectious process. The pathologist also felt that TTP-HUS was unlikely and thus recommended against plasma exchange.

The morning of the next day, the fourth hospital day, the following laboratory studies indicated relatively stable hematological findings and a further increase in serum urea nitrogen and creatinine:

Analyte	Value, conventional units	Reference range, conventional units	Value, SI units	Reference range, SI units
Urea nitrogen (S)	66 mg/dL	8-21	23.6 mmol urea/L	2.9-7.5
Creatinine (S)	7.0 mg/dL	0.8-1.4	619 µmol/L	71-124
Urea nitrogen/creatinine ratio (calculated)	9:1	12-20:1	36.4:1 (urea:creatinine mole ratio)	48.5-80.8:1
Hemoglobin (B)	10.2 g/dL	14-18	6.33 mmol/L	8.69-11.17
Hematocrit (B)	29 %	40-54	0.29	0.40-0.54
Platelet count (B)	67 x 10³/µL	150-450	67 x 10⁹/L	150-450

Dialysis was started, and laboratory results reported on the fifth day were as follows:

Analyte	Value, conventional units	Reference range, conventional units	Value, SI units	Reference range, SI units
Hemoglobin (B)	10.2 g/dL	14-18	6.33 mmol/L	8.69-11.17
Hematocrit (B)	29 %	40-54	0.29	0.40-0.54
Platelet count (B)	94 x 10³/µL	150-450	94 x 10⁹/L	150-450
Bilirubin, total (S)	0.6 mg/dL	0.2-1.1	10 µmol/L	3-19
Haptoglobin (S)	Within normal limits			

Over the next several days the hematological picture improved spontaneously; hemoglobin rose to 12 g/dL (7.45 mmol/L), hematocrit to 36% (0.36), and platelet count to 191 x 10³/μL (191 x 10⁹/μL). Serum electrolytes, acid-base values, and urea nitrogen, determined during this period of hemodialysis, stabilized. The patient remained in acute renal failure until the 22nd hospital day when urine output increased to 500-1000 mL/d. Renal biopsy performed on the 22nd hospital day showed regenerating tubules consistent with improving ATN. By the 27th hospital day, urine output was >1500 mL/d, and serum urea nitrogen and creatinine were decreasing without further dialysis. When serum potassium fell to 3.1 mmol/L, oral potassium supplementation was initiated. After an uneventful diuretic phase, the patient was discharged with only medications for his hypertension.

Differential Diagnosis

This case poses the problem of a febrile illness, anemia, and thrombocytopenia developing into acute renal failure. The combination caused serious consideration to be given to a diagnosis of thrombotic thrombocytopenic purpura–hemolytic uremic syndrome (TTP-HUS). TTP-HUS is treated by plasma exchange (plasmapheresis), a procedure in which whole blood is removed and separated into plasma and cellular components with return of the cellular components to the patient but replacement of the plasma with donor plasma. Once performed manually, plasma exchange is now automated in a continuous flow device that requires extracorporeal circulation and anticoagulation. The risks of plasma exchange for this patient were bleeding due to anticoagulation, infection from the extracorporeal circulation, and most important, infection and adverse reactions from the large amount of donor plasma that would be required. Critical examination of the patient's physical status and laboratory data, as well as the relative rarity of TTP-HUS, led to a choice of hemodialysis as an immediate treatment. During dialysis, spontaneous improvement in the cytopenic state, together with recovery from anuria and the findings of the renal biopsy, finally resolved the diagnostic question in favor of ATN.

Thrombotic Thrombocytopenic Purpura–Hemolytic Uremic Syndrome (TTP-HUS). TTP-HUS was recently reviewed in the case records of the Massachusetts General Hospital.[1] Originally described by Moschowitz in 1925, thrombotic thrombocytopenic purpura (TTP) consists of five classic findings: (1) neurologic deficit, (2) renal dysfunction, (3) fever, (4) thrombocytopenia, and (5) microangiopathic hemolytic anemia. Hemolytic uremic syndrome (HUS), seen predominantly in children, has similar features and an identical pathophysiological process that consists of microvascular hyaline thrombi, and thus it is generally not considered a distinct entity.

This case presents some of the features of TTP-HUS but lacks certain critical laboratory and clinical findings. TTP-HUS is predominantly a disease of the third and fourth decades with only 18% of patients being over age 50.[1] It does, however, occasionally occur in older individuals.[2] Thrombocytopenia with a mean platelet count of 20,500/μL (20.5 x 10⁹/L) is present in 83-93% of patients with TTP-HUS.[1] The drop in platelet count accompanies the formation of microthrombi, the central pathophysiological event. This patient's platelet count remained stable around 52 x 10³/μL (52 x 10⁹/L), while renal function deteriorated. Subsequently, the platelet count rose dramatically as renal function further declined. This pattern is contrary to our current understanding of the pathophysiological mechanism of TTP-HUS.

A second major feature of TTP-HUS is microangiopathic hemolytic anemia secondary to the formation of intraluminal fibrin thrombi in the microvasculature. This finding is present in 96-98% of TTP-HUS patients.[1] A hallmark of this process is the formation of schistocytes, helmet-shaped erythrocyte fragments, seen in 251 of 254 patients in one series.[1]

This patient lacked several key findings of TTP-HUS. First, there was no evidence of intravascular hemolysis, since total serum bilirubin and haptoglobin levels were normal, urine hemosiderin was negative, and serum LDH was only mildly elevated despite coexisting pulmonary disease. Second, schistocytes (the hallmark of TTP-HUS) were not seen on blood smears. Third, the low reticulocyte count suggested an inadequate bone marrow response as a probable cause of the anemia and thrombocytopenia. Failure to find laboratory evidence of hemolysis or evidence of a microangiopathic process in the peripheral blood smear placed the diagnosis of TTP-HUS in serious doubt. Finally, the renal dysfunction seen in 76-88% of the patients with TTP-HUS differs in several important aspects from this patient's findings. TTP-HUS typically is associated with an abnormal urine sediment, hematuria, and moderate proteinuria. This patient's urinalysis was unremarkable initially despite increasing serum urea nitrogen and creatinine levels. When urinalysis results became abnormal, the urine contained renal tubular epithelial cells, a finding more suggestive of acute tubular injury. In addition, the patient's clinical course, characterized by anuria and daily doubling of urea nitrogen and creatinine values, is unusual in TTP-HUS; only 11% of patients present with acute renal failure[1] and even fewer with anuric renal failure.[3]

Although the combination of fever, anemia, thrombocytopenia, and renal failure in this patient initially suggested TTP-HUS, the diagnosis could not be sustained when the laboratory findings were critically examined. Because the anemia and thrombocytopenia were self-limited and could be explained as a secondary effect of bone marrow suppression by the pulmonary infection and drug therapy, the major question remaining was the etiology of anuric acute renal failure.

Prenal Azotemia. This condition is caused by diminished renal function due to poor renal perfusion. In prerenal azotemia there is relative preservation of tubular concentration function. Consequently, renal tubules respond to the decreased glomerular filtration rate (GFR) with sodium and water retention and concentration of the urine.[4] The result is a urine sodium typically <20 mmol/L and an elevated urine osmolality, creatinine, and specific gravity; most characteristic is a fractional excretion* of sodium <1%.[4]

In *acute renal failure* due to intrinsic renal disease, there is loss of tubular function. This loss results in a glomerular filtrate that is little altered by the tubules. Thus, urine may be isosthenuric (specific gravity of urine similar to that of unmodified glomerular filtrate, 1.010 ± 0.002), urine sodium >20 mmol/L, and the fractional excretion of sodium greater than 3%.[4] This patient's urine osmolality, urine sodium, and specific gravity are all typical of intrinsic renal disease and not prerenal azotemia.

Serum findings may also help differentiate prerenal azotemia from intrinsic renal disease. With the reduced GFR of prerenal azotemia, intact tubules will allow back diffusion of urea without creatinine (creatinine is only minimally absorbed by the tubules). Additionally, tubules secrete creatinine but not urea from the blood to the glomerular filtrate, increasing the net excretion of creatinine but not urea. The result is that serum urea concentrations will climb faster than creatinine levels so that the urea nitrogen/creatinine ratio will rise above 20:1. In ATN, the tubule does not exclude creatinine, and a normal or a low ratio is maintained. This

---

* Fractional excretion for sodium is determined from an assay of sodium and creatinine on the same urine and serum specimens. The value is calculated as the sodium clearance divided by the creatinine clearance in an equation simplified by the cancellation of units and flow rate, thus:

$$\text{Fractional excretion (sodium), \%} = \frac{\text{Creatinine (S), mg/dL} \times \text{Sodium (U), mmol/L}}{\text{Creatinine (U), mg/dL} \times \text{Sodium (S), mmol/L}} \times 100$$

patient's ratio remained very close to 10:1 throughout the period of renal dysfunction, favoring the diagnosis of intrinsic renal disease.

The most common cause of acute reversible oliguric renal failure is ATN. The renal tubules are particularly vulnerable to ischemic injury, both because they have a very high metabolic rate and because their blood supply comes from the portal circulation via the efferent arteriole. The portal supply is less oxygenated and under less pressure than a direct arterial supply is. Also, because of their resorptive and concentrating functions, the renal tubular epithelial cells are vulnerable to toxins such as heavy metals and some drugs. Toxic injury and ischemic injury are therefore the two most common causes of ATN.

In this patient there was a well-documented episode of sudden hypotension following the treatment of the patient's hypertensive crisis. Renal function was only very mildly compromised until this event. Subsequently, the patient was anuric with daily doubling of creatinine and urea nitrogen values, a situation indicative of almost complete cessation of renal function. This is a classic picture of ATN secondary to a single ischemic event — in this case, hypotension.

Treatment

Once injured, the renal tubular epithelial cells require three to four weeks to regenerate. During this time the patient must be supported with dialysis as well as fluid and electrolyte management. The most common cause of morbidity is infection. Once regeneration occurs, the patient enters a diuretic phase. The patient must be monitored because there may be wasting of electrolytes such as potassium and sodium. Many patients, such as this one, experience complete recovery of renal function with good supportive care.

References

1. Scully, R.E., Ed.: Case records of the Massachusetts General Hospital. N. Engl. J. Med., *325:* 265, 1991.

2. Knupp, C.L.: Thrombotic thrombocytopenic purpura in older patients. J. Am. Geriatr. Soc., *36:* 331, 1988.

3. Dunea, G., Murhrcke, R.C., Nakamoto, S., and Schwartz, F.D.: Thrombotic thrombocytopenic purpura and acute renal failure. Am. J. Med., *41:* 1000, 1966.

4. Rock, R.C., Walker, W.G., and Jennings, C.D.: Nitrogen metabolites and renal function. *In:* Textbook of Clinical Chemistry. N.W. Tietz, Ed. Philadelphia, W.B. Saunders Co., 1986.

GLOMERULONEPHRITIS, UREMIA, PULMONARY INFILTRATION, AND HEMOPTYSIS

C. Darrell Jennings, Contributor
Richard A. Mc Pherson, Reviewer

A 47-year-old white female developed severe nausea and vomiting four weeks prior to her current hospital admission. There had been no pain, but she had experienced a 7-lb (3.2-kg) weight loss. Her serum urea nitrogen was 40 mg/dL (14.3 mmol urea/L) and her creatinine 3.2 mg/dL (283 µmol/L). Urinalysis revealed numerous erythrocytes and granular casts, but an intravenous pyelogram (IVP) showed no structural abnormalities or obstruction. Five days later the creatinine rose to 6.8 mg/dL (60 µmol/L), the serum urea nitrogen rose to 72 mg/dL (25.7 mmol urea/L), and the creatinine clearance was 13 mL/min (reference range, 72-114). Past history was unrevealing, and there were no abnormal physical findings.

The patient was referred to the University Hospital because of the significant deterioration of renal function. On admission the patient had the following laboratory findings:

Analyte	Value, conventional units	Reference range, conventional units	Value, SI units	Reference range, SI units
Leukocyte count (B)	Within normal limits			
Platelet count (B)	Within normal limits			
Hemoglobin (B)	11.0 g/dL	12-16	6.83 mmol/L	7.45-9.93
Creatinine (S)	6.3 mg/dL	0.7-1.2	557 µmol/L	62-106
Urea nitrogen (S)	70 mg/dL	7-18	25.0 mmol urea/L	2.5-6.4
Sodium (S)	135 mmol/L	136-145	Same	
Potassium (S)	4.6 mmol/L	3.8-5.1	Same	
Chloride (S)	97 mmol/L	98-108	Same	
CO_2, total (S)	21 mmol/L	23-29	Same	
C3 complement (S)	Within normal limits			
Antinuclear antibodies (ANA) (S)	Within normal limits			
Antistreptolysin O (ASO) titer (S)	Within normal limits			
Urinalysis (U)	Specific gravity, 1.010; pH, 6.0; protein, 1+; granular casts and numerous erythrocytes present in sediment; 24-h protein, 518 mg			

A chest X-ray examination revealed a right middle lobe infiltrate.

The patient was treated with intravenous fluids and acid-base and electrolyte management. Subsequently the serum creatinine decreased to 4.4 mg/dL (389 µmol/L). She was discharged with a diagnosis of acute renal failure induced by the IVP and superimposed on renal insufficiency of undetermined cause. Plans were made to determine the etiology of the renal insufficiency on an outpatient basis.

Five days after discharge, the patient presented with increasingly severe nausea and vomiting. Physical examination was unchanged except for an increased temperature of 100.2 °F (37.9 °C). The serum creatinine was now 7.8 mg/dL (690 μmol/L) and the serum urea nitrogen 88 mg/dL (31.4 mmol urea/L). Prothrombin and partial thromboplastin times were normal, and erythrocyte casts were seen on urinalysis.

Shortly after her second admission, a renal biopsy provided findings of crescentic glomerulonephritis. Immunofluorescence studies were indeterminate, and the patient was placed on immunosuppressive therapy. Over a two-week period, the creatinine fell to 1.9 mg/dL (168 μmol/L). An attempt to decrease the immunosuppression therapy resulted in a rise of the serum creatinine to 2.4 mg/dL (212 μmol/L). At this time the patient developed hemoptysis and showed bilateral pulmonary infiltrates on the chest film. Arterial blood gas studies gave the following results:

Analyte	Value, conventional units	Reference range, conventional units	Value, SI units	Reference range, SI units
pH (aB)	7.50	7.35-7.45	Same	
pO_2 (aB)	60 mm Hg	83-108	8.0 kPa	11.1-14.4
pCO_2 (aB)	38 mm Hg	32-45	5.1 kPa	4.3-6.0

Pulmonary function continued to deteriorate with pO_2 falling to 45 mm Hg (6.0 kPa) despite increasing the fraction of inspired oxygen (FI O_2) up to 100%.

Creatinine values continued to rise, urine output decreased progressively, and the creatinine clearance fell to 7 mL/min (0.07 mL/s per m²; reference range, 72-114; 0.69-1.10). By the 29th hospital day recurrent hemoptysis had developed, and aggressive plasmapheresis (plasma exchange) was initiated because open biopsy revealed lung findings that included focal necrosis of alveolar walls with intra-alveolar hemorrhage. Immunofluorescence studies of lung tissue showed linear fluorescence along the alveolar basement membranes.

The patient's respiratory status slowly improved over the next two weeks. However, her renal function improved only minimally as evidenced by a creatinine clearance of 15 mL/min (0.14 mL/s per m²). She was discharged home and, on an outpatient basis, underwent plasmapheresis weekly for one month. Two months later at a clinic visit, she had complaints of nausea and vomiting, diffuse itching, weakness and fatigue, and sharp left-sided pleuritic pain. On physical examination, she was hypertensive and had 1+ to 2+ pedal edema. A pleural friction rub was heard on auscultation. Her skin had a sallow color.

Laboratory tests revealed the following:

Analyte	Value, conventional units	Reference range, conventional units	Value, SI units	Reference range, SI units
Sodium (S)	139 mmol/L	136-145	Same	
Potassium (S)	5.5 mmol/L	3.8-5.1	Same	
Chloride (S)	102 mmol/L	98-108	Same	
CO_2, total (S)	19 mmol/L	23-29	Same	
Urea nitrogen (S)	95 mg/dL	7-18	33.9 mmol urea/L	2.5-6.4
Creatinine (S)	9.1 mg/dL	0.7-1.2	804 μmol/L	62-106
Glucose (S)	105 mg/dL	75-105	5.8 mmol/L	4.2-5.8
Calcium (S)	6.2 mg/dL	8.4-10.2	1.55 mmol/L	2.10-2.54
Phosphorus (S)	5.6 mg/dL	2.7-4.5	1.81 mmol/L	0.87-1.45
Urate (S)	8.8 mg/dL	2.5-6.2	523 μmol/L	149-369
Hemoglobin (B)	9.7 g/dL	12-16	6.02 mmol/L	7.45-9.93

Analyte	Value, conventional units	Reference range, conventional units	Value, SI units	Reference range, SI units
Hematocrit (B)	28 %	37-47	0.28	0.37-0.47
Urinalysis (U)	pH, 6.5; protein, 1+; occasional erythrocytes and leukocytes; rare broad waxy casts			

Erythrocyte indices were as follows: MCV, 91 fL (reference range, 81-99); MCH, 29 pg (reference range, 27-31); MCHC, 35 g Hg/dL (22 mmol Hb/L; reference range, 33-37; 20-23). The corrected reticulocyte count was <1%. The patient was clearly uremic and was considered a candidate for chronic hemodialysis and ultimately renal transplantation.

Discussion

This patient's case presents the problem of rapidly deteriorating renal function, terminating in uremia with coexistent pulmonary hemorrhage and hemoptysis. The presence of erythrocytes in the urine indicated hemorrhage into the urinary tract. Whereas hemorrhage may occur at any point from the glomerulus to the urethra, the presence of erythrocyte casts localizes the process high in the nephron, namely, the glomerulus. Additional evidence of reduced glomerular filtration rate (GFR), i.e., rising serum urea nitrogen and creatinine, further supports the inference that the glomeruli are the site of injury. The combination of hematuria with manifestations of reduced GFR constitutes the nephritic syndrome, which is the result of diffuse injury to the glomeruli.

Most glomerulopathies are the result of immunological injury of either the immune-complex type or antibody-dependent type. The injury may be either a primary manifestation of a disease or part of a systemic disease such as Goodpasture's disease.

A hallmark of glomerulonephritis is severe injury to the glomerular filtration apparatus such that erythrocytes are lost into Bowman's space and then appear in the urine. Less severe forms of glomerular injury may allow loss of protein but not of cellular elements. If protein loss is massive, the nephrotic syndrome may result.

Other features of glomerulonephritis are a reduction of blood flow through the glomeruli and a reduction in GFR because of compromise of the capillaries by the inflammatory process. If the injury involves only a few glomeruli, the result is generally asymptomatic hematuria and proteinuria. Alternatively, if the injury is diffuse, the nephritic syndrome results. The nephritic syndrome consists of hematuria plus evidence of reduced GFR. Reduced GFR is accompanied by hypertension, edema, azotemia, oliguria, and electrolyte and acid-base disturbances, most commonly metabolic acidosis.

When injury to the glomeruli is particularly severe, activated clotting factors enter Bowman's space with resulting deposition of fibrin. The fibrin appears to stimulate a proliferative response from the parietal epithelial cells, infiltrating macrophages, and neutrophils. The capsular proliferation may compress the glomerulus or obstruct the opening into the proximal renal tubule. In either case, severe compromise of nephron function is the result.

Some patients present with the clinical and laboratory findings of acute nephritis and suffer a rapid loss of renal function over a matter of weeks. The clinical term rapidly progressive glomerulonephritis (RPGN) is then used. Frequently these patients have severe oliguria or even anuria. Electrolyte disturbances, particularly hyperkalemia, may become an urgent problem, and metabolic acidosis may develop.

In early glomerulonephritis, tubular function may remain relatively unchanged, and the urine and serum biochemical pattern may resemble prerenal causes of azotemia with concentrated, low-sodium urine and an increased serum urea nitrogen/creatinine ratio. As injury progresses, the urine becomes more isosthenuric (specific gravity of urine similar to that of unmodified glomerular filtrate, 1.010 ± 0.002), and the serum urea nitrogen/creatinine ratio becomes more typical of intrinsic renal disease.

Rapidly progressive glomerulonephritis (RPGN) is a clinical syndrome with many causes. These are generally divided into three groups: postinfectious RPGN, RPGN associated with systemic disease, and idiopathic RPGN. About 50% of RPGN is idiopathic. The most common form occurring after infection is post-streptococcal. Common systemic diseases associated with RPGN include systemic lupus erythematosus, Wegener's granulomatosis, vasculitis, and Goodpasture's syndrome. The pulmonary findings confirm that this patient had Goodpasture's syndrome. Goodpasture's syndrome is associated with antibodies to basement membrane antigens present in pulmonary alveoli and renal glomeruli, and this explains the clinical picture of RPGN with associated pulmonary hemorrhage. In both organs there is an acute necrotizing inflammatory lesion resulting in loss of basement membrane integrity with subsequent hemorrhage.

Patients with Goodpasture's syndrome usually present with pulmonary symptoms. A small number of patients, as in this case, have initial renal findings. Therapy includes immunosuppressive drugs. Although recent reports indicate that there have been dramatic responses to plasma exchange, many patients, as in this case, still eventually require dialysis or transplantation. Transplantation is frequently delayed to reduce the risk of recurrent disease post-transplantation. The diagnosis of Goodpasture's is based on the finding of a linear fluorescent pattern in pulmonary or glomerular basement membrane or both. The demonstration of anti-glomerular basement membrane (anti-GBM) antibodies in peripheral blood is generally the initial laboratory test.

The uremic syndrome is the result of extensive loss of nephron function including both glomerular and tubular components. The full-blown uremic syndrome is generally seen when GFR is less than 20-25% of normal. The cause is inadequately functioning renal mass. It may be thought of as loss of the kidney's normal excretory, regulatory, and endocrine functions.

Failure of excretory function results in retention of nitrogenous wastes, measured as serum urea nitrogen and creatinine concentrations. There is also failure to excrete the daily endogenous acid load with a resulting metabolic acidosis. This acidosis usually results in an elevated anion-gap acidosis secondary to diminished NH_3 production; it is reflected in a decreased serum bicarbonate and pH. The patient may exhibit constitutional symptoms and compensatory hyperventilation. Retention of additional, presently uncharacterized wastes probably contributes to gastrointestinal ulceration; abnormal skin coloration and itching; neuromuscular abnormalities ranging from peripheral neuropathy to seizures, stupor, or coma; and episodes of pleuritis and pericarditis. There is also an acquired deficit of platelet function that may give rise to a prolonged bleeding time and may contribute to gastrointestinal hemorrhage.

Regulatory failure is manifested by failure to regulate electrolytes and water, blood pressure, and acid-base status. Inability to concentrate or dilute the urine adequately leads to inability to handle either a salt load or free water load. An increased salt load results in volume expansion with aggravation of hypertension, edema, and possibly congestive heart failure. An increased free water load causes hyponatremia and may contribute to edema and volume overload. Failure to regulate electrolytes may lead to life-threatening hyperkalemia. Inability to concentrate may give rise to hypovolemia with salt and water deprivation. Poor regulation of the renin-angiotensin system, resulting in salt and water retention with hypervolemia, makes hypertension very common in the uremic syndrome. Hypertension contributes to further renal injury.

Last, failure of important endocrine function also occurs in chronic renal failure with uremia and may help to separate it from acute renal failure. Inadequate secretion of erythropoietin causes a normochromic, normocytic anemia with low reticulocyte count. The uremia may be aggravated by gastrointestinal hemorrhage. Failure of proper synthesis of 1,25-dihydroxyvitamin D and hyperphosphatemia give rise to hypocalcemia with consequent stimulation of parathyroid glands, which ultimately culminates in the complex metabolic bone disease called renal osteodystrophy. The anatomical features of renal osteodystrophy resemble a combination of osteomalacia and osteitis fibrosa cystica.

In summary, this patient presented with acute nephritis with a rapidly progressive course and associated pulmonary hemorrhage. A renal biopsy showed a crescentic glomerulonephritis but indeterminate immunofluorescent staining. A subsequent lung biopsy revealed linear immunofluorescent staining for immunoglobulins characteristic of Goodpasture's syndrome. Although the patient responded to plasma exchange, she ultimately developed end-stage renal disease with uremic syndrome and required hemodialysis; she now awaits renal transplantation.

Additional Reading

Brenner, B.M., and Rector, F.C., Eds.: The Kidney, 4th ed. Philadelphia, W.B. Saunders Co., 1991.

Rock, R.C., Walker, W.G., and Jennings, C.D.: Nitrogen metabolites and renal function. *In:* Textbook of Clinical Chemistry. N.W. Tietz, Ed. Philadelphia, W.B. Saunders Co., 1986.

YOUNG WOMAN WITH EDEMA AND DECREASED URINE OUTPUT

H. William Schnaper, Contributor
David N. Bailey, Reviewer

A 19-year-old woman presented to the hospital complaining of swelling of her ankles, abdomen, and eyelids for the past four days. She had been in good health until several months ago when she noted a "bloating" sensation during her menstrual period. She also thought that she had gained weight recently, noting that her jeans seemed tighter. Four days before presentation, she experienced headaches and mild abdominal pain. At bedtime, there were depressions in her legs at the location of the elastic in her socks. In the morning her legs were less swollen, but her eyes appeared "puffy." These symptoms abated somewhat by evening, but lower extremity swelling recurred. On the morning of the hospital admission, she awoke with her eyes swollen shut. She noticed that her urine appeared a bit darker than usual; on reflection she thought that she also might have been urinating less frequently. Except for some mild upper respiratory congestion, which she had attributed (along with the initial eye "puffiness") to allergies, she reported no other symptoms. She denied blurred vision, rashes, joint pains, fevers, or grossly bloody urine. The past medical history and the rest of the review of systems were noncontributory.

Physical examination revealed a well-nourished, 143-lb (65-kg) black female in no acute distress. Temperature was 99 °F (37.2 °C), heart rate was 78 BPM, respiratory rate was 28/min, and blood pressure was 110/68 mm Hg. There was mild edema of the eyelids. No rashes were seen. The head, eyes, ears, nose, and throat were all normal. The thyroid was not enlarged. There was a 4-cm span of shifting dullness appreciated on percussion of the posterior thorax. No rales or rhonchi were noted on auscultation of the lungs. Cardiac examination was unremarkable. The abdomen was soft without organomegaly; there was a sense of "fullness" to the abdomen, although no fluid wave could be observed. There was 1+ presacral edema. The external genitalia showed trace edema. There was 2-3+ pitting edema two-thirds of the way from the ankle to the knee. The ankles were markedly edematous, with depressions in the edema made by the tops of the patient's shoes. The nail beds were pale, but edema of the hands was minimal. A chest film was obtained and showed bilateral pleural effusions. There was no evidence of infiltration, consolidation, or pulmonary overcirculation.

The following laboratory studies were obtained:

Analyte	Value, conventional units	Reference range, conventional units	Value, SI units	Reference range, SI units
Sodium (S)	135 mmol/L	136-145	Same	
Potassium (S)	4.5 mmol/L	3.5-5.0	Same	
Chloride (S)	97 mmol/L	96-106	Same	
CO_2, total (S)	24 mmol/L	24-30	Same	
Urea nitrogen (S)	25 mg/dL	11-23	8.9 mmol urea/L	3.9-8.2
Creatinine (S)	0.7 mg/dL	0.6-1.2	62 µmol/L	53-106
Glucose (S)	87 mg/dL	70-105	4.8 mmol/L	3.9-5.8
Calcium (S)	7.9 mg/dL	8.4-10.2	1.98 mmol/L	2.10-2.54

Analyte	Value, conventional units	Reference range, conventional units	Value, SI units	Reference range, SI units
Protein, total (S)	4.6 g/dL	6.0-8.0	46 g/L	60-80
Albumin (S)	1.2 g/dL	3.5-5.5	12 g/L	35-55
Urate (S)	4.2 mg/dL	1.5-7.0	250 µmol/L	89-416
Cholesterol, total (S)	322 mg/dL	<200	8.34 mmol/L	<5.18
Triglyceride (S)	270 mg/dL	40-150	3.05 mmol/L	0.45-1.69
pH (U)	6.0	4.5-8.0	Same	
Specific gravity (U)	1.050	1.001-1.036	Same	
Protein (U)	3+ (confirmed by sulfosalicylic acid precipitation)	Negative		
Glucose (U)	Negative	Negative		
Ketones (U)	Negative	Negative		
Microscopic (U)				
Erythrocytes	0-2/hpf	Rare		
Hyaline casts	1-2/hpf	Rare		
Granular casts	None	None		
Erythrocyte casts	None	None		
Other cellular elements, amorphous crystals	None	Rare		

These data indicated that the patient had urinary protein loss, with decreased serum albumin concentration, peripheral edema, and elevated serum cholesterol concentration. This tetrad of findings defines the nephrotic syndrome. Additional tests were performed to elucidate the etiology of the nephrosis:

Analyte	Value, conventional units	Reference range, conventional units	Value, SI units	Reference range, SI units
C3 complement (S)	98 mg/dL	87-150	980 mg/L	870-1500
C4 complement (S)	15 mg/dL	13.8-27.0	150 mg/L	138-270
Antinuclear antibody titer (S)	Negative	<1:20		
Anti-DNA titer (S)	Negative	Negative		
IgM (S)	230 mg/dL	45-145	2.30 g/L	0.45-1.45
IgG (S)	320 mg/dL	550-1900	3.20 g/L	5.50-19.00
IgA (S)	127 mg/dL	60-333	1.27 g/L	0.60-3.33
Protein, quantitative (U)	5.3 g/d	<60 mg/m^2/d or: <100 mg/d		

Along with the previous laboratory results showing normal renal function, the absence of values indicating renal inflammation strongly suggested that the patient did not have an underlying nephritic lesion. Percutaneous renal biopsy was performed, showing very mild mesangial hypercellularity but no other glomerular abnormalities on light microscopy. The tubules and interstitium were unremarkable in appearance. Immunofluorescence microscopy showed trace mesangial staining for IgM but was negative for IgG, IgA, C3, or fibrin. Electron microscopy showed patchy effacement of the glomerular epithelial foot processes but no electron-dense deposits. A diagnosis of minimal change nephrotic syndrome (MCNS) was made.

The patient was started on oral prednisone, 80 mg/d. A sodium-restricted diet with mild fluid restriction was instituted. Because there was no respiratory distress, no attempt was made to induce diuresis pharmacologically. After 11 days, the patient's urine output increased markedly. Her urine protein dropped to 1+ and then to negative within 24 hours. Her weight dropped by 11 lb (5 kg) over the next three days, and fluid restriction was relaxed. The patient was pleased to find that her jeans once again fit easily. However, her appetite increased, and she was cautioned to monitor her caloric intake until the prednisone dose was tapered.

Clinical Findings

This patient had a fairly typical episode of MCNS, a relapsing disease that is most common in children and young adults but that can occur as late as the eighth decade of life. Minimal change disease is characterized by massive urinary loss of albumin, despite the absence of significant histopathological evidence of disruption of the renal glomerular barrier to filtration of macromolecules. Thus, its name is derived from the pathological picture rather than from the degree of clinical changes noted. Patients develop massive edema of insidious onset; it is frequently attributed to nonspecific "fluid retention" (lower extremities) or allergies (eyelids) when it is first noted. Most cases are responsive to treatment with corticosteroids, although some patients require more aggressive therapy or may be entirely unresponsive. This heterogeneity suggests that there may be multiple etiological factors leading to the same histopathological picture.

The most striking finding in nephrotic patients is the peripheral edema that develops first in areas with insufficient tissue turgor to resist infiltration by extravasated fluid (e.g., eyelids or scrotum). Dependent areas, such as the lower extremities (or the presacral region in bedridden patients) may also show prominent pitting edema. Nonspecific complaints reported by the patient that may indicate edema include weight gain, headache or abdominal pain (from swelling of connective tissue), or malaise. The degree of edema and its extent above the ankle correspond to disease severity, the amount of sodium and water intake, and whether the patient has maintained the extremities in an elevated or a dependent position (illustrated by shifting of the edema from the face to the legs as reported by the patient). Pleural effusion, indicated by shifting dullness on thoracic examination in the present case, and abdominal ascites are frequent findings. In the absence of underlying nephritis, evidence of pulmonary overcirculation, such as pulmonary edema, is not found. Additional physical findings that have been observed include softening of the ear cartilage and horizontal lines (Muehrcke's lines) in the nail beds.

Nephrotic patients should be evaluated for a skin rash, which would raise the possibility of a collagen vascular disease such as systemic lupus erythematosus, and also for fever, which would suggest that the patient may have either renal inflammation or intercurrent infection. Upper respiratory illness or other immunogenic stimuli may trigger episodes of MCNS. However, these patients also are susceptible to bacterial infections, mostly pneumococcal. The infections may include otitis, pneumonia, or primary peritonitis. The absence of fever, especially after initiation of corticosteroid treatment, does not rule out infection.

Pathophysiology of Nephrotic Syndrome

It is important to differentiate between the terms *nephrosis* and *nephritis*. Nephrosis is a clinical disorder defined by the following complex of symptoms: (1) proteinuria, (2) hypoalbuminemia, (3) peripheral edema, and (4) hyperlipidemia. In contrast, nephritis is a pathologically defined process involving inflammation in the kidney. It is possible (although not the case for the patient described here) that a patient could be nephrotic because of glomerulonephritis that causes significant urinary protein loss. Thus, *nephritis* and *nephrosis* are different, but not mutually exclusive, diagnoses.

The symptoms of nephrosis represent an "appropriate" physiological response to abnormal circumstances within the body. For example, fluid retention and edema result from an alteration in the normal balance of hydrostatic and oncotic forces in the vascular space. Even under normal circumstances, the capillary wall is not watertight. Fluid is extruded from the proximal part of the capillary but is drawn back in by a combination of oncotic pressure and a reduction in the internal hydrostatic pressure along the length of the capillary. By weight, albumin comprises approximately half of the serum protein mass. However, because it is one of the smaller proteins (M.W. ~68,000) in the serum, it comprises well over half of the number of macromolecules present in the vascular space and is therefore the major oncotic agent contributing to retaining fluid within the vessel. It is thought that urinary loss of albumin alters the balance of pressure ("Starling forces") maintaining capillary integrity (Figure 1). Extravasated fluid is not reabsorbed, leading to peripheral edema. Because vascular volume is reduced, renal perfusion is decreased. This causes the kidney to produce renin, which induces thirst, activates angiotensin to constrict blood vessels and maintain blood pressure, and finally leads to aldosterone activity that stimulates renal tubular reabsorption of sodium. These physiological responses have the effect of leading to further edema. Although all clinical evidence supports this model, it has been difficult to prove experimentally that it is correct.[1]

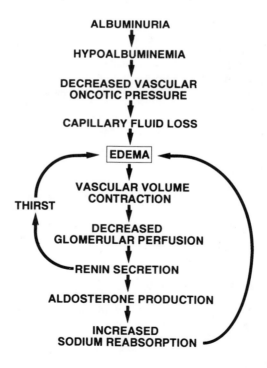

Figure 1. Proposed pathogenesis of the nephrotic syndrome.

The etiology of minimal change disease is uncertain. A significant body of circumstantial evidence, including precipitation of episodes by immunogenic stimuli such as viral illnesses, association with certain extended HLA haplotypes, and transient anergy to skin test antigens during relapse, suggests that an inherited characteristic of the immune system predisposes patients to develop this disease. It has been proposed that in most cases a factor of immune system origin mediates a change in glomerular permeability to albumin.[2] Since proteinuria in MCNS is almost pure albuminuria, and albumin is one of few serum proteins that is negatively charged at plasma pH, it also has been suggested that MCNS represents a disorder of charge selectivity of the glomerular basement membrane.[3] However, this theory remains unproven.

Differential Diagnosis

Hypoalbuminemia may on rare occasions result from congenital analbuminemia, an inherited defect. However, this disorder does not usually cause edema. Patients with acquired hypoalbuminemia have either decreased synthesis, as would be seen in malnutrition or severe hepatic failure, or increased losses. Massive losses most often occur through the gut or the kidney. Thus, in order to confirm a diagnosis of nephrotic syndrome in a patient who has edema, it is essential to establish the presence of proteinuria. If the patient is voiding infrequently because of renal effects of decreased intravascular volume, confirmation may be difficult. It is not unusual for patients with MCNS to go more than 24 hours without voiding, even when normal serum urea nitrogen and creatinine concentrations suggest a normal glomerular filtration rate.

The diseases causing nephrosis can be divided into those that are systemic and those that affect mainly the kidney. Systemic diseases include urologic disorders, cancer (the kidneys may be affected by circulating immune complexes), congestive heart failure, and systemic inflammatory diseases such as systemic lupus erythematosus and Henoch-Schönlein purpura. Immune-mediated diseases of the kidney that cause nephrotic syndrome include membranoproliferative glomerulonephritis (MPGN), membranous nephropathy, or chronic immune-complex glomerulonephritis. Another group of idiopathic renal diseases causing nephrosis is not accompanied by inflammatory changes and may thus be considered as examples of "primary" nephrotic syndrome. These include focal segmental glomerulosclerosis and mild mesangial proliferative glomerulonephritis as well as minimal change disease.

Selection and Interpretation of Laboratory Results

Laboratory tests in nephrotic patients have four purposes: to establish the clinical syndrome, to evaluate renal function, to define the underlying etiological process as well as possible, and to monitor the effects of therapy. In the present case, the protein loss proved to be urinary, as indicated by the positive urine "dipstick" test that was confirmed by the sulfosalicylic acid test. (The "dipstick" test is most sensitive for albumin, whereas the sulfosalicylic acid test is nonspecific and detects all proteins and even radiopaque dyes.) The amount of proteinuria in glomerular disease (including both nephrosis and nephritis) represents the filtered load from the glomerulus minus the protein reabsorbed by the renal tubule. It is usually fairly constant throughout the day and is thus called "fixed" proteinuria. In contrast, the absolute amount of protein excreted in other conditions may vary throughout the day. Since protein determination by dipstick reflects concentration and is affected by urine volume (e.g., results will be lower with effective diuretic therapy), proteinuria is more accurately evaluated by measurements of protein on a timed (12- or 24-h) urine collection. To rule out postural proteinuria, the patient should remain supine during the collection period.

The other findings required for a diagnosis of nephrotic syndrome are low serum albumin and hyperlipidemia. Although findings vary from patient to patient, edema usually becomes apparent when the serum albumin concentration drops to around 2 g/dL (20 g/L). Depending on the glomerular filtration rate and the degree of protein loss, the albumin may even drop below 1 g/dL (10 g/L). When such low concentrations are reached, the amount of albuminuria may decrease because of the lower filtered load. The causes for the elevated plasma cholesterol and triglycerides include increased hepatic synthesis of lipoproteins, abnormal lipid transport, and abnormalities in function of lipolytic enzymes.[4] Lipiduria may lead to the presence of oval fat bodies in the urine.

Decreased renal function in nephrotic patients, as indicated by high serum creatinine and serum urea nitrogen, usually suggests the presence of nephritis or other renal disease. Renal failure is indicated by increased serum urea nitrogen and serum creatinine concentrations and may be accompanied by hyperkalemia, hypertension, and fluid overload culminating in congestive heart failure. Urine output is not a reliable sign of renal failure, since decreased urine volume usually results from the physiological response to hypoalbuminemia. Because of their apparently volume-contracted state, patients with MCNS may have increased recirculation of urea in the kidney and may show mild to moderate increases in serum urea nitrogen concentrations. Rarely, intrarenal edema and low renal blood flow rates may cause a marked decrease in glomerular filtration;[5] this decrease is difficult to differentiate from acute renal failure and is a diagnosis that should be reached only by exclusion of other possibilities such as bilateral renal vein thrombosis or the presence of nephritis.

Once the diagnosis of nephrotic syndrome is established and the patient is stable, it is important to determine whether there is any evidence for inflammatory renal disease. Although a few erythrocytes may be seen in the urine in MCNS, gross hematuria or cylindruria (presence of granular or erythrocyte casts) strongly suggests the presence of nephritis. The urine specific gravity in MCNS should be abnormally high, reflecting both the patient's volume-contracted state and high concentration of protein. Relatively low specific gravity (1.010-1.020) should raise concern about urine concentrating ability and the possibility of renal tubular disease. The type of protein found in the urine is also of potential interest. In MCNS, proteinuria is relatively "selective," with mostly albumin being lost. In patients with nephritic lesions, the larger molecules in the globulin fraction of serum proteins are lost as well. Thus, a low serum globulin, measured by subtracting the albumin from the total protein, is also suggestive of a nephritic lesion. Selectivity can also be demonstrated by comparison of serum and urine electrophoretic patterns.

Antinuclear antibody and anti-DNA antibody titers are obtained to screen for collagen vascular disease, usually lupus. Low serum C4 concentrations reflect activation of the classical complement pathway, and C3 is decreased when either the classical or alternative pathway is activated. Such activation is most common in lupus or membranoproliferative glomerulonephritis. Complement is also consumed in acute glomerulonephritis, which only infrequently causes nephrotic syndrome. Patients with many forms of nephrotic syndrome may lose IgG in the urine; in MCNS, the serum IgM may be elevated, perhaps reflecting an underlying immunogenetic predisposition to development of the disease.[6] In children under the age of seven years, MCNS is so likely to be the cause of nephrosis that patients with no laboratory or clinical evidence supporting an alternative diagnosis are frequently given a therapeutic trial of corticosteroid therapy.[7] In older children and adults, a renal biopsy is often performed to determine the diagnosis and to indicate appropriate therapeutic measures. In the present case, the lack of significant histological changes detectable by light microscopy and absence of evidence for renal inflammation or scarring confirmed the diagnosis of MCNS.

The mildly low serum sodium concentration sometimes seen in nephrotic patients was previously ascribed to plasma water displacement by lipids. However, many laboratories use new methodologies that are not greatly affected by high lipid content. Thus, low serum sodium concentrations usually reflect a combination of decreased urine output with intake of hypotonic fluids.

Treatment

Minimal change disease is usually quite sensitive to corticosteroid therapy. About 90% of children and most adults respond to oral prednisone at a dose of 2 mg/kg or 60 mg/m^2/d (maximum 80 mg). Once the patient's proteinuria remits (usually within four weeks), the dose is tapered over 4-6 weeks, with the patient remaining in remission in about 50% of cases. Corticosteroids have significant side effects, including truncal obesity, acne, hirsutism, bone demineralization, and increased gastric acid secretion leading to hyperphagia and peptic ulceration. These effects eventually abate after discontinuance of the drug. Patients who do not respond, who are steroid-dependent, or who relapse frequently are often given a course of an alkylating agent such as cyclophosphamide or chlorambucil for up to 12 weeks. Cyclosporine may be effective in selected patients, but most of these patients will also respond to steroids. Cyclosporine treatment is thus usually limited to those patients with severe steroid intoxication. All of these other drugs are also more immunosuppressive than are corticosteroids and have significant toxic effects.

Treatments aimed at inducing remission of other forms of nephrosis vary depending upon the etiology in each case. Symptomatic treatment for nephrotic patients includes restriction of sodium and water intake. Bed rest or other means of elevating the lower extremities may help mobilize pedal edema. There are two indications for pharmacological diuresis. In patients with massive ascites or acute respiratory distress from pleural effusions, intravenous infusion of albumin and of furosemide to force diuresis of edema fluid is of some benefit. In patients with steroid-unresponsive disease, oral diuretics may help decrease fluid retention in some patients. However, since the kidneys are responding to a perceived volume-depleted state, diuretics are often less effective than they would be in a patient without nephrosis.

Helpful Notes

All of the findings and problems associated with nephrosis can best be understood when viewed as a consequence of protein loss. Thus, it is important to consider the pathophysiological mechanism of nephrotic syndrome in evaluating the patient. For example, the symptomatic treatments suggested above reflect the need to deplete fluid from the tissue space rather than from the vascular space. Trace minerals that are protein bound (zinc, for instance) may be depleted because of albuminuria. Loss of other proteins may cause alterations in laboratory values, such as the decreased serum calcium concentration that reflects loss of albumin as a binding protein and the decreased serum total thyroxine that reflects loss of thyroxine-binding protein (TBG). These changes are of no physiological consequence since free (ionized) serum calcium concentrations and free thyroxine should be normal. Changes may also occur in concentrations of drugs, such as digoxin, that are mostly bound to circulating proteins; these measurements must be interpreted with care in nephrotic patients.

References

1.   Schnaper, H.W., and Robson, A.M.: Nephrotic syndrome: Minimal change disease, focal glomerulosclerosis, and related disorders. *In:* Diseases of the Kidney, 5th ed. R.W. Schrier and C.W. Gottschalk, Eds. Boston, Little, Brown and Co., 1992, in press.

2. Shalhoub, R.J.: Pathogenesis of lipoid nephrosis: A disorder of T-cell function. Lancet *2:* 556-559, 1976

3. Carrie, B.J., Salyer, W.R., and Myers, B.D.: Minimal change nephropathy: An electro-chemical disorder of the glomerular membranes. Am. J. Med., *70:* 262-268, 1981.

4. Kaysen, G.A.: Hyperlipidemia in the nephrotic syndrome. Am. J. Kidney Dis., *12:* 548-551, 1988.

5. Lowenstein, J., Schacht, R.G., and Baldwin, D.S.: Renal failure in minimal change nephrotic syndrome. Am. J. Med., *70:* 227-233, 1981.

6. Giangiacomo, J., Cleary, T.G., Cole, B.R., et al.: Serum immunoglobulins in the nephrotic syndrome. A possible cause of minimal change disease. N. Engl. J. Med., *293:* 8-12, 1975.

7. International Study of Kidney Disease in Children: The primary nephrotic syndrome in children: Identification of patients with minimal change nephrotic syndrome from initial response to prednisolone. J. Pediatr., *98:* 561-564, 1981.

A 35-YEAR-OLD MAN WITH FULMINANT LIVER FAILURE

Rex B. Conn, Contributor
Steven I. Shedlofsky, Reviewer

This 35-year-old man, a native of Mexico, worked as a food handler at a hotel on the New Jersey shore. He was in good health until one month prior to his admission to a local hospital because of increasing anorexia, weakness, and jaundice. A diagnosis of acute hepatitis B was made on the basis of the clinical and laboratory findings including elevated serum transaminase activities, an elevated serum bilirubin, and a positive test for hepatitis B surface antigen (HBsAg). He was discharged two days later, having what was described as normal mental status, and returned to work. Because of "strange behavior" at work, he was readmitted to the local hospital where the staff noted increasing agitation and progressive obtundation. A diagnosis of acute hepatic failure was made, and the patient was transferred to the University Hospital for possible liver transplantation. No source of the hepatitis B infection was identified; the patient denied contact with prostitutes and homosexual men and denied intravenous drug use.

Physical examination demonstrated the patient to be a well-developed, well-nourished man appearing his stated age. Blood pressure was 126/67 mm Hg, pulse 62 BPM, respirations 18/min, and temperature 98.6 °F (37 °C). The patient was markedly jaundiced, but no cutaneous lesions or needle marks were noted. Examination of the head, neck, eyes, ears, nose, and throat was normal except for markedly icteric sclerae. The lungs were clear to auscultation. The heart was not enlarged, rhythm was regular, and there were no murmurs. The abdomen was soft, nontender, and not distended; the liver and spleen could not be palpated. The cranial nerves were intact, reflexes were 3+, and the patient could move all extremities.

Laboratory data obtained at the time of admission to the University Hospital were as follows:

Analyte	Value, conventional units	Reference range, conventional units	Value, SI units	Reference range, SI units
Leukocyte count (B)	$8.7 \times 10^3/\mu L$	5.0-10.0	$8.7 \times 10^9/L$	5.0-10.0
Hemoglobin (B)	14.3 g/dL	14-18	8.87 mmol/L	8.69-11.17
Platelet count (B)	$396 \times 10^3/\mu L$	150-350	$396 \times 10^9/L$	150-350
Differential count (B)	Unremarkable		Same	
Prothrombin time (PT) (P)	19.1 s (patient) 12.2 s (control)	12.0-14.0	Same	
Partial thromboplastin time (PTT) (P)	50 s	20-35	Same	
Fibrinogen (P)	144 mg/dL	170-410	1.44 g/L	1.70-4.10
Sodium (S)	148 mmol/L	135-146	Same	
Potassium (S)	3.7 mmol/L	3.5-5.0	Same	
CO2, total (S)	32 mmol/L	24-32	Same	
Chloride (S)	104 mmol/L	98-109	Same	
Calcium (S)	8.9 mg/dL	8.5-10.5	2.22 mmol/L	2.12-2.62
Phosphorus (S)	5.2 mg/dL	2.5-4.5	1.68 mmol/L	0.81-1.45

Analyte	Value, conventional units	Reference range, conventional units	Value, SI units	Reference range, SI units
On Fl O$_2$, 40%				
pH (aB)	7.45	7.35-7.45	Same	
pCO$_2$ (aB)	38 mm Hg	35-45	5.1 kPa	4.7-6.0
pO$_2$ (aB)	101 mm Hg	84-100	13.5 kPa	11.2-13.3
O$_2$ saturation (aB)	99 %	95-100	0.99	0.95-1.00
Urea nitrogen (S)	1 mg/dL	10-22	0.4 mmol urea/L	3.6-7.9
Creatinine (S)	0.7 mg/dL	0.7-1.4	62 µmol/L	62-124
Ammonia (B)	260 µmol/L	11-35	Same	
Glucose (S)	102 mg/dL	60-110	5.7 mmol/L	3.3-6.1
Cholesterol (S)	140 mg/dL	Desirable: <200	3.62 mmol/L	Desirable: <5.18
Protein, total (S)	6.7 g/dL	6.0-8.5	67 g/L	60-85
Albumin (S)	2.8 g/dL	3.3-5.2	28 g/L	33-52
Bilirubin, total (S)	26.5 mg/dL	0.2-1.2	453 µmol/L	3-21
Bilirubin, conjugated (S)	15.6 mg/dL	0.0-0.4	266 µmol/L	0-7
ALP (S)	167 U/L	15-115	2.8 µkat/L	0.3-1.9
AST (S)	2331 U/L	7-28	38.86 µkat/L	0.12-0.47
ALT (S)	3080 U/L	1-45	51.34 µkat/L	0.02-0.75
GGT (S)	64 U/L	10-50	1.07 µkat/L	0.17-0.83
LDH (S)	749 U/L	70-186	12.49 µkat/L	1.17-3.10
Drug screen (B, U)	Negative	Negative	Same	
RPR* (S)	Nonreactive			
Urinalysis (U)	Protein, 1+; glucose, negative; ketones, trace; bilirubin, 4+			

Hepatitis serological test results were as follows:

Hepatitis Antigens

Hepatitis B surface antigen (HBsAg)	Positive
Hepatitis B core antigen (HBcAg)	Not available
Hepatitis B e antigen (HBeAg)	Borderline

Hepatitis Antibodies

IgM anti-hepatitis A (IgM anti-HAV)	Negative
IgG anti-hepatitis A (IgG anti-HAV)	Positive
Anti-hepatitis B surface antigen (anti-HBs)	Negative
IgM anti-hepatitis B core antigen (IgM anti-HBc)	Positive
Anti-hepatitis B e antigen (anti-HBe)	Positive
Anti-hepatitis C (anti-HCV)	Negative
IgM anti-hepatitis D (delta agent)	Positive

Other Viral Serology

Anti-human immunodeficiency virus (anti-HIV) (Unable to obtain informed consent)	Not performed
Anti-Epstein-Barr virus (anti-EBV)	Negative
Herpes simplex serology:	
Anti-HSV1 IgG	Mid-positive
Anti-HSV2 IgG	High positive
Anti-varicella IgG	Mid-positive

* Rapid plasma reagin test.

A chest X-ray examination showed a normal-sized heart and clear lung fields. A computed tomographic (CT) scan of the head revealed several hyperdense granulomas interpreted as being consistent with cysticercosis or tuberculosis.

During the patient's brief hospitalization, the major problems were encephalopathy and coagulopathy. The patient became increasingly obtunded, and he was intubated to provide respiratory assistance. His systolic blood pressure decreased to 70 mm Hg, and an intra-venous dopamine drip was started to maintain the systolic pressure above 120 mm Hg. He had one seizure that began in his right arm and spread to the rest of the body. Because of increased intracranial pressure, an intracranial pressure monitor was placed, and pentobar-bital was administered intravenously to induce coma. Intravenous mannitol was also given to induce diuresis. Broad-spectrum antibiotics were given because of suspected sepsis. There was one self-limited episode of hematemesis. The patient's condition continued to deteriorate, and he died on the fourth day of hospitalization.

Types of Hepatitis

Hepatitis is a generic term that is used to describe any type of hepatocellular inflammation and necrosis. It may be caused by any one of a number of viral agents, drug toxicity, alcohol, circulatory failure, or metabolic disorders such as Wilson's disease, or it may be due to an idiopathic autoimmune process. The clinical findings in hepatitis are characteristic but nonspecific and insufficient to identify the cause; laboratory studies are essential to identify the etiological agent.[1-3]

Hepatitis may be acute, subacute, or chronic, and it may range in severity from a completely asymptomatic condition, characterized by elevated serum transaminase activi-ties, to fatal fulminant hepatic failure as occurred in this patient.[4,5] For viral hepatitis, the routes of transmission and the epidemiology, as well as the morbidity and mortality, vary among the agents. An effective vaccine has been developed for only one viral agent, the hepatitis B virus. A vaccine for hepatitis A may be available soon.

Hepatitis A virus (HAV) is found in the blood, stool, and liver only during the acute infection. IgM antibodies (anti-HAV) appear early in the course but disappear within weeks to be replaced by IgG antibodies, which persist for life. Thus, IgM anti-HAV is a marker for acute hepatitis A, whereas presence of IgG anti-HAV indicates previous exposure and immunity to reinfection. There is no carrier state for HAV, and this virus does not produce chronic active hepatitis. Transmission is via the fecal-oral route.

Hepatitis B virus (HBV) has a structure consisting of two concentric protein coats surrounding the viral DNA. The inner coat, the capsid, consists of a single core protein. The outer surface coat is composed of three types of proteins, all of which contain the surface antigen (HBsAg).[6] HBsAg is produced in excess and can be detected in sera of patients with active hepatitis B infection several weeks prior to the onset of symptoms. In a small percentage of patients with active HBV infection, HBsAg may be undetectable, possibly because of immune complex formation with its corresponding antibody. A second antigen, the hepatitis B core antigen (HBcAg), is not found in the blood stream, and tests for it are not routinely performed. A third antigen, the hepatitis B virus e antigen (HBeAg), appears in the blood stream early in HBV infection and correlates with active viral replication in the liver. It disappears within a few weeks in most cases, but it remains present in chronic active hepatitis due to HBV. The chronological profiles of these antigens and antibodies are shown in Figure 1.

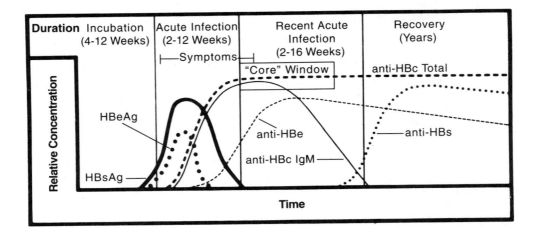

Figure 1. Chronological laboratory test profile in acute hepatitis B infection. (From: Coslett, G.D., and Hojvat, S.A.: Hepatitis Learning Guide. Abbott Diagnostics, Abbott Park, IL, 1988. Used with permission of Abbott Laboratories. All rights reserved.)

Antibodies to each of these antigens appear during the course of the illness. Anti-HBs appears during convalescence, indicating recovery and immunity to reinfection. IgM anti-HBc appears early in the infection and is considered the most useful indicator of acute hepatitis B infection. Occasionally IgM anti-HBc may be detected in chronic carriers of hepatitis B virus during times of active viral replication; however, a negative test for IgM anti-HBc virtually excludes the diagnosis of acute hepatitis B. Anti-HBe appears as HBeAg disappears and indicates a reduction in the rate of viral replication.

Most patients (over 90%) with acute hepatitis B infection recover completely; however, in rare cases (<1%) HBV causes fulminant hepatitis with massive necrosis of the liver. Fulminant hepatitis is not due to a more virulent strain of virus; rather, it appears to be secondary to a stronger immune response by the host in which killer T cells attack hepatocytes containing the virus. Other patients appear to be unable to generate an effective immune response, HBsAg persists in the blood stream indefinitely, and anti-HBs is not produced. These patients become chronic carriers of HBV. The chronic carrier state occurs in 5-10% of adults and 80% of infants infected with HBV. Most chronic carriers are asymptomatic, but many develop chronic persistent hepatitis or chronic active hepatitis that may lead to cirrhosis and hepatocellular carcinoma. Chronic HBV infections affect several hundred million individuals, three-quarters of whom are in Asia.

An HBV-infected mother can pass the virus to her baby during birth or shortly thereafter, a common occurrence in Third World countries. All pregnant women should be tested for HBsAg in the third trimester so that the infants of mothers with positive tests can be vaccinated and be given passive immunization with hepatitis B immune globulin. However, numerous routes of infection exist since the virus is present in blood, saliva, and semen. The epidemiology of HBV infections is similar to that of human immunodeficiency virus (HIV) infections, although HBV is more infectious than HIV is. In the United States the high-risk groups include male homosexuals, intravenous drug users, and individuals having multiple sex partners. Health care workers who must handle blood specimens from HBV-infected patients are not considered a high-risk group, although all should be urged to be immunized against hepatitis B with the currently available recombinant vaccine. Strict adherence to "universal precautions" reduces the risk of health care workers to a negligible level.

Hepatitis D virus (HDV), also called the delta agent, is an incomplete-RNA virus that can replicate only in the presence of HBV. It circulates in the plasma coated with surface antigen from HBV.[7] Superinfection with HDV can occur in either acute or chronic HBV infection, and simultaneous infections with both HBV and HDV may occur. In acute hepatitis due to HBV, superinfection with HDV does not affect the course or outcome of the disease process;[3] however, HDV infection in a chronic HBV carrier may cause an acute, florid hepatitis that may progress rapidly to acute liver failure, as seen in this patient, or it may lead to cirrhosis. While it appears more common that superinfection with HDV in a chronic carrier of HBV causes an exacerbation of the hepatitis, it has been reported that infection with HDV may cause all clinical and laboratory evidence of HBV infection to disappear.[8] The laboratory findings in coinfection and in superinfection are shown in Figure 2.

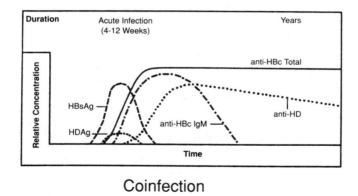

Coinfection

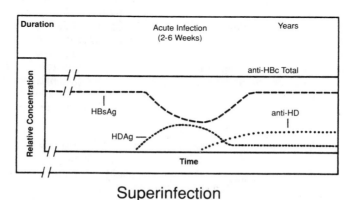

Superinfection

Figure 2. Laboratory test profiles in acute hepatitis B with concurrent or superinfection by hepatitis D virus. (From: Coslett, G.D., and Hojvat, S.A.: Hepatitis Learning Guide. Abbott Diagnostics, Abbott Park, IL, 1988. Used with permission of Abbott Laboratories. All rights reserved.)

No vaccine to HDV exists; however, immunization against HBV is protective since the former cannot replicate in the absence of the latter. Combined infection with HBV and HDV cannot be distinguished from that due to HBV alone on clinical or laboratory grounds; the diagnosis of hepatitis D depends upon detecting acute antibodies to this agent (IgM anti-HDV).

Hepatitis C virus (HCV) remains a cause of transfusion-associated hepatitis after precautions have been implemented in blood donor centers to exclude the possibility of hepatitis A and hepatitis B in donors. The condition was called non-A, non-B hepatitis. Recently, a test for antibodies to the principal non-A, non-B virus was developed, the virus was named the hepatitis C virus (HCV), and the antibody was named anti-hepatitis C (anti-HCV). The test was made mandatory for all blood donors as soon as it became available.

Hepatitis E virus (HEV) is one of the non-A, non-B hepatitis viruses. Tests for HEV are available only in research laboratories. Apparently this virus has not been found in the United States except in immigrants and travelers from endemic areas.[3]

Discussion

When admitted to the University Hospital, this patient had substantial evidence of fulminant liver failure. The striking increases in serum AST and ALT indicated substantial liver necrosis was occurring. ALT is invariably higher than AST in all types of acute hepatitis except alcoholic hepatitis; however, the degree of elevation correlates poorly with the degree of liver damage, and late in the course of hepatic failure both may decline, presumably because there are few hepatocytes left as the source. Both the total and conjugated bilirubin concentrations are markedly increased as well, providing further evidence of the degree of liver failure.

Failure of the protein synthetic functions of the liver is indicated by the decreased serum albumin and the very prolonged prothrombin and partial thromboplastin times. The decreased plasma fibrinogen concentration is a result of the same defects in protein synthesis.

Perhaps the most striking evidence of liver failure is the serum urea nitrogen of 1 mg/dL (0.36 mmol urea/L) accompanied by a normal serum creatinine indicating normal renal function. Urea is synthesized in the liver from ammonia derived from protein degradation, and this function is usually maintained until late in the course of liver failure. The marked increase in blood ammonia is also related to failure of urea synthesis, and it is a valid sign of hepatic encephalopathy in fulminant liver failure. However, it is not a reliable index in patients with chronic liver disease. Other laboratory findings in severe liver failure are a low serum cholesterol (140 mg/dL [3.62 mmol/L] in this patient) and hypoglycemia (not seen because the patient was on intravenous fluids containing glucose). The granulomas noted on CT scan of the head should be considered an incidental finding; laboratory studies to detect mycobacteria were performed and were negative.

The hepatitis serological tests indicate that the patient had hepatitis A sometime previously because of the presence of IgG anti-HAV and absence of IgM anti-HAV. The positive test for HBsAg does not by itself indicate the patient had acute hepatitis B; the patient might have had chronic hepatitis B, which was then complicated by superinfection with HDV. However, the presence of IgM anti-HBc indicates the patient had acute hepatitis B and concurrently or subsequently acquired the hepatitis D infection. The data are insufficient to determine if HDV was acquired as a coinfection or as a superinfection. The absence of anti-HBs is not inconsistent with the other data; it usually appears late in the illness as HBsAg disappears, but it is found in only 90-95% of patients with acute hepatitis B.[3]

The tests for other viruses were obtained to investigate possible causes for the hepatitis other than the hepatitis viruses. The results indicate immunity to both types of *Herpes simplex* as well as to varicella. In some geographical regions, tests for the yellow fever virus would be indicated as well.

Treatment

The treatment of acute hepatitis, with or without liver failure, is supportive. The patient should be put on a low fat, high carbohydrate diet because fat absorption is compromised and hypoglycemia may occur in some patients. The patient should be followed carefully after apparent recovery to determine if the acute infection progresses to chronic persistent hepatitis or chronic active hepatitis.

References

1. Alter, H.J., Ed.: Hepatitis. Semin. Liver Dis., *6:* 1, 1986.

2. Zuckerman, A.J., Ed.: Viral Hepatitis and Liver Disease. New York, Alan R. Liss, 1988.

3. Verhille, M.S., and Friedman, L.S.: Viral hepatitis and its differential diagnosis. *In:* Current Diagnosis, 8th ed. R.B. Conn, Ed. Philadelphia, W.B. Saunders Co., 1991.

4. McIntyre, N.: Clinical presentation of acute viral hepatitis. Br. Med. Bull., *46:* 533-547, 1990.

5. Garcia, G., and Gentry, K.R.: Chronic viral hepatitis. Med. Clin. North Am., *73:* 971-983, 1989.

6. Tiollais, P., Pourcel, C., and Dejean, A.: The hepatitis B virus. Nature, *317:* 489-495, 1985.

7. Di Bisceglie, A.M., and Negro, F.: Diagnosis of hepatitis delta virus infection. Hepatology, *10:* 1014-1016, 1989.

8. Pastore, G., Monno, L., Santantonio, T., et al.: Hepatitis B virus clearance from serum and liver after acute hepatitis delta virus superinfection in chronic HBsAg carriers. J. Med. Virol., *31:* 284-290, 1990.

A NURSE WITH METASTATIC CANCER

Rex B. Conn, Contributor
Steven I. Shedlofsky, Reviewer

A 41-year-old nurse who was born in the Philippines was admitted for a liver biopsy. She complained of weight loss, abdominal swelling, and a constant, sharp, nonradiating pain in the right upper quadrant that had been present for one month. The pain was not affected by meals or position, but the patient had frequent nausea and vomiting. The patient had previously been in good health except for a long history of irritable bowel syndrome.

On physical examination, the blood pressure was 170/90 mm Hg; the other vital signs were normal. There was slight scleral icterus. The lungs were clear to percussion, but scattered inspiratory rales were noted. The abdomen was soft with tenderness to palpation in the right upper quadrant. The liver was firm and extended 3 cm below the right costal margin. The spleen was not palpable. A moderate amount of ascitic fluid (later confirmed by ultrasonography) was present as demonstrated by shifting dullness. The remainder of the examination was unremarkable.

A chest X-ray examination showed numerous nodules throughout both lung fields; the nodules were interpreted as consistent with tumor metastases. Ultrasonographic studies revealed a mass in the right lobe of the liver, portal vein thrombosis, and a moderate amount of ascitic fluid. A computed tomographic (CT) scan confirmed the presence of an inhomogeneous mass 10.4 cm in diameter, and an arteriogram verified its vascular nature.

Admission laboratory data were as follows:

Analyte	Value, conventional units	Reference range, conventional units	Value, SI units	Reference range, SI units
Leukocyte count (B)	$6.0 \times 10^3/\mu L$	5.0-10.0	$6.0 \times 10^9/L$	5.0-10.0
Differential count (B)	Unremarkable			
Hemoglobin (B)	12.2 g/dL	12-16	7.57 mmol/L	7.45-9.93
Prothrombin time (P)	12.3 s	12-14	Same	
Partial thromboplastin time (P)	37 s	20-35	Same	
Electrolytes (S)	Within normal limits			
Urea nitrogen (S)	7 mg/dL	10-22	2.5 mmol urea/L	3.6-7.9
Creatinine (S)	0.7 mg/dL	0.7-1.4	62 μmol/L	62-124
Glucose (S)	108 mg/dL	60-110	6.0 mmol/L	3.3-6.1
Protein, total (S)	8.5 g/dL	6.0-8.5	85 g/L	60-85
Albumin (S)	4.0 g/dL	3.3-5.2	40 g/L	33-52
Bilirubin, total (S)	4.3 mg/dL	0.2-1.2	74 μmol/L	3-21
Bilirubin, conjugated (S)	1.9 mg/dL	0.0-0.4	32 μmol/L	0-7
ALP (S)	235 U/L	15-115	3.9 μkat/L	0.3-1.9
AST (S)	106 U/L	7-28	1.77 μkat/L	0.12-0.47
ALT (S)	30 U/L	1-30	0.50 μkat/L	0.02-0.50
GGT (S)	79 U/L	7-40	1.32 μkat/L	0.12-0.67
LDH (S)	246 U/L	70-186	4.10 μkat/L	1.17-3.10

Analyte	Value, conventional units	Reference range, conventional units	Value, SI units	Reference range, SI units
Protein electrophoresis (S)				
Gamma globulin	2.4 g/dL	0.5-1.6	24 g/L	50-160
Other protein fractions	Within reference limits			
Immunoglobulins (S)				
IgG	2910 mg/dL	723-1685	29.10 g/L	7.23-16.85
IgA	474 mg/dL	69-382	4.74 g/L	0.69-3.82
IgM	220 mg/dL	63-277	2.20 g/L	0.63-2.77
α-Fetoprotein (S)	210 ng/mL	<20	210 µg/L	<20
HBsAg (S)	Positive	Negative	Same	
Anti-HCV (S)	Negative	Negative	Same	
Urinalysis (U)	Protein, 2+; glucose, trace; ketones, trace; bilirubin, 3+			

A percutaneous needle biopsy of the liver was performed under ultrasonographic guidance, and the pathology report was hepatocellular carcinoma with increased fibro-connective tissue and chronic inflammation. A diagnosis of underlying cirrhosis could not be made on the basis of the biopsy findings. The patient was discharged on oral narcotics.

Further questioning of the patient elicited a significant event in the patient's history, namely, a finger stick with an infected needle nine years previously. Tests for hepatitis B surface antigen (HBsAg) were found to be positive the next day. Except for a mild increase in serum AST, subsequently there was no evidence of active liver disease. The test for HBsAg remained positive, although the patient felt well and continued to work until the onset of the present illness.

Comments

This unfortunate woman had been infected with hepatitis B virus (HBV) at a time earlier than the needle-stick injury nine years previously because the test for HBsAg was positive at the time of the injury. It is likely that she acquired HBV at birth or shortly thereafter from her mother who was a chronic HBV carrier. This is known as "vertical transmission." (See *Case 9*.) Vertical transmission of HBV is common in Asia because of the high prevalence of the HBV carrier state. Of course, this mode of transmission could not be documented at the time of the patient's birth because HBsAg was not identified until 20 years later. HBsAg was initially known as the Australia antigen because it was first isolated from serum from an Australian aborigine, and Dr. Baruch Blumberg received the Nobel Prize in 1976 for this discovery.

Hepatocellular carcinoma (HCC) may invade the portal veins and cause portal vein thrombosis, as occurred in this patient; it also may metastasize to regional lymph nodes and to the lungs. The concentration of α-fetoprotein (AFP) in this patient was significantly elevated; however, only if values are over 500 ng/mL (500 µg/L) or if they are increasing can this test contribute to a diagnosis of hepatocellular carcinoma that can be accepted with any degree of confidence. The low diagnostic specificity of the imaging studies and of the AFP at the concentration found made it necessary to perform the liver biopsy to arrive at a definitive diagnosis.

The laboratory findings, other than the biopsy results, indicate the presence of underlying liver disease that is probably secondary to the portal vein thrombosis, although cirrhosis as the cause cannot be excluded. The significant findings include elevated total and conjugated serum bilirubin and increased activity of alkaline phosphatase (ALP), aspartate aminotransferase (AST), γ-glutamyltransferase (GGT), and lactate dehydrogenase (LDH). Serum protein electrophoresis revealed a polyclonal gammopathy; increased IgG and IgA were demonstrated by immunonephelometry.

The Hepatitis B Virus

The genome of HBV is circular and contains 3200 base pairs; HBV is one of the smallest known animal viruses. There are four genes, but the genome does not contain an oncogene. The viral DNA may become incorporated into the genome of the host hepatocyte at several different sites. The exact mechanism through which HBV produces HCC is not known, but it may activate hepatocyte oncogenes and thus initiate uncontrolled cell growth.[1,2] HBV also causes abnormalities such as chromosome deletions and translocations, abnormalities that are frequently seen in malignant tumors. Current research on the oncogenic properties of HBV is focused on the mechanisms of malignant transformation.[3] Because of the high incidence of HCC in Japan, research emphasis in that country is on development of effective screening programs to detect HCC in the early and more treatable stages.[4,5]

Hepatocellular Carcinoma

The association between chronic HBV infection and hepatocellular carcinoma (HCC) is well established; HBV is one of a few viruses that causes cancer in humans. HCC may also be associated with hepatitis C virus (HCV) infection, but the data on this association are incomplete because diagnostic tests for HCV infection have only recently been widely available. A recent study from Italy of HCC in patients with cirrhosis found 45% had HCV infection, whereas 11% had HBV infection.[6] There is a much higher prevalence of chronic HBV infection in patients with HCC than in the general population, and the incidence of HCC worldwide parallels the prevalence of the HBV carrier state.[7] In the United States, HCC is a relatively rare malignant tumor (HBV carrier state <1%), but in sub-Saharan Africa, Southeast Asia, and Japan it is one of the most frequent (HBV carrier state 10-20%). On a worldwide basis, HCC may be the most prevalent malignant tumor.

HCC usually arises in a cirrhotic liver, the most frequent cause for the cirrhosis on a worldwide basis being HBV infection. Other risk factors include alcoholic cirrhosis, hemochromatosis (10% of patients develop HCC), exposure to aflatoxins, use of oral contraceptives, and presence of a benign adenoma. A single tumor mass, as seen in this patient, is more common in noncirrhotic livers, whereas a multinodular tumor mass is more frequent in cirrhotic livers. A histological variant, the fibrolamellar type, is seen in young adults and appears to have a better prognosis. Males have an incidence of HCC 4-8 times that of females. The duration of the carrier state until HCC develops is quite variable and may range up to 50 years.

Numerous abnormal *laboratory findings* have been described in HCC; however, it may be difficult to determine if they are due to the HCC or to underlying liver disease. α-Fetoprotein (AFP) is an oncofetal glycoprotein present in the plasma during fetal life, but it disappears rapidly after birth. Serum concentrations of AFP are increased in 70% of patients with HCC, and AFP is considered the most useful tumor marker in this condition.[8] AFP is also produced by teratocarcinomas and yolk sac tumors, and slightly increased serum concentrations may be found in patients with benign liver disease or with gastrointestinal malignancies with hepatic metastases. It is not useful in screening programs or as an indicator of tumor burden; however, changes in serum concentration can be used as an indicator of the results of treatment. Recent research on the degree of fucosylation of AFP (the fucosylation index) may provide a more effective screening test for HCC.[9]

Treatment of HCC is usually not effective. Radiation therapy, chemotherapy, local resection, and liver transplantation have all been used, but the median survival time after diagnosis remains about six months.

References

1. Tiollais, P., and Buendia, M.-A.: Hepatitis B virus. Sci. Am., April 1991, 116-123.

2. Lampertico, P., Malter, J.S., Colombo, M., et al.: Detection of hepatitis B virus DNA in formalin-fixed, paraffin-embedded liver tissue by the polymerase chain reaction. Am. J. Pathol., *137:* 253-258, 1990.

3. Ogata, N., Tokino, T., Kamimura, T., et al.: A comparison of the molecular structure of integrated hepatitis B virus genomes in hepatocellular carcinoma cells and hepatocytes derived from the same patient. Hepatology, *11:* 1017-1023, 1990.

4. Heyward, W.L., Lanier, A.P., McMahon, B.J., et al.: Early detection of primary hepatocellular carcinoma. JAMA, *254:* 3052-3054, 1985.

5. Liaw, Y.-F., Tai, D.-I., Chu, C.-M., et al.: Early detection of hepatocellular carcinoma in patients with chronic type B hepatitis: A prospective study. Gastroenterology, *90:* 263-267, 1986.

6. Colombo, M., de Franchis, R., del Ninno, E., et al.: Hepatocellular carcinoma in Italian patients with cirrhosis. N. Engl. J. Med., *325:* 675-680, 1991.

7. Beasley, R.P., Hwang, L.Y., Lin, C.C., et al.: Hepatocellular carcinoma and hepatitis B virus: A prospective study of 22,707 men in Taiwan. Lancet, *2:* 1129-1133, 1981.

8. Di Bisceglie, A.M., moderator: NIH conference: Hepatocellular carcinoma. Ann. Intern. Med., *108:* 390-401, 1988.

9. Aoyagi, Y., Suzuki, Y., Igarashi, K., et al.: The usefulness of simultaneous determinations of glucosaminylation and fucosylation indices in alpha-fetoprotein in the differential diagnosis of neoplastic diseases of the liver. Cancer, *67:* 2390-2394, 1991.

ADULT MALE WITH NEW ONSET ASCITES

Steven I. Shedlofsky, Contributor

A 56-year-old white male presented with abdominal and ankle swelling of several months' duration. There was no history of chronic medical problems, except for impotence over the past 3-4 years; the patient was on no medications. He was a successful accountant, married with three children. He was a 1/2 pack/day smoker and a social drinker. His father had been killed during World War II, and he had an uncle who died of liver cirrhosis 10-15 years previously. He was an only child.

On physical examination the patient was well developed, looked tanned even though it was winter, weighed 196 lb (89 kg), and had normal vital signs. The patient had several prominent stigmata of chronic liver disease, including spider angiomata on his chest, palmar erythema, Dupuytren's contractures, testicular atrophy, and female escutcheon; however, he was anicteric. He had normal chest and normal cardiac findings, but his abdomen was protuberant with a fluid wave and shifting dullness. There was no palpable or ballotable liver edge, but his spleen was felt just under the left costal border. On digital rectal examination he had prominent hemorrhoids and a normal prostate. A stool sample was brown and negative for occult blood. He had 2+ pitting ankle edema.

Initial laboratory results were as follows:

Analyte	Value, conventional units	Reference range, conventional units	Value, SI units	Reference range, SI units
Hemoglobin (B)	14.5 g/dL	14-18	9.0 mmol/L	8.69-11.17
Hematocrit (B)	43 %	40-54	0.43	0.40-0.54
Leukocyte count (B)	4.9 x 10³/µL	4.8-10.8	4.9 x 10⁹/L	4.8-10.8
MCV (B)	92 fL	80-94	Same	
Platelet count (B)	103 x 10³/µL	150-450	103 x 10⁹/L	150-450
Ethanol (B)	0.0 mg/dL	0	0.0 mmol/L	0
Prothrombin time (P)	13.2 s (patient) 11.9 s (control)	11-15	Same	
Sodium (S)	134 mmol/L	136-145	Same	
Potassium (S)	3.6 mmol/L	3.8-5.1	Same	
Chloride (S)	99 mmol/L	98-107	Same	
CO₂, total (S)	27 mmol/L	23-31	Same	
Urea nitrogen (S)	8 mg/dL	8-21	2.8 mmol urea/L	2.8-7.5
Creatinine (S)	0.8 mg/dL	0.7-1.3	71 µmol/L	62-115
Glucose (S)	148 mg/dL	80-115	8.2 mmol/L	4.4-6.4
Protein, total (S)	6.4 g/dL	6.2-7.6	64 g/L	62-76
Albumin (S)	2.9 g/dL	3.2-4.6	29 g/L	32-46
Cholesterol (S)	182 mg/dL	140-220	4.70 mmol/L	3.62-5.69
Bilirubin, total (S)	1.3 mg/dL	0.2-1.0	22 µmol/L	3-17
AST (S)	62 U/L	19-48	1.03 µkat/L	0.32-0.80
ALT (S)	71 U/L	13-40	1.18 µkat/L	0.22-0.67
LDH (S)	170 U/L	110-210	2.83 µkat/L	1.83-3.50
ALP (S)	82 U/L	56-119	1.4 µkat/L	0.9-2.0

Analyte	Value, conventional units	Reference range, conventional units	Value, SI units	Reference range, SI units
GGT (S)	27 U/L	10-50	0.45 μkat/L	0.17-0.83
Urinalysis (U)	Within normal limits			
Sodium, random (U)	5 mmol/L		Same	

An ultrasonographic scan of the abdomen and right upper quadrant showed marked ascites with a nonhomogeneous liver not containing any intrahepatic masses and an intact gallbladder without gallstones. Peritoneal fluid was aspirated and found to have a total leukocyte count of 75 x 10^3/μL (75 x 10^9/L), 20% of which were granulocytes; total protein, 1.9 g/dL (19 g/L); albumin, 0.2 g/dL (2 g/L); glucose, 120 mg/dL (6.7 mmol/L); amylase, 81 U/L (1.35 μkat/L); and LDH, 80 U/L (1.33 μkat/L). The Gram stain was negative, as was cytological examination for malignant cells.

The patient was started on spironolactone (50 mg q.i.d.) and placed on a diet of 2 g sodium/d. There was a gradual diuresis of 20 lb (9 kg) over the next two weeks with resolution of his ankle edema as well as most of his ascites. Further laboratory studies to evaluate causes for chronic liver disease were reported as follows:

Analyte	Value, conventional units	Reference range, conventional units	Value, SI units	Reference range, SI units
HBsAg (S)	Negative	Negative	Same	
Anti-hepatitis C Ab (S)	Negative	Negative	Same	
Antinuclear Ab (S)	Negative	Negative	Same	
Anti-smooth muscle Ab (S)	Negative	Negative	Same	
α_1-Antitrypsin (S)	132 mg/dL	78-200	1.3 g/L	0.8-2.0
Ceruloplasmin (S)	30 mg/dL	18-45	300 mg/L	180-450
Iron, total (S)	316 μg/dL	65-170	57 μmol/L	12-30
Transferrin (S)	322 mg/dL	220-400	3.22 g/L	2.20-4.00
Transferrin saturation (S)	98 %	20-50	0.98	0.20-0.50
Ferritin (S)	2675 ng/mL	17-270	2675 μg/L	17-270

Because of his abnormal serum iron values, a tentative diagnosis of genetic hemochromatosis (GH) causing cirrhosis and portal hypertension was made. Confirmation depended on the results of a liver biopsy, which could not be performed until the patient's ascites was resolved. After several more weeks of diuresis and a repeat ultrasonographic examination that showed no residual ascites, his liver biopsy revealed cirrhosis with marked iron deposition (4+) in hepatocytes and Kupffer cells. A quantitative iron determination on the biopsy sample showed 360 μmol/g dry weight (reference range, 5-22), and his "iron index" (liver iron divided by age) was 360/56 = 6.4 (see *Discussion*). His serum α-fetoprotein concentration was 1.2 ng/mL (1.2 μg/L; reference range, <15). Finally, to determine whether any of his three children might have GH, human leukocyte antigen (HLA) typing was performed on the patient and his family. The patient was found to have an A3, B7, B8 phenotype; but his wife lacked A3 and B7, and his three children were heterozygous for the A3, B7 or A3, B8 phenotype. None of his children had transferrin saturations above 40%.

Weekly phlebotomies of 500 mL were begun. After 17 months, 68 units of blood having been removed, the patient's serum ferritin was 194 ng/mL (194 μg/L), and his hematocrit had fallen to 36% (0.36). His AST and ALT returned to normal. Although his initial glucose had been high on presentation, he never developed overt diabetes, and a glucose tolerance test performed a year after therapy was normal. Although some of the signs of chronic liver disease resolved, he never regained sexual potency.

After several years of taking spironolactone (25 mg b.i.d.), the patient discontinued the drug. His ascites recurred, and a repeat paracentesis again showed a transudate. He responded to reinstitution of therapy but required much larger doses. A repeat liver biopsy showed cirrhosis, but there was no parenchymal cell iron staining. He continued to donate blood 3-5 times a year and has remained relatively stable, eight years after his diagnosis was made. Unfortunately he has been unable to work for the past five years owing to weakness and difficulty concentrating. Results of yearly determinations of α-fetoprotein have remained low.

Discussion

Evaluation of New Onset Ascites. Although cirrhosis of the liver with resulting portal hypertension is the most common cause of ascites, there are many other possible etiological factors, such as right-sided heart failure, constrictive pericarditis, malignancies, chronic peritoneal infection (especially tuberculosis), pancreatic duct leak, and hypothyroidism. Therefore, every patient with ascites should have an examination of the ascitic fluid obtained by paracentesis that assesses cell and differential count, cytology, glucose, LDH, amylase, total protein, and albumin.[1] Determining the difference between serum and ascitic fluid albumin concentrations (the "albumin gradient") has been found particularly useful for differential diagnosis; a "wide gradient" (>1.1 g/dL) suggests a transudate due to chronic liver disease or cardiac failure, whereas a "narrow gradient" (<1.2 g/dL) suggests peritoneal carcinoma, peritoneal inflammation, or a hollow organ leak.

The goal of therapy in patients with ascites is to eliminate the peritoneal fluid accumulation, which not only is uncomfortable for the patient and can cause some respiratory compromise but also puts the patient at increased risk of a peritoneal infection. Indeed, the most important reason for performing a paracentesis on all patients who present with ascites is to determine whether they have "spontaneous bacterial peritonitis."[2] Spontaneous bacterial peritonitis has a very poor prognosis unless aggressively treated with antibiotics. Recent studies have even suggested the prophylactic use of antibiotics in selected patients with recurrent infections.[3] A diagnosis of spontaneous bacterial peritonitis is made immediately if the peritoneal fluid *granulocyte* count (not total leukocyte count) is >250 x 10^3/μL (>250 x 10^9/L). Culture of peritoneal fluid can be 91% sensitive for diagnosis of spontaneous bacterial peritonitis; but the culture medium must be inoculated at the bedside,[2] and results are not available for several days. Gram stain of peritoneal fluid is not very sensitive for detecting and identifying organisms.

Fortunately for the patient under discussion, his ascites was a noninfected transudate with a low granulocyte count and was relatively easily resolved with diuretics and a sodium-restricted diet.

Pathophysiology and Diagnosis of Genetic Hemochromatosis. Genetic hemochromatosis (GH) is a relatively common homozygous recessive disorder with variable penetrance affecting approximately 1:250 to 1:400 Caucasians.[4] The incidence in non-Caucasian populations is very low. In GH there is abnormally high intestinal absorption of dietary iron over the subject's lifetime, which leads to iron deposition and damage to a number of organs.[4] Despite its high frequency in the population, GH frequently goes undiagnosed because most manifestations are ascribed to other causes, and iron studies are not routinely ordered. Early diagnosis of GH is important because the end-organ damage can be easily prevented or halted by simple phlebotomy therapy. Furthermore, family studies can identify other siblings or children "at risk," so that early therapy can be instituted. Treated precirrhotic GH patients have been shown to have a normal life expectancy; but once cirrhosis or diabetes develops, GH patients have markedly shortened life spans.[5]

The nature of the genetically determined pathological defect that causes increased intestinal iron absorption in GH still is not known. The genetic defect is closely linked to the HLA-A locus, and most subjects with GH have either A3, B7 or A3, B14 haplotypes.[6] However, even if A3 is absent, once a proband is identified by clinical, biochemical, and histological studies, then comparison of his or her HLA alleles with those in siblings and children can identify which relatives are homozygous for the GH defect and therefore at risk. Although heterozygotes usually have mild iron-loading, they are not at risk for developing end-organ damage. A high percentage of homozygotes, but not all, slowly accumulate iron over their lifetime to manifest end-organ damage in their 40's to 60's. The majority of probands with GH are men; women with GH are somewhat protected since they lose iron over many years with menses.

Iron-loading in GH affects several organs.[4] In the liver, it leads first to occult, then clinically evident cirrhosis, and eventually to development of hepatomas. In the pancreas, iron-loading of the islets of Langerhans causes glucose intolerance or frank diabetes. Cardiomyopathies and arrhythmias can develop. Testicular atrophy and impotence occur as a result of decreased gonadotropin production by the pituitary. Chondrocalcinosis develops in joint synovia. Hyperpigmentation of skin may be observed but is due to increased melanin rather than iron deposition. Because the clinical picture has varied aspects secondary to causes other than GH, a physician must cultivate a high index of suspicion for the disease and utilize screening tests.

The appropriate way to screen for GH is to determine *fasting* serum iron and transferrin, with calculation of the percent transferrin saturation.[4] An alternative test to the serum transferrin is the total iron-binding capacity (TIBC), which is then used to calculate the percent saturation. Using serum iron and transferrin to make a diagnosis in very sick, cirrhotic GH patients who have infected ascites or bleeding esophageal varices is usually unrewarding — the diagnosis in these patients is often made at autopsy. However, one should not forget to screen siblings and children.

Ferritin, an important iron-binding and intracellular iron-storage protein, should also be measured in the serum of patients with suspected GH. However, serum ferritin does not become elevated early in GH and only increases with heavy iron-loading when iron spills over from hepatocytes into reticuloendothelial cells. In non-GH patients, serum ferritin is increased with acute hepatocyte damage (hepatitis) or if there is a systemic inflammatory reaction. Therefore, a serum ferritin value should be interpreted with caution. HLA typing should never be used as a screening test for GH because the vast majority of people with A3, B7, or B14 alleles will not have GH, and many patients with GH will not have any of these alleles.[6] HLA typing is also expensive.

Upon finding a high percent saturation of transferrin, a diagnosis of GH is confirmed with a liver biopsy, followed by staining with special stains for iron deposits (Prussian blue or Perls' stain) and by quantitative determination of iron content of liver tissue. It is important to distinguish heterozygotes from homozygotes, since heterozygotes have lesser risk of end-organ damage despite increased iron-loading. An "iron index"[7] is calculated from the iron content of liver (in µmol/g of dry liver) divided by the age of the subject and is useful for making the distinction between homozygote and heterozygote or normal individuals. An index >1.9 indicates homozygosity for GH.

The importance of identifying GH in patients who present with cirrhosis, diabetes, cardiomyopathy, chondrocalcinosis, or impotence cannot be overstressed because iron removal therapy is safe and generally effective if instituted early. Usually cirrhosis, diabetes, and impotence are not reversible.[5] If homozygotes are recognized early, prior to development of symptoms of end-organ effect, preventive (prophylactic) treatment is easily initiated by prescribing regular blood donation to reduce the rate of iron-loading. Whether random serum iron determination as part of a chemistry screening panel will help in early identification of homozygotes is not yet known. Screening with *fasting* serum iron and transferrin tests, however, appears to be practical at this time.

References

1. Hoefs, J.C.: Diagnostic paracentesis, a potent clinical tool. Gastroenterology, *98:* 230-236, 1990.

2. Runyon, B.A.: Spontaneous bacterial peritonitis: An explosion of information. Hepatology, *8:* 171-175, 1988.

3. Gines, P., Rimola, A., Planas, R., et al.: Norfloxacin prevents spontaneous bacterial peritonitis recurrence in cirrhosis: Results of a double-blind, placebo controlled trial. Hepatology, *12:* 716-724, 1990.

4. Tavill, A.S., and Bacon, B.R.: Hereditary hemochromatosis: Pathogenesis and clinical features of a common disease. *In:* Hepatology: A Textbook of Liver Disease. D. Zakim and T.D. Boyer, Eds. Philadelphia, W.B. Saunders Co., 1990.

5. Niederau, C., Fischer, R., Sonnenberg, A., et al.: Survival and causes of death in cirrhotic and in noncirrhotic patients with primary hemochromatosis. N. Engl. J. Med., *313:* 1256-1262, 1985.

6. Simon, M., Le Mignon, L., Fauchet, R., et al.: A study of 609 HLA haplotypes marking for the hemochromatosis gene. Am. J. Hum. Genet., *41:* 89-105, 1987.

7. Summers, K.M., Halliday, J.W., and Powell, L.W.: Identification of homozygous hemochromatosis subjects by measurement of hepatic iron index. Hepatology, *12:* 20-25, 1990.

Additional Reading

Weintraub, L.R., Edwards, C.Q., and Krikker, M., Eds.: Hemochromatosis: Proceedings of the First International Conference. Ann. N.Y. Acad. Sci., *526:* 1-368, 1988.

ADOLESCENT FEMALE WITH TREMOR, DEPRESSION, AND HEPATITIS

Steven I. Shedlofsky, Contributor

A 16-year-old white female presented to her pediatrician with tremor and depression. Approximately eight months previously, her mother noted mild muscle incoordination, which slowly progressed. As a result the patient failed to be re-elected as a school cheerleader just one month prior to presentation. A depressed affect with fatigue and malaise had developed and was thought to be secondary to this failure. However, when a tremor was noted along with mild dysarthria, the patient's mother decided to seek medical attention for her. Prior to this time, the patient had been healthy except for an appendectomy at age nine. There was no history of head trauma or neonatal jaundice, nor was there a history of neurological disease in her family.

On initial examination, the patient had a flat affect. She weighed 108 lb (49 kg) and had normal vital signs. There was a fine tremor of both hands and arms, worse with voluntary actions, but no focal neurological deficits. Mild scleral icterus was noted, and the patient had several spider angiomata on her chest and several ecchymoses on each of her shins. Her liver was palpable 2 cm below the right costal margin with a dull edge, and there was tenderness to fist percussion. Her spleen was barely palpable under the left costal margin.

The following initial laboratory results were obtained:

Analyte	Value, conventional units	Reference range, conventional units	Value, SI units	Reference range, SI units
Hemoglobin (B)	10.2 g/dL	12-16	6.33 mmol/L	7.45-9.93
Hematocrit (B)	32 %	37-47	0.32	0.37-0.47
Leukocyte count (B)	12.0 x 10^3/µL	4.8-10.8	12.0 x 10^9/L	4.8-10.8
MCV (B)	98 fL	80-94	Same	
Platelet count (B)	78 x 10^3/µL	150-450	78 x 10^9/L	150-450
Prothrombin time (P)	18.2 s (patient) 12.1 s (control)	11-15	Same	
Sodium (S)	137 mmol/L	136-145	Same	
Potassium (S)	4.7 mmol/L	3.8-5.1	Same	
Chloride (S)	99 mmol/L	98-107	Same	
CO$_2$, total (S)	23 mmol/L	23-31	Same	
Urea nitrogen (S)	10 mg/dL	8-21	3.6 mmol urea/L	2.9-7.5
Creatinine (S)	0.8 mg/dL	0.7-1.3	71 µmol/L	62-115
Glucose (S)	118 mg/dL	80-115	6.5 mmol/L	4.4-6.4
Calcium (S)	4.7 mEq/L	4.2-5.1	2.35 mmol/L	2.10-2.55
Phosphorus (S)	2.1 mg/dL	2.7-4.5	0.68 mmol/L	0.87-1.45
Protein, total (S)	6.8 g/dL	6.2-7.6	68 g/L	62-76
Albumin (S)	2.9 g/dL	3.2-4.6	29 g/L	32-46
Cholesterol (S)	152 mg/dL	120-210	3.94 mmol/L	3.11-5.44
Urate (S)	2.1 mg/dL	2.5-6.2	125 µmol/L	149-369
Bilirubin, total (S)	7.7 mg/dL	0.2-1.0	131 µmol/L	3-17
AST (S)	211 U/L	19-48	3.52 µkat/L	0.32-0.80
ALT (S)	122 U/L	13-40	2.03 µkat/L	0.22-0.67

Analyte	Value, conventional units	Reference range, conventional units	Value, SI units	Reference range, SI units
ALP (S)	128 U/L	30-100	2.1 μkat/L	0.5-1.7
GGT (S)	62 U/L	10-50	1.03 μkat/L	0.17-0.83
Urinalysis (U)	Negative for protein, blood, and cells; but 2+ glucose, 2+ bilirubin, and amorphous phosphate and urate crystals were noted	Negative for protein, blood, cells, glucose, and bilirubin		

Because of the patient's anemia and elevated bilirubin, further studies were ordered to rule out hemolytic disease.   The patient's conjugated bilirubin was 5.0 mg/dL (85 μmol/L), and a corrected reticulocyte count was 4.2% (reference range, 0.5-1.5). Despite her glycosuria, a 2-h postprandial serum glucose was only 114 mg/dL (6.3 mmol/L). Ultrasonographic examination of her liver and biliary system showed a normal gallbladder without stones and no dilated intra- or extrahepatic ducts. However, her liver was inhomogeneous and slightly enlarged with a prominent portal vein, suggesting cirrhosis with active inflammation. A small amount of ascitic fluid was noted. Further evaluation of the abnormal liver studies included the following:

Analyte	Value, conventional units	Reference range, conventional units	Value, SI units	Reference range, SI units
HBsAg (S)	Negative	Negative	Same	
IgM anti-HB core Ab (S)	Negative	Negative	Same	
IgM anti-HA Ab (S)	Negative	Negative	Same	
Anti-hepatitis C Ab (S)	Negative	Negative	Same	
α_1-Antitrypsin (S)	182 mg/dL	78-200	1.82 g/L	0.78-2.00
Ceruloplasmin (S)	16 mg/dL	18-45	160 mg/L	180-450
Antinuclear Ab (S)	Negative	Negative	Same	
Anti-smooth muscle Ab (S)	Negative	Negative	Same	

The slightly low ceruloplasmin level raised the suspicion of hepatolenticular degeneration (Wilson's disease). A more careful eye examination showed a golden brown band of pigment encircling the posterior cornea near the limbus on both eyes. An ophthalmologist performed a slit-lamp examination confirming the presence of Kayser-Fleischer rings. Due to the patient's poor coagulation status, a liver biopsy could not be performed. A 24-h urine collection was assayed for copper in order to confirm the presumptive diagnosis of Wilson's disease; copper excretion was markedly elevated, 1154 μg/d (18.2 μmol/d; reference range, 20-65; 0.30-1.02). The serum copper, 171 μg/dL (26.9 μmol/L), was within the normal range of 60-190 (9.4-29.9).

On the basis of the clinical and laboratory findings, therapy with D-penicillamine and a low copper diet was initiated. Although abdominal distention due to ascites developed, the patient responded to a low sodium diet and spironolactone. Her bilirubin decreased to 2.4 mg/dL (41 μmol/L) after two months, and her AST and ALT levels decreased to normal. Her hematocrit increased to 36% (0.36), and the reticulocytosis disappeared. Several 24-h urine specimens obtained during the first six months of her D-penicillamine therapy showed marked cupruresis of 3000-5000 μg/d (47.2-78.7 μmol/d).

The patient's neurological findings resolved completely, but after 10 months of therapy she developed a rash, arthralgias, and proteinuria. These symptoms were believed to indicate a lupus-like syndrome secondary to her D-penicillamine therapy. She was then switched to trientine therapy, which she has followed for the last two years without problems. When her prothrombin time became normal one year after the diagnosis of Wilson's disease, a percutaneous liver biopsy was performed. She required platelet infusions for the liver biopsy because her platelet count remained low at 65 x 10³/µL (65 x 10⁹/L). The liver biopsy showed inactive cirrhosis. An orcein stain for copper was slightly positive, and her hepatic copper level was slightly elevated (132 µg/g dry weight liver, normal being <50 µg/g), but this value was much lower than published values[1] of hepatic copper in patients with untreated Wilson's disease and chronic active hepatitis (530-1531 µg/g dry weight).

Because of her cirrhosis with its continued evidence of portal hypertension, the patient was placed on a waiting list for elective liver transplantation.

Definition of Disease

Pathophysiology of Wilson's Disease. Wilson's disease, also called hepatolenticular degeneration, is a rare autosomal recessive disorder of copper metabolism.[2] The incidence of Wilson's disease in the general population is estimated to be only 0.5-3 per 100,000, but the disease is invariably fatal unless the patient is identified and copper accumulation prevented. Although the nature of the defect has not yet been clarified, it appears that the liver is unable to excrete excess copper into bile so that copper accumulates first in the liver and then undergoes periods of release from the liver and redistribution into other organs such as brain, eyes, kidneys, and circulating red blood cells.

The physiological process of normal copper absorption, utilization, and excretion is complex. There is usually a large excess of dietary copper, most of which is absorbed in the intestine and rapidly transported to the liver. Once in the liver cell, copper can be either temporarily sequestered by various cytosolic proteins or stored in lysosomes. Some of the copper is loaded onto a glycoprotein, ceruloplasmin, that is secreted into the blood stream and has several important serum pro-oxidase functions. Some of the copper is incorporated into cellular enzymes such as cytochrome *c* oxidase, cytosolic superoxide dismutase, and monoamine oxidase. All excess copper is excreted into the bile tightly bound to as yet poorly described, high-molecular-weight proteins that prevent intestinal reabsorption and promote fecal elimination. In Wilson's disease, there is an inability to excrete excess copper into the bile as well as a decreased ability to secrete ceruloplasmin into the circulation. Copper accumulates in the liver from birth, and 85-95% of patients have low serum ceruloplasmin levels.

Manifestations of Wilson's Disease. Wilson's disease patients[3,4] present after age 6 (usually between the ages of 12 and 30) with either neurological or psychiatric problems, or at slightly earlier ages with manifestations of liver disease. Fifteen percent have acute intravascular hemolytic anemia, renal disease (Fanconi-like syndrome), or bone disease (osteomalacia). Approximately 25% of cases present with two or more manifestations,[3] as did this patient.

The hepatic involvement of Wilson's disease can take several forms, including the insidious onset of cirrhosis, chronic active hepatitis, or fulminant liver failure. In the first and most common presentation, patients develop complications of *cirrhosis* such as ascites, bleeding esophageal varices, and liver failure (e.g., coagulopathy, spider angiomata, hyperbilirubinemia, encephalopathy). The liver is usually small and not palpable; often there is little hepatocellular necrosis, and serum aminotransferases may be normal. When patients present with a *chronic active hepatitis*-like picture,[1] the liver is usually enlarged, but there is minimal aminotransferase elevation. Histological examination of the liver often cannot distinguish between wilsonian chronic active hepatitis and other causes (e.g., viral or autoimmune diseases or drugs). Copper studies are essential for the differential diagnosis of patients with chronic active hepatitis who are <30 years old. *Fulminant liver failure* due to Wilson's disease is also often difficult to differentiate from other causes since serum ceruloplasmin can be low and urinary copper excretion high in other forms of fulminant liver disease. However, in Wilson's disease, liver failure appears to be associated with relatively low serum alkaline phosphatase activities and very high bilirubin values, so that an alkaline phosphatase/bilirubin ratio* of <2.0 has been proposed as good evidence for wilsonian fulminant liver failure.[5]

The neurological and psychiatric presentations of Wilson's disease are also insidious and often misdiagnosed.[4] Poor coordination, resting and intention tremor, excessive salivation, and dysarthria are commonly seen. The more severe dystonic manifestations are now rarely seen because of earlier diagnosis and institution of therapy.[2] Psychiatric manifestations can be quite varied but are always progressive. Unfortunately, once well established, psychiatric manifestations do not respond as well to copper removal.[4]

The hemolytic anemia of Wilson's disease is often episodic, probably owing to intermittent release of free copper from the liver that affects red blood cell membranes.[2] An intravascular hemolytic anemia often accompanies fulminant hepatic failure and should strongly suggest Wilson's disease as the cause of the liver failure. Renal involvement can be significant with a Fanconi-like syndrome characterized by aminoaciduria, glycosuria, phosphaturia, hypercalciuria, and high uric acid excretion with low serum urate levels (as occurred in the case presented). It is probably this chronic renal involvement that leads to the osteomalacia sometimes seen.

Diagnosis

The most commonly used laboratory study to diagnose this entity is serum ceruloplasmin assay; a value of <18 mg/dL (<180 mg/L) suggests the diagnosis. A low ceruloplasmin is found in 95% of Wilson's disease patients with neurological manifestations but in only 85% of those who present with hepatic disease.[2] Looking for Kayser-Fleischer rings is the next most important step; they will be seen in almost all patients with neurological symptoms if carefully sought with a slit-lamp examination. However, Kayser-Fleischer rings are absent 50% of the time when there is only hepatic involvement. Their absence is probably due to copper's first accumulating in the liver, where it initiates either major or minor damage, and only after there is substantial hepatic release of copper do other organs like the brain and eye accumulate the metal.

Confirmation of the diagnosis of Wilson's disease usually requires a liver biopsy with quantitation of the liver copper. All patients with Wilson's disease will have a markedly elevated hepatic copper, >250 μg/g dry weight. Heterozygotes for the Wilson's disease gene often have low serum ceruloplasmin but usually have intermediate hepatic copper concentration.[4] However, other cholestatic liver disorders such as primary biliary cirrhosis, sclerosing cholangitis, biliary obstruction or atresia, and Indian childhood cirrhosis can also display high liver copper concentrations. These entities are usually associated with normal or high serum ceruloplasmin.[2]

With severe liver disease and coagulopathy, liver biopsy often cannot be performed at initial presentation, as was the case for this patient. In the absence of Kayser-Fleischer rings,

---

*Alkaline phosphatase in U/L
 Bilirubin, total in mg/dL

determining 24-h urinary excretion of copper helps to confirm the clinical diagnosis. However, high urine copper values can also be seen with other causes of cirrhosis and chronic active hepatitis.[2] Serum copper levels, either total levels or the so-called "non-ceruloplasmin" copper,* have not been considered useful for the differential diagnosis.[2]

If significant doubt exists concerning the diagnosis of Wilson's disease, a copper incorporation test [6] has been promoted as a sensitive and specific test. A 2-mg dose of ^{64}Cu is administered orally, and serum is drawn at 1, 2, 4, 24, and 48 hours. In non-wilsonian liver disease there is a progressive increase in serum radioactivity that reflects ^{64}Cu-ceruloplasmin secretion by the liver, whereas in Wilson's disease there is very little radioactivity detected at 24 and 48 hours.

Treatment

Because Wilson's disease is invariably fatal if untreated and because effective treatment resolves most problems and allows prolonged survival, every patient with Wilson's disease must undergo uninterrupted therapy. A low copper diet is important, with avoidance of such foods as shellfish, nuts, mushrooms, legumes, and organ meats such as liver. The drug D-penicillamine, at doses of 2-5 g/d, chelates hepatic copper and allows rapid urinary excretion. Although most patients tolerate D-penicillamine, it often has hypersensitivity-type side effects, some of which are too serious to allow its continued use. In such cases another effective chelating agent, trientine, can be used. Recently there have been studies of the effect of oral zinc supplements to block intestinal absorption of dietary copper in Wilson's patients who have been de-coppered.[7]

Liver transplantation has been performed in a number of Wilson's disease patients, usually for fulminant liver failure. Transplantation is also indicated in patients who do not respond to chelation therapy or who cannot be managed with oral chelation therapy because of either noncompliance or drug sensitivities. The fact that liver transplantation completely resolves copper accumulation is further evidence that the defect of Wilson's disease is primarily one of hepatic excretion. Liver transplantation is nevertheless the therapy of last resort.

References

1. Schilsky, M.L., Scheinberg, I.H., and Sternlieb, I.: Prognosis of wilsonian chronic active hepatitis. Gastroenterology, *100:* 762-767, 1991.

2. Gollan, J.L.: Copper metabolism, Wilson's disease, and hepatic copper toxicosis. *In:* Hepatology, A Textbook of Liver Disease. D. Zakim and T.D. Boyer, Eds. Philadelphia, W.B. Saunders Co., 1990.

3. Sternlieb, I., and Scheinberg, I.H.: Wilson's disease. *In:* Liver and Biliary Disease. R. Wright, K.G.M. Alberti, S. Karran, et al., Eds. London, W.B. Saunders Co., 1985.

4. Cartwright, G.E.: Diagnosis of treatable Wilson's disease. N. Engl. J. Med., *298:* 1347-1350, 1978.

---

*The difference between total Cu^{2+} expressed in µg/dL minus 5.5 × ceruloplasmin in mg/dL (reference range, 6-19 µg/dL).[5]

5.   Berman, D.H., Leventhal, R.I., Gavaler, J.S., et al.: Clinical differentiation of fulminant wilsonian hepatitis from other causes of hepatic failure. Gastroenterology, *100:* 1129-1134, 1991.

6.   Sternlieb, I., and Scheinberg, I.H.: The role of radiocopper in the diagnosis of Wilson's disease. Gastroenterology, *77:* 138-142, 1979.

7.   Hill, G.M., Brewer G.J., Prasad, A.S., et al.: Treatment of Wilson's disease with zinc. 1. Oral zinc therapy regimens. Hepatology, *7:* 522-528, 1987.

MIDDLE-AGED ALCOHOLIC WITH JAUNDICE AND ASCITES

Albert I. Rubenstone, Contributor
Steven I. Shedlofsky, Contributor

A 51-year-old white male came to the Emergency Department complaining of weakness, lack of appetite, shortness of breath, and abdominal distention. He was a known alcoholic who had failed detoxification programs several times in the past and continued to drink approximately one pint of vodka or gin per day. Eight months before presentation he had been admitted to another hospital with alcoholic hepatitis and at that time had suffered severe withdrawal symptoms. Soon after discharge, however, he resumed drinking. Two weeks prior to the current presentation, he developed a "cold" and lost his appetite. He began taking over-the-counter ibuprofen for nonspecific pains and continued to drink. When he experienced profound weakness, shortness of breath, and abdominal bloating, he asked his girl-friend to take him to the hospital.

Physical examination revealed his wasted appearance, alcohol on his breath, icterus, and a protuberant abdomen. Vital signs included temperature, 98 °F (36.8 °C); respiratory rate, 24/min; pulse, 70 BPM; and blood pressure, 140/70 mm Hg without orthostasis. He had bilateral gynecomastia and sparse axillary hair; spider angiomata were present on his anterior chest. Cardiac examination revealed a hyperdynamic precordium with normal heart sounds; the lungs were normal to percussion and auscultation. The abdomen was tense with a fluid wave and shifting dullness. Liver and spleen were neither palpable nor ballotable, and the abdominal venous pattern, although prominent, drained normally. The testes were atrophic, and the legs showed petechial hemorrhages and 3+ edema. Palmar erythema was noted. Rectal examination provided a soft, brown stool that was positive for occult blood. Neurological examination disclosed poor concentration, but the patient was not disoriented. No asterixis was observed, but pain and light touch perception and proprioception were diminished in both lower extremities.

The patient's mother had died of a heart attack, and his father was an alcoholic. The patient had no history of previous operations or blood transfusion. He was divorced and childless.

On admission, laboratory values were as follows:

Analyte	Value, conventional units	Reference range, conventional units	Value, SI units	Reference range, SI units
Blood alcohol	97 mg/dL	0	21 mmol/L	0
Hemoglobin (B)	9.5 g/dL	14-18	5.90 mmol/L	8.69-11.17
Hematocrit (B)	30 %	40-54	0.30	0.40-0.54
Leukocyte count (B)	11.5 x 10³/µL	4.8-10.8	11.5 x 10⁹/L	4.8-10.8
MCV (B)	106 fL	80-94	Same	
Platelet count (B)	97 x 10³/µL	150-450	97 x 10⁹/L	150-450
Prothrombin time (P)	16.2 s (control: 11.9 s)	11-15	Same	
Sodium (S)	131 mmol/L	136-145	Same	

Analyte	Value, conventional units	Reference range, conventional units	Value, SI units	Reference range, SI units
Potassium (S)	4.0 mmol/L	3.8-5.1	Same	
Chloride (S)	108 mmol/L	98-107	Same	
CO2, total (S)	13.8 mmol/L	23-31	Same	
Urea nitrogen (S)	7 mg/dL	8-21	2.5 mmol urea/L	2.9-7.5
Creatinine (S)	0.9 mg/dL	0.7-1.3	80 µmol/L	62-115
Glucose (S)	110 mg/dL	70-105	6.1 mmol/L	3.9-5.8
Calcium (S)	9.2 mg/dL	8.4-10.2	2.30 mmol/L	2.10-2.54
Phosphorus (S)	4.5 mg/dL	2.7-4.5	1.45 mmol/L	0.87-1.45
Protein, total (S)	5.6 g/dL	6.2-7.8	56 g/L	62-78
Albumin (S)	2.3 g/dL	3.2-4.6	23 g/L	32-46
Cholesterol (S)	126 mg/dL	140-220	3.25 mmol/L	3.62-5.69
Urate (S)	6.1 mg/dL	2.6-7.2	363 µmol/L	155-428
Bilirubin, total (S)	6.5 mg/dL	0.2-1.0	111 µmol/L	3-17
AST (S)	210 U/L	10-42	3.50 µkat/L	0.17-0.70
ALT (S)	56 U/L	10-60	0.93 µkat/L	0.17-1.00
ALP (S)	180 U/L	42-121	3.0 µkat/L	0.7-2.0
GGT (S)	320 U/L	7-64	5.33 µkat/L	0.12-1.07
Urinalysis (U)	Specific gravity, 1.005; pH, 5.0; negative for glucose, protein, blood, and cells; bilirubin, 2+			

Ultrasonographic scan of the abdomen and right upper quadrant showed an intact gallbladder without gallstones; marked ascites was present with a slightly enlarged, inhomogeneous liver. Intrahepatic ducts were not dilated, and the common bile duct was normal size. The scan therefore did not suggest biliary obstruction.

The patient was treated with thiamine, folate, multivitamins, and vitamin K and was placed on a diet restricted to sodium <2 g/d and fluid <1.5 L/d. An intravenous line was placed to infuse 5% dextrose. Six liters of peritoneal fluid were removed by paracentesis, and the patient received 50 g of albumin immediately after paracentesis.

Laboratory results on the peritoneal fluid were as follows:

Analyte	Value, conventional units	Noninfected ascites, reference range	Value, SI units	Reference range, SI units
Leukocyte count, total	105 x 10³/µL	<350	105 x 10⁹/L	<350
Protein, total	1.5 g/dL	0.5-2.8	15 g/L	5-28
Albumin	0.3 g/dL	0.1-1.8	3 g/L	1-18
Glucose	95 mg/dL	70-105	5.3 mmol/L	3.9-5.8
Amylase	22 U/L	20-170	0.37 µkat/L	0.33-2.83
Gram stain	Negative			
Cytological examination	No malignant cells			

On the second hospital day, the patient began hallucinating, became violent, and had to be physically restrained. These withdrawal symptoms were successfully treated with oral oxazepam. On the fourth hospital day, spironolactone for treatment of his ascites was added to his drug regimen. A week after admission, his pedal edema and abdominal girth were improved; the liver became palpable 3 cm below the right costal margin and the spleen as well under the left costal margin. Serum electrolytes became normal. However, AST remained elevated (275 U/L; 4.58 µkat/L), and bilirubin had increased (9.7 mg/dL; 166 µmol/L). Despite three doses of vitamin K, his prothrombin time was still prolonged (15.6 s). Other liver tests were performed:

Analyte	Value, conventional units	Reference range, conventional units	Value, SI units	Reference range, SI units
HBsAg (S)	Negative	Negative	Same	
Anti-hepatitis C Ab (S)	Negative	Negative	Same	
α-Fetoprotein (S)	<5.0 ng/mL	<8.5	<5.0 µg/L	<8.5
α₁-Antitrypsin (S)	194 mg/dL	78-200	1.9 g/L	0.8-2.0
Ceruloplasmin (S)	39 mg/dL	18-45	390 mg/L	180-450
Iron, total (S)	27 µg/dL	65-170	5 µmol/L	12-30
Transferrin (S)	123 mg/dL	220-400	1.23 g/L	2.20-4.00
% Transferrin saturation (S)	22 %	20-50	0.22	0.20-0.50
Ferritin (S)	117 ng/mL	30-270	117 µg/L	30-270

The patient remained mildly confused even after oxazepam was stopped. Plasma ammonia of 88 µmol/L (reference range, 11-35 µmol/L) suggested portosystemic encephalopathy. The patient responded to lactulose therapy. Presence of anemia and blood in the stool led to esophagogastroduodenoscopy (EGD); the examination showed large esophageal varices without evidence of a recent bleeding site. Flexible sigmoidoscopy showed no abnormality.

After two weeks, the patient was stable with minimal ascites, mild encephalopathy, and persistent jaundice. He was discharged after being scheduled for an outpatient clinic visit the next week. He failed to keep the appointment but returned two weeks later after an alcoholic binge. He was readmitted with a temperature of 100.2 °F (39 °C), massive ascites, a serum bilirubin of 22 mg/dL (376 µmol/L), and a hematocrit of 32% (0.32). Repeat paracentesis showed spontaneous bacterial peritonitis; the leukocyte count was 2.3 x 10³/µL (2.3 x 10⁹/L), and 95% of cells were granulocytes. Intravenous antibiotics were started, but the patient had a massive hematemesis and his hematocrit dropped to 17% (0.17). Emergency EGD showed ruptured esophageal varices. Despite successful sclerotherapy and supportive transfusions, the patient lapsed into coma and died two days later.

Definition of Alcoholic Liver Disease

This case is classic for alcohol-induced cirrhosis with its three major complications: ascites, portosystemic encephalopathy, and bleeding from esophageal varices. This patient suffered also from many of the other complications of persistent alcohol abuse: acute alcoholic hepatitis, peripheral neuropathy, withdrawal syndrome, and spontaneous bacterial peritonitis. These manifestations in any patient further complicate management of the cirrhosis and darken the prognosis.

Alcoholic liver disease (ALD) is usually divided into three stages: Stage 1, hepatic steatosis; Stage 2, alcoholic hepatitis; and Stage 3, alcoholic cirrhosis.[1,2] Almost all heavy users of alcohol develop steatosis, but only 10-15% of abusers actually progress to acute alcoholic hepatitis or develop cirrhosis. Despite these statistics, ALD is still the fourth most common cause of death in males between the ages of 25 and 64.

Three theories of the mechanism by which ethanol causes damage in the liver and other tissues are current.

1. Oxidation of ethanol in the liver by the enzyme alcohol dehydrogenase produces acetaldehyde, which is rapidly dehydrogenated with the reduction of NAD to NADH. Excess aldehyde may accumulate and act as a hepatotoxin. The highly reduced environment of cytoplasm and mitochondria inhibits fatty acid oxidation and the citric acid cycle so that lipogenesis is stimulated (leading to steatosis). Hyperuricemia and hyperlactacidemia may also develop. Ethanol induces one of the hepatic cytochromes P-450, CYP2E1, and thus might affect metabolism of steroids and many drugs.

2. Damage may be mediated by immune mechanisms involving antibodies or sensitized T cells with specificities directed against hepatic antigens or both. One lesion often seen in hepatocytes in ALD is the "Mallory body,"[2,3] a perinuclear mass of dense, eosinophilic material. Mallory bodies and other proteins altered in response to ethanol toxicity might represent neoantigens that stimulate an autoimmune response.

3. Ethanol, or the damage it causes, may activate collagen synthesis by the perisinusoidal fat-storing (Ito) cells and may serve as an initiator for perivenular fibrosis and eventually for bridging fibrosis and cirrhosis.

Alcoholic Hepatitis. The diagnosis of alcoholic hepatitis is usually based on a history of prolonged alcohol intake and clinical findings of abdominal pain, anorexia, nausea, vomiting, fever, leukocytosis, and tender hepatomegaly.[2] Serum AST is characteristically elevated but <300 U/L (<5.00 µkat/L); AST is, however, usually much higher than ALT, which may even be normal. Low ALT appears to be due to a relative pyridoxine (vitamin B_6) deficiency that causes diminished activity to be measured in serum assays that are not supplemented with pyridoxal-5'-phosphate.[4]

Liver biopsy can provide a histological diagnosis based on steatosis, lobular granulocyte infiltrates, and degenerating hepatocytes with or without Mallory bodies. However, liver biopsy is generally performed only in patients who seem to have a protracted course and fail to respond to alcohol abstinence, rehydration, and nutritional replacement of thiamine, folate, and protein. Alcoholic hepatitis is a serious lesion, and mortality rates of 17%, 23%, and 44% for mild, moderate, and severe cases, respectively, have been observed.[5] Often, as in this patient, alcoholic hepatitis is accompanied by an underlying alcoholic cirrhosis.

Alcoholic Cirrhosis. Micronodular cirrhosis can develop in ALD because of repeated episodes of alcoholic hepatitis with necrosis followed by fibrosis and regeneration. It is characterized by small (<3 mm in diameter), uniform nodules. In quiescent cirrhosis without active hepatitis, the liver shrinks and hardens. Patients can develop one or more of the manifestations of portal hypertension (ascites, esophageal varices, hypersplenism) or of liver failure (jaundice, prolonged prothrombin time, hypoalbuminemia, portosystemic encephalopathy, sensitivity to hepatically cleared medications). Only a few of these manifestations can be discussed here.

Ascites. Ascites in alcoholic cirrhotics is due both to obstruction of hepatic lymphatic flow and to avid renal retention of sodium. Sodium retention arises because of marked peripheral vasodilation with a hyperdynamic circulation, high cardiac output, and low peripheral vascular resistance; this situation leads to contraction of the central plasma volume.[6] Spider angiomata and palmar erythema are probably manifestations of the peripheral arterial vasodilation. Reduced renal blood flow stimulates renin and aldosterone production, and despite total body sodium overload, very little sodium is excreted. Because renal cortical blood flow is maintained by prostaglandins, nonsteroidal anti-inflammatory drugs (such as ibuprofen), which inhibit cyclo-oxygenase, can lead to functional renal failure (the so-called hepatorenal syndrome) and exacerbation of sodium retention, and thus cause or worsen ascites.

Evaluation of ascites by paracentesis is very important in alcoholic cirrhotics in order to rule out spontaneous bacterial (or secondary) peritonitis and to differentiate cirrhotic ascites from malignant ascites.[7,8] In alcoholic cirrhosis, levels of protein and albumin in the fluid are very low. With bacterial peritonitis, the granulocyte count will be very high, >350 x $10^3/\mu L$ (>350 x 10^9/L). Antibiotic treatment of the infection is imperative.

Treatment of ascites decreases the likelihood of spontaneous bacterial peritonitis, improves patient comfort and respiration, and permits percutaneous liver biopsy if the procedure is needed. More than 90% of compliant patients will respond to dietary sodium restriction and K^+-sparing diuretics such as spironolactone. However, diuretics take several weeks to eliminate ascites, and large-volume paracentesis (6-8 L/d until "dry") with intravenous administration of 40-50 g of albumin is now routine prior to starting a diuretic regimen. In patients with recalcitrant ascites, placement of a LeVeen peritoneovenous shunt may also be effective but does not improve survival any more than does frequent paracentesis.[9]

Esophageal Varices. Increased portal pressures with a gradient of >12 mm Hg between the portal and hepatic venous systems lead to varices in the stomach and lower esophagus. These varices may bleed massively. Despite various approaches to prevention of variceal bleeding (prophylactic propranolol, portosystemic shunts of various types) and different ways to staunch bleeding (sclerotherapy, Sengstaken-Blakemore tubes, shunts, administration of vasopressin or nitrates), patients with bleeding varices have a very poor prognosis. When an alcoholic patient presents with hematemesis or melena, orthostasis, and a falling hematocrit, variceal rupture should not be immediately assumed. Endoscopy should be routinely performed to rule out other causes such as ulcers or alcoholic gastritis. If bleeding varices are found, sclerotherapy is the usual treatment.

Hypersplenism. With portal hypertension, the spleen enlarges and sequesters both platelets and leukocytes. Peripheral thrombocytopenia contributes to coagulopathy, and leukopenia to susceptibility to infection.

Anemia. Causes of anemia in ALD are complex; they include ethanol or acetaldehyde suppression of bone marrow function, vitamin deficiencies (e.g., folate), inflammation causing an "anemia of chronic disease," and acute and chronic blood loss leading eventually to iron deficiency. In most cases, the anemia that appears is macrocytic.

Liver Function Tests in ALD. Causes of jaundice in adults are numerous, among them, viral hepatitis, drug-induced hepatitis or cholestasis, biliary obstruction, or hemolytic anemia. With problems unrelated to the hepatobiliary systems, serum bilirubin is rarely >7 mg/dL (>120 µmol/L), and determination of conjugated (direct) bilirubin is unnecessary. Alcoholics presenting with jaundice should be promptly examined with ultrasonography of the right upper quadrant; if biliary obstruction is present, aggressive therapy to decompress the biliary tract is necessary.

In alcoholic hepatitis, AST and ALT are only mildly elevated, and AST more so than ALT. Because these enzyme assays evaluate hepatocellular necrosis, levels may actually be normal in quiescent cirrhosis. Alkaline phosphatase (ALP) and γ-glutamyltransferase (GGT) are synthesized in excess by biliary ductular cells reacting to irritation or inflammation of the intra- or extrahepatic biliary system; levels are commonly increased in many liver and biliary diseases, including ALD, biliary obstruction, and metastatic tumor. The GGT level is especially sensitive to alcohol-induced liver disease and may be increased when ALP is still normal. On the other hand, increased ALP with normal GGT is reason to look for a nonhepatobiliary cause for ALP elevation, e.g., bone disease.

Coagulation Tests. There are several reasons for disturbances of coagulation in ALD. Thrombocytopenia and prolonged prothrombin and partial thromboplastin times (PT and PTT) are the most commonly seen. Hypersplenism causes most cases of thrombocytopenia, but platelet consumption in a diffuse intravascular coagulopathy (DIC-like) syndrome can also occur. PT and PTT are prolonged owing to impaired hepatic production of factors II, VII, IX, X, protein C, and protein S, all of which require vitamin K for γ-carboxylation and activity. Liver failure alone may account for abnormal PT and PTT, but inadequate nutritional intake of vitamin K is also a possibility. A good test for liver reserve in ALD patients is to see whether PT is corrected by administration of parenteral vitamin K (10 mg subcutaneously each day for three days).

Hypoalbuminemia. Low albumin contributes to ascites and edema in ALD patients. Liver failure, poor nutrition, inflammatory conditions and infections, and protein loss from the gut or kidneys are all factors that can cause or intensify hypoalbuminemia.

Encephalopathy. The encephalopathy of liver failure has been termed portosystemic encephalopathy (PSE). Current theories explain PSE as an inability of the compromised liver to convert ammonia into urea, coupled with accumulation in plasma of aromatic amino acids (AAA) and depletion of branched-chain amino acids (BCAA). BCAA depletion is the result of their preferential utilization instead of AAA by muscle. The postulate is that the combination of increased plasma ammonia and an altered ratio of BCAA to AAA leads to generation of false neurotransmitters responsible for encephalopathy. The measurement of plasma ammonia (collected on ice and run immediately) has often been used to determine whether a patient has PSE. However, plasma ammonia concentrations are often unreliable, and it is not recommended that such measurements be used to follow a patient's course. To treat PSE, the removal of ammonia with oral lactulose therapy is usually effective. Lactulose is a nonabsorbable sugar that is fermented by colonic bacteria. This process acidifies the colon and sequesters the ammonia in the colon lumen as NH_4^+. The use of dietary supplements or parenteral infusions of BCAA have not been shown to be beneficial.[10] In general, restriction of protein intake is contraindicated for patients with ALD since it may enhance existing nutritional deficiency. It may, however, be invoked should sensitivity to protein loads develop.

Drug Sensitivity and Feminization in Men. Patients with cirrhosis often have decreased activity of hepatic cytochromes P-450 and can be very sensitive to medications that require hepatic metabolism. This is especially true for certain sedatives, hypnotics, and psychoactive drugs. A good principle to follow is to avoid medication whenever possible; when medication cannot be avoided, use discretion in choosing the drugs and dosages. Male alcoholics often manifest feminization because estrogenic steroids, normally cleared by hepatic oxidative systems, accumulate. On the other hand, acute alcohol ingestion suppresses testosterone formation by the gonads, and this mechanism can be more important than estrogen accumulation in causing feminization.

Treatment

The many manifestations of ALD require therapy that is directed both at avoiding all alcohol ingestion and at treating the specific complications of portal hypertension, liver failure, and nutritional depletion. Liver transplantation is rarely considered for these patients, since the liver damage is considered by many to be self-inflicted. Transplantation has, however, been successful in medically and psychosocially stable and abstinent patients with end-stage ALD but no other alcohol-related problems.[11]

References

1. Lieber, C.S.: Biochemical and molecular basis of alcohol-induced injury of liver and other tissues. N. Engl. J. Med., *319:* 1639-1650, 1988.

2. Zakim, D., Boyer, T.D., and Montgomery, C.: Alcoholic liver disease. *In:* Hepatology, A Textbook of Liver Disease, 2nd ed. D. Zakim and T.D. Boyer, Eds. Philadelphia, W.B. Saunders Co., 1990.

3. French, S.W.: The Mallory body: Structure, composition, and pathogenesis. Hepatology, *1:* 76-83, 1981.

4. Ludwig, S., and Kaplowitz, N.: Effect of pyridoxine deficiency on serum and liver transaminases in experimental liver injury in the rat. Gastroenterology, *79:* 545-549, 1980.

5. Mendenhall, C.L., and the VA Cooperative Study Group on Alcoholic Hepatitis: Alcoholic hepatitis. Clin. Gastroenterol., *10:* 417-441, 1981.

6. Schrier, R.W., Arroyo, V., Bernardi, M., et al.: Peripheral vasodilation hypothesis. A proposal for the initiation of renal sodium and water retention in cirrhosis. Hepatology, *8:* 1151-1157, 1988.

7. Hoefs, J.C.: Diagnostic paracentesis, a potent clinical tool. Gastroenterology, *98:* 230-236, 1990.

8. Runyon, B.A.: Spontaneous bacterial peritonitis: An explosion of information. Hepatology, *8:* 171-175, 1988.

9. Gines, P., Arroyo, V., Vargas, V., et al.: Paracentesis with intravenous infusion of albumin as compared with peritoneovenous shunting in cirrhosis with refractory ascites. N. Engl. J. Med., *325:* 829-835, 1991.

10. Eriksson, L.S., and Conn, H.O.: Branched-chain amino acids in the management of hepatic encephalopathy: An analysis of variants. Hepatology, *10:* 228-246, 1989.

11. Starzel, T.L., van Thiel, D., and Tsakis, H.G.: Orthotopic liver transplantation for alcoholic cirrhosis. JAMA, *260:* 2542-2544, 1988.

PATIENT WITH ABDOMINAL PAIN

Avram M. Cooperman, Contributor
Susan A. Fuhrman, Reviewer

A 32-year-old nonpregnant woman, gravida 2 para 2, was seen in the Emergency Department because of recurrent epigastric pain and colicky pain in the right upper quadrant. The current episode began four hours after a "heavy" dinner and was characteristic of previous episodes that had occurred several times a year for the past three years. The pain had become more severe during the more recent episodes, and the patient developed an intolerance for fatty foods. At this time, the vital signs were normal, and the patient was afebrile. There was tenderness without rebound in the right upper quadrant. Bowel sounds were normal. The urine was slightly dark.

On admission, the following laboratory values were obtained:

Analyte	Value, conventional units	Reference range, conventional units	Value, SI units	Reference range, SI units
Leukocyte count (B)	$8.6 \times 10^3/\mu L$	4.8-10.2	$8.6 \times 10^9/L$	4.8-10.2
Hemoglobin (B)	13.1 g/dL	12.0-14.8	8.13 mmol/L	7.45-9.18
Hematocrit (B)	40 %	36-44	0.40	0.36-0.44
Sodium (S)	138 mmol/L	138-145	Same	
Potassium (S)	4.5 mmol/L	4.1-5.3	Same	
Chloride (S)	109 mmol/L	98-107	Same	
CO$_2$, total (S)	22 mmol/L	20-28	Same	
Urea nitrogen (S)	11 mg/dL	5-18	3.9 mmol urea/L	1.8-6.4
Creatinine (S)	0.4 mg/dL	0.4-1.1	35 µmol/L	35-97
Glucose (S)	99 mg/dL	60-100	5.5 mmol/L	3.3-5.6
Protein, total (S)	6.1 g/dL	6.2-8.0	61 g/L	62-80
Albumin (S)	3.6 g/dL	3.8-5.4	36 g/L	38-54
Urate (S)	3.4 mg/dL	2.0-5.5	202 µmol/L	119-327
Cholesterol (S)	86 mg/dL	140-200	2.22 mmol/L	3.62-5.17
Bilirubin, total(S)	2.4 mg/dL	0.2-1.0	41 µmol/L	3-17
Bilirubin, conjugated (S)	1.4 mg/dL	0.0-0.2	24 µmol/L	0-3
AST (S)	80 U/L	9-30	1.33 µkat/L	0.15-0.50
ALT (S)	28 U/L	10-28	0.47 µkat/L	0.17-0.47
LDH (S)	450 U/L	180-430	7.50 µkat/L	3.00-7.17
ALP (S)	400 U/L	124-255	6.7 µkat/L	2.1-4.3
GGT (S)	120 U/L	5-85	2.00 µkat/L	0.08-1.42
Bile (U)	Positive	Negative		

X-ray examination of the abdomen showed a normal gas pattern. Ultrasonographic examination revealed gallstones in a normal-sized gallbladder, which contracted with a fatty meal, and showed no dilation of the common duct. The pancreas was normal. A diagnosis of cholelithiasis was made.

Definition of the Disease

Cholelithiasis affects about 25 million people per year in the United States, 8-10% of the population. One million new cases are diagnosed annually. The risk of developing gallstones is increased in individuals who are elderly, female, diabetic, or obese. When a gallstone obstructs the cystic duct, the gallbladder contracts and pain is produced. Inflammation (cholecystitis) and other manifestations of gallstones are due to migration of stones into the common duct (cholangitis, pancreatitis) or erosion into the bowel (gallstone ileus). Most commonly stones obstruct the cystic duct.

Development of Gallstones. In about 85% of gallstones, cholesterol is the predominant constituent. In the others, bilirubin is the primary component; these stones are called pigmented. The process of lithogenesis is driven by saturation of the bile with cholesterol or by hemolysis. Bile is an aqueous secretion containing bile acids and salts, phospholipids, and cholesterol. When the constituents occur in their normal proportions, micelles of cholesterol and bile salts are formed and thus keep cholesterol, a water-insoluble compound, in solution. Supersaturation of bile with excessive cholesterol is a key factor in cholesterol stone formation. Bilirubin, degraded from hemoglobin released as a consequence of systemic hemolytic events, conjugated in the liver, and then secreted into the bile in the conjugated form, is readily combined into insoluble calcium bilirubinate. Microcrystals of any type serve as nucleation promoters and act as a nidus for stone formation in the gallbladder. Cholelithiasis is not simply a consequence of crystallization of insoluble compounds in bile. Other factors include biliary stasis and possibly abnormalities in composition or secretion of mucus in the biliary tract. Stones in the gallbladder may remain *in situ* or migrate wholly or in part into the common duct.

Clinical Features. The spectrum of clinical manifestations of gallstone disease includes a wide range of presentations, varying from no symptoms at all to recurrent acute biliary colic. Gallstones frequently remain silent for a long time; only 2% of individuals with gallstones develop symptoms. The evolution of symptoms may be chronic. Initial presentation in 20% of affected patients is acute biliary colic; in 10% of the cases, the colic is due to a stone's obstructing the common duct and causing cholangitis (chills, fever, or jaundice) or to pancreatitis. Biliary colic is the most common and significant symptom of biliary disease. The classic symptom is epigastric or right upper quadrant pain, occurring after meals and lasting for minutes or hours. The cause of the pain is the impacted stone and the contraction of the distended, obstructed gallbladder.

Nonspecific symptoms such as belching, bloating, and abdominal fullness sometimes prompt gastrointestinal workup in which silent gallstones are disclosed. However, mere finding of the gallstones may not explain these symptoms, which are commonplace in the population with or without gallstones. Recurrence or persistence of the symptoms, in the absence of any other explanation, may suggest cholelithiasis more strongly and lead to therapeutic measures.

Diagnosis

Definitive diagnosis of gallstones is made by imaging procedures such as ultrasonography, by oral cholecystography, or by isotope scanning. Biochemical tests such as conjugated bilirubin, ALP, and GGT have ancillary benefit. Ultrasonography of the right upper quadrant utilizes sound waves to display densities and acoustic shadowing. The procedure is the most popular diagnostic test because it is least expensive, has a high accuracy rate (95%), is painless, and requires no preparation.

An oral cholecystogram outlines the gallbladder wall and its contents. The "dye" is excreted into the bile and then concentrated in the gallbladder. Nonvisualization (failure to visualize) of the gallbladder indicates gallbladder disease; on the other hand, visualization may outline the stones.

Radionuclide scanning (cholescintigraphy) can also be used to make the diagnosis. This test utilizes intravenous administration of technetium-labeled iminodiacetic acid, which when secreted into the biliary tract outlines the extrahepatic biliary system. If the gallbladder is not visualized, acute cholecystitis and obstruction of the cystic duct is confirmed. The test is rapid and definitive.

Laboratory tests diagnosing gallbladder disease include tests for total and conjugated bilirubin or its metabolites in serum, urine, and stool. Determination of *total and conjugated (direct) bilirubin* in serum may be helpful for evaluating both the ability of the liver to conjugate bilirubin with glucuronic acid and the patency of the biliary tract for delivery of conjugated bilirubin into the intestine. Increase of serum *total* bilirubin may occur for either reason, but in obstruction uncomplicated by hepatic disease or damage, increase in the *conjugated* form (glucuronides, the so-called direct forms) has particular significance. Unconjugated bilirubin in plasma is almost entirely bound to plasma albumin; the conjugated form is not bound and can be excreted in the urine. Thus, elevation of conjugated bilirubin in serum is responsible for bilirubinuria, which is a feature of obstructive jaundice. Another diagnostic feature is absence of urobilinogen from the stool, because bile duct obstruction prevents conjugated bilirubin from reaching the distal ileum where it is normally degraded to urobilinogen and urobilin. Absence of urobilinogen from the stool occurs only with complete biliary obstruction, as is seen in carcinoma of the head of the pancreas. Gallstones usually do not produce complete obstruction, and therefore some bile gets into the intestine. These urine and stool tests have become less popular for diagnosis of obstructive jaundice as imaging procedures have become more definitive. In some patients, after correction of an obstruction, the rate of decrease of serum bilirubin approximates the half-life of the albumin (14 days) to which it is largely bound.

The increase of *serum alkaline phosphatase* (ALP) activity in cholestasis is due to increased synthesis of the liver isoenzyme in the sinusoids, the endothelium of the central and periportal veins, and the biliary canaliculi and its release into the circulation. The stasis of bile in the tract is believed to induce the synthesis of liver ALP. Elevation of ALP is the earliest manifestation of biliary obstruction; after correction of obstruction, return to normal levels occurs in line with the half-life (7 days) of the enzyme. Two other serum enzymes, γ-*glutamyltransferase* (GGT) and *5'-nucleotidase* (5'-NT), may also be elevated in hepatobiliary diseases. Their increases usually parallel those of ALP.

The patient in this case displayed mild elevations of bilirubin and of ALP and GGT. The laboratory and imaging data suggested that stones may have migrated from the gallbladder and may have obstructed the common duct.

Treatment

Immediate Treatment. Immediate care calls for analgesics to comfort the patient and maintenance of hydration by means of intravenous fluids. Administration of systemic antibiotics directed against the flora of the biliary tract limits the chances of development of sepsis. In 90% of patients, acute colic with or without cholecystitis resolves spontaneously. In this patient, immediate measures were effective pending definitive treatment.

Definitive Treatment. A number of alternatives are available for the treatment of gallstones. Nonoperative therapy attempts to *solubilize bile and to decrease cholesterol saturation* in bile. Agents such as chenodeoxycholic acid (CDCA) and ursodeoxycholic acid (UDCA), taken orally, are effective in about one-third of the patients. These agents work best for single, small, cholesterol stones. However, patients may need to take these drugs after dissolution of the stones to prevent reformation.

Lithotripsy has been adapted for breaking up gallstones, but it was supplanted by other methods before a complete evaluation of its effectiveness had been achieved.

Cholecystectomy has been the definitive treatment for gallstones. Its disadvantages include the risks of surgery and the pain of an incision; but it has been the only certain way to forestall the complications of gallstones. Recently, laparoscopic cholecystectomy, i.e., removal of the gallbladder guided by video monitors and through a minimally invasive incision, has become the procedure of choice. Performed on an ambulatory basis, it is associated with minimal morbidity and little discomfort and allows rapid return to full activity. Laparo-scopic cholecystectomy is replacing other treatment methods because of its low risks and certainty of effectiveness. It was applied in this patient's case, in conjunction with an intraoperative cholangiogram; no stones were seen in the duct.

Additional Reading

Cooperman, A.M.: Laparoscopic Cholecystectomy — Difficult Cases — Creative Solutions. St. Louis, Quality Medical Publishing, 1991.

Grace, W.C.A., and Ransohoff, D.B.: The natural history of silent gallstones. N. Engl. J. Med., *307:* 798-800, 1983.

Kaplan, M.: Use of liver function tests. *In:* Diseases of the Liver. L. Schiff and E.R. Schiff, Eds. Philadelphia, J. B. Lippincott Co., 1987.

YOUNG WOMAN WITH RECURRENT ABDOMINAL PAIN

Steven I. Shedlofsky, Contributor

A 22-year-old white female presented to the Emergency Department with severe abdominal pain and profound generalized weakness. Milder episodes of similar abdominal pains had been occurring intermittently since age 17. When the patient was 18, an appendectomy was performed during one episode, but her appendix and terminal ileum were normal. Episodes occurred, on the average, every three months. Because her pain usually began four to seven days before onset of her menstrual period and resolved with menses, a gynecological cause was suspected. However, numerous pelvic examinations, ultrasonographic examinations of her ovaries, tubes, and uterus, and even a laparoscopy revealed normal anatomy. At age 20, she underwent a cholecystectomy, but there were no gallstones and the gallbladder was normal.

The patient's pains were usually dull, aching, and poorly localized and would last for hours without relief. Often there would be nausea but rarely vomiting. Frequently the patient developed abdominal distention and constipation and complained of leg weakness, but she was usually able to walk. When seen in the Emergency Department or office during these episodes, she was tachycardic but otherwise had a nonrevealing examination. Her stool was always negative for occult blood. Over the years, she had maintained a stable weight of 103-107 lb (47-48 kg). All of her routine laboratory studies, including complete blood counts, pancreatic enzymes, liver function tests, antinuclear antibodies, and urinalyses, were normal. The patient and her boyfriend were using condoms for contraception, and urine pregnancy tests were always negative. An upper gastrointestinal X-ray examination with a small bowel study, an endoscopic examination of her stomach and duodenum, a barium enema, and a computed tomographic (CT) scan of her abdomen and pelvis had all been performed within the last year and were normal.

Prior to age 17, the patient never had any significant illnesses, although she had required phototherapy for neonatal jaundice. She was the eldest of four children (two sisters and one brother) who, along with her parents, were in good health. There was no history of gastrointestinal or gynecological problems in her family, although an aunt on her father's side had suffered with unexplained abdominal pain.

To manage the pain, the patient would take oral meperidine and acetaminophen with some relief. Only once in the past two years did she have to visit the Emergency Department because of dehydration due to an inability to eat or drink. The patient had been referred to a psychiatrist two years previously and was still seeing him occasionally. Although the psychiatrist had expressed concern about her narcotic use, he discovered no affective or thought disorder and had recommended a variety of antianxiety drugs, which the patient would not take.

Just three days prior to the patient's current presentation, her physician had prescribed trimethoprim and sulfamethoxazole for a urinary tract infection. When the patient arrived in pain this time, she was complaining of much more severe abdominal pain, nausea with vomiting, bilateral leg pain with paresthesias, and generalized weakness such that she could not stand. She was a well-nourished but dehydrated young woman in obvious pain and very weak with a pulse of 125 BPM and a blood pressure of 142/105 mm Hg. Although she complained of abdominal pain, there was no localized tenderness or rebound pain. Her abdomen was distended and revealed scars from her appendectomy and cholecystectomy as well as laparoscopy incisions. Neurological examination showed decreased motor strength in both legs and absent reflexes. Responses to pin-prick, light touch, and proprioception were decreased.

Initial laboratory results were as follows:

Analyte	Value, conventional units	Reference range, conventional units	Value, SI units	Reference range, SI units
Hemoglobin (B)	13.4 g/dL	12-16	8.32 mmol/L	7.45-9.93
Hematocrit (B)	39 %	37-47	0.39	0.37-0.47
Leukocyte count (B)	9.4 x 10^3/μL	4.8-10.8	9.4 x 10^9/L	4.8-10.8
MCV (B)	85 fL	80-94	Same	
Platelet count (B)	381 x 10^3/μL	150-450	381 x 10^9/L	150-450
Sodium (S)	151 mmol/L	136-145	Same	
Potassium (S)	3.2 mmol/L	3.8-5.1	Same	
Chloride (S)	97 mmol/L	98-107	Same	
CO_2, total (S)	36 mmol/L	23-31	Same	
Urea nitrogen (S)	27 mg/dL	8-21	9.6 mmol urea/L	2.9-7.5
Creatinine (S)	0.8 mg/dL	0.7-1.3	71 μmol/L	62-115
Glucose (S)	106 mg/dL	80-115	5.8 mmol/L	4.4-6.4
Calcium (S)	8.8 mg/dL	8.4-10.2	2.20 mmol/L	2.10-2.55
Phosphorus (S)	3.2 mg/dL	2.7-4.5	1.03 mmol/L	0.87-1.45
Protein, total (S)	6.6 g/dL	6.2-7.6	66 g/L	62-76
Albumin (S)	3.4 g/dL	3.5-5.0	34 g/L	35-50
AST (S)	44 U/L	16-48	0.73 μkat/L	0.27-0.80
ALT (S)	37 U/L	13-40	0.63 μkat/L	0.22-0.67
ALP (S)	88 U/L	30-100	1.46 μkat/L	0.50-1.67
GGT (S)	33 U/L	10-50	0.56 μkat/L	0.17-0.83
β-hCG pregnancy test (S)	Negative	Negative		
Urinalysis (U)	Negative for glucose, protein, bilirubin, blood, and leukocytes; pH, 5.2; specific gravity, 1.033			

Abdominal X-ray films showed some distended loops of bowel but no air-fluid levels or free air. The patient was admitted, and her dehydration was treated with intravenous fluids. Shortly after admission, the patient's physician was contacted by the clinical laboratory and told that her urine sample had turned a deep red-wine color after standing at room temperature on the laboratory bench. The laboratory had taken the initiative to perform a qualitative test for urine porphobilinogen, which was strongly positive. This test is also known as a Hoesch test, a modification of the classic Watson-Schwartz test. The laboratory results suggested a possible diagnosis of acute porphyria, but the physician also wondered if the patient had been on phenazopyridine (Pyridium) for her urinary tract infection, which could cause a false positive test. The patient, however, was not on phenazopyridine.

The patient's physician quickly obtained information on how to diagnose and treat the acute hepatic porphyrias. He stopped her sulfamethoxazole and began therapy with intravenous glucose (total of ~300 g/d), meperidine and promethazine for pain and nausea, propranolol for the tachycardia, and a stool softener with laxatives for constipation. The patient responded with some relief, but her pain did not totally resolve until she started her menstrual period.

Further studies were obtained to elucidate her suspected porphyria. A 24-h urine specimen for the quantitative determination of porphyrins and porphobilinogen (PBG) was collected while she was still having pain. (The specimen was collected with sodium bicarbonate, kept on ice, and protected from light.) Another 24-h urine specimen for quantitative analysis of δ-aminolevulinate (ALA) was collected the next day. The specimen bottle contained hydrochloric acid, was kept on ice, and was protected from light. A random stool was collected after her attack and constipation had abated. In addition, the erythrocyte porphobilinogen deaminase activity was determined. The test results were as follows:

Analyte	Value, conventional units	Reference range, conventional units	Value, SI units	Reference range, SI units
24-h Urine (Sodium Bicarbonate)				
Volume	750 mL			
Creatinine	945 mg/d	600-1600	8.4 mmol/d	5.3-14.1
Porphobilinogen (PBG)	12.4 mg/d	0.0-1.5	54.8 μmol/d	0.0-6.6
Uroporphyrin	64 μg/d	0-22	77 nmol/d	0-26
Heptacarboxyporphyrin	16 μg/d	0-9	20 nmol/d	0-11
Hexacarboxyporphyrin	2 μg/d	0-4	3 nmol/d	0-5
Pentacarboxyporphyrin	13 μg/d	0-3	18 nmol/d	0-4
Coproporphyrin	122 μg/d	0-60	186 nmol/d	0-92
24-h Urine (Hydrochloric Acid)				
Volume	625 mL			
Creatinine	956 mg/d	600-1600	8.5 mmol/d	5.3-14.1
ALA	8.4 mg/d	0.0-3.0	64 μmol/d	0-23
Random Stool Specimen				
Weight	64 g			
Uroporphyrin	127 μg	<1000 μg/d	152 nmol	<1200 nmol/d
Coproporphyrin	188 μg	<200 μg/d	285 nmol	<300 nmol/d
Protoporphyrin	383 μg	<1500 μg/d	674 nmol	<2600 nmol/d
Porphobilinogen deaminase (Uro-1-synthase) (Ercs)	7.0 nmol/(s · L)	8.1-16.8	7.0 nkat/L	8.1-16.8

The markedly elevated urinary PBG excretion confirmed that the patient had one of the *acute hepatic porphyrias*. Since the PBG excretion was much greater than the ALA excretion, lead poisoning could be ruled out as a cause of the symptoms. (In lead poisoning, ALA excretion is greater than PBG excretion.) The normal stool porphyrin studies ruled out variegate porphyria (VP) and hereditary coproporphyria (HCP) and confirmed that the patient must have acute intermittent porphyria (AIP). This diagnosis was further supported by the decreased erythrocyte PBG deaminase activity and the fact that she never experienced any photosensitivity or skin lesions in sun-exposed areas (see *Diagnosis of the Acute Hepatic Porphyrias*).

The physician surmised that the recent sulfamethoxazole therapy for the patient's urinary tract infection had induced this rather severe attack of AIP in coincidence with one of her milder, hormonally induced premenstrual attacks. Because of the diagnosis of AIP, the patient was instructed to avoid a number of potentially dangerous medications. (See Bonkovsky[1] for a listing of safe and risky drugs.) She continued to have mild, painful attacks two to three times per year, almost always prior to menses; the attacks responded to glucose and analgesics. She was given intravenous hematin (Panhematin) early on during a few of her attacks in an effort to abort the attack, but whether the hematin was really effective remained unclear.

After her marriage, the patient became pregnant and her attacks abated until six months postpartum. Despite being told that AIP was a genetic disorder, the patient realized that it was inherited only when her youngest sister began having similar intermittent attacks of abdominal pain. Although the patient had a healthy daughter, she requested tubal ligation. By age 28, six years after the diagnosis of AIP was made, the patient had stopped having premenstrual pain attacks and has remained in good health since that time.

Definition of Porphyrias

The Heme Pathway and the Porphyrias. The group of metabolic disorders collectively called the porphyrias is a diverse group of diseases that are caused by defects in the heme metabolic pathway. Recent excellent in-depth reviews have been published,[1-4] so the following brief discussion will only highlight those facts that will help reach appropriate diagnosis, avoid inducing porphyric attacks, and promote an understanding of various therapeutic measures. Figure 1 shows a simplified schematic of the heme pathway, and Table 1 summarizes the urine, feces, and erythrocyte abnormalities for diagnosing more frequently seen porphyrias.

The first important concept to understand is that a porphyria presents either as an acute, neurologically mediated pain crisis or as a porphyrin-induced cutaneous photosensitivity reaction, depending upon which heme precursors are being produced in excess. The heme precursors, δ-aminolevulinate (ALA) and porphobilinogen (PBG), are small water-soluble molecules that are rapidly excreted in the urine if overproduced; neither is photosensitizing. Porphyrins, on the other hand, are carboxylated tetrapyrroles that absorb light of 400 nm (Soret wavelength) with subsequent locally damaging release of energy. In vivo, only the reduced porphyrinogens actually pass through the biochemical pathway; excess porphyrinogens are rapidly oxidized to become photosensitizing porphyrins. Porphyrins become less water-soluble as they are decarboxylated from 8-COOH (uroporphyrin) to 4-COOH (coproporphyrin) to 2-COOH (protoporphyrin). As porphyrins lose water solubility, they are excreted by the liver into bile and are found in stool rather than in urine. A high concentration of PBG in the urine will spontaneously form a red-colored tetrapyrrole, especially if the urine is exposed to light.

The next important concept to understand is that there are only three genetic acute porphyric disorders that have pain and neurological manifestations, namely, acute intermittent porphyria (AIP), variegate porphyria (VP), and hereditary coproporphyria (HCP). The neuropathy responsible for the acute pain crisis in each of these disorders can also involve peripheral nerves and the central nervous system. The neuropathic manifestations are *always* associated with an elevation in PBG. Because all these disorders are called porphyrias, the common and unfortunate mistake made by most clinicians is to order tests for porphyrins when the clinician really wants to know if there is PBG overproduction. It is always best to screen for acute hepatic porphyria *during* the painful attack, since urinary PBG concentration in latent (asymptomatic) porphyria may be below the detection level of a screening test.

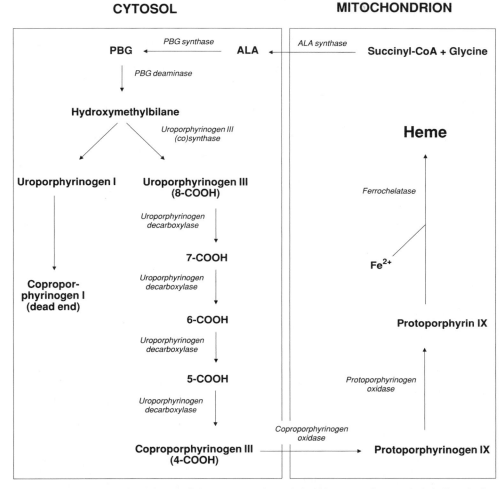

Figure 1. Heme metabolic pathway. Substrates are shown in bold letters and enzymes in italics. In the three acute hepatic porphyrias (AIP, VP, and HCP) there is inappropriate induction of ALA synthase. The enzyme deficiencies for each porphyria are as follows: acute intermittent porphyria (AIP): PBG deaminase; congenital erythropoietic porphyria (CEP): uroporphyrinogen III (co)synthase; porphyria cutanea tarda (PCT): uroporphyrinogen decarboxylase; hereditary coproporphyria (HCP): coproporphyrinogen oxidase; variegate porphyria (VP): protoporphyrinogen oxidase; erythrocytic protoporphyria (EPP): ferrochelatase.

Because ALA has a structure similar to certain neurotransmitters (e.g., γ-aminobutyric acid [GABA]), one theory explaining the acute neurological painful attacks of the acute porphyrias proposes that excess ALA is responsible.[5] In general, conversion of ALA to PBG by the enzyme PBG synthase (ALA dehydratase) is very rapid, so that urinary PBG is higher than ALA in the acute porphyric attack. This is in contradistinction to lead poisoning, hereditary tyrosinemia, and homozygous PBG synthase deficiency in which the enzyme is inhibited (Figure 1) and ALA builds up with no PBG excess. These last three disorders can also present with painful crises, but usually in childhood.

Table 1. LABORATORY FINDINGS FOR THE DIAGNOSIS OF THE MOST FREQUENTLY SEEN PORPHYRIAS

	URINE*				FECES			ERYTHROCYTES	
	ALA	PBG	Uro	Copro	Uro	Copro	Proto	Proto[†]	PBG deaminase
Acute Hepatic Porphyrias									
Acute Intermittent Porphyria									
Manifest	↑↑	↑↑	↑	↑	→↑	→↑	↑	N	Low
Latent	↑	↑	→↑	→↑	N	N	→↑	N	Low
Hereditary Coproporphyria									
Manifest	↑↑	↑↑	↑	↑↑	→↑	↑↑	↑	N	N
Latent	N	N	→↑	↑↑	N	↑	→↑	N	N
Variegate Porphyria									
Manifest	↑↑	↑↑	↑	↑↑	→↑	↑	↑↑	N	N
Latent	N	N	N	↑	N	↑	↑	N	N
Lead Poisoning[‡]	↑↑	→↑	N	→↑	N	→↑	→↑	→↑[‡]	
Porphyria Cutanea Tarda									
Manifest	→↑	N	↑↑	↑	↑	↑	N	N	
Latent	N	N	↑	→↑	↑	→↑	N	N	
Erythrocytic Protoporphyria									
Manifest	N	N	→↑	→↑	N	→↑	↑↑	↑↑	
Latent	N	N	N	N	N	N	↑	↑	

ALA = δ-aminolevulinate; PBG = porphobilinogen; Uro = uroporphyrin; Copro = coproporphyrin; Proto = protoporphyrin. N = normal; →↑ = might be mildly elevated; ↑ = elevated; ↑ ↑ = markedly elevated.

*Urine for ALA should be collected in acid, whereas for PBG and porphyrins in alkali.

†Erythrocyte study to diagnose erythrocytic protoporphyria is the "free erythrocyte protoporphyrin."

‡Although lead poisoning is not a "porphyria," abnormalities in heme precursors are seen, and erythrocytes may contain Zn-protoporphyrin.

ALA production and subsequent heme biosynthesis is tightly regulated by the first and *inducible* enzyme in the heme pathway, ALA synthase. All the acute hepatic porphyrias are characterized by an inappropriate induction of ALA synthase in the liver that then leads to ALA and PBG excess. Therefore, any drug, hormone, or foreign compound that increases the need for hepatic heme (e.g., drugs like phenobarbital, sulfonamides, and phenytoin that induce hepatic cytochromes P-450) can induce ALA synthase and precipitate an attack. For as yet unknown reasons, increasing hepatic glucose tends to blunt ALA synthase activity.

Therefore, a mainstay of management is to avoid fasting and administer glucose (>300 g/d) in the event of an attack. Hormonal changes that occur during menstrual cycles often affect ALA synthase activity such that many women with acute porphyria tend to have premenstrual attacks as in the case presented. Finally, with regard to ALA synthase, it has been shown that administration of heme itself can exert feedback inhibition of ALA synthase induction.[6] Therefore, hematin (heme hydroxide) (an "orphan" drug called Panhematin made by Abbott) and heme arginate (Normosang, made in Finland and not available in the United States) have been used to abort severe attacks of acute porphyria and have been proposed as a way to prevent onset of attacks in selected patients.[7]

Whereas AIP presents only with neurological manifestations, VP and HCP can also have porphyrin overproduction and present with photosensitivity. This is because the enzyme defect in AIP (PBG deaminase) is a defect prior to uroporphyrinogen formation, whereas the enzyme defect in VP (protoporphyrinogen oxidase) can cause accumulation of protoporphyrin and in HCP (coproporphyrinogen oxidase) can cause accumulation of coproporphyrin. VP and HCP, like AIP, are autosomally dominant inherited disorders.

However, the most common porphyria to cause photosensitive skin lesions is porphyria cutanea tarda (PCT) in which there is a defect in decarboxylating 8-COOH uroporphyrinogen and 7-COOH uroporphyrinogen; both accumulate, oxidize to their corresponding porphyrins, and are overexcreted in the urine. Patients with PCT *never* have acute neurological manifestations and often develop photosensitivity because of alcoholism, use of estrogens, or mild iron-overloading of the liver. There are both inherited (familial) forms and sporadic (acquired) forms of PCT.

The photosensitivity of VP, HCP, and PCT leads to blistering skin lesions, ulcerations, marked skin fragility, increased pigmentation, and hypertrichosis in light-exposed areas. This photosensitivity is different from that seen in erythrocytic protoporphyria (EPP), another autosomal-dominant genetic defect, in which red blood cells have markedly elevated free protoporphyrin concentrations due to deficient ferrochelatase activity. EPP patients tend to present in childhood with a burning, stinging sensation during light exposure and with erythema and edema that can lead to scarring and thickening of the dermis. Although EPP patients never have acute neurological attacks, they can develop cholestatic liver failure due to hepatic accumulation of very insoluble protoporphyrin deposits.

Final mention should be made of a very rare and severe porphyria called *congenital erythropoietic porphyria* that is caused by a defect in uroporphyrinogen III (co)synthase. These unfortunate patients produce huge amounts of excess porphyrins in bone marrow and liver that accumulate in all tissues and lead to severe photomutilation. Acute attacks do not occur.

Diagnosis of the Acute Hepatic Porphyrias

When a patient presents with acute, recurrent abdominal pain without clear source, especially accompanied by neurological abnormalities such as mental status changes, seizures, and peripheral neuropathies, the possibility of one of the acute hepatic porphyrias should be entertained and evaluated by qualitatively screening a fresh, random urine specimen of the patient for PBG (not porphyrins). The qualitative screening test for PBG uses *p*-dimethylaminobenzaldehyde (Erhlich's reagent) for both the Hoesch test and the classic Watson-Schwartz test. If the screen is positive, then a quantitative analysis for PBG and porphyrins in a 24-h urine specimen should be undertaken immediately, while the patient is still symptomatic. The urine should be collected in the presence of sodium bicarbonate, kept on ice, and protected from light.

Even if the symptoms have passed or if clinical suspicion for acute porphyria remains high despite a negative *qualitative* PBG test, the *quantitative* urine test may still demonstrate PBG overproduction. A quantitative determination of ALA on another 24-h urine specimen collected with hydrochloric acid, kept cold, and protected from light can further confirm the diagnosis and can rule out disorders in which PBG synthase is inhibited (e.g., occult lead poisoning). However, very often quantitative urine porphyrin studies can cause diagnostic confusion because of minor increases in coproporphyrin and/or uroporphyrin excretion of uncertain clinical significance. The increases are most likely due to hepatic dysfunction causing more of these porphyrins to be excreted by the kidneys into urine rather than by the liver into bile. This confusion has often led to an inappropriate diagnosis of "porphyria."

Once diagnosis of an acute hepatic porphyria is made by quantitative PBG and ALA assays, then an analysis of stool for porphyrins is important in order to distinguish an AIP variant from VP or HCP. A marked increase in stool protoporphyrin indicates VP, whereas an increase in coproporphyrin indicates HCP. With VP and HCP, protective measures against sun exposure may be required. AIP can also be confirmed by determining erythrocyte PBG deaminase (also called uroporphyrinogen-1-synthase) activity. There is considerable variability in values for PBG deaminase activity in normals and AIP patients. However, within a family, those persons having half the activity of the others will usually be shown to carry the defective gene.

When patients present initially with photosensitive skin lesions and skin fragility, urinary qualitative screening or quantitative analysis for porphyrins is appropriate; the tests may then be followed with quantitative stool porphyrin analysis to diagnose PCT, VP, or HCP. Diagnosis of EPP is usually made by analysis of erythrocyte free protoporphyrin.

Management of the Acute Hepatic Porphyrias

There are only a few important principles for managing these patients. First and most important, exacerbating drugs must be avoided.[1] In South Africa, where VP is relatively common, certain barbiturate sedatives have been responsible for many severe and often fatal attacks of acute porphyria. Second, patients must avoid fasting and crash dieting. Third, because infections can precipitate attacks, the patient should be evaluated and infections treated with safe antibiotics such as penicillins, cephalosporins, or tetracyclines. Once into an attack, ingestion or infusion of glucose (>300 g/d) should be instituted. Pain, nausea, anxiety, and tachycardia can be treated with meperidine, acetaminophen, phenothiazines, and propranolol (all "safe" drugs for the porphyric patient). Intravenous hematin therapy is generally reserved for relatively severe or recurrent attacks.

As demonstrated in this case, porphyric women often have menstrually related attacks. There have been reports of some success with luteinizing hormone-releasing hormone (LH-RH) analogues in these women,[8] but generally attacks are mild and can be managed conservatively.

Conclusions. Although the porphyrias have diverse clinical presentations arising from defects in complex biochemical pathways, all clinicians should understand the need to check for excess PBG excretion in cases of acute pain crises and check for porphyrins *only* if there are photosensitive skin lesions present. For the acute pain crises, avoiding drugs that can exacerbate the biochemical defect and administering glucose, appropriate pain and anxiety medications, and possibly hematin are the primary principles of management.

References

1. Bonkovsky, H.L.: Porphyrin and heme metabolism and the porphyrias. *In:* Hepatology, A Textbook of Liver Disease. D. Zakim and T.D. Boyer, Eds. Philadelphia, W.B. Saunders Co., 1990.

2. Bloomer, J.R., and Straka, J.G.: Porphyrin metabolism. *In:* The Liver, Biology and Pathobiology, 2nd ed. I.M. Arias, W.B. Jakoby, H. Popper, et al., Eds. New York, Raven Press, 1988.

3. Kushner, J.P.: Laboratory diagnosis of the porphyrias. N. Engl. J. Med., *324:* 1432-1434, 1991.

4. Elder, G.E., Smith, S.G., and Smyth, S.J.: Laboratory investigation of the porphyrias. Ann. Clin. Biochem., *27:* 395-412, 1990.

5. Bonkovsky, H.L., and Schady, W.: Neurologic manifestations of acute porphyria. Semin. Liver Dis., *2:* 108-124, 1982.

6. Lamon, J.M., Frykholm, B.C., Hess, R.A., and Tschudy, D.P.: Hematin therapy for acute porphyria. Medicine, *58:* 252-269, 1979.

7. Mustajoki, P., Tenhunen, R., Pierach, C., and Volin, L.: Heme in the treatment of porphyrias and hematologic disorders. Semin. Hematol., *26:* 1-9, 1989.

8. Anderson, K.E.: LHRH analogues for hormonal manipulation in acute intermittent porphyria. Semin. Hematol., *26:* 10-15, 1989.

SEVERE EPIGASTRIC PAIN

A. Ralph Henderson, Contributor
Steven I. Shedlofsky, Reviewer

A 43-year-old man presented early one morning with a ten-hour history of acute abdominal pain that followed an all-day alcoholic binge. He had no history of hepatobiliary disease but did admit to many years of alcoholic overindulgence. On admission, the patient was noted to be sitting on the stretcher with his trunk flexed and his knees drawn up, since this posture diminished the intensity of the pain. He described the pain as the worst he had ever experienced, as steady and intensely "boring" in nature, located in the epigastrium and radiating through to his back. He felt nauseated but had not vomited.

Blood pressure was normal, but a rapid pulse was noted. Temperature was 101.3 °F (38.5 °C). The patient was in severe pain, and his pain increased when he was supine. He was not jaundiced. There was tenderness and rigidity in the left upper quadrant. Bowel sounds were absent. X-ray examination showed no air under the diaphragm, and there was no evidence of pleural effusion.

Laboratory results upon admission were reported as follows:

Analyte	Value, conventional units	Reference range, conventional units	Value, SI units	Reference range, SI units
Sodium (S)	136 mmol/L	135-145	Same	
Potassium (S)	3.1 mmol/L	3.5-5.0	Same	
Chloride (S)	107 mmol/L	95-105	Same	
Bicarbonate (S)	22 mmol/L	22-32	Same	
Anion gap (S)	7 mmol/L	8-16	Same	
Creatinine (S)	2.5 mg/dL	0.8-1.6	220 mmol/L	70-140
Urea nitrogen (S)	36 mg/dL	7-18	13 mmol urea /L	3.0-6.5
Glucose (S)	198 mg/dL	61-126	11 mmol/L	3.4-7.0
Calcium (S)	7.5 mg/dL	8.5-10.5	1.88 mmol/L	2.12-2.62
Protein, total (S)	7.3 g/dL	6-8	73 g/L	60-80
Albumin (S)	2.8 g/dL	3.5-4.9	28 g/L	35-49
Urate (S)	3.6 mg/dL	4.5-8.0	210 µmol/L	270-480
Cholesterol (S)	120 mg/dL	154-268	3.10 mmol/L	4.00-6.95
Triglycerides (S)	203 mg/dL	44-320	2.29 mmol/L	0.50-3.61
Bilirubin, total (S)	0.6 mg/dL	0.4-1.3	10 µmol/L	7-22
CK (S)	356 U/L	38-174	5.93 µkat/L	0.63-2.90
CK-MB (S)	2 U/L	0-10	0.03 µkat/L	0.00-0.17
ALT (S)	34 U/L	5-30	0.57 µkat/L	0.08-0.50
AST (S)	32 U/L	10-30	0.53 µkat/L	0.17-0.50
ALP (S)	97 U/L	18-113	1.6 µkat/L	0.3-1.9
Amylase, total (S)	950 U/L	30-220	15.84 µkat/L	0.50-3.67
Amylase, P-type (S)	893 U/L	16-115	14.89 µkat/L	0.27-1.92
% of total	94 %	45-50	0.94	0.45-0.50
Lipase (S)	1800 U/L	30-190	30.01 µkat/L	0.50-3.17
pH (aB)	7.34	7.35-7.45	Same	

Analyte	Value, conventional units	Reference range, conventional units	Value, SI units	Reference range, SI units
pCO_2 (aB)	42 mm Hg	35-45	5.6 kPa	4.7-6.0
pO_2 (aB)	52 mm Hg	75-100	6.9 kPa	10.0-13.3
Hematocrit (B)	49 %	40-54	0.49	0.40-0.54
Leukocyte count (B)	19.2 x 10^3/μL	4.0-10.0	19.2 x 10^9/L	4.0-10.0
Urinalysis (U)	Within normal limits			

The following laboratory results were obtained 12 hours post-admission:

Amylase, total (S)   701 U/L (11.69 μkat/L)
Lipase (S)   976 U/L (16.27 μkat/L)

Amylase returned to normal within three days and lipase within five days after admission.

Differential Diagnosis

The differential diagnosis of the acute abdomen includes a number of diseases.[1] However, there are a few major, and common, diagnoses that must always be considered. These are perforated viscus, acute cholecystitis and biliary colic, acute intestinal obstruction, mesenteric vascular obstruction, renal colic, myocardial infarction, dissecting aortic aneurysm, and diabetic ketoacidosis.[2] The nature and location of this patient's pain suggest an intra-abdominal crisis that is not colicky and thus not indicative of intestinal obstruction, biliary colic, or renal colic; or that does not involve the peritoneum and thus a perforated viscus; or that does not suggest myocardial infarct, since CK-2 (CK-MB) activity is normal relative to time of onset of pain. Mesenteric vascular obstruction and dissecting aortic aneurysm are both unlikely because of a normal hematocrit and absence of signs of shock. Diabetic ketoacidosis is excluded by the normal serum bicarbonate and pCO_2 despite the slightly increased glucose.

Striking features of the laboratory data are marked elevations of serum amylase and lipase. Total amylase activity is more than threefold the upper reference limit. Causes of hyperamylasemia are shown in Table 1. With this level of amylase activity and the very high (94%) proportion of P-type isoamylase, the two most likely diagnoses are a perforated viscus or acute pancreatitis. Absence of air under the diaphragm makes the former unlikely, and elevation of serum lipase activity reinforces the latter diagnosis. The admission diagnosis was recorded as acute pancreatitis and was supported by computed tomographic (CT) scan, which showed an enlarged, edematous pancreas with calcifications.

Discussion

Because of ready availability, serum amylase assay is the most widely used test in the diagnosis of acute pancreatitis.[3] Amylase arises principally from the salivary glands and the pancreas but is also found in a variety of other tissues. Consequently, there are many causes for hyperamylasemia (see Table 1). Serum amylase activity usually rises within 24 hours of the onset of acute pancreatitis and returns to normal within five days, unless complications ensue. Complications are discussed later. Amylase has a molecular weight of about 50,000. It is filtered by the renal glomerular membrane and can be detected in the urine, even after the serum level has returned to normal. Estimates of diagnostic sensitivity* of amylase assay in acute pancreatitis vary widely, chiefly because the disease has often been defined by the

---

* Diagnostic sensitivity, or just sensitivity, is the proportion of those subjects who are positive by the target test (in this case, amylase assay) relative to the number of subjects who actually have the disorder.

elevation of amylase itself. Only recently have studies been performed in which the diagnosis of acute pancreatitis was established by systematic early CT scan, independent of the amylase activity. These studies show that up to 20% of all proven cases of acute pancreatitis have normal serum amylase levels, thus indicating a diagnostic sensitivity of only 80%.[4] Normoamylasemia in the face of pancreatitis may result from hyperlipidemia. Lipemia commonly occurs in acute pancreatitis associated with alcohol abuse, but the cause is uncertain. There is also an association between Type I and Type V hyperlipidemia and nonalcoholic pancreatitis (see *Causes of Pancreatitis*).

Table 1. CAUSES OF HYPERAMYLASEMIA[5]

Pancreatic disease (P-type ↑)*
    Pancreatitis
        Acute
        Chronic
        Complications
            Pseudocyst; ascites and pleural effusion; abscess
        Pancreatic trauma, including investigative maneuvers
        Pancreatic carcinoma

Disorders of nonpancreatic origin (mechanism unknown)
        Renal insufficiency (mixed ↑)
        Neoplastic hyperamylasemia - usually bronchogenic or ovarian (S-type ↑)
        Salivary gland lesions, e.g., mumps, calculus disease (S-type ↑)
        Macroamylasemia (predominantly S-type)

Disorders of complex origin (mechanism unknown or uncertain)
        Biliary tract disease
        Intra-abdominal disease (other than pancreatic diseases; see above)
            Perforated peptic ulcer (P-type ↑)
            Intestinal obstruction (P-type ↑)
            Mesenteric infarction (P-type ↑)
            Peritonitis (mixed ↑ ; depends on cause)
            Acute appendicitis
            Ruptured ectopic pregnancy (S-type ↑)
            Aortic aneurysm with dissection
        Cerebral trauma (type depends on other organ damage)
        Burns and traumatic shock
        Postoperative hyperamylasemia (usually S-type ↑)
        Diabetic ketoacidosis (mixed ↑)
        Renal transplantation (S-type ↑)
        Acute alcoholism (mixed ↑)
        Drugs
            Medicinal opiates (P-type ↑)
            Heroin addiction → ? heroin lung (S-type ↑)

---

*Predominant isoenzyme type is shown in parentheses: P-type (pancreatic); S-type (salivary); mixed (either or both isoenzymes may be present).

After Salt and Schenker's classification (Salt, W.B., and Schenker, S.: Amylase — its clinical significance: A review of the literature. Medicine, *55:* 269-289, 1976).

Assays to differentiate the isoamylase arising from the pancreas (P-type) and from the salivary glands (S-type) are now available. Although distinction of P- and S-types does not appear to improve diagnostic sensitivity of the amylase assay in acute pancreatitis, it does increase specificity when it excludes S-type isoenzyme as the cause of hyperamylasemia.

Assay of serum lipase activity is now more reliable because of recent improvements in formulation of assay reagents. Lipase originates principally from the pancreas but also, to a lesser extent, from the stomach, tongue, and some other tissues. Probably because of its limited origin, its assay appears to have a diagnostic sensitivity superior to serum amylase assay in acute pancreatitis. In addition, the lipase level has other features that enhance its diagnostic value: it rises more than serum amylase in alcoholic pancreatitis; it may remain elevated for a longer period; and it is often increased in the presence of normoamylasemia. Indeed, a recent study has shown that both assays used together increase the diagnostic sensitivity for acute pancreatitis from about 80% for amylase alone to more than 94%.[4]

Pancreatitis may develop multisystem complications, and some of these are illustrated in the present case. The slight metabolic acidosis (serum bicarbonate of 22 mmol/L) probably results from both a lactic acidosis, a consequence of overindulgence in alcohol, and a mild ketoacidosis of starvation. If the patient had been in diabetic ketoacidosis, the bicarbonate would have been <15 mmol/L, and his pCO_2 would have been very low because of respiratory compensation of his metabolic acidosis. The pO_2 may be low because of an impending adult respiratory distress syndrome. The serum glucose is elevated for many reasons, including a reduced insulin output from an inflamed pancreas and increased catecholamines and glucocorticoid levels.

Decreased serum calcium is characteristic, but the cause is unknown. Postulated mechanisms are damage to the cell membrane from the increased concentration of free fatty acids and enhanced influx of calcium into cells; end-organ unresponsiveness to parathyroid hormone; or sequestration of calcium in the retroperitoneal tissue by saponification of tissue lipids. However, recent experimental work[6] suggests that hypocalcemia is a specific consequence of active pancreatic inflammation and is unrelated to an increase in serum concentration of free fatty acids. An important index of disease severity is the hematocrit as an indicator of hemorrhage; in the present case, the hematocrit was normal. The patient's mild fever was compatible with inflammation, which is supported by an elevated leukocyte count.

In this case, histological changes in the pancreas would be expected to include an inflammatory reaction and destruction of the pancreatic substance and fat tissue, as a result of proteolytic or lipolytic action, as well as necrosis of blood vessels in some cases with hemorrhage.[7] However, in a clinical setting, pancreatic tissue is never biopsied because of the danger of provoking more severe pancreatitis and hemorrhage.

Causes of Pancreatitis

In the United States, the annual incidence of acute pancreatitis is about 30 per 100,000, with a mortality rate of about 10%. Incidence is directly related to the extent of alcohol consumption and is approximately equal for males and females.

The mechanisms that precipitate pancreatic inflammation are uncertain. Several have been proposed: acinar cell injury, pancreatic duct obstruction, or deranged intracellular transport of pancreatic enzymes.[7] Cell injury could be initiated by alcohol, bile acids, viral infection, drugs, ischemia, or traumatic injury. Duodenal reflux could allow intraductal phospholipase to generate lysolecithin, which may cause acinar cell necrosis. Pancreatic duct obstruction could occur from stone or obstructive lesions that raise the intraductal pressure and cause intracellular leakage of activated proteolytic and lipolytic enzymes. Deranged intracellular transport of pancreatic enzymes may allow their intracellular activation by lysosomal hydrolases; this mechanism has been demonstrated only in experimental animals.

Although the mechanisms causing acute pancreatitis remain uncertain, several causative factors are well recognized (Table 2). Most cases, about 80%, occur in cases of alcoholic overindulgence or cholelithiasis.

Table 2. POSSIBLE CAUSES OF ACUTE PANCREATITIS

Alcohol and gallstones (about 80% of all cases)
Trauma, post-surgical, and following ductal manipulation
Infection
Drugs
Penetrating duodenal ulcer
After renal transplantation
Metabolic (hypertriglyceridemia or hypercalcemia)
Congenital

Patients with hypertriglyceridemia are at increased risk for acute pancreatitis, although the mechanism for this is uncertain. Hydrolysis of triglycerides by pancreatic lipase in the pancreatic microcirculation may damage small vessels and produce ischemic injury. Hypertriglyceridemia is often associated with alcoholism, may persist even after abstention from alcohol, and may play a causal role in the pancreatitis or may be caused by the pancreatitis. Hypertriglyceridemia also occurs in familial hyperlipoproteinemia Type I (hyperchylomicronemia due to deficiency of either lipoprotein lipase or apolipoprotein CII) and Type V (increased very low density lipoproteins), both of which disorders are associated with pancreatitis.

In the case of hypercalcemia, the mechanism by which pancreatitis might occur was originally thought to be formation of multiple microcalculi and obstruction of the smaller pancreatic ducts. However, because the hypercalcemia of hyperparathyroidism is not a major risk factor for acute pancreatitis, this hypothesis is not currently favored.

Clinical Manifestations

Abdominal pain is the most common symptom; it is usually epigastric and continuous in nature. About a third of all patients describe the pain as radiating to the back. It may be so severe that the patient adopts the posture described in this case history. Half of all patients vomit following the attack; 25% display mental confusion. The patient is often distressed and anxious. Clinical signs include fever, abdominal distention, and hypotension. Shock may be present. Pleural effusion, if present, is usually left-sided.

Complications of Pancreatitis

Acute pancreatitis may range from the mild, self-limiting pathological process of edematous pancreatitis to the much more severe, often fatal, necrotizing pancreatitis. Certain clinical features, such as Ranson's criteria[8] (Table 3) or others, are recognized as predictors of less than favorable outcome, especially when three or more of them occur together. Additional factors have been identified by other authors. These include age over 55 years; findings upon admission of hypotension, abnormal pulmonary function, presence of an abdominal mass, hypocalcemia, hyperglycemia, or hypoxemia; findings during the first 48 hours of hospitalization of hypoalbuminemia, azotemia, encephalopathy, or coma; and need for massive replacement of fluid and colloids. In the present case, a number of risk factors were present: decreased serum albumin and calcium, low pO_2, and elevated creatinine and urea nitrogen. Fortunately, the outcome for this patient was complete recovery.

Table 3. UNFAVORABLE PROGNOSTIC INDICES IN PANCREATITIS

(Three or more positive factors indicate severe disease.)

On admission:	Age	>55 y
	Leukocyte count (B)	>16 x 10^3/μL (>16 x 10^9/L)
	Glucose (S)	>180 mg/dL (>10 mmol/L)
	LDH (S)	>600 U/L (>10 μkat/L)
	AST (S)	>120 U/L (>2 μkat/L)
During first 48 h:	Hematocrit (B)	decrease of >10% (>0.10)
	Calcium (S)	<8 mg/dL (<2 mmol/L)
	Urea nitrogen (S)	rise of >2.5 mg/dL (>0.9 mmol urea/L)
	pO_2 (aB)	<60 mm Hg (<7.98 kPa)
	Base deficit (B)	>4 mmol/L
	Fluid sequestration	>6000 mL

Modified from Ranson.[8]

Within a week or more following the attack, other serious complications may develop: pancreatic phlegmon, abscess, or pseudocyst. A *phlegmon* is a mass of swollen, inflamed pancreatic tissue that can become necrotic or infected and form an abscess. *Abscess* formation should be suspected when fever, leukocytosis, and signs of toxicity persist. A *pseudocyst*, so called because unlike a true cyst it has no epithelial lining, is a fluid collection of tissue, liquefied pancreatic enzymes, and blood within the substance of the pancreas; its walls consist of granulation and fibrous tissue. Pseudocyst formation should be suspected when there is a palpable abdominal mass or when clinical signs of pancreatitis or the hyperamylasemia does not subside within a week. If the pseudocyst does not resolve spontaneously, it may require surgical drainage. Amylase and lipase activity may remain increased for prolonged periods of time.

Treatment

The majority of patients respond to conservative medical treatment consisting of alleviation of pain, maintenance of normal intravascular volume by intravenous infusions, nasogastric suction, and withholding of oral alimentation to reduce physiological pancreatic activity. Antibiotic therapy is required for complications such as secondary infection of necrotic pancreatic tissue or of an obstructed biliary tract. Surgical debridement of necrotic pancreatic tissue in the post-acute phase may be necessary.

References

1. Silen, W.: Cope's Early Diagnosis of the Acute Abdomen, 15th ed. New York, Oxford University Press, 1979.

2. Greenberger, N.J., Toskes, P.P., and Isselbacher, K.J.: Diseases of the pancreas. *In:* Harrison's Principles of Internal Medicine, 11th ed.   E. Braunwald, K.J. Isselbacher, R.G. Petersdorf, et al., Eds. New York, McGraw-Hill, Inc., 1987.

3. Clavian, P.-A., Robert, J., Meyer, P., et al.: Acute pancreatitis and normoamylasemia, not an uncommon combination. Ann. Surg., *210:* 614-620, 1989.

4. Clavian, P.-A., Burgan, S., and Moosa, A.R.: Serum enzymes and other laboratory tests in acute pancreatitis. Br. J. Surg., *76:* 1234-1243, 1989.

5. Moss, D.W., Henderson, A.R., and Kachmar, J.F.: Enzymes. *In:* Textbook of Clinical Chemistry. N.W. Tietz, Ed. Philadelphia, W.B. Saunders Co., 1986.

6. Rattner, D.W., Napolitano, L.M., Corsetti, J., et al.: Hypocalcemia in experimental pancreatitis occurs independently of changes in serum nonesterified fatty acid levels. Int. J. Pancreatol., *6:* 249-262, 1990.

7. Cotran, R.S., Kumar, V., and Robbins, S.L.: Robbins Pathologic Basis of Disease, 4th ed. Philadelphia, W.B. Saunders Co., 1989.

8. Ranson, J.H.C.: Etiological and prognostic factors in human acute pancreatitis: A review. Am. J. Gastroenterol., *77:* 633-638, 1982.

WOMAN WITH JAUNDICE

Paul A. Luce, Contributor
George F. Gray, Jr., Contributor
Fred Gorstein, Reviewer

The patient was a 49-year-old obese white woman with a four-week history of nonbilious emesis, fever, and chills. She attributed her symptoms to the flu and sought no medical attention. However, her nausea and vomiting persisted, and she visited her local physician two weeks prior to admission complaining of jaundice, crampy mid-abdominal pain, "cola-colored" urine, and clay-colored stools. At the time of admission, the patient was in no acute distress. Scleral icterus was present. Physical examination revealed a soft, nontender abdomen without hepatosplenomegaly or masses. Well-healed surgical scars were present from umbilicus to pubic symphysis and at McBurney's point. No lymphadenopathy was evident. She specifically denied any history of hepatitis, transfusions, gallstones, alcohol abuse, or drug abuse. She took no medications and had no allergies. Her past medical history was significant for bilateral salpingo-oophorectomy five years before with subsequent radiation and chemotherapy for a tumor involving both ovaries and the peritoneum. Exploratory laparotomy two years ago demonstrated no gross evidence of recurrent tumor. The clinical picture of "cola-colored" urine, light brown stools, and jaundice were clear signs of intrahepatic or extrahepatic biliary obstruction.

The laboratory values on admission were as follows:

Analyte	Value, conventional units	Reference range, conventional units	Value, SI units	Reference range, SI units
Electrolytes (S)	Within normal limits			
Glucose (S)	141 mg/dL	60-100	7.8 mmol/L	3.3-5.6
Urea nitrogen (S)	5 mg/dL	5-18	1.8 mmol urea/L	1.8-6.4
Creatinine (S)	0.9 mg/dL	0.2-1.4	80 µmol/L	18-124
Bilirubin, total (S)	3.9 mg/dL	0.2-1.2	67 µmol/L	3-21
Bilirubin, conjugated (S)	3.2 mg/dL	0-0.3	55 µmol/L	0-5
Bilirubin, unconjugated (S)	0.7 mg/dL	0-0.9	12 µmol/L	0-15
Protein, total (S)	7.0 g/dL	6-8	70 g/L	60-80
Albumin (S)	3.9 g/dL	3.5-5	39 g/L	35-50
AST (S)	120 U/L	4-40	2.0 µkat/L	0.07-0.67
ALT (S)	130 U/L	4-40	2.2 µkat/L	4-40
ALP (S)	712 U/L	35-120	11.9 µkat/L	0.6-2.0
Amylase (S)	107 U/L	30-90	1.78 µkat/L	0.50-1.50
Carcinoembryonic antigen (CEA) (S)	<3.0 ng/mL	0-3	<3.0 µg/L	0-3
Prothrombin time (P)	16 s	12-15	Same	
Differential count (B)				
Neutrophils	80 %	42-77	0.80	0.42-0.77
Lymphocytes	12 %	25-40	0.12	0.25-0.40
Monocytes	6 %	2-10	0.06	0.02-0.10
Eosinophils	1 %	0-5	0.01	0.00-0.05
Basophils	1 %	0.0-1.2	0.01	0.00-0.012

Analyte	Value, conventional units	Reference range, conventional units	Value, SI units	Reference range, SI units
Hematocrit (B)	34 %	37-44	0.34	0.37-0.44
Hemoglobin (B)	11 g/dL	12-16	6.8 mmol/L	7.45-9.93
Leukocyte count (B)	$5.4 \times 10^3/\mu L$	4-11	$5.4 \times 10^9/L$	4-11
Urinalysis (U)	Bilirubin 4 +			

Serum and urine bilirubin levels confirmed conjugated hyperbilirubinemia, thus eliminating a hemolytic basis for jaundice from the differential diagnosis. Elevation of ALP to greater than fivefold normal (712 U/L) was highly suggestive of extrahepatic biliary obstruction. Furthermore, the serum AST was too low to suggest intrahepatic cholestasis due to hepatocellular disease, i.e., viral or toxic hepatitis was unlikely. The elevation of AST and ALP as well as presence of fever and chills was suggestive of cholangitis. Although CEA was not elevated, a primary liver cancer or recurrent ovarian cancer could not be excluded by this test.

In an effort to locate the level of the obstruction within the biliary tree, abdominal ultrasonography was performed. The intrahepatic and extrahepatic biliary systems were dilated, with the common bile duct measuring 13 cm in diameter. The duct of Wirsung was also dilated. The gallbladder showed a small collection of sludge, 7 mm in diameter, on its wall; however, no stones were visualized. There was no evidence of a mass in the head of the pancreas.

Since the nature of the obstruction remained unknown, endoscopic retrograde cholangiopancreatography (ERCP) was carried out to visualize the papilla. The intramural portion of the common bile duct was found to be dilated. Biopsy of the orifice demonstrated carcinoma of the ampulla of Vater.

A radical pancreatoduodenectomy, or Whipple's resection, was performed on this patient following endoscopic biopsy. Gross examination of the sectioned specimen revealed a firm, pale mass approximately 1 cm in diameter. Histological examination demonstrated a well-differentiated adenocarcinoma with invasion of the submucosa. Regional and vena caval lymph nodes were negative for tumor. There was no similarity to the poorly differentiated carcinoma of the ovary removed five years previously.

Jaundice

Jaundice, a yellow color of the skin, mucous membranes, and sclera, is a manifestation of hyperbilirubinemia that becomes clinically evident at serum bilirubin levels of ≥ 2.0-2.5 mg/dL (≥ 34-43 µmol/L). The primary source of bilirubin is from the metabolism of hemoglobin. The destruction of erythrocytes by reticuloendothelial cells yields iron, heme, and globin protein. The iron and globin are salvaged; however, the heme moiety is converted to water-insoluble bilirubin. The bilirubin is transported to the liver bound to albumin, taken up, and conjugated to form mainly water-soluble diglucuronides before excretion into the bile. Bilirubin diglu-curonide and the metabolite urobilinogen are eliminated in the stool and further converted to urobilin, which imparts the dark brown color to feces.

Hyperbilirubinemia may be classified as either conjugated or unconjugated, based on the type of bilirubin found by laboratory investigations. Hemolytic anemia and neonatal jaundice are common examples in which the conjugation system is unable to keep pace with bilirubin formation and thus cause unconjugated hyperbilirubinemia.

Conjugated hyperbilirubinemias result from interference with the excretion of conjugated bilirubin into the bile ducts and are the major causes of jaundice. Cholestasis can occur at any level of the biliary system and is further subdivided into intrahepatic (hepatocellular or "medical") jaundice or extrahepatic (obstructive or "surgical") jaundice. Either type can take an acute or chronic form. Hepatocellular cholestasis may occur in viral hepatitis and drug-induced hepatitis, whereas obstructive jaundice most often results from mechanical obstruction of the biliary tree by a calculus or tumor. Many mechanisms have been proposed for the re-entry of unconjugated bilirubin into the systemic circulation; however, it is probably due to the combination of back diffusion of bile with canalicular compression, canalicular rupture, and impaired excretion.

Differential Diagnosis

Bilirubin, alkaline phosphatase, aminotransferases, and prothrombin time provide the foundation for the laboratory assessment of liver function. Unconjugated hyperbilirubinemia indicates a possible hemolytic process. Conjugated hyperbilirubinemia occurs in both intrahepatic and extrahepatic cholestasis and is of limited diagnostic importance in separating mechanical duct obstruction from hepatocellular cholestasis. Demonstration of bilirubin in the urine is clinically important and is present only with conjugated bilirubinemia. However, serum conjugated and unconjugated bilirubin levels should be measured to determine if a mixed hyperbilirubinemia is present.

Alkaline phosphatase (ALP) and aminotransferases (AST and ALT) are used to distinguish obstructive cholestasis from hepatocellular cholestasis. ALP is markedly elevated with obstructive jaundice, and its elevation is out of proportion to the elevation of AST or ALT values. Increase in ALP activity is frequently more than sixfold in the presence of gallstones but may increase 10-fold with carcinoma of the head of the pancreas and 30-fold in primary biliary cirrhosis. Incomplete obstruction may occur with choledocholithiasis, and ALP activity may be more characteristic of hepatocellular cholestasis. Marked increases in AST and ALT activity occur with hepatocellular cholestasis, including viral and toxic hepatitis. It is not uncommon for these enzymes to reach activities 20- to 50-fold normal in the early stages of the disease. These intracellular enzymes reflect hepatocellular necrosis and may rise with obstructive cholestasis due to ascending cholangitis. ALP levels remain only slightly elevated (<3 times the upper reference limit).

It is important to remember that overlap in enzyme levels is common in both obstructive and hepatocellular cholestasis. Therefore, interpretation of liver function tests must be done in the context of careful history and physical examination. Furthermore, ALP, AST, and ALT are nonspecific markers of liver disease and may be elevated in other disease processes. For example, ALP is commonly elevated in bone disease, whereas AST values rise in myocardial or pulmonary infarction. Although not performed in this patient, determination of γ-glutamyltransferase (GGT) may be useful in some circumstances; it parallels ALP in liver disease and intra- or extrahepatic obstruction but not in bone disease, in which it is normal.

Finally, prothrombin time may be a useful test in evaluating a patient with cholestasis. Inability to secrete bile acids for two weeks or more due to cholestasis results in depletion of vitamin K stores, since the lipid-soluble vitamin is not absorbed. Parenteral vitamin K will not correct prolonged prothrombin times associated with hepatocellular cholestasis if liver function is severely impaired. In obstructive jaundice, prolonged prothrombin times can be corrected with parenteral vitamin K, since synthetic function of clotting factors is not impaired.

Although these liver function tests are important, other studies are required to make a firm diagnosis. If obstructive jaundice is suspected, imaging procedures are performed to visualize the biliary tree. Noninvasive techniques such as ultrasonography and abdominal CT detect dilation of the biliary tree in up to 95% of patients with proven obstruction. CT has a great ability to detect mass lesions in the head of the pancreas, but it is more expensive and involves the risk of radiation exposure. If CT and ultrasonographic findings are equivocal, cholangiography may be used to visualize the biliary tree. Percutaneous transhepatic cholangiography (PTC) and ERCP are used when indicated. However, morbidity and mortality associated with these procedures may expose the patient to additional risk of complications. Unfortunately, these procedures are of limited benefit for diagnosing hepatocellular cholestasis. If viral or toxic hepatitis is suspected, antibody titers, viral serology, and drug levels should be assessed.

Carcinoma of the biliary system is uncommon. However, this presentation with jaundice, bilirubinuria, clay-colored stools, elevated ALP, and prolonged prothrombin time that corrects with parenteral vitamin K is classic. These tumors become symptomatic owing to obstruction of the flow of bile, but approximately 75% have metastasized to liver, lungs, and lymph nodes at the time of diagnosis. Prognosis is dismal for all biliary tract carcinomas except those of the ampulla of Vater, which have five-year survival rates of up to 40%.

Additional Reading

LaMont, J.T.: Cholestasis: Medical or surgical. Hosp. Pract., *20:* 82A-82EE, 1985.

Olen, R., Pickleman, J., and Freeark, R.J.: Less is better: The diagnostic workup of the patient with obstructive jaundice. Arch. Surg., *124:* 791-794, 1989.

Scharschmidt, B.F., Goldber, H.I., and Schmid, R.: Approach to the patient with cholestatic jaundice. N. Engl. J. Med., *308:* 1515-1519, 1983.

Zimmerman, H.J., and Deschner, K.W.: Differential diagnosis of jaundice. Hosp. Pract., *22:* 99-122, 1987.

ABDOMINAL PAIN AND POLYURIA

Dennis G. Karounos, Contributor
Susan A. Fuhrman, Reviewer

A 10-year-old Caucasian boy was brought to the Pediatric Clinic by his parents who were alarmed by his complaints of abdominal pain, polyuria (excessive urination), and polydipsia (excessive thirst). He had been in good health, energetic, and active in sports, until eight weeks prior to presentation when he developed fever, cough, and nasal congestion that his family physician attributed to a viral upper respiratory infection (URI). The symptoms of URI had resolved four weeks ago, but the patient then developed polydipsia and polyuria that in the past 24 hours had intensified and were now accompanied by nausea, fatigue, and right lower quadrant abdominal pain.

On physical examination the boy weighed 60 lb (27 kg) and was 56 in (1.42 m) tall. The physician noted a weight loss of 5 lb (2.2 kg) since a previous examination six months ago. His temperature was 100 °F (37.8 °C), pulse 100 BPM, blood pressure (supine) 110/76 mm Hg, blood pressure (upright) 98/70 mm Hg, and respiration 28/min. His skin was thin, dry, and without lesions. Examination of the abdomen revealed decreased bowel sounds and right lower quadrant tenderness. The examination was otherwise entirely normal. He was admitted to the University Hospital for further evaluation and treatment; the preliminary diagnosis was dehydration, with possible acute appendicitis.

Upon admission, laboratory tests were obtained, intravenous fluid (normal saline) was started, and a general surgery consultation was initiated. Laboratory results were as follows:

Analyte	Value, conventional units	Reference range, conventional units	Value, SI units	Reference range, SI units
Sodium (S)	143 mmol/L	136-145	Same	
Potassium (S)	5.0 mmol/L	3.8-5.1	Same	
Chloride (S)	102 mmol/L	98-108	Same	
CO_2, total (S)	14 mmol/L	23-29	Same	
Urea nitrogen (S)	18 mg/dL	7-18	6.4 mmol urea/L	2.5-6.4
Creatinine (S)	0.8 mg/dL	0.3-0.7	71 µmol/L	27-62
Glucose (S)	290 mg/dL	75-105	16.1 mmol/L	4.2-5.8
Leukocyte count (B)	$16 \times 10^3/\mu L$	4.5-11.0	$16 \times 10^9/L$	4.5-11.0
Hemoglobin (B)	14 g/dL	11-16	8.69 mmol/L	6.83-9.93
Urinalysis (U)				
Specific gravity	1.025			
Glucose	3+ reducing substances; positive glucose oxidase test strip			
Ketone bodies	Moderate			
Protein, nitrite, heme	Negative			
Sediments	No abnormal findings			

Differential Diagnosis

This child presented with right lower quadrant abdominal pain as well as symptoms of polyuria and polydipsia several weeks after a febrile illness. Abdominal pain and right lower quadrant tenderness as well as leukocytosis suggested a diagnosis of acute appendicitis. Other causes of acute abdominal pain, such as inflammatory bowel disease, small bowel obstruction, and ureteral obstruction, were considered. Urinary tract infection was excluded by the results of urinalysis, which revealed no leukocytes, bacteria, or nitrite (a chemical indicator of bacterial infection). Appendicitis appeared to be a possible diagnosis, but several important issues needed to be resolved before any surgical intervention. Symptoms of polyuria and polydipsia and significant weight loss, together with laboratory evidence of hyperglycemia, acidosis, glucosuria, and ketonuria, commanded consideration of a diagnosis of diabetes mellitus (criteria are discussed later). Decreased serum total CO_2 and ketonuria indicated a metabolic acidosis, most likely diabetic ketoacidosis (DKA) due to insulin deficiency. Since evaluation of serum glucose levels alone did not adequately indicate the severity of the metabolic derangement (up to 20% of patients with DKA may have serum glucose <300 mg/dL [<16.7 mmol/L]), arterial blood gas and serum ketone determinations were requested.

Analyte	Value, conventional units	Reference range, conventional units	Value, SI units	Reference range, SI units
pH (aB)	7.31	7.35-7.45	Same	
pCO_2 (aB)	32 mm Hg	35-48	4.3 kPa	4.7-6.4
pO_2 (aB)	108 mm Hg	83-108	14.4 kPa	11.1-14.4
Oxygen saturation (aB) (on room air)	98 %	95-98	0.98	0.95-0.98
Ketones (S)	Moderate in diluted plasma (nitroprusside test)		Same	

In DKA, the blood pH can range from 6.8 to 7.3. The findings in this case strongly indicate DKA as a diagnosis. Ketoacidosis results from insulin deficiency and the associated decreased utilization of carbohydrates. Under these conditions, lipids are mobilized and increased amounts of fatty acids are produced. Fatty acids are converted to acetoacetate, which accumulates beyond the capacity of the peripheral tissues to metabolize this compound. Some of the acetoacetate is spontaneously converted to acetone (which can be detected by the odor of some patients with ketonemia), and the greater part is converted to β-hydroxybutyrate. Average proportions of the compounds are β-hydroxybutyrate 78%, acetoacetate 20%, and acetone 2%. Ketonemia causes metabolic acidosis and leads to ketonuria. In DKA, three to five times more β-hydroxybutyrate is produced than is acetoacetate. Consequently, the nitroprusside test (which is sensitive only to acetoacetate) does not reflect the full extent of the ketosis.

The metabolic acidosis seen with DKA is accompanied by an increased anion gap. The anion gap, reflecting the amount of unmeasured anions in the serum, is calculated by the formula: serum $[Na^+] - ([Cl^-] + [CO_2])$, and the normal value is 6-15 mmol/L. In this patient the anion gap is 27 mmol/L and suggests that the patient has a metabolic ketoacidosis. If the anion gap had been elevated but the serum ketones normal, then other causes of acidosis would have been investigated such as uremic acidosis, the presence of exogenous drugs or poisons, or lactic acidosis.

The drain on cations caused by excretion of the keto acids causes depletion of sodium and potassium. A further decrease in these ions may be seen as a result of hyperosmolality, with the associated vascular expansion. Osmotic diuresis may result in loss of body water. Evaluation of electrolyte and acid-base status is therefore essential to acute management. This patient was started on insulin, in addition to intravenous saline, and monitored hourly for four hours for serum glucose, bicarbonate, sodium, potassium, chloride, phosphate, urea nitrogen, and creatinine levels. As his status improved, monitoring was reduced to 2-h and then 4-h intervals. Laboratory results were recorded on a DKA flow sheet so that laboratory indices could be more readily followed and therapy altered accordingly.

Surprisingly, as this patient's metabolic acidosis improved, his abdominal pain resolved. An endocrinology consultation was obtained, and the consultant pointed out that severe abdominal pain as a result of gastric stasis and distention may be a presenting symptom in DKA and that it resolves with treatment of the DKA. The possibility of acute appendicitis was therefore dismissed, and attention was focused on diabetes mellitus (DM).

The patient was started with twice daily subcutaneous injections of intermediate-acting and regular human insulin. Although he and his family were shocked by the diagnosis, they quickly learned the basic survival skills of insulin injection, blood glucose monitoring, and urine ketone measurement. On the fourth hospital day, the boy was discharged with a fasting plasma glucose of 110 mg/dL (6.1 mmol/L).

Clinical Features of Diabetes Mellitus

Diabetes is a prevalent disease. Approximately 11 million people in the United States have diabetes, and the estimated annual incidence in the individuals under 20 years of age is 15 per 100,000.[1]

Type I diabetes mellitus (previously referred to as insulin-dependent diabetes or juvenile diabetes) is characterized by low or undetectable levels of serum insulin, associated with β-cell depletion; the onset is usually prior to age 30. There is no family history of the disease, but there is a relationship between tissue typing (or major histocompatibility) genes and susceptibility to the disease. Exogenous insulin is the primary treatment considered necessary to sustain life and health. Type I disease is caused by autoimmune destruction of the islets of Langerhans, the insulin-producing or β-cells of the pancreas.[2] It is interesting to note that Type I is often associated with other immunologically mediated disorders. Approximately 10% of individuals with diabetes have the Type I disorder; 90% have Type II diabetes. In Type II diabetes (previously called maturity-onset or noninsulin-dependent diabetes) there is a derangement in insulin secretion or decreased response to insulin (insulin resistance), possibly due to decreased or abnormal insulin receptors or a postreceptor defect. Thus, in Type II diabetes, serum insulin levels may be low, normal, or elevated, and these levels have little diagnostic value. The primary treatment for Type II diabetes is diet and exercise.

Complications of Diabetes. Longstanding DM, regardless of type, may lead to cardiovascular disease, renal disease, blindness, and neuropathy. Vascular changes include microangiopathy, accelerated atherosclerosis with resulting myocardial infarction, stroke, gangrene, and hypertension. Retinopathy may lead to blindness. A worrisome acute complication of DKA is the development of cerebral edema, which may lead to cerebral damage or death. Three renal lesions are common in DM, nephrosclerosis, pyelonephritis, and intercapillary glomerulosclerosis (Kimmelstiel-Wilson disease).

Renal complications were unlikely in this patient who had only recently developed diabetes. However, as the duration of disease approaches 10-15 years, the incidence of diabetic nephropathy increases. Some 30-40% of patients with Type I diabetes will develop end-stage renal disease. To monitor for deterioration of renal function, tests for urinary protein are invoked. A positive dipstick reaction should lead to collection and testing of a 24-h urine specimen for protein and creatinine.   Urine protein concentration <15 mg/dL (<0.15 g/L) or excretion <150 mg/d (<0.15 g/d) for adults is normal, as is urine creatinine excretion >600 mg/d (>5.3 mmol/d); values are lower in children. A more sensitive indicator of earlier nephropathy is microalbuminuria,* excretion of such small amounts of albumin that radioimmunoassay or another assay of similar sensitivity must be used to measure it. The specimen is a timed urine (e.g., overnight collection), and the reference range for albumin excretion is <15 µg/min. Because of variations in excretion from day to day, at least three separate urine collections should be made and tested. Without treatment, approximately 80% of patients with microalbuminuria progress to frank proteinuria or to overt diabetic nephropathy. When microalbuminuria is confirmed, efforts are directed toward close control of hypertension (if it exists) and toward tighter control of blood glucose levels. Recent studies, still in progress, suggest that microalbuminuria resolves when these cases are treated with either intensive insulin therapy or with angiotensin-converting enzyme inhibitors.[3]

Diagnostic Criteria for Diabetes Mellitus

The diagnosis of diabetes is based on plasma or serum glucose values obtained under appropriate conditions and on the clinical symptoms at the time of presentation. The diagnosis of diabetes in children should be restricted to *one* of the following criteria as recently summarized by the American Diabetes Association:[1,4]

1.   a random plasma (serum) glucose level ≥200 mg/dL (≥11.1 mmol/L) *plus* the classic symptoms of diabetes mellitus, among them polyuria, polydipsia, and weight loss;

2.   two fasting plasma (serum) glucose values >140 mg/dL (>7.8 mmol/L), obtained on at least two occasions, *and* at least two oral glucose tolerance tests showing sustained elevated plasma glucose, i.e., two values ≥200 mg/dL (≥11.1 mmol/L) between 0 and 2 hours and at 2 hours postchallenge.

An oral glucose tolerance test used for diagnosis should be performed after an overnight fast; the challenge should be oral administration of 1.75 g glucose/kg ideal body weight, up to a total dose of 75 g. If a child's fasting glucose is <140 mg/dL (<7.8 mmol/L) *but* the 2-h glucose is >140 mg/dL (>7.8 mmol/L), the diagnosis is *impaired glucose tolerance*.

The diagnostic criterion for adults is any *one* of the following:

1.   a random plasma (serum) glucose level (≥200 mg/dL (≥11.1 mmol/L) *plus* classic symptoms of diabetes;

2.   fasting plasma glucose ≥140 mg/dL (≥7.8 mmol/L) on at least *two* occasions;

3.   fasting plasma glucose <140 mg/dL (<7.8 mmol/L) *plus* sustained elevated plasma glucose of ≥200 mg/dL (≥11.1 mmol/L) at 2 hours and one additional value ≥200 mg/dL (≥11.1 mmol/L) between 0 and 2 hours after 75 g of glucose taken orally. These findings should be observed during at least two glucose tolerance tests.

In adults the diagnosis of *impaired glucose tolerance* is limited to individuals with fasting plasma glucose <140 mg/dL (<7.8 mmol/L) *and* a 2-h postchallenge glucose value between 140 and 200 mg/dL (7.8-11.1 mmol/L) *and* at least one glucose value >200 mg/dL (>11.1 mmol/L) obtained between 0 and 2 hours postchallenge. Since up to 25% of individuals with impaired glucose tolerance go on to develop

---

* Microalbuminuria indicates the presence of a very low, but normal, amount of albumin; it does not refer to a micromolecular species.   Thus, the term is somewhat of a misnomer.

overt diabetes mellitus, they should be screened with fasting glucose tests every 6 to 12 months or whenever symptoms of hyperglycemia appear.

The diagnostic criteria for gestational diabetes (diabetes during pregnancy) are

fasting glucose ≥105 mg/dL (≥5.8 mmol/ L); *and* a 1-h glucose value, following an oral dose of 100 g glucose, of ≥190 mg/dL (≥10.5 mmol/L).

These criteria are more stringent than those for other types of diabetes since studies have shown that the incidence of neonatal morbidity and mortality is greatly increased by poorly controlled maternal diabetes. Early diagnosis and control of gestational diabetes is therefore essential to minimizing complications in both mother and infant.

The boy presenting in this case history had Type I diabetes meeting the first criterion for diabetes in children: random plasma glucose >200 mg/dL (>11.1 mmol/L) and classic symptoms of diabetes mellitus.

Treatment

This patient presented with a mild metabolic acidosis that resolved rapidly upon treatment with insulin and intravenous fluid. The fact that he was evaluated and treated promptly when symptoms first developed contributed to successful therapy. Since this is a case of Type I (insulin-dependent) diabetes, the patient will always have to be maintained on insulin therapy to avoid hyperglycemia and ketosis. The only exception to this prediction is that some patients, early in the course of Type I diabetes, display a "honeymoon" phase in which their insulin requirements decrease dramatically. The cause of this remission is unknown and the remission is temporary, usually lasting for less than one year.

The patient did exceptionally well on his insulin regimen; dosage was gradually tapered off and then stopped completely. At this time, a serum C-peptide test was requested in order to determine the child's endogenous insulin reserve.[5] C-peptide is the fragment of the proinsulin molecule, which is cleaved off during the insulin biosynthesis. C-peptide and insulin are secreted by the pancreatic β-cells in equimolar amounts. Since C-peptide has a longer serum half-life than does insulin, it is a better measure of β-cell function. In addition, measurement of C-peptide has the advantage that it can be measured directly, whereas a measurement of serum insulin does not distinguish between insulin given exogenously and that produced endogenously. Therefore, C-peptide levels give a better estimate of endogenous insulin reserve.

The patient's fasting value was 0.8 ng/mL (0.26 nmol/L; reference range 0.7-2.8, 0.23-0.92). The patient's parents were advised that a "honeymoon" period had occurred and that it could last six months to a year, during which time blood glucose must be monitored at home. Eventually, the patient will have to go back on insulin.

Screening Tests for Diabetes

Prior to leaving the hospital, the parents expressed concern that their other two children might develop diabetes and they inquired about screening tests for diabetes. Two to five percent of siblings of children with Type I diabetes will develop the disorder. The appropriate screening test is a fasting plasma glucose; a result ≤140 mg/dL (≤7.8 mmol/L) excludes overt disease. Other tests utilized in screening, but still considered research techniques, are determinations of islet-cell or insulin autoantibodies or both and assessment of serum insulin response to intravenously administered glucose.

Monitoring Diabetes Control

Home or self-monitoring of blood glucose has proved invaluable in assessing diabetic control and adjustment of insulin therapy.[6] A variety of instruments are available for testing capillary (fingerstick) blood with reagent-impregnated strips that are inserted into a reading chamber. Proper instruction of the patient as to correct techniques and maintenance of the monitoring equipment is essential for accurate results and success in self-adjustment of regimen. Some instruments automatically record and store quality control data as well as the test result and the date and time it was obtained. Digital readout provides real-time information for the patient.

Self-monitoring and immediate feedback of results relative to dietary or insulin therapy allow the patient to react quickly with intelligent and informed measures to maintain or regain diabetic control.

This patient and his parents were instructed by the diabetes clinic staff in the various aspects of self-monitoring. They were also instructed how to test urine for ketones with appropriate test strips and to do so during any acute illness or whenever the boy's blood glucose was persistently elevated (>250 mg/dL; >13.9 mmol/L). The parents were cautioned that persistent ketonuria is a marker of ketosis and an indicator that an increase in insulin dosage is required to forestall ketoacidosis. The staff stressed specific high-risk situations in which contact with the attending physician was important.

An important tool for assessing **long-term control** of glycemia is the measurement of *glycosylated (glycated) hemoglobin*.[7,8] This test capitalizes on the fact that glucose becomes attached to a number of blood proteins by a nonenzymatic and largely irreversible reaction. The degree to which stable bonding between a protein and glucose occurs is a function of the average concentration of plasma glucose during the life of that protein in the circulation. Glycosylation (glycation) of hemoglobin A (Hb A) to form the subspecies Hb A_1 occurs very slowly during the entire 120-day life span of the erythrocytes, and the number of Hb A molecules affected is proportional to the degree and duration of exposure of the erythrocytes to glucose. Hb A_1 consists of Hb A_{1a}, Hb A_{1b}, and Hb A_{1c}.* The last subspecies makes up about 80% of all Hb A_1.

Determination of concentrations of Hb A_{1c} in the blood of a diabetic can be used to monitor the average level of blood glucose maintained over a preceding period of 6-12 weeks. In some laboratories, the concentration of Hb A_{1c} is reported in terms of percentage of total hemoglobin, and reference ranges related to level of control are as follows:

The reference range for Hb A_{1c} for nondiabetic individuals	<6% of total hemoglobin
Control of blood glucose	
Excellent	4-6%
Good	6-8%
Fair	8-10%
Poor	>10%

* Note: A labile fraction called pre-Hb A_{1c} can form as a result of rapid changes in blood glucose. If this fraction is not removed, Hb A_{1c} values may not accurately reflect longer time-averaged glucose concentrations.

This test is not reliable in every diabetic patient. Persistence of fetal hemoglobin (infants up to 1 year and patients with β-thalassemia) can cause an apparent increase in Hb A_{1c}, suggesting less control than may be true. Increased life span of erythrocytes, as in post-splenectomy or polycythemia, has the same effect. Decreased life span of erythrocytes, as in hemolytic anemia, has the opposite effect. Genetically determined hemoglobin variants have variable effects.

The *fructosamine assay* is another test useful for monitoring glycemic control, but over a shorter period. The test measures total glycosylated serum protein and is technically easier to perform than the test for glycohemoglobin. Since the predominant serum protein is albumin, which has a shorter half-life than hemoglobin, the serum fructosamine level correlates well with mean blood glucose values over the previous 2-3 weeks.[9] The advantage is that the test responds relatively rapidly to changes in therapy. The disadvantage is that change in the serum fructosamine level may reflect change in serum albumin and globulin levels rather than in glucose levels; consequently, the test cannot be used in a variety of concurrent diseases that alter concentrations of serum proteins. The fructosamine assay is not yet widely utilized.

References

1.   Physician's guide to insulin-dependent (Type I) diabetes diagnosis and treatment. American Diabetes Association, Alexandria, VA, 1988.

2.   Cahill, G.F., and McDevitt, H.O.: Insulin-dependent diabetes mellitus: The initial lesion. N. Engl. J. Med., *304:* 1454-1466, 1981.

3.   Bell, D.S.H.: Diabetic nephropathy: Changing concepts of pathogenesis and treatment. Am. J. Med. Sci., *301:* 195-200, 1991.

4.   Singer, D.E., Coley, C.M., Samet, J.H., and Nathan, D.M.: Test of glycemia in diabetes mellitus. Ann. Intern. Med., *110:* 125-137, 1989.

5.   Clarson, C., Daneman, D., Drash, A.L., et al.: Residual beta-cell function in children with IDDM: Reproducibility of testing and factors influencing insulin secretory reserve. Diabetes Care, *10:* 33-38, 1987.

6.   Goldstein, D.E., Hoepen, M.R., Hirsch, I., and Voluck, J.: Glucose monitoring: Home and office. Diagnosis, *7:* 35-46, 1985.

7.   Nathan, D.M., Singer, D.E., Hurxthal, K., and Goodson, J.D.: The clinical information value of the glycosylated hemoglobin assay. N. Engl. J. Med., *310:* 341-346, 1984.

8.   Baynes, J.W., Bunn, H.F., Goldstein, D., et al.: National Diabetes Data Group: Report of expert committee on glycosylated hemoglobin. Diabetes Care, *7:* 602-608, 1984.

9.   Cefalu, W.T., Parker, T.B., and Johnson, C.R.: Validity of serum fructosamine as index of short-term glycemic control in diabetic outpatients. Diabetes Care, *11:* 662-664, 1988.

RECURRENT DIARRHEA

Z. Myron Falchuk, Contributor
David N. Bailey, Reviewer

A 25-year-old woman presented to her doctor with a three-week history of diarrhea, malaise, and a 5-lb (2.3-kg) weight loss. Two weeks prior to the onset of her illness she had been camping in the mountains and had drunk water from the local stream, which appeared "quite clear." She was having six bowel movements per day and was occasionally waking up at night with diarrhea. There was no blood in the stool, but it was foul smelling and had mucus in it. She denied any fever, nausea, or vomiting. There was no history of arthritis, difficulty with vision, or rashes. She had not taken antibiotics in the past three months.

On physical examination she appeared pleasant and in no distress. The skin turgor was normal, the liver and spleen were not enlarged, and there was no ascites or peripheral edema. Heart sounds were normal, and no murmurs were heard.

Laboratory tests included a chemistry profile and complete blood count; all results were within reference limits. Stool specimens were collected for culture of *Salmonella*, *Shigella*, *Campylobacter*, enteropathogenic *Escherichia coli*, and *Yersinia*; the cultures were negative. Stool samples were also submitted to examination for ova, cysts, and parasites. *Giardia lamblia* organisms were found, and the patient was treated with metronidazole. Within seven days all of her symptoms abated, and she regained her sense of well-being as well as her weight.

Four months after this initial episode, the patient returned to her doctor with recurrence of diarrhea. She was having eight to ten bowel movements per day, consisting of liquid, foul-smelling stool. There was neither blood nor mucus in her stool. She denied any travel history since her last camping trip. Her roommates were well and without diarrhea. She denied any rash, joint aches, or fever. However, she had some swelling about her ankles, had been bruising easily, and was having difficulty driving at night. On close questioning, the patient recalled having been told by her mother that she was a "colicky child" who frequently had bouts of diarrhea when growing up.

At the time of the physical examination, the patient was in no distress. Her mucous membranes were dry. Cheilosis was noted; the fundal examination was normal. The chest was clear upon auscultation, and heart sounds were normal with no murmurs. The liver spanned 9 cm on percussion, and the spleen was not palpable. Bowel sounds were active but not high-pitched, and no abdominal masses were palpated. There was trace pedal edema. The stool was also negative for occult blood. Neurological examination was normal. Stool was sent for bacteriological cultures and for examination for ova, cysts, and parasites; all results were negative.

Laboratory data included the following:

Analyte	Value, conventional units	Reference range, conventional units	Value, SI units	Reference range, SI units
Sodium (S)	146 mmol/L	135-148	Same	
Potassium (S)	4.3 mmol/L	3.5-5.0	Same	

Analyte	Value, conventional units	Reference range, conventional units	Value, SI units	Reference range, SI units
Chloride (S)	105 mmol/L	95-107	Same	
CO_2, total (S)	20 mmol/L	21-31	Same	
Urea nitrogen (S)	9 mg/dL	7-18	3.2 mmol urea/L	2.5-6.4
Glucose (S)	104 mg/dL	70-105	5.8 mmol/L	3.9-5.8
Protein, total (S)	5.8 g/dL	6.1-8.0	58 g/L	61-80
Albumin (S)	2.8 g/dL	3.5-5.0	28 g/L	35-50
Cholesterol (S)	115 mg/dL	100-200	2.98 mmol/L	2.59-5.18
AST (S)	25 U/L	10-35	0.42 µkat/L	0.17-0.58
ALP (S)	90 U/L	16-106	1.5 µkat/L	0.3-1.8
Iron (S)	30 µg/dL	40-160	5 µmol/L	7-29
Iron-binding capacity (S)	250 µg/dL	250-440	45 µmol/L	45-79
Vitamin A (S)	20 µg/dL	25-70	0.70 µmol/L	0.87-2.44
IgA (S)	420 mg/dL	40-350	4.20 g/L	0.40-3.50
IgG (S)	1100 mg/dL	500-1500	11.00 g/L	5.00-15.00
IgM (S)	65 mg/dL	40-250	0.65 g/L	0.40-2.50
Hematocrit (B)	39 %	38-44	0.39	0.38-0.44

The presence of severe diarrhea with a foul smell, weight loss, and peripheral edema along with low values for serum cholesterol, albumin, iron, and vitamin A suggested the presence of malabsorption. Stool fat excretion was measured and found to be 21 g/d (reference range, <7 g/d). A gastrointestinal series was performed; it showed a dilated, fluid-filled small bowel consistent with malabsorption. In the absence of small bowel stasis, pancreatic calcification, or other evidence of pancreatic disease, small bowel mucosal abnormality was suspected as the cause for the problem. Serum was sent for measurement of antigliadin antibodies as well as antireticulin and antiendomysial antibodies since these are present in a high proportion of patients with gluten-sensitive enteropathy (GSE).[1,2] All of these antibodies were demonstrated in the patient's serum.

A small bowel biopsy showed diffuse villus flattening with loss of the villus architecture. The crypts were hypertrophied, and the mitotic index in the crypts was increased. The surface epithelial cells were cuboidal and vacuolated, lacking brush borders as well as the basal orientation of the tall columnar epithelial cells of the normal small bowel mucosa. The lamina propria was infiltrated with round cells — plasma cells and lymphocytes.

The patient was placed on a gluten-free diet and promptly felt better as resolution of the diarrhea and associated symptoms occurred. A follow-up biopsy of the small bowel performed three months later was normal.

Definition of the Disease

Gluten-sensitive enteropathy, also known as celiac disease, is a disease of the small intestine in which ingestion of gluten causes a serious injury of the intestinal mucosa and consequent inability to absorb nutrients.[3,4] Gluten is a glycoprotein found in wheat, rye, barley, and oats. The injurious portion of gluten is an alcohol-soluble moiety called gliadin. Patients with this disease may manifest difficulty in infancy soon after weaning and along with introduction of dietary cereals. However, they may also be totally asymptomatic until later in adult life. Although it is unclear why this bimodal peak of age presentation exists, the clinical syndromes of the infant and the adult can be identical.

The predominant manifestation of malabsorption is steatorrhea with diarrhea. Patients may have the entire spectrum of malabsorption symptoms with weight loss, hypoalbuminemia and pedal edema, vitamin A deficiency and night blindness, vitamin D deficiency and osteomalacia or tetany, vitamin K deficiency and bleeding, and iron deficiency with anemia. Otherwise, patients may present with a single element of malabsorption, e.g., iron deficiency anemia. Such patients can be a diagnostic enigma for the physician. On occasion, as with the patient described, the disease seems to be triggered by some gastrointestinal event such as an infection or an operation for ulcers.

Differential Diagnosis

The differential diagnosis of malabsorption includes distinguishing those diseases in which the defect is in the lumen of the small bowel from those in which the defect is in the membrane or epithelium of the small bowel. Pancreatic insufficiency — which may be due to alcoholism, familial pancreatitis, or cystic fibrosis — causes maldigestion and malabsorption. Loss of bile salts as in bacterial overgrowth syndrome or in dysfunction of the terminal ileum (e.g., Crohn's disease) will cause steatorrhea. All of these are disorders in which the defect is in the lumen and results in malabsorption. The other major diseases to consider in differential diagnosis of malabsorption syndrome are primarily disorders of membrane or epithelium; they include gluten-sensitive enteropathy (GSE), tropical sprue, and Whipple's disease.

Certain characteristics of laboratory findings are common to all malabsorption syndromes. Steatorrhea (quantitative increase in fat content of stool) is the hallmark. Specific nutritional deficiencies may be detected: vitamin D deficiency by low serum calcium levels or by osteomalacia confirmed by X-ray evidence; vitamin K deficiency by prolonged prothrombin time; iron deficiency by microcytic anemia. The D-xylose absorption test is useful for screening for membrane defects since it provides normal results in malabsorption due to luminal defects.

It has been known for a long time that antigliadin as well as antiendomysial antibodies occur in patients with GSE, but recent advances in technique have improved the sensitivity and specificity of these tests, so that they can be used as screening tests. However, these antibodies may occur in the absence of GSE. Testing is therefore valuable only for screening and not for diagnosis.

The "gold standard" for diagnosis of GSE remains the small bowel biopsy, which can be easily accomplished with any of the peroral or endoscopic instruments available today. The patient described had the findings typical for the disease. The biopsy is not pathognomonic for the disease, however, since certain other conditions such as tropical sprue, viral gastroenteritis, lactose deficiency, and intestinal lymphoma can have biopsy findings that mimic those of GSE. Thus, follow-up biopsies after institution of a gluten-free diet, and sometimes after an appropriate gluten challenge, are crucial to avoid making an incorrect diagnosis in a specific patient.

The entire small bowel is sensitive to the deleterious effect of gluten, but the distal small bowel is usually histologically normal. As gluten travels down the small intestine, digestion by pancreatic proteases renders it progressively more innocuous.

Gluten-sensitive enteropathy has features of a recessive form of inheritance. Families of index cases should be screened with some of the routine blood tests outlined, e.g., antigliadin antibodies, and if tests are positive, small bowel biopsy should be performed.

Pathogenesis

Gluten-sensitive enteropathy is associated with genetic markers of the major histocompatibility complex (MHC). Up to 90% of patients have HLA-B8 and HLA-DR3, in comparison to an incidence of 30% in the general population.[5,6] In addition, patients with GSE produce antigluten antibodies in the mucosa, the site of the pathological change. Mucosal organ culture studies have shown that lymphokines are produced by intestinal biopsy specimens in vitro in response to gluten addition to the culture medium. Treatment of patients with prednisone, an immune-modulating drug, results in remission of symptoms even while patients continue to ingest gluten.

It thus appears that immunological events are central to the pathogenic events in GSE. Recently the early region Elb protein of adenovirus Ad12, a known human gastroenteritis virus, has been shown to possess homology with certain regions of the gliadin molecule. It is possible that immunological cross-reactivity between this virus and gluten generates, in the appropriately predisposed patient (e.g., one with the MHC-HLA gene), an immunological response that results in the damage seen in GSE. The presence of specific antibodies (antigliadin) and the production of lymphokines in the intestinal mucosa of these patients mean that the mucosa contains the necessary elements of the effector arm of the immune response that could produce immunological damage.

Treatment

Treatment with a gluten-free diet is lifelong. Patients must be apprised of the many ways gluten is used in foods; opportunity for its inadvertent ingestion is great and often results in the patient remaining ill. Intestinal lymphoma is a complicating feature in longstanding, untreated GSE and is a most important reason to emphasize the importance of gluten-free diet to the patient.

References

1. Levenson, D., Austin, R., Dietler, M., et al.: Specificity of antigliadin antibody in celiac disease. Gastroenterology, *89:* 1-5, 1985.

2. Hallstrom, O.: Comparison of IgA-class reticulin and endomysium antibodies in celiac disease and dermatitis herpetiformis. Gut, *30:* 1225-1232, 1989.

3. Falchuk, M.: Gluten-sensitive enteropathy. Clin. Gastroenterol., *12:* 475-494, 1983.

4. Kelly, C., Fegery, C., Gallagher, R., et al.: Diagnosis and treatment of gluten-sensitive enteropathy. Adv. Intern. Med., *35:* 341-364, 1990.

5. Falchuk, M., Rogentine, N., and Strober, W.: Predominence of histocompatibility antigen HLA-8 in patients with gluten-sensitive enteropathy. J. Clin. Invest., *51:* 1602-1605, 1974.

6. Keuning, J., Pena, S., Leeuwen, J., et al.: HLA-DW3 association with celiac disease. Lancet, *1:* 506-508, 1976.

Additional Reading

Trier, J.S.: Celiac sprue. N. Engl. J. Med., *325:* 1709-1719, 1991.

WOMAN WITH CHRONIC DIARRHEA AND WEIGHT LOSS

Donald C. Bondy, Contributor

The patient, a 44-year-old black woman, was admitted to University Hospital with severe diarrhea. Her history was extensive. In 1980 she had weighed 407 lb (185 kg) and was unable to continue working as a registered nurse. In 1981 she had a horizontal banded gastroplasty and, over the following years, lost weight down to 130 lb (59 kg). She returned to work full time in 1983. Early in 1987 she began to gain weight very rapidly, and by August she weighed 293 lb (133 kg). Investigation revealed that the gastric pouch above the staple line was now very large, the staple line itself had disrupted, and the stomach was functioning almost normally without limiting food intake. The patient's psychiatrist believed that she was potentially suicidal should her weight gain continue. Her surgeon agreed to revise the gastroplasty in July 1989. A new staple line was placed across the stomach to fashion a smaller fundal pouch excluding the distal stomach entirely. A gastroenterostomy with a small stoma about 12 mm in diameter was made to drain the stomach.

After a difficult postoperative course, the patient left the hospital in August 1989 weighing 198 lb (90 kg). Her weight loss continued; by August 1990, she weighed 148 lb (67 kg). Three months later, she began to feel weak and fatigued. She increased her dietary intake in an attempt to overcome her weakness. She gained some weight but felt no better. Severe diarrhea developed, with up to 20 bowel movements daily. A considerable amount of gas accompanied the diarrhea, and both stools and flatus were very malodorous. Her inability to control the flatus proved very embarrassing to her when both her family and coworkers complained about the odor. The problem seriously curtailed her social activities. The diarrhea finally became so severe that she was unable to continue working. She developed severe swelling in her legs and feet and could no longer wear her shoes. She became very short of breath on exertion. At this juncture she was admitted to the University Hospital for thorough study.

Upon admission, physical examination revealed marked pallor of conjunctivae and buccal mucosa, multiple abdominal scars, and pitting edema of the legs without evidence of tenderness or heat in the legs. Other than tachycardia, there were no findings to suggest heart disease.

Initial laboratory work provided the results given below. Note that the grouping of tests reflects their relationship to various probable and observed features of the patient's disorder. Because of the gastrojejunostomy with bypass of the duodenum, where iron and folate are best absorbed, those deficiencies were suspected.

Analyte	Value, conventional units	Reference range, conventional units	Value, SI units	Reference range, SI units
Hemoglobin (B)	6.2 g/dL	11.5-16.0	3.85 mmol/L	7.14-9.93
MCV (B)	72 fL	79-97	Same	
MCH (B)	21 pg	27-34	Same	
Iron (S)	11 µg/dL	67-173	2 µmol/L	12-31
TIBC (S)	262 µg/dL	251-408	47 µmol/L	45-73
Transferrin saturation (S)	4 %	20-55	0.04	0.20-0.55
Folate (S)	2.5 ng/mL	2.5-17.0	6 nmol/L	6-39

Analyte	Value, conventional units	Reference range, conventional units	Value, SI units	Reference range, SI units
Vitamin B_{12} (S)	52 pg/mL	149-895	38 pmol/L	110-660
Albumin (S)	2.3 g/dL	2.9-4.8	23 g/L	29-48
Calcium (S)	7.9 mg/dL	8.5-10.5	1.96 mmol/L	2.12-2.62
Phosphorus (S)	1.8 mg/dL	2.5-4.1	0.58 mmol/L	0.81-1.32
Occult blood (F)	Negative	Negative	Same	

A serum ferritin assay was requested to verify the apparent iron deficiency; the result was <5 ng/mL (<5 µg/L; reference range, 15-200). Because of the severe anemia and the shortness of breath, she was transfused with packed red blood cells. Hemoglobin increased to 8.5 g/dL (5.28 mmol/L). Therapy to deal with deficiencies of folate, vitamin B_{12}, and iron was instituted. Impedance plethysmography was performed and was normal in both legs. The chest film and electrocardiogram were within normal limits.

The hypoalbuminemia, the edema, the severe anemia, and the diarrhea suggested maldigestion or malabsorption. Thus, the following additional laboratory tests were performed on feces and urine:

Analyte	Value, conventional units	Reference range, conventional units	Value, SI units	Reference range, SI units
Weight, 48 h (F)	724 g/d	<200	Same	
Fat, 48 h (F)	85.9 g/d	1.7-5.1	302 mmol/d	6-18
Ova and parasites (F)	Negative	Negative	Same	
Culture (F)	Negative for enteric pathogens	Negative	Same	
Leukocytes (U)	10/hpf	0-5	Same	
Erythrocytes (U)	20/hpf	0-3	Same	
Oxalate (U)	53 mg/d	10-40	589 µmol/d	111-444

The pyuria and hematuria raised the question of urinary tract infection and nephrolithiasis. Urine culture and an ultrasonographic examination of the kidneys and ureters were invoked. Culture grew Escherichia coli >1 x 10^5 colony-forming units/L; the organisms were sensitive to ampicillin, with which the infection was then treated. Ordinarily oxalate is bound to calcium in the small intestine, the calcium oxalate passing out in the stool; but in the presence of steatorrhea the calcium binds to the fatty acids to form soaps, leaving the oxalate ion to pass into the colon, where it is absorbed. Once absorbed, oxalate is excreted into the urine, in which it binds to calcium and may precipitate out as a calcium oxalate stone. This is known as enteric hyperoxaluria. Ultrasonography revealed a stone in the left kidney; it was successfully broken up with lithotripsy, and fragments were passed without difficulty. Gross steatorrhea was evident, more than would be expected with a gastrojejunostomy.[1] Additional tests were done to further define the nutritional deficiencies and to determine the cause of the steatorrhea.

Analyte	Value, conventional units	Reference range, conventional units	Value, SI units	Reference range, SI units
Sodium (S)	140 mmol/L	135-145	Same	
Potassium (S)	4.0 mmol/L	3.5-5.0	Same	
Chloride (S)	106 mmol/L	95-102	Same	
Bicarbonate (S)	21 mmol/L	24-32	Same	
Magnesium (S)	1.8 mg/dL	1.7-2.3	0.75 mmol/L	0.70-0.95

Analyte	Value, conventional units	Reference range, conventional units	Value, SI units	Reference range, SI units
Vitamin A (S)	46 µg/dL	34-80	1.61 µmol/L	1.19-2.79
Vitamin E (S)	0.30 mg/dL	0.78-1.25	7 µmol/L	18-29
Prothrombin time (PT) (P)	11 s	9.0-11.5	Same	

Esophagogastrojejunostomy

Jejunal biopsy	Normal
Culture of jejunal aspirate	A mixture of anaerobic organisms <1.0 x 10³ colony-forming units/L (within normal limits)

These results excluded small intestinal disease and bacterial overgrowth. Tests of pancreatic exocrine secretion were considered, but the exclusion of the distal stomach by the band of staples in the upper stomach made it impossible to do either the secretin, Lundh, or PABA tests for pancreatic exocrine insufficiency.[2] A therapeutic trial with pancreatic enzymes added to her diet, followed by repeat fecal fat analysis, was done to assess possible maldigestion due to pancreatic exocrine insufficiency. Testing to evaluate hepatic status was appropriate and was requested. Results were as follows:

Analyte	Value, conventional units	Reference range, conventional units	Value, SI units	Reference range, SI units
Weight, 48 h (F)	610 g/d	<200	Same	
Fat, 48 h (F)	70.6 g/d	1.7-5.1	248 mmol/d	6-18
Glucose, fasting (S)	94 mg/dL	60-110	5.2 mmol/L	3.3-6.1
ALT (S)	13 U/L	5-30	0.22 µkat/L	0.08-0.50
AST (S)	15 U/L	10-30	0.25 µkat/L	0.17-0.50
GGT (S)	10 U/L	0-30	0.17 µkat/L	0.00-0.50
ALP (S)	303 U/L	18-113	5.1 µkat/L	0.3-1.9

Although liver damage was essentially excluded by the results of these tests, the elevation of ALP with a normal GGT indicated that the ALP was likely of skeletal origin.[3] This raised the possibility of osteomalacia occurring as a consequence of impaired absorption of calcium and dietary vitamin D. The low calcium was consistent with the albumin level.[4] Skeletal X-ray studies were requested and showed some osteopenia of the spine but no obvious evidence of osteomalacia.

The failure of pancreatic enzymes to affect the steatorrhea to any great extent left the attending staff perplexed. There was no pancreatic exocrine insufficiency, no malabsorption syndrome, and no bacterial overgrowth to explain the massive steatorrhea.

At this stage of investigation, the operation notes of the surgeon who had performed the revised gastroplasty and gastrojejunostomy became available. To achieve maximal weight loss, the surgeon had placed the distal end of the jejunal loop in the ileum, 100 cm from the cecum, thus reducing the total small intestinal length from gastrojejunostomy to cecum to only 130 cm. The effect was massive loss of the patient's small intestinal absorbing surface; it ensured poor mixing of pancreatic and biliary secretions with her food. As a result of the drastic alteration of anatomy, the patient had both malabsorption and maldigestion. Upon learning of this anatomical situation, attending physicians at the University Hospital recommended that she have the intestinal bypass taken down. The patient, however, refused, stating that she was certain that improving her absorptive capacity would lead to return of her obesity. She preferred the present discomfort to obesity.

On discharge she was given oral calcium preparations to treat hyperoxaluria and prevent hypocalcemia. Water-soluble preparations as oral supplements of fat-soluble vitamins (A, D, and K) were prescribed as prophylaxis against bone and coagulation problems. She was urged to eat frequent small meals of a lower fat content. Her local physician wrote that with the lower fat diet, the problem of odor improved but the diarrhea continued. Her serum iron levels did not improve on oral iron, and she now receives parenteral iron injections. Her anemia is improving. She has not gained weight but has not returned to work.

References

1. Radziuk, J., and Bondy, D.C.: Gastric surgery. *In:* Current Therapy in Nutrition. K.N. Jeejeebhoy, Ed. Philadelphia, B C Decker, Inc., 1988.

2. Tietz, N.W., Rinker, A.D., and Henderson, A.R.: Gastric, pancreatic, and intestinal function. *In:* Textbook of Clinical Chemistry. N.W. Tietz, Ed. Philadelphia, W.B. Saunders Co., 1986.

3. Moss, D.W., Henderson, A.R., and Kachmar, J.F.: Enzymes. *In:* Textbook of Clinical Chemistry. N.W. Tietz, Ed. Philadelphia, W.B. Saunders Co., 1986.

4. Tietz, N.W., Ed.: Clinical Guide to Laboratory Tests. Philadelphia, W.B. Saunders Co., 1990.

PERSISTENT JAUNDICE IN INFANT

Drora Berkowitz, Contributor
William F. Balistreri, Contributor

A six-week-old infant boy was admitted to Children's Hospital Medical Center for evaluation of jaundice. He was born at term, Apgar scores 9/10, birth weight 7 lb 11 oz (3500 g). His mother noticed that he was icteric when he was three weeks old, but her pediatrician had made the diagnosis of "prolonged physiological jaundice due to breast-feeding" and had suggested that breast-feeding be discontinued. Ten days after his last office visit, the serum total bilirubin level had increased from 9.2 mg/dL (157 µmol/L) to 11.6 mg/dL (198 µmol/L). Throughout this time the baby continued to eat and gain; however, during the last few weeks the mother had noticed that the stool had become "lighter" in color.

The parents were young and healthy, and this was their first child. The father had had "bronchitis" as a child, and the mother was anemic during her pregnancy. There was no family history of liver disease.

Physical examination on admission showed a well-nourished, active, icteric baby. No cataracts were evident. The heart and lungs were normal, and the abdomen was not distended. The liver was palpated 2 cm below the right costal margin, the span was 5 cm, and the edge was soft and smooth. The spleen was not enlarged. Neonatal reflexes were normal. On rectal examination, acholic stools, negative for occult blood, were present.

Laboratory results upon admission were as follows:

Analyte	Value, conventional units	Reference range, conventional units	Value, SI units	Reference range, SI units
Hemoglobin (B)	10.2 g/dL	10-15	6.33 mmol/L	6.20-9.31
Leukocyte count (B)	7.6 x 10³/µL	5-19.5	7.6 x 10⁹/L	5-19.5
Platelet count (B)	350 x 10³/µL	135-466	350 x 10⁹/L	135-466
MCV (B)	90 fL	83-97	Same	
MCH (B)	28 pg	27-34	Same	
MCHC (BErcs)	35 g Hb/dL	31.5-34.5	22 mmol Hb/L	19.5-21.4
Prothrombin time (PT) (P)	13.9 s	11-15	Same	
Partial thromboplastin time (PTT) (P)	33.2 s	23.1-33.3	Same	
Bilirubin, total (S)	12.2 mg/dL	<0.2-1.0	209 µmol/L	<3-17
Bilirubin, conjugated (S)	10.1 mg/dL	<0.2	173 µmol/L	<3
AST (S)	90 U/L	9-80	1.50 µkat/L	0.15-1.33
ALT (S)	50 U/L	10-28	0.83 µkat/L	0.17-0.47
ALP (S)	350 U/L	124-255	5.8 µkat/L	2.1-4.3
Ammonia (S)	50 µmol/L	50-80	Same	
Bile acids, total (S)	28 µmol/L	0.1-7.0	Same	
Calcium (S)	9.8 mg/dL	9-11	2.45 mmol/L	2.25-2.75
Phosphorus (S)	4.9 mg/dL	4.5-6.7	1.58 mmol/L	1.45-2.16
α₁-Antitrypsin phenotype (S)	MM			
Reducing substances (U)	Within normal limits			
Chloride (Sw)	Within normal limits			

Analyte	Value, conventional units	Reference range, conventional units	Value, SI units	Reference range, SI units
Blood and urine cultures	Negative			
TORCH battery (includes: *TO*xoplasmosis titers; *R*ubella titers; *C*ytomegalovirus titers; *H*erpes simplex titers)	Negative			

Abdominal ultrasonography was unremarkable (no gallbladder was seen). Hepatobiliary scintigraphy showed no excretion after 24 hours. Percutaneous liver biopsy revealed bile duct proliferation, bile plugs, and portal fibrosis. Laparotomy with intra-operative cholangiography was carried out.

Discussion

Hyperbilirubinemia is a very common problem in neonates. Since conjugated hyperbilirubinemia is always pathological, the initial evaluation should be directed toward determining if any degree of conjugated hyperbilirubinemia is present. Conjugated hyperbilirubinemia is defined as a serum concentration >2 mg/dL (>34 μmol/L) or >20% of total bilirubin. *Unconjugated* hyperbilirubinemia at this age is most often due to benign causes such as physiological jaundice or breast milk jaundice.

Causes of Cholestasis in the Neonate. The list of causes is extensive (Table 1); however, two entities, idiopathic neonatal hepatitis and extrahepatic biliary atresia, account for >75% of all causes of neonatal cholestasis. When cholestatic liver disease (conjugated hyperbilirubinemia) is diagnosed, an effort should be made to first identify the *treatable* causes, since many of them require prompt therapy: (1) urinary tract infection; (2) metabolic disorders such as galactosemia, hypothyroidism, hypopituitarism, or disorders of bile acid metabolism; and (3) extrahepatic biliary atresia.

Table 1. **CLASSIFICATION OF DISORDERS ASSOCIATED WITH NEONATAL CHOLESTASIS**

Cholestasis Associated with Infection
    Bacterial
        Generalized sepsis
        Syphilis
        Toxoplasmosis
        Tuberculosis
        Listeriosis
    Congenital viral infection
        Cytomegalovirus
        Herpes virus
        Coxsackievirus
        ECHO virus
        Hepatitis B virus (? hepatitis C and other non-A, non-B viruses)
        HIV

Metabolic Disorders
    Metabolic disease in which the defect is uncharacterized
        α_1-Antitrypsin deficiency
        Cystic fibrosis
        Familial erythrophagocytic lymphohistiocytosis
        Endocrine disorders
            Idiopathic hypopituitarism
            Hypothyroidism
        Neonatal iron storage disease
        Infantile copper overload
        Multiple acyl-CoA dehydrogenation deficiency (glutaric acid Type II)

Disorders of bile acid metabolism
    Primary enzyme deficiencies
        3β-hydroxysteroiddehydrogenase/isomerase
        Δ4-3-oxosteroid 5β-reductase
    Secondary (peroxisomal disorders)
        Zellweger syndrome (cerebrohepatorenal syndrome)
        Specific peroxisomal enzymopathies
Disorders of carbohydrate metabolism
    Galactosemia
    Fructosemia
    Glycogenosis Type IV
Disorders of amino acid metabolism (tyrosinemia)
Disorders of lipid metabolism
    Wolman's disease
    Cholesteryl ester storage disease (CESD)
    Niemann-Pick disease
    Gaucher's disease

Toxic
    Cholestasis associated with parenteral nutrition
    Sepsis with possible endotoxemia (urinary tract infection, gastroenteritis)
    Drugs

Genetic or Chromosomal

Miscellaneous
    Histiocytosis X
    Shock or hypoperfusion
    Intestinal obstruction
    Polysplenia syndrome
    Neonatal lupus erythematosus
    Congenital hepatic fibrosis or infantile polycystic disease
    Caroli's disease (cystic dilation of intrahepatic ducts)

Extrahepatic (Anatomical) Disorders
    Choledochal cyst
    Spontaneous perforation of bile duct
    Obstruction associated with bile or mucous plug or stone mass neoplasia
    Neonatal sclerosing cholangitis
    Bile duct stenosis
    Anomalous choledochal-pancreatic-ductal junction

Idiopathic Obstructive Cholangiopathies
    Extrahepatic biliary atresia
    Idiopathic neonatal hepatitis
    Intrahepatic cholestasis, persistent
        With intrahepatic bile duct paucity
            Arteriohepatic dysplasia (Alagille syndrome)
            Nonsyndromic paucity
        Progressive familial intrahepatic cholestasis
            Byler disease
            Nielsen's (Greenland)
            Microfilament dysfunction
        Familial benign chronic intrahepatic cholestasis (Eriksson/Larson)
    Intrahepatic cholestasis, recurrent
        Familial benign recurrent cholestasis
        Hereditary cholestasis with lymphedema (Aagenaes)

Modified from: Balistreri, W.F., and Schubert, W.K.: Liver disease in infancy and childhood. *In:* Disease of the Liver, 7th ed. L. Schiff and E.R. Schiff, Eds. Philadelphia, J.B. Lippincott Co., in press.

    History and clinical examination often help to make the diagnosis. Initial history should include a careful family history, seeking previously affected infants and lung disease.

Delineation of the clinical course should determine the time of onset of jaundice, the type of feeding received, growth pattern, and stool color. The physical examination should be directed toward abdominal findings (liver, spleen, ascites) but should also identify other abnormalities that may be associated with specific entities, such as cataracts, retinal changes, wandering nystagmus, heart murmurs, microphallus, and stigmata of chromosomal abnormalities. It is extremely important to examine the stool, since the presence or absence of bile pigment may help in differentiating between intra- and extrahepatic obstruction.

The initial laboratory and radiographical studies (Table 2) should be directed at detection of treatable causes of cholestasis. If no specific cause of cholestasis has been identified, the differential diagnosis focuses on two conditions, extrahepatic biliary atresia and idiopathic neonatal hepatitis.

Table 2. WORKUP FOR NEONATAL CHOLESTASIS

Fractionated serum bilirubin
Stool pigment
Hepatic function (PT, albumin)
Cultures (blood, urine)
Metabolic screen
    Urine reducing substances
    Serum amino acids
Viral serology (TORCH)
α_1-Antitrypsin phenotype
T_4; TSH
Sweat chloride
Abdominal ultrasonography

The modalities to differentiate between these diagnoses include hepatobiliary scintigraphy, liver biopsy, and intubation to obtain duodenal fluid that can be examined for presence of bilirubin and bile acids. It is important to diagnose extrahepatic ductal obstruction as promptly as possible because the prognosis for successful surgery is dependent upon an early age at operation.

In this case, the initial laboratory tests did not identify a specific etiological factor for the cholestasis. Therefore, the focus was on differentiating between extrahepatic biliary atresia and idiopathic neonatal hepatitis. History and physical examination of this infant gave few clues to support the diagnosis of biliary atresia. He was born at term with normal birth weight; in neonatal hepatitis, the infants often are born preterm or small for gestational age (SGA). In biliary atresia, jaundice develops at three to six weeks of age in otherwise well-appearing, thriving infants, and eventually the stools become acholic. Approximately 15-30% of infants with biliary atresia may have associated defects such as polysplenia, cardiovascular anomalies, or malrotation of the bowel. The family history in patients with biliary atresia is negative; there is no documented genetic predisposition and no familial recurrence. Another important clue is the consistent absence of stool pigment. One must examine the center of the stool for pigment since bilirubin is excreted through the intestinal mucosa, and sloughed cells will coat the surface and give it a faint yellow appearance.

For differentiation of biliary atresia from neonatal hepatitis, additional techniques to demonstrate patency of the biliary tract were used. Duodenal fluid was collected and assayed for the presence of bilirubin and bile acids; but both were absent. The hepatobiliary scintigraphy showed uptake of isotope into the liver but no excretion into the intestine. This finding is most consistent with biliary atresia. Conversely, in neonatal hepatitis, uptake is slow but excretion does occur. The abdominal ultrasonogram also supports the diagnosis of biliary atresia, since the gallbladder is often absent. This finding, however, is not pathognomonic of biliary atresia.

Percutaneous hepatic biopsy is of great value in the differentiation of neonatal hepatitis from extrahepatic biliary atresia. Findings that favor the diagnosis of extrahepatic biliary atresia include bile ductal proliferation, bile plugs, and portal and perilobular fibrosis. The biopsy provides the correct diagnosis in 95% of cases, as in this patient. In the 5% in whom the diagnosis is not clear, operative exploration and cholangiography should be performed.

Surgical Treatment of Extrahepatic Biliary Atresia

The obstructed segment may be localized to any portion of the extrahepatic biliary system. In only 15-25% of cases, the obstruction occurs as a discrete distal lesion and thus allows surgical drainage of the patent portion proximal to the atresia, with subsequent cure. In 75-85% of cases, the atretic area extends to above the level of the porta hepatis, making surgical drainage difficult. The surgical approach (hepatoportoenterostomy-Kasai operation) consists of transection of the porta hepatis with positioning of an intestinal loop to drain the bile ducts. The rationale is to drain any small, persisting bile duct remnants. The success of the operation depends on the patient's age and the size of bile ducts found in the porta hepatis. The success rate is 90% under the age of two months, but decreases to less than 20% in patients older than three months. Patients whose ducts exceed 150 μm in diameter are likely to have good postoperative bile flow.

Postoperative bacterial cholangitis may lead to reobstruction of a previously patent conduit of bile and worsen the prognosis. Most medical centers report five-year survival rates of 30-60%, but in a large proportion of the survivors there is evidence of ongoing liver disease. The beneficial effect of the Kasai procedure is often to provide adequate time for growth prior to hepatic transplantation. Biliary atresia without intervention is almost always fatal, with a mean age of death at less than one year.

Additional Reading

Balistreri, W.F.: Neonatal cholestasis — medical progress. J. Pediatr., 106: 171-184, 1985.

Balistreri, W.F.: Neonatal cholestasis: Lessons from the past, issues for the future. In: Seminars in Liver, Vol. 7: Neonatal Cholestasis. W.F. Balistreri, Ed. New York, Thieme Medical Publishers, Inc., 1987.

Ryckman, F.C., and Noseworthy, J.: Neonatal cholestatic conditions requiring surgical reconstruction. In: Seminars in Liver, Vol. 7: Neonatal Cholestasis. W.F. Balistreri, Ed. New York, Thieme Medical Publishers, Inc., 1987.

Sokol, R.J.: Medical management of neonatal cholestasis. In: Pediatric Hepatology. W.F. Balistreri and J.T. Stoker, Eds. New York, Hemisphere Publishing Corp., 1990.

A THREE-WEEK-OLD INFANT WITH VOMITING

Douglas J. Schneider, Contributor
Carol M. Cottrill, Contributor

A three-week-old male infant was brought to the clinic because of vomiting. He had been born at term by an uncomplicated vaginal delivery after a benign prenatal course. His birth weight was 7 lb 4 oz (3.3 kg). He did well until 10 days of age when he began spitting up after his feedings. At his two-week check-up, he weighed 7 lb 8 oz (3.4 kg). An examination was normal, but his diet was changed to a soy-based formula because of his vomiting. Over the next several days emesis progressed to projectile vomiting of nonbilious material after every feeding, but he appeared hungry and continued to eat. He had not had fever, cough, diarrhea, or rash.

Physical examination revealed a weight of 7 lb 6 oz (3.35 kg), a heart rate of 124 BPM, a respiratory rate of 28/min (normal for a three-week-old awake infant would be 40 ± 10), and a temperature of 98.8 °F (37.1 °C). The child was alert, active, and very fussy. His eyes were sunken, and his mucous membranes were dry. Skin turgor was poor. His anterior fontanelle was sunken, the neck supple and without masses, and the chest clear to auscultation. The cardiac examination, when the infant was lying quietly, was unremarkable. An occasional "wave" of movement was noted in the left upper quadrant of the abdomen. When palpating deeply just above the umbilicus, the examining physician noted a small, firm mass. Edema and cyanosis were absent from the child's extremities.

The following laboratory results were reported:

Analyte	Value, conventional units	Reference range, conventional units	Value, SI units	Reference range, SI units
Glucose (S)	95 mg/dL	50-100	5.3 mmol/L	2.8-5.6
Urea nitrogen (S)	24 mg/dL	5-18	8.6 mmol urea/L	1.8-6.4
Creatinine (S)	0.5 mg/dL	0.2-0.4	44 µmol/L	18-35
Sodium (S)	139 mmol/L	139-146	Same	
Potassium (S)	3.1 mmol/L	4.1-5.3	Same	
Chloride (S)	89 mmol/L	98-108	Same	
Bicarbonate (S)	37 mmol/L	20-28	Same	
pH (aB)	7.54	7.35-7.45	Same	
pCO_2 (aB)	46 mm Hg	27-41	6.1 kPa	3.6-5.5
pO_2, room air (aB)	90 mm Hg	83-108	12.0 kPa	11.1-14.4
Oxygen saturation (aB)	97 %	95-98	0.97	0.95-0.98
Leukocyte count (B)	11.3 x 10³/µL	6-17.5	11.3 x 10⁹/L	6-17.5
Differential count (B)				
Neutrophils	70 %	18-54	0.70	0.18-0.54
Bands	4 %	0-5	0.04	0-0.05
Lymphocytes	24 %	28-90	0.24	0.28-0.90
Monocytes	2 %	0-17	0.02	0-0.17
Hematocrit (B)	46 %	30-40	0.46	0.30-0.40
Platelet count (B)	280 x 10³/µL	150-450	280 x 10⁹/L	150-450

X-ray examination was unremarkable except for a large stomach bubble; ultrasonographic examination of the abdomen was normal except for a small mass at the pylorus. Upper gastrointestinal (GI) contrast study disclosed narrowing and elongation of the pylorus with a "string sign" composed of a thin line of contrast medium passing through the hypertrophied pylorus.

Discussion

The spectrum of possibilities for differential diagnosis in an infant with vomiting is quite broad since emesis is a symptom of many diseases, including bowel-obstructing malformations, gastroesophageal reflux, central nervous system abnormalities, and metabolic derangements. In addition, "spitting up" (regurgitation) is commonly seen in normal infants with no demonstrable disease. A careful history, physical examination, and selected initial laboratory tests can often lead to a diagnosis before expensive and invasive tests are performed. The infant in this case had hypertrophic pyloric stenosis, and his presentation demonstrates many of the typical features of this disease.

Pyloric stenosis can be strongly suspected in this infant from the history alone. The quality, timing, and severity of the vomiting are important. Usually the onset of vomiting is between the second and fourth weeks of age, and there is gradual progression from small amounts of regurgitation to forceful projectile vomiting. The infant usually is active and hungry, which helps to differentiate this disorder from neurological or primary metabolic problems, in which the infant would likely be lethargic. A nonbilious (clear, milky, or yellow rather than green) vomitus in this case pointed to obstruction proximal to the entrance of bile into the intestine.

As might be expected, the physical findings depend largely upon the degree and severity of the vomiting. In this infant, the weight loss and signs of dehydration (sunken fontanelle, dry mucous membranes, sunken eyes, poor skin turgor, and tachycardia) indicate significant volume depletion that could occur from many causes of vomiting other than pyloric stenosis. Of interest is his respiratory rate of 28/min, which is low for an awake infant his age, especially a sick one. This relatively low respiratory rate resulted from hypoventilation to compensate for the metabolic alkalosis (discussed later). Other important physical signs are the visible peristaltic wave, which is suggestive of pyloric stenosis but not specific, and the palpable mass of the hypertrophied pylorus, called the "olive." Palpation of the olive is sometimes a difficult task in a fussy, hungry baby but, when possible, confirms the diagnosis of pyloric stenosis.

The initial laboratory evaluation can be quite helpful in making or excluding the diagnosis of pyloric stenosis, especially since many patients do not present with such typical findings as in this case. Laboratory features of pyloric stenosis include evidence of volume depletion, hypochloremia, metabolic alkalosis, and hypokalemia. Loss of gastric juices from vomiting initiates these abnormalities.

Volume depletion was evident on physical examination and was responsible for this patient's elevated urea nitrogen, creatinine, and hematocrit. Not only was the infant unable to ingest and absorb fluids, he was losing water and electrolytes because of the vomiting of gastric secretions. Hypovolemia stimulates the renin-angiotensin system and results in an elevated aldosterone level and renal conservation of sodium and water.

Hypochloremia results from large losses of chloride ion in vomited gastric juices. The chloride concentration in the vomitus is usually 130-160 mmol/L, compared with a sodium concentration of 70-110 mmol/L and a potassium concentration of 7-15 mmol/L. Thus, electrolyte loss in vomited gastric juice is non-isotonic, a situation different from losses occurring because of almost all other types of abdominal surgical conditions.

The excessive loss of chloride and hydrogen ions in the vomitus leads to metabolic alkalosis. Note the bicarbonate level of 37 mmol/L and pH of 7.54. The pCO_2 was slightly elevated as a result of respiratory compensation for the alkalosis. During volume depletion, renal sodium resorption takes precedence over homeostatic correction of alkalosis. Since chloride ion is depleted out of proportion to sodium losses, much of the reabsorbed sodium is paired with bicarbonate rather than chloride; the alkalosis that follows is sustained until sodium chloride is administered to correct the volume depletion and replenish the chloride. Other factors contributing to the metabolic alkalosis are the elevated aldosterone and the potassium depletion, both of which result in increased secretion of hydrogen ions in the distal tubules.

The elevated aldosterone also contributes to the hypokalemia seen in patients with pyloric stenosis. Although some potassium is lost in the vomitus, most is lost through the kidneys. Alkalosis causes a shift of potassium into the cells, and aldosterone, increased because of the hypovolemia, stimulates potassium secretion into the urine; the result is potassium deficiency. Severe hypokalemia occurs only after the intracellular potassium stores are greatly depleted and therefore occurs relatively late in the course of this illness.

In the case described, both an upper GI contrast study and an ultrasonographic examination were performed to confirm the diagnosis, although either study alone would have been adequate to make the diagnosis. In fact, when the olive is palpable, the diagnosis is confirmed, and no further studies are necessary.

Treatment

Management of pyloric stenosis involves surgery to relieve the obstruction. Preoperative care consists mainly of fluid and electrolyte replacements with normal saline and potassium chloride. Restoring volume, chloride, and potassium will allow the kidneys to correct the alkalosis. A nasogastric tube is placed to remove gastric juice and to minimize the risk of aspiration pneumonia. The operation, or pyloromyotomy, involves cutting the hypertrophied pylorus longitudinally down to the mucosa, thereby relieving the obstruction. This procedure has an extremely high success rate and low risk.

The infant in this case had his pyloromyotomy on the day following admission, after his fluid and electrolyte status was stable. On the following day he was allowed to resume feeding, and within 48 hours he was taking his formula vigorously without any difficulty.

Additional Reading

Benson, C.D.: Stomach and duodenum. *In:* Pediatric Surgery, 3rd ed. M.M. Ravitch, K.J. Welch, C.D. Benson, et al., Eds. Chicago, Year Book Medical Publishers, Inc., 1979.

Dudgeon, D.L., Colombani, P.M., and Beaver, B.L.: Disorders of the stomach and duodenum. *In:* Pediatrics, 18th ed. A.M. Rudolph, Ed. Norwalk, Appleton and Lange, 1987.

Raffensperger, J.G.: Pyloric stenosis. *In:* Swenson's Pediatric Surgery, 5th ed. Norwalk, Appleton and Lange, 1990.

Shuman, F.I., Darling, D.B., and Fisher, J.H.: The radiographic diagnosis of congenital hypertrophic pyloric stenosis. J. Pediatr., *71:*70, 1967.

ANTERIOR NECK MASS

Kenneth B. Ain, Contributor
Nelson B. Watts, Reviewer

A 50-year-old writer discovered an enlargement of his left anterior neck while attempting to button his shirt collar. Over the past month he had noticed a significant increase in his appetite without any apparent change in weight. In addition, although he usually used a laxative to stimulate alternate-day bowel movements, his bowel movements had increased to twice daily over the past three weeks without the aid of medication. He felt well otherwise, yet was concerned enough about his neck enlargement to consult his physician.

Physical examination revealed a well-developed man, 68 inches (1.7 m) in height, whose weight was 150 lb (68 kg). The pulse rate was 82 BPM and the blood pressure 110/76 mm Hg. On visual inspection, he appeared to have an ocular stare with a slight lid lag. There was no evidence of proptosis or chemosis, and the extraocular movements were intact and conjugate. The thyroid was asymmetrically enlarged to an estimated 40 g with a prominent, firm nodule (3 by 2.5 cm) in the middle of the left lobe.

The initial clinical impression was that of mild to moderate thyrotoxicosis with a uninodular goiter. Although the lid retraction suggested a state of increased adrenergic responsiveness, there was no evidence at that time of autoimmune ophthalmopathy. The following serum values were reported:

Analyte	Value, conventional units	Reference range, conventional units	Value, SI units	Reference range, SI units
Glucose (S)	122 mg/dL	75-105	6.8 mmol/L	4.2-5.8
Urea nitrogen (S)	7 mg/dL	7-18	2.5 mmol urea/L	2.5-6.4
Creatinine (S)	0.5 mg/dL	0.7-1.3	44 µmol/L	62-115
Potassium (S)	3.5 mmol/L	3.8-5.1	Same	
Calcium, total (S)	10.6 mg/dL	8.4-10.2	2.64 mmol/L	2.10-2.54
Phosphorus (S)	4.8 mg/dL	2.7-4.5	1.55 mmol/L	0.87-1.45
Albumin (S)	3.2 g/dL	3.4-4.7	32 g/L	34-47
Cholesterol (S)	142 mg/dL	140-240	3.67 mmol/L	3.62-6.21
LDH (S)	80 U/L	100-190	1.33 µkat/L	1.67-3.17
CK (S)	35 U/L	55-200	0.58 µkat/L	0.92-3.33
ALP (S)	160 U/L	49-120	2.7 µkat/L	0.8-2.0
T_4, total (S)	12.2 µg/dL	5-11.5	157 nmol/L	64-148
T_3 resin uptake (S)	35 %	25-35	0.35	0.25-0.35
T_3, total (S)	311 ng/dL	100-215	4.8 nmol/L	1.5-3.3
TSH (S)	<0.1 µU/mL	0.7-7.0	<0.1 mU/L	0.7-7.0
T_4-binding ratio*	1.2	0.9-1.1	Same	
Free thyroxine index (FTI) †	14.6	6-11.5	Same	
Antithyroglobulin antibodies	Negative	Negative		
Antimicrosomal antibodies	+ 1:1280	Negative		

* T_4 resin uptake divided by the mean of a reference population.
† The product of the T_4-binding ratio and the total T_4.

The laboratory results for TSH, FTI, and total T_3 confirmed the impression of thyrotoxicosis and suggested the coexistence of autoimmune thyroid disease (thyroid antibodies). The abnormal values in the chemistry panel are the consequence of thyrotoxicosis, as discussed later. However, the cause was still unclear. The differential diagnosis included an autonomously functioning toxic nodule (Plummer's disease), Graves' disease with a thyroid nodule, or exogenous thyrotoxicosis due to overtreatment of a hypothyroid goiter. In each of these conditions, the patient is thyrotoxic with suppressed TSH levels. The discriminating test is a nuclear medicine study of thyroid uptake and imaging. An autonomous toxic nodule concentrates isotope with great avidity while uptake by surrounding thyroid tissue is suppressed. Graves' disease exhibits increased uptake in a generally diffuse and homogeneous pattern. Thyrotoxicosis due to exogenous levothyroxine therapy results in a very low isotope uptake of the thyroid gland. The choice of isotope for this study may be important. ^{99m}Tc-pertechnetate has the advantage of minimizing radiation exposure, but it is trapped without organification, occasionally leading to falsely increased uptake in parts of the thyroid gland. ^{131}I and ^{123}I are more physiological tracers, but ^{123}I is preferred because of significantly lower radiation exposure. A ^{123}I uptake and scan was performed.

The 6-h uptake was 68%, and the 24-h uptake was 54% (5-28%). The scan image revealed an area in the middle of the left lobe that had decreased functional uptake of ^{123}I corresponding to the palpable nodule. The remainder of the gland demonstrated homogeneous distribution of ^{123}I.

The results of this study excluded both Plummer's disease and exogenous thyrotoxicosis as diagnostic possibilities. These results were most consistent with a diagnosis of Graves' disease with a hypofunctioning nodule. Although the cause of the hyperthyroidism had become clear, it was important to evaluate the thyroid nodule in order to determine whether it was malignant. This would determine the mode of therapy to be implemented.

Fine-needle aspiration biopsy of the left thyroid nodule revealed the features of papillary thyroid carcinoma. This prompted the selection of surgical thyroidectomy as a therapy for both the carcinoma and Graves' disease. Had the nodule been benign, ^{131}I therapy or antithyroid medication would have been considered as therapeutic options. Near-total thyroidectomy was performed with preservation of the parathyroid glands and the recurrent laryngeal nerves. Intraoperative frozen section analysis of the resected nodule showed papillary thyroid carcinoma, and examination of the permanent sections revealed the tumor of 2.1 by 3.4 cm to be intrathyroidal. Two out of four ipsilateral cervical nodes were positive for metastatic papillary thyroid carcinoma.

The patient was placed on liothyronine sodium (Cytomel) therapy for four weeks in preparation for ^{131}I whole-body scanning to evaluate the presence and extent of thyroid cancer. The scan was performed six weeks after the surgery to provide time for clearance of endogenous thyroid hormones and maximal stimulation of TSH. At that time, his laboratory studies revealed total T_4, 1.3 µg/dL (17 nmol/L); FTI, 1.6; TSH, 65.2 µU/mL (65.2 mU/L); and thyroglobulin, 10 ng/mL (10 µg/L). Whole-body scanning revealed ^{131}I uptake in the thyroid bed, consistent with remnant thyroid tissue. One hundred millicuries ^{131}I was administered to ablate the thyroid remnant, and the patient was placed on 175 µg levothyroxine daily. Two months later the patient felt well, and laboratory studies showed the following:

Analyte	Value, conventional units	Value, SI units
T_4, total (S)	10.2 µg/dL	131 nmol/L
T_4-binding ratio (S)	1.2	Same
FTI (S)	12.2	Same
TSH (S)	<0.1 µU/mL	<0.1 mU/L
Thyroglobulin (S)	<1.0 ng/mL	<1.0 µg/L

These results were interpreted to show adequate suppression of endogenous TSH to reduce stimulation of the carcinoma by this growth factor, with minimal elevation of the free thyroxine index to minimize thyrotoxic symptoms. The thyroglobulin level was consistent with good control of the tumor since, in the absence of normal thyroid tissue, it should be the only source of thyroglobulin.

Follow-up ^{131}I scans and thyroglobulin levels remained negative over the next two years, and the patient had not demonstrated any recurrences of tumor by physical or X-ray examination. The most recent office visit revealed the recent occurrence of tearing and itching of his eyes. On physical examination, the left eye was proptotic at 18 mm and the right eye at 20 mm.

Presentation of Thyrotoxicosis

The presence of thyrotoxicosis should be suspect as a clinical entity before laboratory tests are ordered. Thyroid hormone is necessary for the proper functioning of nearly every organ and acts as an essential cellular regulatory factor by interacting with nuclear DNA via T_3-receptors. Consequently, thyrotoxicosis can produce symptoms relating to nearly every major organ system. Cutaneous alterations include erythema, hyperhidrosis, onycholysis (Plummer's nails), and increased warmth. Pulmonary effects are less obvious and occasionally present as exertional dyspnea. The clinical consequences of thyrotoxicosis on the cardiovascular system are frequently of major significance. These are results of induction of tachyarrhythmia or atrial fibrillation, high-output cardiac failure, or exacerbation of cardiac ischemia. Mineral effects are usually evident as a mild hypercalcemia, hyperphosphatemia, and increased alkaline phosphatase, a reflection of accelerated bone turnover. Gastrointestinal hypermotility in thyrotoxicosis results in increased frequency of stools and occasional steatorrhea. Polycythemia may occur as a consequence of increased erythropoietin in response to the hypermetabolic oxygen demands of the thyrotoxic state. Thyrotoxicosis may produce a myopathy that is responsible for weakness and easy fatigability. Thyroid hormone excess enhances β-adrenergic response to endogenous catecholamines, which is responsible for lid lag, lid retraction, tremor, hyperreflexia, and many cardiac symptoms. Behavioral changes include anxiety, emotional lability, and insomnia.

Definition of the Disease

Many of the features described are often found in thyrotoxic Graves' disease, but some additional findings are related to the autoimmune process, which is the primary pathogenetic mechanism. Pretibial myxedema and thyroid acropachy appear specific to thyroid autoimmunity. Likewise, Graves' ophthalmopathy is an autoimmune ocular disorder that may result in conjunctival edema and injection, restriction and infiltration of extraocular muscles, proptosis, corneal ulceration, and optic nerve dysfunction. Although etiologically linked, the temporal occurrences of Graves' thyrotoxicosis and ophthalmopathy do not always coincide, as in this example.

Laboratory features of thyrotoxic Graves' disease are illustrated by the serum studies obtained on this patient. Estimation of the free fraction of thyroxine using the free thyroxine index (a product of the T_4-binding ratio and the total T_4) usually reveals an elevated value, but the total T_4 may not necessarily be high. In unusual cases, the free thyroxine index may be normal with an elevated total T_3. The suppression of pituitary secretion of TSH by elevated thyroid hormones is reflected by a low serum TSH value, often below the detection limits of presently available TSH assays. Autoantibodies to microsomal antigen (which is thyroid peroxidase) or thyroglobulin are associated with thyroid autoimmunity. However, their presence is neither diagnostic nor specific for Graves' disease. Although thyroid-stimulating immunoglobulins that bind to the TSH receptors are considered to be causative agents of this disorder, their measurement is unnecessary for the diagnostic evaluation of most patients with Graves' disease. Once the diagnosis of thyrotoxicosis is established, the presence of Graves' disease is supported by the demonstration of a palpable goiter, increased radioiodine uptake in a diffuse distribution on scan, and suppressed serum TSH values. The increased uptake excludes conditions such as thyroiditis and exogenous levothyroxine administration, which show thyrotoxicosis without increased function of the thyroid gland. The suppressed TSH excludes states of TSH excess such as TSH-secreting pituitary tumors and pituitary resistance to thyroid hormone. Only the exceedingly rare cases of thyroid stimulation by human chorionic gonadotropin from trophoblastic tumors would not be distinguished with the use of this approach.

Treatment

The most frequently used therapeutic modality for long-term management of thyrotoxicosis of Graves' disease in the United States is radioablation using ^{131}I. There is a modest rate of remission attained in some patients with thionamide drugs such as propylthiouracil and methimazole. Although subtotal thyroidectomy has been less frequently utilized in recent times, it is an effective therapeutic option in selected patients. In the presence of nodular goiters with hypofunctioning areas on ^{131}I scans or suspicious cytological findings, thyroidectomy is the preferred modality. It is important to note that none of these therapies treats the underlying immune disorder, but rather, they deal with the end-organ effects of TSH-receptor stimulation.

Graves' Disease and Thyroid Cancer

TSH is considered to be an important growth factor for both normal and neoplastic thyroid tissues. Likewise, it is possible that the TSH-receptor-stimulating immunoglobulins of Graves' disease would also stimulate the growth of thyroid cancers. It is questionable whether the prevalence of thyroid tumor is increased in Graves' disease.[1] However, the aggressive behavior of these tumors has been noted.[2]

References

1.   Mazzaferri, E.L.: Thyroid cancer and Graves' disease. J. Clin. Endocrinol. Metab., *70:* 826-829, 1990.

2.   Belfiore, A., Garofalo, M.R., Giuffrida, D., et al.: Increased aggressiveness of thyroid cancer in patients with Graves' disease. J. Clin. Endocrinol. Metab., *70:* 830-835, 1990.

Additional Reading

DeGroot, L.J., Larsen, P.R., Refetoff, S., and Stanbury, J.B.: The Thyroid and Its Diseases, 5th ed. New York, Wiley Medical Publication, 1984.

Ingbar, S.H., and Braverman, L.E., Eds.: Werner's The Thyroid, 5th ed. Philadelphia , J.B. Lippincott Co., 1986.

THE FATIGUED ATTORNEY

Kenneth B. Ain, Contributor

A 28-year-old attorney reported for her yearly physical examination complaining of tiredness, difficulty concentrating on her work, and a noticeable decline in her memory over the past several months. She attributed many of these symptoms to the severe stress generated by her legal case-load. Further questioning by her physician revealed that the frequency of her bowel movements had decreased from once daily, six months ago, to once every two or three days. She was having difficulty avoiding a gain in weight, and despite warm weather, she felt chilled without a light sweater. Her only medication was an oral contraceptive. Family history was significant for hypothyroidism in her mother and older sister.

Physical examination revealed a well-proportioned woman, 65 inches (1.65 m) in height, 125 lb (56.7 kg) in weight, and with sparse eyebrows (particularly at the lateral margins). Her facial features appeared slightly puffy in comparison to the photograph on her driver's license taken three years before. The pulse rate was 58 BPM and the blood pressure 138/88 mm Hg. Examination of her neck disclosed a small goiter of 25 g (normal, 15-20 g) with a palpable pyramidal lobe and a firm, bosselated texture. Her deep tendon reflexes were normally contractive but showed a delayed relaxation phase.

The initial clinical impression was that of moderate hypothyroidism of several months' duration. The texture of her thyroid gland and the occurrence of hypothyroidism in her family suggested an autoimmune etiological factor. The following serum values were reported:

Analyte	Value, conventional units	Reference range, conventional units	Value, SI units	Reference range, SI units
T_4, total (S)	7.0 μg/dL	5-11.5	90 nmol/L	64-148
T_3 resin uptake (S)	19 %	25-35	0.19	0.25-0.35
T_3, total (S)	134 ng/dL	100-215	2.1 nmol/L	1.5-3.3
T_4-binding ratio (THBR)*	0.6	0.9-1.1	Same	
Free thyroxine index (FTI)[†]	4.3	6-11.5	Same	
TSH (S)	22.0 μU/mL	0.7-7.0	22.0 mU/L	0.7-7.0
Antithyroglobulin antibodies (S)	Positive, 1:640	Negative		
Antimicrosomal antibodies (S)	Positive, 1:5120	Negative		
Cholesterol (S)	230 mg/dL	140-225	5.95 mmol/L	3.62-5.82

The laboratory results (low FTI and increased TSH) confirmed the clinical impression of hypothyroidism. The inadequacy of the total T_4 value alone, as a measure of metabolically

---

*T_4 resin uptake divided by the mean of a reference population.

[†]The product of the T_4-binding ratio and the total T_4.

active thyroxine, is demonstrated in this case study.* This patient's low THBR reflects the increased levels of thyroxine-binding globulin caused by the estrogen content of her oral contraceptive pills. The FTI actually represents the amount of T_4 circulating as free hormone.

The cause of hypothyroidism may be primary (thyroid dysfunction), secondary (pituitary dysfunction), or tertiary (hypothalamic dysfunction). In this case the elevated TSH with a concordantly low FTI indicates primary hypothyroidism. The etiology of this thyroid dysfunction appears likely to be autoimmune thyroiditis (Hashimoto's thyroiditis) as evidenced by the positive titers of antimicrosomal and antithyroglobulin antibodies. The patient was started on 112 µg L-thyroxine (levothyroxine) daily and two months later reported resolution of all of her symptoms. Laboratory studies at that time showed the following:

Analyte	Value, conventional units	Reference range, conventional units	Value, SI units	Reference range, SI units
T_4, total (S)	11.4 µg/dL	5-11.5	147 nmol/L	64-148
T_3 resin uptake (S)	21 %	25-35	0.21	0.25-0.35
T_4-binding ratio (THBR)	0.7	0.9-1.1	Same	
Free thyroxine index (FTI)	8.0	6-11.5	Same	
TSH (S)	3.2 µU/mL	0.7-7.0	3.2 mU/L	0.7-7.0

Presentation of Hypothyroidism

Thyroid hormone is a general name describing both thyroxine (T_4) and triiodothyronine (T_3), although T_4 functions only as a prohormone, requiring cellular mono-deiodination to T_3 for functional activity. Intranuclear T_3 binds to specific receptor proteins, which in turn bind to specific T_3-response elements of DNA in order to regulate transcriptional activity. In this way, deficiency of thyroid hormone can have protean manifestations and, if severe, mortal results.

In adults, the characteristic signs and symptoms of hypothyroidism may have an insidious onset. Cutaneous changes include dry, puffy skin with a yellowish complexion as well as a thickening of the subcutaneous tissues due to accumulation of mucopolysaccharides. The hair becomes dry and brittle and is often sparse. The voice may deepen in pitch, and hypoventilation has been observed. Hypothyroid patients can show decreased pulse

---

* Only 0.03% of the total T_4 represents the portion of T_4 that circulates free in the serum (free T_4) and is available to the tissues. The majority of circulating T_4 is protein-bound to thyroxine-binding globulin, thyroxine-binding prealbumin, and albumin. Protein-bound T_4 (PB-T_4) is related to total T_4 by the following expression:

$$[\text{free } T_4] \times [T_4\text{-binding sites on serum proteins}] \Leftrightarrow [\text{PB-}T_4] .$$

Since >99.9% of the total T_4 is PB-T_4, this value may be substituted and the expression can be arranged as follows:

$$[\text{free } T_4] = [\text{total } T_4] / K \text{ (binding constant)} \times [T_4\text{-binding sites on serum proteins}] .$$

Using the T_3 or T_4 resin uptake or the T_4-binding ratio (THBR) as a measure of the distribution of T_4 between the bound and free fractions, in a product with the [total T_4] , permits an estimation of [free T_4], expressed as the free thyroxine index (FTI):

$$FTI = [\text{total } T_4] \times THBR .$$

rate, decreased cardiac stroke volume, and decreased myocardial contractility that causes decreased cardiac output. Since peripheral metabolism is slowed, arteriovenous oxygen may not show a significant difference. Pleural and pericardial effusions may develop as a result of increased capillary permeability to serum proteins. This leakage of protein, as well as possibly decreased renal free water clearance, may contribute to generalized edema and hyponatremia. Gastrointestinal hypomotility with associated constipation is frequently seen, and the effects of hypothyroidism on hepatic metabolism may be reflected in the decreased degradation rate of certain drugs as well as by the degree of hypercholesterolemia. Neuromuscular effects are evidenced by increased muscular volume and stiffness with slow contractility and relaxation. Mental symptoms include decreased ability to concentrate, impaired memory, and hypersomnolence; behavioral manifestations range from depression to frank psychosis. Severe hypothyroidism may result in coma with significant associated mortality.

The incidence of congenital hypothyroidism (cretinism) is approximately one in 4000 births and may be associated with the most severe neuropsychological abnormalities. This high incidence has resulted in the institution of neonatal screening programs in many developed countries. Clinical features include feeding problems, hypotonia, umbilical hernia, constipation, enlarged tongue, dry skin, characteristic facies, and open posterior fontanelle. On radiological examination, poor skeletal maturation can be seen as retardation in the appearance of ossification centers. Failure to institute early treatment with thyroid hormone leads to significant brain damage. Even with early therapy there may still be a residual effect to lower the intelligence quotient.

Definition of the Disease

Hashimoto's thyroiditis (lymphocytic thyroiditis) is the most frequent cause of primary hypothyroidism in developed countries, occurring with a prevalence of approximately 3-4%, and is more common in women. In most of the underdeveloped countries, iodine deficiency is still the most common cause of hypothyroidism; an estimated 400 million people are currently at risk. Hashimoto's thyroiditis is characterized by lymphocytic infiltration of the thyroid gland and the production of antibodies that recognize thyroid-specific antigens. It is currently thought that the disease occurs as a consequence of abnormalities in suppressor T-lymphocyte function that cause a localized cell-mediated immune response, although the pathogenesis is still not completely understood. The study of Hashimoto's thyroiditis has served as a general model for inquiry into the mechanisms of autoimmune disease.

Most patients with Hashimoto's thyroiditis present with some degree of thyroid enlargement (goiter) that has a bosselated texture on palpation. There is usually some degree of hypothyroidism, although transient hyperthyroidism may result from inflammatory release of pre-formed thyroid hormones. The immune processes underlying Hashimoto's disease are similar to the processes causing hyperthyroidism from thyroid-stimulating antibodies in Graves' disease. Both conditions show a significant concordance with other autoimmune disease as well as frequent familial concordance. Findings that are associated with this condition include the presence of circulating autoantibodies directed against thyroid microsomal antigen (thyroid peroxidase) and thyroglobulin. Histopathological diagnosis is not usually necessary, although fine-needle aspiration biopsy may provide diagnostic cellular material if needed.

Treatment

Patients presenting with hypothyroidism should be treated with L-thyroxine (levothyroxine) at dosages sufficient to normalize the TSH level. In patients with normal thyroid function, the size of a goitrous thyroid may be reduced by such replacement therapy. However, TSH levels should be prospectively monitored, even if replacement therapy is not used, since there is a significant rate of development of hypothyroidism.

Additional Reading

DeGroot, L.J., Larsen, P.R., Refetoff, S., and Stanbury, J.B.: The Thyroid and Its Diseases, 5th ed. New York, Wiley Medical Publication, 1984.

Ingbar, S.H., and Braverman, L.E., Eds.: Werner's The Thyroid, 5th ed. Philadelphia, J.B. Lippincott Co., 1986.

THE RELUCTANT CHEF

Kenneth B. Ain, Contributor

A general internist in the community referred a 42-year-old woman to an endocrinologist for evaluation of a newly discovered 1.0 cm right-sided thyroid nodule. The patient failed to appear for her appointment and for two rescheduled visits. Ten months later, she appeared at the clinic, apprehensive because she had noticed the appearance of another neck mass lateral to the thyroid nodule. The patient was employed as a pastry chef at a local hotel and otherwise felt well. She was healthy except for recently diagnosed mild diastolic hypertension, under current treatment with a small, daily dose of captopril.

Physical evaluation revealed a thin, nervous woman with a blood pressure of 136/86 mm Hg and a pulse rate of 96 BPM. Examination of her neck disclosed a firm nodule, 3.6 by 2.4 cm, in the medial aspect of the right thyroid lobe. Two lymph nodes, 2.0 cm, were palpable in the right anterior cervical triangle. Other features of the examination disclosed no further abnormalities. Fine-needle aspiration biopsies of the thyroid nodule and both lymph nodes were performed at this initial visit, and blood was drawn for the following studies:

Analyte	Value, conventional units	Reference range, conventional units	Value, SI units	Reference range, SI units
T$_4$, total (S)	9.5 µg/dL	5.0-11.5	122 nmol/L	64-148
T$_3$ resin uptake (S)	28 %	25-35	0.28	0.25-0.35
T$_3$, total (S)	141 ng/dL	100-215	2.2 nmol/L	1.5-3.3
T$_4$-binding ratio*	0.93	0.9-1.1	Same	
Free thyroxine index (FTI)[†]	8.9	6.0-11.5	Same	
TSH (S)	1.4 µU/mL	0.7-7.0	1.4 mU/L	0.7-7.0
Antithyroglobulin antibodies (S)	Negative	Negative		
Antimicrosomal antibodies (S)	Negative	Negative		

These laboratory results confirmed the clinical impression of euthyroidism and gave no serological evidence for autoimmune thyroid disease. Evaluation of the thyroid biopsy smears revealed clusters of pleomorphic cells with eccentrically located nuclei and presence of intranuclear cytoplasmic inclusions. Immunoperoxidase staining identified calcitonin granules in the cytoplasm. The cytological diagnosis was medullary carcinoma of the thyroid. Biopsies of the cervical lymph nodes revealed the presence of cells identical to those seen on the thyroid biopsy. With these results in mind, the physician obtained the following studies:

Analyte	Value, conventional units	Reference range, conventional units	Value, SI units	Reference range, SI units
Calcitonin, basal (P)	98 pg/mL	<20	98 ng/L	<20
Calcitonin, stimulated (P)[‡]	2100 pg/mL	<120	2100 ng/L	<120

* T$_4$ resin uptake divided by the mean of a reference population.

[†] The product of the T$_4$-binding ratio and the total T$_4$.

[‡] Measured as maximal value after intravenous pentagastrin injection (0.5 µg/kg body weight over 90 s).

Analyte	Value, conventional units	Reference range, conventional units	Value, SI units	Reference range, SI units
Carcinoembryonic antigen (S)	12.0 ng/mL	0-3.0	12.0 µg/L	0-3.0
Calcium, total (S)	9.2 mg/dL	8.4-10.2	2.30 mmol/L	2.10-2.55
Calcium, ionized (P)	4.62 mg/dL	4.48-4.92	1.16 mmol/L	1.12-1.23
Epinephrine (U)	3.1 µg/d	<10	17 nmol/d	<55
Norepinephrine (U)	12.5 µg/d	<80	74 nmol/d	<473
Vanillylmandelic acid (U)	2.4 mg/d	<6.8	12 µmol/d	<34
Normetanephrines (U)	0.8 mg/d	<2.0	4.4 µmol/d	<11.0

The patient underwent total surgical thyroidectomy and modified radical right cervical node resection. All detectable tumor was removed, and her recovery was uneventful. Pathological analysis of the operative specimen confirmed the diagnosis of medullary thyroid carcinoma with an intrathyroidal primary tumor, 4.0 by 2.5 cm in size, and 7 of 24 resected lymph nodes containing metastatic tumor. Follow-up evaluation with biyearly physical examination, chest X-ray, and stimulated serum calcitonin measurement was planned.

Definition of the Disease

Medullary thyroid carcinoma (MTC) is a malignancy of the parafollicular cells of the thyroid gland and represents 5-10% of thyroid cancers. Parafollicular cells are derived from the embryonic neural crest and do not concentrate iodine or secrete thyroid hormones. MTC cells may produce calcitonin, prostaglandins, serotonin, histaminase, carcinoembryonic antigen (CEA), and occasionally corticotropin (ACTH). Eighty percent of cases of MTC are sporadic; the remaining cases are familial, presenting either as multiple endocrine neoplasia (MEN) syndromes 2a or 2b or as isolated medullary thyroid carcinoma. The familial forms are inherited as an autosomal dominant trait, which has recently been linked to a locus near the centromere of chromosome 10. Inherited MTC is frequently bilateral; it may be diagnosed in the precursor stage (C-cell or calcitonin-secreting parafollicular cell hyperplasia) in affected relatives of an index case by provocative testing for elevated calcitonin. Sporadic (nonhereditary) MTC more often presents as a unilateral thyroid mass not associated with the features that characterize MEN syndromes. The MTC of MEN 2a is associated with hyperparathyroidism, often presenting as four-gland hyperplasia, and with pheochromocytoma, the adrenal medullary tumor that secretes catecholamines. The MTC of MEN 2b is usually a more aggressive malignancy and is associated with pheochromocytoma, marfanoid body habitus, mucosal neuromas, and intestinal ganglioneuromas.

Differential Diagnosis

In this patient, MTC became evident as a unilateral thyroid mass with local lymph node involvement. The key determinations at the time of presentation were tests for pheochromocytoma and hyperparathyroidism so that probability of a MEN syndrome could be assessed. This approach is important for two reasons. First, surgical removal of a thyroid mass in a patient with untreated pheochromocytoma is risky and potentially fatal. Second, if the patient has a familial form of MEN, evaluation of asymptomatic relatives is central to their early diagnosis and cure. Normocalcemia in this patient tended to rule out hyperparathyroidism, and normal urinary catecholamine values suggested absence of pheochromocytoma. Some physicians recommend computed axial tomography of the adrenal glands for additional evidence of absence of pheochromocytoma. The familial connection for this patient was impossible to pursue since she was an adopted child and knew of no blood relatives to be screened.

The basal calcitonin level served in this case as a tumor marker for MTC and would serve after primary resection of the tumor as an index for recurrence or progression of neoplasia. Detection of MTC is made more sensitive by use of stimulation tests utilizing intravenous calcium gluconate, pentagastrin (as in this case), or both. Because a definitive diagnosis for this case was already recorded, based on an elevated basal calcitonin level and biopsy findings, a stimulation test was actually unnecessary. Nevertheless, the results illustrate a strongly positive response, which — had it occurred in an asymptomatic blood relative — would have been important evidence of a precursor stage to MTC. A similar response occurring in the patient after apparently successful surgical treatment would raise concern for local recurrence or metastatic dispersal of tumor. Elevation of CEA as seen in this patient is not surprising in view of the diagnosis but would not of itself be sufficient to support a diagnosis of MTC.

Treatment

Once associated pheochromocytoma has been either excluded or recognized and surgically treated, treatment of MTC requires total thyroidectomy and appropriate lymph-adenectomy. Since efficacy of chemotherapeutic agents has not been well established for this disease, as complete as possible surgical removal of tumor is critical. Although there is no evidence that survival is improved, some clinicians treat postoperative thyroid remnants with ^{131}I in an effort to eradicate residual tumor foci adjacent to follicular cells. ^{131}I treatment for distant, unresectable, metastatic MTC is totally ineffective since the tumor cells cannot concentrate iodine. Radiation therapy may be used to treat locally recurrent, unresectable tumor, but this therapy usually proves merely palliative and has not been shown to improve survival. The patient with apparently successful surgical ablation must be followed indefinitely with stimulated calcitonin testing as well as other examinations. Onset of manifestations of MEN syndromes may not be synchronous; consequently, patients without hyper-parathyroidism or pheochromocytoma at their initial presentation must be regularly screened for development of these conditions.

When diagnosed, sporadic MTC is usually more advanced than is familial MTC detected by screening. Thyroidectomy performed in the earliest stages of C-cell hyperplasia may be curative. Survival in MTC after treatment is approximately 80% at five years, although persons with more advanced tumors do worse and those with less advanced tumors at the time of diagnosis do better.

Additional Reading

Deftos, L.J.: Medullary Thyroid Carcinoma. Basel, Karger, 1983.

Ingbar, S.H., and Braverman, L.E., Eds.: Werner's The Thyroid, 5th ed. Philadelphia, J.B. Lippincott Co., 1986.

Robbins, J., Merino, M.J., Boice, J.D., Jr., et al.: Thyroid cancer: A lethal neoplasm. Ann. Intern. Med., *115:*133-147, 1991.

CHILD WITH RAPID GROWTH AND PRECOCIOUS SEXUAL MATURATION

Phyllis W. Speiser, Contributor

The patient, a six-year-old boy, was admitted to the Medical Center with a four-year history of rapid somatic growth and a six-month history of pubic hair growth. The patient was the full-term product of a normal vaginal delivery following an uncomplicated first gestation in a 34-year-old healthy female. Birth weight was 8 lb 9 oz (3.9 kg) and length 21.5 inches (54.6 cm). There were no neonatal problems. The mother ceased breast-feeding the infant at 10 days of life and changed to formula because he did not seem to gain weight. Thereafter, weight gain was normal. Between 9 and 18 months of age, the patient's linear growth was just above the 95th percentile, but by 2-1/2 years of age, his height was average for a 4-1/2-year-old child. His tall stature was disregarded by his family and pediatrician, who considered this normal since his parents were tall (father 74 inches [1.90 m] and mother 66 inches [1.68 m]). When the patient was three years old, his mother observed that his penis was larger than that of age-matched peers, and by the age of four some acne had developed. Pubic hair developed at 5-1/2 years of age, at which time he was referred to a pediatric endocrinologist for evaluation.

Physical examination revealed a tall, well-proportioned, muscular boy with mild facial acne. His height at 54.6 inches (1.39 m) was average for a boy of 10 years 3 months; his weight of 68 lb (31 kg) was average for 9 years 10 months. Blood pressure was normal (100/64 mm Hg). Dentition was advanced for age. The thyroid was not palpable. Examination of the chest and abdomen was unremarkable. The penis measured 7 cm semi-erect; fine, dark pubic hair was observed at the base of the phallus (Tanner Stage II). Testes were each 3 mL in volume, without palpable masses. There were no pigmented cutaneous lesions. Neurological examination was normal.

Laboratory results were as follows:

Analyte	Value, conventional units	Reference range, conventional units	Value, SI units	Reference range, SI units
Sodium (S)	138 mmol/L	135-145	Same	
Potassium (S)	4.0 mmol/L	3.5-4.7	Same	
Chloride (S)	103 mmol/L	99-108	Same	
Bicarbonate (S)	25 mmol/L	24-32	Same	
Luteinizing hormone (LH), basal (S)	1.7 mU/mL	<2 (pre-puberty)	1.7 U/L	<2 (pre-puberty)
Follicle-stimulating hormone (FSH), basal (S)	<1 mU/mL	<1	<1 U/L	<1
Testosterone (S)	172 ng/dL	2-12	5968 pmol/L	69-416
17-Hydroxyprogesterone, basal (S)	11,690 ng/dL	<100	354,207 pmol/L	<3030
17-Hydroxyprogesterone, 60 min after ACTH stimulation (S)	22,000 ng/dL	<250	666,600 pmol/L	<7575
Cortisol, basal (S)	7 µg/dL	5-20	193 nmol/L	138-552
Cortisol, after ACTH stimulation (S)	10 µg/dL	2-3 x basal	276 nmol/L	2-3 x basal

Computed tomography of the head was normal. Bone age based on X-ray examination of the wrist was read as compatible with a maturation of 12 years 9 months. Ultrasonographic examination of the testes showed no masses. Serotyping for antigens of the major histocompatibility complex revealed the HLA haplotypes B39,DR4 and Bw47,DR7.

The history of chronic accelerated growth velocity accompanied by signs of sexual maturation, the presence of relatively small testes for the degree of masculinization, and markedly elevated levels of serum 17-hydroxyprogesterone, the principal substrate for 21-hydroxylase, led to the diagnosis of congenital adrenal hyperplasia due to 21-hydroxylase deficiency (21-OHD).

The patient was started on treatment with hydrocortisone. Re-evaluation following three months of medical therapy indicated that linear growth was still accelerated, the testes had enlarged slightly, and the testosterone level had further increased. Repeat measurement of serum gonadotropins during sleep showed an LH of 19.9 mU/mL (19.9 U/L) and an FSH of 3.5 mU/mL (3.5 U/L), indicating pituitary stimulation of the testes. A gonadotropin-releasing hormone analogue was added to the medical regimen to suppress central puberty.

Definition of the Disease

Congenital adrenal hyperplasia (CAH) is a group of diseases that result from reduced or absent activity of one of the five enzymes of cortisol synthesis in the adrenal cortex (see Figure 1).[1,2] Each enzyme deficiency produces characteristic alterations in the levels of the particular steroid hormones that are substrates for, or products of, metabolism by the defective enzyme. Approximately 90% of cases of CAH are attributable to deficiency of 21-hydroxylase, a microsomal cytochrome P-450 enzyme required in the pathways leading to cortisol and aldosterone but not required in the production of sex steroids. In the presence of a defect in 21-hydroxylase, the synthesis of cortisol is blocked. This leads to disruption of the normal feedback mechanisms and overproduction of ACTH. The result is adrenal hyperplasia, the oversecretion of precursors of potent androgens such as androstenedione, and pre- and postnatal virilization. Deficiency of 21-hydroxylase may also interfere with the synthesis of aldosterone, which leads to salt-wasting.

The disease has an autosomal recessive mode of inheritance. The gene (termed CYP21) encoding the 21-hydroxylase enzyme and a highly homologous pseudogene are located on the short arm of the sixth chromosome in the midst of the HLA complex. Thus, the antigens produced by closely linked HLA genes serve as useful genetic markers for the 21-hydroxylase, with several characteristic HLA antigens in linkage disequilibrium with various alleles of CYP21. The strongest of these associations are HLA-Bw47,DR7 and deletion of CYP21, and HLA-B14,DR1 and a point mutation in the seventh exon (Val-281→Leu).

A combination of two severe mutations in CYP21 on each of the two sixth chromosomes produces the classic form of the disease (i.e., deletion/deletion), whereas two milder mutations (exon 7 Val-281→Leu/exon 7 Val-281→Leu) or a combination of a severe and a mild deficiency allele produces a *forme fruste* (mild) or nonclassic variant. Eight other mutations, aside from the two mentioned, have been detected in patients with 21-OHD. Interestingly, these have all arisen by transfer of deleterious sequence from the nonfunctional pseudogene to the active gene. Heterozygotes have reduced enzyme activity that is detectable only by the mildly elevated 17-hydroxyprogesterone level after ACTH stimulation.[3]

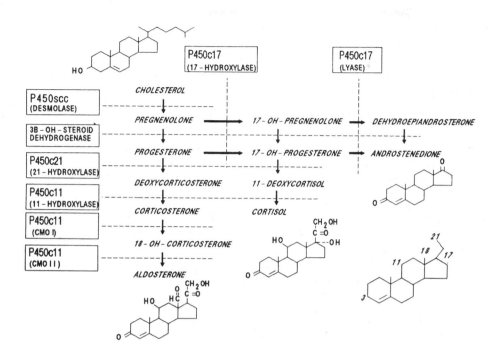

Figure 1. Pathways of steroidogenesis within the adrenal gland.
Enzyme nomenclature is given inside boxes; common names of steroid intermediates are listed. Steroid structures are shown for cholesterol (upper left), and for the three terminal steroids: aldosterone, cortisol, and androstenedione. At lower right a skeletal steroid molecule is shown with carbon positions numbered. Note that androstenedione, a weak androgen, is converted to a more potent androgen, testosterone, in several nonadrenal organs by the enzyme 17β-hydroxysteroid dehydrogenase. (Reprinted, by permission of the New England Journal of Medicine, from: White, P.C., New, M.I., and Dupont, B.: N. Engl. J. Med., *316:* 1519-1524, 1580-1586, 1987.)

Clinical Features. The most prominent feature of 21-OHD is progressive virilism with advanced somatic development. In the classic or severe form of the disease, this process begins *in utero*, manifesting in affected females as varying degrees of genital ambiguity that range from mild clitoral enlargement, through fusion of the labioscrotal folds and urogenital sinus (common opening onto the perineum of both urethra and vagina), to a penile urethra. Internal genitalia, including upper vagina, cervix, uterus, fallopian tubes, and ovaries, are structurally normal. Because male fetuses are normally exposed to androgen *in utero*, both internal and external genital formation are normal in males affected with 21-OHD.

Approximately 75% of cases of classic 21-OHD have the "salt-wasting" phenotype.[4] These patients have neonatal onset of hyponatremia and hyperkalemia, inappropriately high urinary sodium, and low serum and urinary aldosterone with concomitantly high plasma renin activity (PRA). Hypovolemia and shock often are present at the time of diagnosis. The remaining 25% of classic cases have sufficient 21-hydroxylase activity to produce adequate aldosterone in response to sodium deprivation; these patients are termed simple virilizers. Whereas the diagnosis is usually flagged in newborn females with both phenotypic forms of classic 21-OHD by their genital ambiguity, males with this form of the disease can easily escape detection in early childhood. The case presented here is entirely typical of the clinical history of a male with simple virilizing 21-OHD.

The nonclassic form of 21-OHD presents with less severe virilization of postnatal onset and may be distinguished from the classic form of the disease by lesser elevation of serum 17-hydroxyprogesterone, different HLA associations, and different mutations.[5]

Diagnosis

The hormonal diagnosis of 21-OHD is straightforward: baseline and ACTH-stimulated serum levels of 17-hydroxyprogesterone are abnormally high. It is important to measure a panel of several adrenocortical hormones in order to rule out other forms of virilizing adrenal hyperplasia (see Table 1). Normative data for both the basal and ACTH-stimulated values of these hormones are age- and sex-specific. A reference nomogram for identifying classic versus nonclassic patients and heterozygotes is available.[3] Adjunctive tests include elevated urinary levels of the 17-hydroxyprogesterone metabolite pregnanetriol as well as androgen metabolites measured as 17-ketosteroids.

Administration of glucocorticoids to the patient with advanced bone age due to chronic hypersecretion of adrenal androgens will rapidly suppress ACTH and thereby adrenal secretion of these hormones. Such vacillations in adrenal sex steroid hormones may release the hypothalamic-pituitary axis from tonic suppression. Therefore, if testicular enlargement or breast development indicative of ovarian estrogen secretion is observed in young children, gonadotropins should be measured to ascertain whether central puberty is in progress.

The salt-wasting form of 21-OHD is accompanied by the metabolic derangements described in the preceding. Normal individuals or patients affected with the simple virilizing form of 21-OHD, when stressed with severe sodium deprivation (dietary intake of 10 mmol/d), excrete more than 22 mmol/m^2/d of aldosterone (measured as the urinary 18-glucuronide metabolite). Salt-wasting patients, however, excrete negligible aldosterone despite markedly elevated levels of plasma renin activity and angiotensin II, which are the primary stimuli of *de novo* aldosterone synthesis. A patient with 21-OHD who demonstrates signs of virilism, but has no history of electrolyte abnormalities or dehydration, such as in this case, is likely to have normal aldosterone synthesis.

HLA serotyping or genotyping may serve as an adjunct to hormonal diagnosis, particularly in the genetic counseling of family members with equivocal hormone levels suggesting either heterozygote or unaffected status. With the advent of polymerase chain reaction to amplify DNA, it has become easier to perform allele-specific hybridization to detect CYP mutations in known patients, provide genetic counseling for family members, and perform prenatal diagnosis.[6]

Treatment

The aim of medical treatment is to replace cortisol and thus reduce ACTH secretion, thereby suppressing adrenal androgens and restoring normal somatic growth and sexual maturation. The drug of choice in young children is hydrocortisone given in slightly larger than physiological doses. Hydrocortisone is preferred over more potent and long-acting steroids such as prednisone or dexamethasone, because the hydrocortisone is less likely to result in growth suppression. Patients with evidence of precocious central puberty may also require pituitary suppression with a gonadotropin-releasing hormone analogue.

Table 1. FORMS OF ADRENAL HYPERPLASIA WITH CLINICAL AND LABORATORY FINDINGS*

Deficiency	Syndrome	Ambiguous genitalia	Postnatal virilization	Salt metabolism	Steroids increased	Steroids decreased	Frequency
Cholesterol desmolase	Lipoid hyper-plasia	Males	No	Salt-wasting	None	All	Rare
3β-OH-steroid dehydrogenase	Classic	Males	Yes	Salt-wasting	DHEA, 17-OH-preg-nenolone	Aldo, T, cortisol	Rare
	Non-classic	No	Yes	Normal	DHEA, 17-OH-preg-nenolone	---	? Fre-quency
17α-Hydroxylase	---	Males	No	Hyper-tension	DOC, cortico-sterone	Cortisol, T	Rare
17,20-Lyase	---	Males	No	Normal	---	DHEA, T, Δ^4-A	Rare
21-Hydroxylase							1/14,000
	Salt-wasting	Females	Yes	Salt-wasting	17-OHP, Δ^4-A	Aldo, cortisol	75%
	Simple virilizing	Females	Yes	Normal	17-OHP, Δ^4-A	Cortisol	25%
	Non-classic	No	Yes	Normal	17-OHP, Δ^4-A	---	0.1-1% (3% in European Jews)
11-Hydroxylase	Classic	Females	Yes	Hyper-tension	DOC, 11-deoxy-cortisol (S)	Cortisol, ± aldo	1/100,000
	Non-classic	No	Yes	Normal	11-deoxy-cortisol, ± DOC	---	? Fre-quency
Corticosterone methyl oxidase Type II	Salt-wasting	No	No	Salt-wasting	18-OH-cortico-sterone	Aldo	Rare (except in Iranian Jews)

NOTE: Aldo = aldosterone; T = testosterone; Δ^4-A = Δ^4-androstenedione; DHEA = dehydroepi-androsterone; DOC = 11-deoxycorticosterone; 17-OHP = 17α-hydroxyprogesterone.

*Information on other rare forms of congenital adrenal hyperplasia can be obtained from: Fernandes, J., Saundubray, J.M., and Tada, K. (Eds.): Inborn Metabolic Diseases: Diagnosis and Treatment. Berlin, Springer-Verlag, 1990.

In salt-wasting patients with deficiency of aldosterone, mineralocorticoid replacement must be added. The drug of choice is oral 9α-fludrocortisone, often given with oral sodium chloride supplements. If life-threatening shock ("adrenal crisis") should occur, both hydro-cortisone and isotonic sodium chloride are administered intravenously until normotension is restored.

Surgical treatment is necessary to correct the genital ambiguity in females with classic disease. A first stage procedure is usually done within the first few months of life; it consists of clitoroplasty to reduce the size of the erectile tissue. A second stage procedure is required if there is a urogenital sinus. In this operation, the surgeon separates the distal urethra and vagina, dilating the vaginal orifice to permit sexual intercourse. Unless there is evidence of urinary tract infection or other complications at an early age, the second procedure is best left until late adolescence, since without periodic dilation the vagina may undergo stenosis.

Helpful Diagnostic Notes

Ambiguous genitalia in the newborn may be caused by a number of different conditions,[7] including the incomplete form of androgen resistance syndrome (testicular feminization), gonadal dysgenesis, and inability to convert testosterone to its active metabolite, dihydrotestosterone, due to deficiency of the nonadrenal enzyme 5α-reductase. Initial evaluation of all such patients should include karyotype analysis, radiographical imaging of the pelvis to identify internal genital anatomy, and basal and appropriately stimulated levels of hormones in the mineralocorticoid, glucocorticoid, and sex-steroid pathways. The diagnosis of 21-hydroxylase deficiency is strongly suspected in a female when the karyotype is 46,XX and there are no male (wolffian) internal genital structures. In newborn males, the first manifestation of the disease is salt-wasting adrenal crisis. Clues to the diagnosis in older males are usually rapid linear growth and signs of androgen excess with disproportionately small testes. The latter sign differentiates gonadal from extragonadal pseudopuberty, as in congenital adrenal hyperplasia.

References

1. White, P.C., New, M.I., and Dupont, B.: Congenital adrenal hyperplasia. N. Engl. J. Med., *316:* 1519-1524, 1580-1586, 1987.

2. New, M.I., White, P.C., Pang, S., et al.: The adrenal hyperplasias. *In:* The Metabolic Basis of Inherited Disease, 6th ed. C.R. Scriver, A.L. Beaudet, W.S. Sly, and D. Valle, Eds. New York, McGraw-Hill, 1989.

3. New, M.I., Lorenzen, F., Lerner, A.J., et al.: Genotyping steroid 21-hydroxylase deficiency: Hormonal reference data. J. Clin. Endocrinol. Metab., *57:* 320-326, 1983.

4. Pang, S., Wallace, M.A., Hofman, L., et al.: Worldwide experience in newborn screening for classical congenital adrenal hyperplasia due to 21-hydroxylase deficiency. Pediatrics, *81:* 866-874, 1988.

5. Speiser, P.W., New, M.I., and White, P.C.: Molecular genetic analysis of nonclassic steroid 21-hydroxylase deficiency associated with HLA-B14,DR1. N. Engl. J. Med., *319:* 19-23, 1988.

6. Mornet, E., Crete, P., Kuttenn, F., et al.: Distribution of deletions and seven point mutations on CYP21B genes in three clinical forms of steroid 21-hydroxylase deficiency. Am. J. Hum. Genet., *48:* 79-88, 1991.

7. Lanes, R.L.: Ambiguous genitalia, micropenis, cryptorchidism. *In:* Pediatric Endocrinology. F. Lifshitz, Ed. New York, Marcel Dekker, Inc., 1990.

SUDDEN ONSET OF POLYURIA AND POLYDIPSIA

Robert M. Carey, Contributor
Michael J. Kelner, Reviewer

A 66-year-old man was admitted to the University Hospital for evaluation of increasing polyuria (10 L/d) and polydipsia over six weeks. He had a history of noninsulin-dependent diabetes mellitus (NIDDM), which had been stable for several years, but had experienced a weight loss of 31 lb (14 kg) over the previous six months; otherwise he had been in good health.

Physical examination on admission revealed a chronically ill, cachectic man. His blood pressure was 140/74 mm Hg and his temperature was 96.9 °F (36.1 °C). The lungs were clear on auscultation. The liver was enlarged at 15 cm below the right costal margin with a firm nodular edge, and ascites was present. The prostate gland was moderately enlarged but without nodules. The remainder of the physical examination, including neurological evaluation, was normal.

The results of laboratory studies performed on admission were as follows:

Analyte	Value, conventional units	Reference range, conventional units	Value, SI units	Reference range, SI units
Hematocrit (B)	34 %	37-51	0.34	0.37-0.51
Glucose (S)	177 mg/dL	80-115	9.8 mmol/L	4.4-6.4
Sodium (S)	149 mmol/L	136-145	Same	
Potassium (S)	3.1 mmol/L	3.5-5.1	Same	
Chloride (S)	102 mmol/L	98-107	Same	
Bicarbonate (S)	27 mmol/L	18-23	Same	
AST (S)	118 U/L	10-25	1.97 µkat/L	0.17-0.42
LDH (S)	1423 U/L	140-280	23.72 µkat/L	2.33-4.67
ALP (S)	678 U/L	25-100	11.3 µkat/L	0.4-1.7
Acid phosphatase, prostatic (S)	0.7 ng/mL	0.1-1.8	0.7 µg/L	0.1-1.8
Bilirubin, total (S)	2.1 mg/dL	<0.2-1.0	36 µmol/L	<3-17

Interpretation: Weight loss, cachexia, hepatic enlargement with ascites, mild anemia, and abnormal liver function tests suggested the possibility of neoplastic disease. Physical examination of the prostate suggested the possibility of carcinoma of the prostate. Increasing polyuria and polydipsia suggested the possibility of diabetes insipidus or, together with elevated serum glucose, diabetes mellitus. Therefore, a formal evaluation of water balance was conducted.

Evaluation of water balance

Analyte	Value, conventional units	Reference range, conventional units	Value, SI units	Reference range, SI units
No fluid restriction				
Osmolality (P)	298 mOsm/kg	280-301	298 mmol/kg	280-301
Osmolality (U), 24 h	143 mOsm/kg	300-900	143 mmol/kg	300-900
Volume (U), 24 h	6 L/d			

Analyte	Value, conventional units	Reference range, conventional units	Value, SI units	Reference range, SI units
Water deprivation test, at 3 h				
Osmolality (P)	310 mOsm/kg	280-301	310 mmol/kg	280-301
Osmolality (U), 24 h	131 mOsm/kg	300-900	131 mmol/kg	300-900
Reduction of body weight	4 %		0.04	
After vasopressin, 5 IU IV, at 2 h				
Osmolality (U), 24 h	461 mOsm/kg	300-900	461 mmol/kg	300-900

Interpretation: Results were compatible with a diagnosis of central diabetes insipidus. Subsequent treatment of the patient with intranasal 1-desamino-8-D-arginine vasopressin (DDAVP) led to reduction of urine volume to 1-2 L/d. In light of the central vasopressin deficiency, a full evaluation of hypothalamic-pituitary function was then conducted.

Endocrinological studies gave the following values:

Analyte	Value, conventional units	Reference range, conventional units	Value, SI units	Reference range, SI units
Cortisol (P), 0800 h	41 μg/dL	7-25	1132 nmol/L	193-690
Prolactin (S)	6.9 ng/mL	3-20	6.9 μg/L	3-20
Luteinizing hormone (LH; lutropin) (S)	3.2 mU/mL	7.9-18.1	3.2 U/L	7.9-18.1
Follicle-stimulating hormone (FSH; follitropin) (S)	<1.5 mU/mL	1.5-22.6	<1.5 U/L	1.5-22.6
Testosterone, total (P)	82 ng/dL	300-1000	2.85 nmol/L	10.41-34.70
Thyroxine (T_4) (S)	1.7 μg/dL	4.5-11.5	22 nmol/L	58-148
Triiodothyronine (T_3) (S)	55 ng/dL	80-200	0.85 nmol/L	1.23-3.08
T_3 resin uptake (S)	33 %	30-40	0.33	0.30-0.40
Thyroid-stimulating hormone (TSH; thyrotropin) (S)	0.1 μU/mL	0.7-7.0	0.1 mU/L	0.7-7.0
Insulin challenge test (0.1 U/kg insulin)				
Glucose (S), baseline	281 mg/dL	80-115	15.6 mmol/L	4.4-6.4
Glucose (S), 30 min	67 mg/dL		3.7 mmol/L	
Cortisol (P), baseline	53 μg/dL	7-25	1463 nmol/L	193-690
Cortisol (P), 30 min	No change			
Growth hormone (S), baseline	<2 ng/mL	0-10	<2 μg/L	0-10
Growth hormone (S), 30 min	No change			
Thyrotropin-releasing factor challenge (400 μg TRH, IV)				
TSH (S)	Minimal change from baseline			

Interpretation: Results demonstrated a deficiency of growth hormone and TSH. Decreased levels of LH, FSH, and testosterone established the diagnosis of hypogonadotropic hypogonadism. Thus, deficiencies of vasopressin, growth hormone, TSH, and the pituitary gonadotropins suggested panhypopituitarism, possibly due to hypothalamic disease from metastatic tumor. However, ACTH deficiency was not demonstrated. Instead, elevation of plasma cortisol and failure of insulin challenge to stimulate an increase in plasma cortisol suggested the possibility of Cushing's syndrome.

Tests of the adrenocortical-pituitary axis were initiated, with the following results:

Analyte	Value, conventional units	Reference range, conventional units	Value, SI units	Reference range, SI units
ACTH (P)	165 pg/mL	<80	36 pmol/L	<18
Cortisol (P)	45 µg/dL	7-25	1242 nmol/L	193-690

Day	Dexamethasone challenge	17-OHCS (U), mg/g creatinine	Cortisol, free (U), pg/g creatinine	Cortisol (P), µg/dL
1	Pre-administration	24	690	41
2	Pre-administration	24	560	40
3	Low-dose (0.5 mg q 6 h x 48h)	18	932	42
4	Low-dose	18	930	44
5	High-dose (2.0 mg q 6 h x 48h)	22	800	44
6	High-dose	24	730	40
7	High-dose	21	920	36

Normal response to this pattern of challenge by day 6 would be a serum cortisol <10 µg/dL (<276 nmol/L), and urine 17-OHCS and cortisol <50% of baseline.

Interpretation: Results confirmed hypercortisolism (Cushing's syndrome); nonsuppressibility by both low- and high-dose dexamethasone indicated that pituitary origin of the hypercortisolism was unlikely. High levels of ACTH in this context suggested presence of an ectopic ACTH-producing tumor. Hypokalemic alkalosis, which occurs often in the ectopic ACTH syndrome, is also consistent with this diagnosis.

A high resolution computed axial tomographic (CAT) scan of the head demonstrated a small area of enhancement immediately beneath the floor of the third ventricle anteriorly. This image was consistent with metastatic tumor. There was no evidence of an enhancing intrasellar mass. Cerebrospinal fluid analysis was normal. Bone marrow biopsy performed two weeks after admission showed small-cell carcinoma possibly due to metastatic carcinoma of the prostate. CAT scans of chest and abdomen revealed a solid mass (2.5 cm) in the lower lobe of the right lung and massive hepatic enlargement with multiple hypodense areas, both of which suggested metastatic carcinoma.

The patient was thought to have widely metastatic small-cell carcinoma possibly of prostatic origin. Chemotherapy with doxorubicin and cyclophosphamide was initiated, but the patient died on the 22nd hospital day, soon after his first dose. A diagnosis of ectopic CRF (corticotropin-releasing factor) production was suggested retrospectively by demonstration of immunoreactive plasma CRF level of 52 pg/mL (reference range, <2). This case was the first well-established case of the ectopic CRF syndrome.[1]

Cushing's Syndrome

Definition and Metabolic Features.[2] Cushing's syndrome is a group of diseases characterized by hypercortisolism. Cortisol, produced and secreted by the adrenal cortex, is the major human glucocorticoid. It stimulates hepatic gluconeogenesis by enhancing amino acid uptake and protein synthesis but decreases glucose utilization by extrahepatic tissue. The effect is to enhance glycogen storage in the liver while increasing the blood glucose level. It also enhances protein catabolism in extrahepatic tissue by inhibiting amino acid uptake and protein synthesis. Excess of the hormone affects lipid metabolism by a paradoxical combination of lipolytic and lipogenic actions that lead to abnormal but characteristic distribution of body fat. Cortisol increases diuresis and natriuresis by stimulating glomerular filtration rate while inhibiting the effect of vasopressin on the distal nephron. It may stimulate hematopoiesis in the bone marrow while inhibiting antibody production. An excess of cortisol inhibits allergic and inflammatory reactions by stabilizing lysosomal membranes, thus inhibiting release of intracellular proteolytic enzymes. Cortisol's effect to suppress leukocyte migration in tissue interferes with expression of delayed hypersensitivity and with host responses to bacterial infection.

Clinical Features.[3]* Prolonged elevation of cortisol is associated with obesity, muscular weakness, and mental disorder. Cortisol may act at the renal mineralocorticoid receptor to produce hypokalemic alkalosis. Weight gain and lipid accumulation in nuchal, truncal, and girdle areas provide the descriptive phrases of "moon facies," "buffalo" or "dowager's" hump, and centripetal obesity. Obesity is largely due to cortisol's effect to spare fat; in this patient, however, the effect was overriden by the wasting caused by malignant tumor. Muscular weakness is associated with proximal myopathy and muscular wasting, and there is a decrease in total lean body mass; thin extremities are characteristic. Most patients with Cushing's syndrome suffer from psychological complications, most commonly depression.

High blood pressure is a common feature in patients with Cushing's syndrome due to excessive cortisol or mineralocorticoid production. Impaired glucose tolerance or clinical diabetes mellitus with polyuria and polydipsia may occur. In females, hypercortisolism can cause menstrual irregularities by inhibiting release of gonadotropins. In males, low levels of testosterone and low sperm count may be due to a direct inhibiting effect of cortisol on the testes. In contrast, females may develop elevated testosterone, acne, and hirsutism. In both sexes, cutaneous manifestations include thin, fragile, easily bruised skin; facial plethora; and purple abdominal striae. Because of the effect of cortisol excess on the immune system, patients are more susceptible to infection.

As with the present case, most patients with ectopic ACTH or CRF secretion from fast-growing tumors (e.g., oat or small cell tumors) do not present with the usual features of Cushing's syndrome. These patients usually present with a rapidly progressive course including weight loss and cachexia. Slower growing ACTH-secreting tumors, such as thymic carcinoid and pancreatic islet cell tumors, may produce typical features of Cushing's syndrome. Cutaneous hyperpigmentation often signifies high levels of ACTH, which may have a tropic effect on melanocytes.

Diagnosis[4-7]

This patient presented with a complicated illness that posed difficulties in diagnosis. In an elderly individual with recent advent of cachexia and weight loss, the most likely possibility is neoplastic disease. The large, nodular liver, in conjunction with abnormal liver function tests and in the absence of a significant history of ethanol ingestion, suggested metastatic carcinoma as a most likely diagnosis. This consideration, taken with prostatic enlargement, suggested a primary prostatic carcinoma, even though benign prostatic hypertrophy is the more common explanation when enlargement is the only sign.

The sudden onset of central diabetes insipidus in this patient suggested neoplastic infiltration of the neural tracts through which vasopressin is transported from the supraoptic and paraventricular nuclei in the hypothalamus to the pituitary stalk. Such infiltration accounts for >10% of central diabetes insipidus. The diagnosis of central diabetes insipidus was made on the basis of a combination of findings: a relatively high plasma osmolality in the face of a low urine osmolality, failure of urine osmolality to rise to values greater than plasma osmolality in response to water deprivation, and a rise in urine osmolality after exogenous vasopressin administration.

---

* See also *Cases 28 and 30.*

In light of the presence of central diabetes insipidus, the patient underwent a complete evaluation of the hypothalamic-pituitary axis. A combination of low serum testosterone and low gonadotropins (LH and FSH) suggested hypogonadotropic hypogonadism. A combination of low thyroid hormone levels (T_4 and T_3) and low TSH suggested secondary (pituitary) hypothyroidism. Low basal growth hormone concentrations and failure of growth hormone to rise in response to insulin-induced hypoglycemia suggested growth hormone deficiency. Thus, the patient appeared to have panhypopituitarism, and deficiency of these anterior pituitary hormones together with central diabetes insipidus suggested an infiltrative process in the suprasellar region blocking synthesis or transport of multiple hypothalamic hormones (vasopressin, thyrotropin-releasing hormone, gonadotropin-releasing hormone, and growth hormone-releasing hormone).

However, it was surprising that there was no deficiency of ACTH. In contrast, elevation of plasma and urinary free cortisol suggested Cushing's syndrome. This diagnosis was further suggested by absence of suppression of cortisol values to low-dose dexamethasone and by absence of plasma cortisol response to insulin-induced hypoglycemia. In normal individuals, there is a rise in cortisol within 30 minutes of an insulin challenge. These findings prompted a workup for the cause of the hypercortisolism according to the following algorithm:

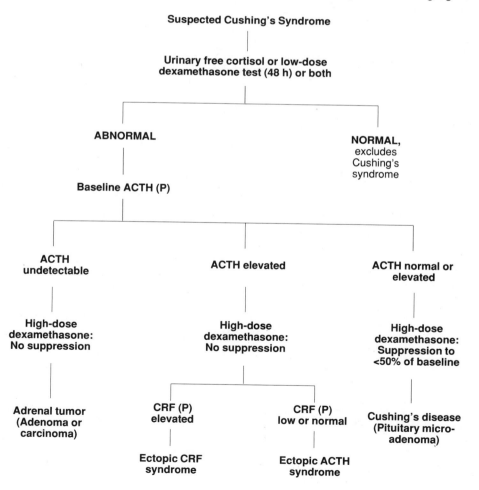

The patient was found to have nonsuppressible cortisol values with the high-dose dexamethasone, and plasma ACTH was elevated. Plasma corticotropin-releasing hormone (CRF) then was measured and found to be elevated. Thus, the patient had the ectopic CRF syndrome.

With all of the preceding information, then, the patient was thought to have probable prostatic carcinoma with metastasis to the liver, bone marrow, and hypothalamus, median eminence, or upper pituitary stalk. The infiltrative process in the pathway of hypothalamic hormones blocked transport to the pituitary, resulting in hypopituitarism and diabetes insipidus. However, the infiltrative neoplastic cells were synthesizing CRF, leading to stimulation of ACTH and the pituitary-adrenocortical axis that resulted in Cushing's syndrome.

The diagnosis was verified at postmortem examination. Large areas of the median eminence and pituitary stalk were replaced by tumor, creating an anatomical barrier for hypothalamic releasing-hormone transport to the pituitary. However, the pituitary corticotrophs were markedly hyperplastic. The presence of CRF and absence of ACTH in the tumor were demonstrated by assay of tumor material and by immunocytochemistry.

Treatment

The treatment of Cushing's syndrome depends upon the established etiology. Ideal treatment lowers cortisol secretion to normal, eradicates any tumor threatening the health of the patient, and avoids overt endocrine deficiency and permanent dependence on medication. A surgical approach is usually used for tumors: transsphenoidal hypophysectomy for ACTH-secreting pituitary microadenoma, adrenalectomy for glucocorticoid-secreting adrenal tumors, or tumor resection for the ACTH or CRF syndromes. When surgery is contraindicated, radiotherapy is considered, especially in the case of pituitary microadenoma. If these methods of therapy are impossible or are ineffective, drug therapy to lower steroid secretion may be used.

References

1. Carey, R.M., Varma, S.K., Drake, C.R., Jr., et al.: Ectopic secretion of corticotropin-releasing factor as a cause of Cushing's syndrome. N. Engl. J. Med., *311:* 13-20, 1984.

2. Vaughan, E.D., Jr., and Carey, R.M.: Adrenal Disorders. New York, Thieme Medical Publishers, Inc., 1989.

3. Cushing, H.: The basophil adenomas of the pituitary body and their clinical manifestations (pituitary basophilism). Bull. Johns Hopkins Hosp., *50:* 137-195, 1932.

4. Liddle, G.W.: Tests of pituitary-adrenal suppressibility in the diagnosis of Cushing's syndrome. J. Clin. Endocrinol. Metab., *20:* 1539-1560, 1960.

5. Crapo, L.: Cushing's syndrome. A review of diagnostic tests. Metabolism, *28:* 955-977, 1979.

6. Oldfield, E.H., Doppman, J.L., Nieman, L.K., et al.: Petrosal sinus sampling with and without corticotropin-releasing hormone for the differential diagnosis of Cushing's syndrome. N. Engl. J. Med., *325:* 897-905, 1991.

7. Orth, D.N.: Differential diagnosis of Cushing's syndrome. N. Engl. J. Med., *325:* 957-959, 1991.

WOMAN WITH IRREGULAR MENSES, HIRSUTISM, AND DEPRESSION

Ted L. Anderson, Contributor
Fred Gorstein, Reviewer

This 27-year-old female was in good health until she delivered a normal baby boy nine months prior to admission. The pregnancy and delivery seemed uncomplicated, but soon thereafter she became depressed and required hospitalization for an acute psychotic episode. After several medication trials, she was discharged on lithium with some control of her anorexia and insomnia. Recently, a relative who was a physician but had not seen her for ten months noted a change in her appearance, including facial fullness and increased facial hair.

At the time of the current admission, the patient complained of continued depression and insomnia. She denied easy bruising, voice change, significant weight change, edema, headache, visual disturbances, memory loss, or arthritis. She noted that menstrual periods, which were regular prior to pregnancy, had become irregular; she was not breast-feeding. Although she had always had some facial hair, for the past 3-4 months she needed bleaching and electrolysis because of an increasing moustache.

On examination, she was afebrile with a blood pressure of 146/110 mm Hg, pulse of 90 BPM, and respiratory rate of 16/min; she appeared in no acute distress. Her face was puffy (moon facies) and hirsute with a ruddy color. No truncal obesity, peripheral wasting, or striae were noted. There were numerous acne lesions on the chest and back but few on the face. She had a normal female escutcheon. Her eyes appeared slightly prominent, movements and pupillary reactions were normal, and visual fields were grossly intact. Her neck was supple without thyromegaly. Heart sounds were regular in rhythm without murmurs. No tenderness or masses were noted on abdominal or pelvic examination. Neurological examination was within normal limits. Minimal loss of strength was noted in the pelvic girdle.

On admission the following laboratory values were reported:

Analyte	Value, conventional units	Reference range, conventional units	Value, SI units	Reference range, SI units
Sodium (S)	144 mmol/L	135-145	Same	
Potassium (S)	5.2 mmol/L	4.0-5.3	Same	
Chloride (S)	105 mmol/L	98-107	Same	
CO_2, total (S)	26 mmol/L	20-28	Same	
Calcium, total (S)	10 mg/dL	8.5-10.5	2.5 mmol/L	2.12-2.62
Urea nitrogen (S)	16 mg/dL	5-18	5.7 mmol urea/L	1.8-6.4
Creatinine (S)	0.8 mg/dL	0.7-1.2	72 µmol/L	63-122
Glucose (S)	92 mg/dL	70-110	5.1 mmol/L	3.9-6.1
Protein, total (S)	7.5 g/dL	6-8	75 g/L	60-80
Albumin (S)	4.9 g/dL	3.5-5.0	49 g/L	35-50
Bilirubin (S)	0.6 mg/dL	0.2-1.2	10.3 µmol/L	3-21
ALP (S)	38 U/L	35-120	0.63 µkat/L	0.6-2.0
AST (S)	15 U/L	10-42	0.25 µkat/L	0.2-0.7

Analyte	Value, conventional units	Reference range, conventional units	Value, SI units	Reference range, SI units
Hematocrit (B)	43 %	37-44	0.43	0.37-0.44
Hemoglobin (B)	13.6 g/dL	12-16	8.44 mmol/L	7.45-9.93
Erythrocyte count (B)	$5.5 \times 10^6/\mu L$	4.7-6.1	$5.5 \times 10^{12}/L$	4.7-6.1
Leukocyte count (B)	$7.7 \times 10^3/\mu L$	4-11	$7.7 \times 10^9/L$	4-11
Differential count (B)	Within normal limits			
Urinalysis (U)	Within normal limits			

Menstrual irregularities can result from several endocrine and nonendocrine disorders, but the presence of virilizing features implicates androgen excess as part of the cause. Measuring serum testosterone in this patient with hirsutism and acne would probably have little diagnostic value, since elevation of testosterone could already be inferred from the phenotypic expression as hirsutism. For diagnosis and clinical intervention, distinction between adrenal and ovarian origin of elevated androgens is important. Furthermore, endocrinopathy involving corticosteroids or thyroid function has been linked with depression, both during and aside from the postpartum interval;[1] hyperthyroidism has also been shown to cause elevated androgens.[2] Consequently, a thorough evaluation of endocrine-related symptoms in this patient was appropriate. The following laboratory tests were obtained:

Analyte	Value, conventional units	Reference range, conventional units	Value, SI units	Reference range, SI units
TSH (S)	3.2 µU/mL	0.7-7.0	3.2 mU/L	0.7-7.0
T_3, total (S)	160 ng/dL	75-200	2.5 nmol/L	1.2-3.1
T_4, total (S)	6.2 µg/dL	4.6-12	80 nmol/L	59-154
Prolactin (S)	14 ng/mL	Nonpreg.: <20	14 µg/L	<20
LH, mid-follicular (S)	6 mU/mL	5-20	6 U/L	5-20
FSH, mid-follicular (S)	10 mU/mL	2.6-16	10 U/L	2.6-16
Cortisol, 2400 h (S)	37 µg/dL	5-25	1021 nmol/L	138-690
0800 h (S)	49 µg/dL	5-25	1352 nmol/L	138-690
ACTH, 0800 h (P)	135 pg/mL	<100	30 pmol/L	<22
Cortisol (U)	160 µg/d	20-90	441 nmol/d	56-252
17-Hydroxycortico-steroids (U)	11.9 mg/d	3.0-8.0	32.8 µmol/d	8.3-22.1
17-Ketosteroids (U)	18.8 mg/d	5-15	65 µmol/d	17-52

The observed normal values for thyroid screening tests diminished the likelihood of thyroid dysfunction in this patient. Similarly, a normal (nonpregnant) prolactin level in the absence of breast-feeding discounted postpartum (lactational) anovulation as a primary concern. Normal gonadotropin levels ruled out increased ovarian androgens due to polycystic ovarian (Stein-Leventhal) syndrome, in which LH/FSH ratios can be elevated to as much as 3:1.[3] The clinical presentation of this patient, together with elevated levels of plasma ACTH, serum and urinary cortisol, and urinary hydroxycorticosteroids and ketosteroids, supported a diagnosis of Cushing's syndrome.

Definition of the Disease

Pathophysiology. Cushing's syndrome refers to hypercortisolism and its clinical sequelae. The term Cushing's syndrome implies no definition of etiological categories, of which there are at least four.[4] The first category involves ACTH excess of pituitary origin, whether due to an adenoma of corticotrophs (*Cushing's disease*) or to increased hypothalamic corticotropin-releasing factor (CRF) secretion. A second category involves intrinsic adrenal cortisol excess related to adrenal adenoma, carcinoma, or nodular hyperplasia. The tumors are often unilateral and usually result in the most marked elevation of serum cortisol. The third category involves ectopic ACTH production by neoplasms. This reflects only a small number (10-15%) of cases, including small cell carcinomas of the lung; thymomas; islet cell tumors of the pancreas; and carcinoid tumors or paragangliomas in a variety of locations. The fourth category is iatrogenic, resulting from steroid therapy of asthma or autoimmune disorders or immunosuppressive therapy of patients with organ transplants.

Clinical Features. The clinical presentation of patients with Cushing's syndrome is similar regardless of the underlying cause for hypercortisolism. Cushing's syndrome is more common in women than in men and most often emerges in mid-adult life. A unique pattern of adipose deposition results in truncal obesity, moon facies, and a buffalo hump at the nuchal base. Abdominal striae and increased susceptibility for bruising are due to thinning of the skin with collagen breakdown in the dermis. Compromised immunocompetence is a frequent finding with cortisol excess (this is the original therapeutic objective in iatrogenic Cushing's syndrome), and thromboembolic phenomena are occasionally observed. If adrenal cortical hyperfunction includes increased aldosterone secretion, sodium retention may lead to hypertension. Similarly, urinary potassium loss may result in metabolic (hypokalemic) alkalosis. Other common features of Cushing's syndrome include weakness and fatigue, edema, glucosuria (rarely overt diabetes), hyperpigmentation (if ACTH excess is present), osteoporosis, and mental disturbances such as insomnia, irritability, and psychotic depression.[5] In females, androgen excess can result in menstrual dysfunction, acne, severe hirsutism with development of a male escutcheon, and other signs of virilization including voice changes, temporal baldness, and clitoromegaly.

Diagnosis

Clearly, the symptoms manifested by this patient have no iatrogenic cause since steroid administration is not a part of the medical history. Furthermore, ectopic ACTH production is unlikely in the absence of primary signs and symptoms that would be expected if neoplasms were present. Thus, we are left to distinguish between adrenal and pituitary (or hypothalamic) etiological factors. A useful laboratory test in the differential diagnosis of Cushing's syndrome involves suppression of ACTH secretion, as measured by the decreased output of urinary 17-hydroxycorticosteroids (17-OHCS). Depression of ACTH secretion is attempted with dexamethasone, a potent synthetic glucocorticoid, after a low-dose (0.5 mg q 6 h $\times$ 48 h) and a high-dose (2.0 mg q 6 h $\times$ 48 h) challenge.[6] Results of 24-h urinary 17-OHCS determinations obtained after dexamethasone were as follows:

	Patient	*Reference Range*
Baseline	11.9 mg/d	3.0-8.0
Low-dose	8.0 mg/d	<3
High-dose	3.1 mg/d	See below

In normal individuals, a precipitous fall in urinary 17-OHCS to levels approaching zero is not uncommon, even during the first day of low-dose administration. However, only moderate (if any) suppression is evident in patients with Cushing's syndrome of adrenal etiology. These patients show consistently markedly reduced ACTH levels (due to negative feedback of cortisol), and their tumors usually are not ACTH-dependent. As such, they generally fail to exhibit 17-OHCS suppression even after high-dose dexamethasone challenge. Conversely, most patients with *Cushing's disease (pituitary etiology)* exhibit at least

50% suppression of plasma and urinary corticosteroids after high-dose dexamethasone, but little or no suppression after the low dose. The response of patients with tumors producing ectopic ACTH is not predictable. In light of the clinical and laboratory findings in this patient, computed tomography of the brain was performed. Thinning of the floor of the sella turcica and increased sella volume were detected, which is consistent with a diagnosis of pituitary microadenoma.

It is noteworthy that development of Cushing's disease in temporal proximity to pregnancy probably delayed the diagnosis in this patient. Indeed, increased urinary 17-OHCS excretion, loss of diurnal variation in serum cortisol levels, and absence or failure of normal response to dexamethasone suppression during pregnancy make the diagnosis of adrenal cortical hyperfunction more difficult.[7] Further, hirsutism and acne are not uncommon during pregnancy, nor are menstrual irregularities and depression uncommon during the postpartum interval.[1]

In establishing a diagnosis of Cushing's syndrome, it is of paramount importance to determine the etiological category in order to effect appropriate therapeutic intervention. Iatrogenic Cushing's syndrome is generally an anticipated side effect of glucocorticoid therapy, and such a diagnosis is most often based on clinical, rather than laboratory, findings. However, in the case of pituitary, adrenal, and ectopic (ACTH-producing) tumors, logical selection and interpretation of key laboratory tests prove beneficial in establishing diagnosis and etiology. Further, the presence of primary symptoms of ectopic tumors may aid in the diagnosis. The table below outlines the salient laboratory findings expected in Cushing's syndrome due to different tumors.

Test	Pituitary Microadenoma	Adrenal Tumor	Ectopic ACTH Production
ACTH (P)	N to ↑↑	↓	↑ to ↑↑↑
Cortisol (S, U)	↑ to ↑↑	↑↑ to ↑↑↑	↑↑ to ↑↑↑
17-OHCS (U) after high-dose dexamethasone	>50% decrease (often >70%)	<10% decrease (often none)	<10% decrease (often none)

N = normal; (↓) = decreased; (↑) = slightly increased; (↑↑) = moderately increased; (↑↑↑) = greatly increased.

Note that the pituitary tumor described in this patient was a microadenoma that was found by gross and histological examination to be <10 mm in diameter. In contrast, macroadenomas of the pituitary are far less common and result in ACTH and cortisol values that are increased significantly greater than in this patient. Additionally, although a comparable percentage reduction of 17-OHCS would be expected after high-dose dexamethasone, the observed results may be less sensitive to the standard suppression test. Ectopic ACTH-producing tumors do not usually exhibit negative feedback by cortisol and, as such, would not be expected to respond dramatically to dexamethasone suppression. However, actual clinical observations may be less predictable.

Finally, computed tomography and magnetic resonance imaging studies offer further resolution in distinguishing among the tumors listed in the above table as etiological factors for Cushing's syndrome. Pituitary and ectopic ACTH-producing tumors typically result in bilateral adrenal cortical hyperplasia, whereas adrenal tumors are most frequently unilateral. Whereas pituitary macroadenomas may be difficult to detect by these methods, the tumors associated with ectopic ACTH production are usually less obscure.

Treatment

Treatment of Cushing's syndrome is aimed at reducing pituitary ACTH production. It may employ surgical removal of an adenoma, radiation of a tumor, or medication with a hypothalamic serotonin antagonist. An additional goal is elimination of adrenal corticosteroid secretion by adrenalectomy or metabolic inhibition of corticosteroid synthesis. This patient was treated with metyrapone to block adrenal 11β-hydroxylation, which is the final step in cortisol synthesis.[8] Following transsphenoidal removal of her adenoma,[9] histopathological and immunohistochemical analysis of the lesion confirmed the diagnosis of an ACTH-producing microadenoma of the pituitary (Cushing's disease).

References

1. Pop, V.J.M, deRooy, H.A.M., Vader, H.L., et al.: Postpartum thyroid dysfunction and depression in an unselected population. N. Engl. J. Med., *324:* 1815-1816, 1991.

2. Gordon, G.G., Southren, A.L., Rochimoto, S., et al.: Effect of hyperthyroidism and hypothyroidism on the metabolism of testosterone and androstenedione in man. J. Clin. Endocrinol. Metab., *29:* 164-170, 1969.

3. Rebar, R.W.: Practical evaluation of hormonal status. *In:* Reproductive Endocrinology, 2nd ed. S.S.C. Yen and R.B. Jaffe, Eds. Philadelphia, W.B. Saunders Co., 1986.

4. Gold, E.M.: The Cushing syndromes: Changing views of diagnosis and treatment. Ann. Intern. Med., *90:* 829-844, 1979.

5. Orth, D.N.: The old and the new in Cushing's syndrome. N. Engl. J. Med., *310:* 649-651, 1984.

6. Liddle, G.W.: Tests of pituitary adrenal suppressibility in the diagnosis of Cushing's syndrome. J. Clin. Endocrinol. Metab., *20:* 1539-1560, 1960.

7. Grimes, E.M., Fayez, J.A., and Miller, G.L.: Cushing's syndrome and pregnancy. Obstet. Gynecol., *42:* 550-559, 1973.

8. Liddle, G.W., Island, D., and Meador, C.K.: Normal and abnormal regulation of corticotropin secretion in man. Recent Prog. Horm. Res., *18:* 125-166, 1962.

9. Mampalam, T.J., Tyrell, J.B., Wilson, C.B., et al.: Transsphenoidal microsurgery for Cushing's disease: A report of 216 cases. Ann. Intern. Med., *109:* 487-493, 1988.

INTERMITTENT RIGHT FLANK PAIN

Margie A. Scott, Contributor
Fred Gorstein, Reviewer

A 59-year-old, previously healthy, white male office manager presented to his local physician complaining of intermittent right-sided flank pain. He described a 10-day history of awaking at night with sharp stabbing pain in his right side, a pain that often radiated from his abdomen to his flank. The pain would last from seconds to minutes and was relieved by sitting upright or by lying in a fetal position. There was no history of fever, chills, nausea, vomiting, diarrhea, melena, bloody stools, dysuria, or hematuria. He did mention a 15-lb (6.8-kg) weight loss over the last six months that he attributed to dieting.

Physical examination revealed a tall, well-developed, pleasant white male in no apparent distress. Vital signs were within normal limits. The lungs were clear to auscultation, and cardiac examination revealed a regular rate and rhythm without murmurs, gallops, or rubs. The abdominal examination was significant for an easily palpable, nontender, right-sided mass. There was no peripheral adenopathy. The extremities were negative for cyanosis, clubbing, and edema. Rectal examination was negative for palpable masses; stool was negative for occult blood.

The patient agreed to an immediate hospital admission to determine the nature of his right abdominal mass.

Chest X-ray examination was negative for effusions, infiltrates, and masses. A plain abdominal X-ray film confirmed the presence of a large, partially cystic, right abdominal mass. The lesion was thought to be arising from liver, adrenal gland, or superior pole of the kidney.

Laboratory data were as follows:

Analyte	Value, conventional units	Reference range, conventional units	Value, SI units	Reference range, SI units
Leukocyte count (B)	$8.8 \times 10^3/\mu L$	4.8-10.8	$8.8 \times 10^9/L$	4.8-10.8
Hemoglobin (B)	15.5 g/dL	14-18	9.62 mmol/L	8.69-11.17
Platelet count (B)	$357 \times 10^3/\mu L$	130-400	$357 \times 10^9/L$	130-400
Prothrombin time (B)	12 s	10-13	Same	
Urinalysis (U)	Within normal limits			
Sodium (S)	138 mmol/L	135-145	Same	
Potassium (S)	4.5 mmol/L	4.1-5.3	Same	
Chloride (S)	100 mmol/L	98-108	Same	
CO_2, total (S)	27 mmol/L	20-28	Same	
Urea nitrogen (S)	13 mg/dL	5-18	4.6 mmol urea/L	1.8-6.4
Creatinine (S)	1.1 mg/dL	0.4-1.4	97 μmol/L	35-124
Glucose (S)	86 mg/dL	60-110	4.8 mmol/L	3.3-6.1
Protein, total (S)	6.8 g/dL	6.2-8.0	68 g/L	62-80
Albumin (S)	3.8 g/dL	3.8-5.0	38 g/L	38-50
Cholesterol (S)	164 mg/dL	167-240	4.24 mmol/L	4.32-6.21
Calcium, total (S)	8.9 mg/dL	8.4-10.2	2.22 mmol/L	2.10-2.54
Bilirubin, total (S)	0.5 mg/dL	0.1-1.2	9 μmol/L	2-21

Analyte	Value, conventional units	Reference range, conventional units	Value, SI units	Reference range, SI units
ALP (S)	85 U/L	20-90	1.42 µkat/L	0.33-1.50
LDH (S)	935 U/L	100-190	15.59 µkat/L	1.67-3.17
AST (S)	37 U/L	8-38	0.62 µkat/L	0.13-0.63
Cortisol, 0800 h (S)	12 µg/dL	5-23	331 nmol/L	138-635
Cortisol, 1600 h (S)	7 µg/dL	3-13	193 nmol/L	83-359

Differential Diagnosis

At this point, renal cell carcinoma, adrenal cortical neoplasm, pheochromocytoma, and a hepatic tumor were considered possible causes. Laboratory data gave no indication of hematopoietic dysfunction, renal impairment, or electrolyte imbalance. Studies that supported normal liver function included the prothrombin time, total protein, albumin, total bilirubin, ALP, and AST. The markedly elevated LDH was thought to reflect probable tumor necrosis from the abdominal mass. Based on physical examination, absence of an endocrinopathy, and normal serum chemistry studies reflecting no evidence of hepatic injury, renal impairment, or electrolyte imbalance, the favored diagnoses included renal cell carcinoma, oncocytoma, and a nonfunctioning adrenal neoplasm.

An intravenous pyelogram (IVP) highlighted an inferiorly displaced right kidney with a normal filling time. Abdominal computed tomography (CT) favored a right adrenal mass with extension to the right hemidiaphragm, liver, kidney, and inferior vena cava (IVC). Laboratory results for a 24-h urine specimen were as follows:

Analyte	Value, conventional units	Reference range, conventional units	Value, SI units	Reference range, SI units
Total volume	2.0 L /d	0.6-1.6	Same	
Creatinine	1888 mg/d	995-1990	16.7 mmol/d	8.8-17.6
17-Ketosteroids	37 mg/d	8-20	128 µmol/d	28-69
11-Ketoandrosterone	0.9 mg/d	0.21-1.01	3.0 µmol/d	0.7-3.3
Catecholamines, total	83 µg/d	0-100	491 nmol/d	0-591
Metanephrines, total	0.4 mg/d	0-1.6	2.2 µmol/d	0.0-8.7
Vanillylmandelic acid	7.7 mg/d	1.5-7.5	39 µmol/d	8-38

Elevation of urinary 17-ketosteroids was suggestive of an adrenal cortical neoplasm. Secreting adrenal cortical tumors are generally accompanied by some of the greatest increases in 17-ketosteroids (may be up to 70 mg/d). Moderate elevations, as seen in this patient, can also be observed in silent tumors. If such elevations occur in adult males, clinical presentations related to 17-ketosteroid excess may not be apparent. Urinary catecholamines, metanephrines, and vanillylmandelic acid levels reflected normal adrenal medullary function.

An arteriogram revealed a moderately vascular neoplasm deriving its vascular supply from the right middle adrenal artery. A venogram confirmed extrinsic compression of the IVC by the mass but no gross intraluminal involvement. A preoperative bone scan was negative.

Based on IVP, abdominal CT, and arteriography, this was an adrenal neoplasm; 24-h urine studies were more suggestive of an adrenal cortical neoplasm with mild 17-ketosteroid excess than of a medullary process. The final preoperative differential diagnosis included a clinically silent adrenal cortical carcinoma and a nonfunctioning pheochromocytoma.

The patient underwent successful surgical resection of a well-encapsulated 1700-g adrenal cortical carcinoma. There was no gross invasion of the kidney, hemidiaphragm, liver, or IVC. Grossly, the tumor was composed of soft tan-pink parenchyma with central cystic degeneration and scattered necrosis and hemorrhages. On microscopical examination, poorly organized alveolar nests and diffuse sheets of polygonal cells demonstrated eosinophilic cytoplasm and moderate nuclear pleomorphism. There was no invasion of the capsule or vasculature.

The patient recovered rapidly, declined adjuvant therapy, and was followed closely in the outpatient clinic.

This case demonstrates the diagnostic dilemma of dealing with a clinically silent or nonfunctioning adrenal cortical carcinoma. Fortunately, these account for 50% or less of all cases. The majority of patients with adrenal cortical carcinoma present with Cushing's syndrome secondary to uncontrolled cortisol production nonsuppressible by high-dose dexamethasone administration. Plasma cortisol and free urinary cortisol levels are markedly elevated. Clinical virilism is associated with marked elevation of urinary 17-ketosteroids. Feminization secondary to estrogen excess is rare and is associated with a dismal prognosis.

Discussion

Adrenal cortical carcinomas are relatively uncommon neoplasms accounting for only 0.02-0.2% of all malignancies.[1,2] Patients may present at any age; however, composite studies demonstrate a bimodal age distribution with most children presenting before age five and most adults presenting in the 5th and 6th decades. Functional tumors are more common in females, whereas nonfunctional tumors are more common in males. Approximately 20-50% of patients present with no evident endocrinopathy. Clinical symptoms in this group are limited to an abdominal mass that may or may not be painful. The remainder of patients present with Cushing's syndrome secondary to nonsuppressible cortisol excess, clinical virilism secondary to plasma androgen excess, or (least commonly) feminization.

Adrenal cortical carcinomas vary in size from 100 g to >5000 g, in contrast to adrenal cortical adenomas, which rarely exceed 50 g. The carcinomas appear as well-encapsulated, soft, fleshy, tan-brown to yellow masses that may demonstrate areas of necrosis, cystic degeneration, or hemorrhage. Adrenal carcinomas tend to grow in an expansile fashion, often "pushing aside" adjacent structures rather than infiltrating them.

These tumors are often composed microscopically of polygonal to round cells with cytoplasm varying from granular eosinophilic to clear character and with variable nuclear pleomorphism. Adrenal cortical carcinomas vary in histological patterns from diffuse to alveolar to distinctly trabecular. Coalescent necrosis, a brisk mitotic rate, and unequivocal vascular invasion (when present) are helpful criteria in assessing malignancy. Occasional borderline lesions will evade even the most experienced pathologist.

Treatment

The treatment of choice is surgical excision. Local recurrence and distant metastasis to the liver, lung, and lymph nodes are common. Approximately 25% of patients present with metastatic disease, and up to 95% will return with recurrent or metastatic disease within two years of diagnosis.[1-3] Currently adjuvant therapy may include local radiation or multiple chemotherapeutic agents or a combination of both.[4,5] Success of these therapies, however, is not yet established.

References

1. Page, D., DeLellis, R., and Hough, A.: Tumors of the adrenal. *In:* Atlas of Tumor Pathology, ser. 2, fascicle 23. Washington, D.C., AFIP, 1986.

2. Gruhn, J., and Gould, V.: The adrenal gland. *In:* Anderson's Pathology. J. Kissane, Ed. St. Louis, C.V. Mosby Co., 1990.

3. Venkatesh, S., Hickey, R., Sellin, R., et al.: Adrenal cortical carcinoma. Cancer, *64:* 765-769, 1989.

4. Markoe, A., Serber, W., Micaily, B., et al.: Radiation therapy for adjunctive treatment of adrenal cortical carcinoma. Am. J. Clin. Oncol., *14:* 170-174, 1991.

5. Schlumberger, M., Brugieres, L., Gicquel, C., et al.: 5-Fluorouracil, doxorubicin, and cisplatin as treatment for adrenal cortical carcinoma. Cancer, *67:* 2997-3000, 1991.

MIDDLE-AGED MAN WITH WEAKNESS AND WEIGHT GAIN

David G. Elliott, Contributor

A 42-year-old white man presented with a five-month history of muscle weakness, fatigue, weight gain, polydipsia, and polyuria. Physical examination revealed predominantly truncal and facial obesity with plethoric facies and moderate acne. Height was 67 inches (1.70 m), weight 262 lb (119 kg); blood pressure was 190/110 mm Hg and pulse rate 95 BPM.

A chest X-ray examination showed no active disease, and laboratory evaluation showed the following values:

Analyte	Value, conventional units	Reference range, conventional units	Value, SI units	Reference range, SI units
Sodium (S)	137 mmol/L	136-145	Same	
Potassium (S)	2.6 mmol/L	3.8-5.1	Same	
Chloride (S)	92 mmol/L	98-107	Same	
CO$_2$, total (S)	32 mmol/L	23-29	Same	
Urea nitrogen (S)	22 mg/dL	7-18	7.9 mmol urea/L	2.5-6.4
Creatinine (S)	0.8 mg/dL	0.7-1.3	71 μmol/L	62-115
Glucose (S)	220 mg/dL	75-105	12.2 mmol/L	4.2-5.8
pH (aB)	7.51	7.35-7.45	Same	
pCO$_2$ (aB)	48 mm Hg	35-48	6.4 kPa	4.7-6.4
pO$_2$ (aB)	81 mm Hg	83-108	10.8 kPa	11.1-14.4
Urinalysis (U)	Glucose, 3+; ketones, 2+; otherwise within normal limits			

The initial clinical impression was that the patient suffered from adult onset diabetes mellitus. However, in consideration of facial acne and centripetal fat distribution and of the improbability of hypokalemic metabolic alkalosis being associated with diabetes, additional tests were ordered to explore the possibility of hypercortisolism (Cushing's syndrome). The results were as follows:

Analyte	Value, conventional units	Reference range, conventional units	Value, SI units	Reference range, SI units
Cortisol (P), 0800 h	53 μg/dL	5-23	1463 nmol/L	138-635
Cortisol (P), 1600 h	47 μg/dL	3-13	1297 nmol/L	83-359
Cortisol, free (U)	625 μg/d	20-90	1725 nmol/d	55-248
ACTH (S)	320 pg/mL	<50	70 pmol/L	<11
Dexamethasone suppression, low-dose (2 mg/d)	Urinary free cortisol excretion and plasma cortisol not suppressed			
Dexamethasone suppression, high-dose (8 mg/d)	Minimal reduction in urinary free cortisol excretion and plasma cortisol			

Analyte	Value, conventional units	Reference range, conventional units	Value, SI units	Reference range, SI units
Metyrapone test	No significant increase in plasma 11-deoxycortisol			

In view of plasma and baseline urine cortisol values, adrenal hyperfunction appeared to be present. Absence of suppression of cortisol production by low-dose dexamethasone and elevation of serum ACTH were consistent with hyperadrenocorticism secondary to increased ACTH production. Lack of suppression of cortisol with the high-dose dexamethasone suppression test (8 mg/d) and the metyrapone test results were interpreted to indicate Cushing's syndrome due to ectopic ACTH production, i.e., a paraneoplastic syndrome.

The initial chest film had been unremarkable. Computed tomographic (CT) scans of head, chest, and abdomen were done, and no intrasellar abnormalities were found. An abdominal scan was within normal limits with the exception of bilaterally enlarged adrenal glands. A small nodule, identified in the right lower lobe of the lungs adjacent to the hilum, was suspected as a possible source of ectopic hormone production. After bronchoscopy failed to find a discrete intraluminal lesion, lobectomy was performed. A tan nodule, 0.9 cm in diameter, was found underlying the bronchial mucosa. Light microscopy revealed features of a carcinoid tumor, and electron microscopy demonstrated dense core neurosecretory granules consistent with carcinoid. Immunohistochemistry for ACTH was strongly positive; there was no evidence of metastasis in the resected lymph nodes. Following surgery, serum ACTH and urine cortisol levels returned to normal, and the patient's symptoms gradually disappeared.

Definition of the Syndrome

Cushing's syndrome may arise from autonomous adrenal neoplasms or nodular hyperplasia, ACTH-producing adenomas of the pituitary (Cushing's disease), iatrogenic glucocorticoid administration, or ectopic ACTH production by various neoplasms. Ectopic ACTH-producing tumors account for ~15% of cases of Cushing's syndrome, and a variety of neoplasms have been associated with ectopic ACTH production.[1] The most common tumors involve the lung and include bronchial carcinoids and small cell carcinoma.[2] Less commonly, thymic carcinoids, medullary thyroid carcinoma, pancreatic islet tumors, pheochromocytomas, and a wide array of adenocarcinomas have been implicated as ectopic sources of ACTH. That these various tumors produce ACTH suggests that the amplification of certain oncogenes may be associated with de-repression of the hormone genes with resultant ACTH elaboration.[3] Although the overt clinical manifestations of Cushing's syndrome due to ectopic ACTH are uncommon, a significant percentage of neoplasms release the ACTH precursor pro-opiomelanocortin (POMC) or a larger, inactive form of ACTH ("big ACTH"). However, these tumors apparently lack the necessary enzymes to convert the precursor into the appropriate hormonally active form and thus are not accompanied by clinical features of Cushing's syndrome.

Ectopic production of corticotropin-releasing hormone (CRH) by neoplasms may also occur and may give misleading test profiles when a patient is evaluated for Cushing's syndrome (see *Diagnosis*).[4]

Clinical Features. Regardless of the underlying etiological factor, patients with Cushing's syndrome demonstrate certain characteristic physical features after the disorder has been present for a prolonged period of time. The cushingoid habitus includes obesity (predominantly centripetal), buffalo hump on the back and moon facies due to abnormal fat deposition, and abdominal striae. Other findings include acne, hirsutism, loss of libido, menstrual irregularities, impotence, muscular atrophy and weakness, osteoporosis, thin skin with easy bruisability, premature cataract formation, hyperpigmentation, and psychological disorders. Patients are often hypertensive, and glucose intolerance with overt diabetes is frequently evident. Elevated levels of glucocorticoids are lympholytic and thus impair the cell-mediated arm of the immune system. Also, wound healing may be impaired.

Hypercortisolism arising on the basis of ectopic ACTH production by a highly malignant tumor, such as small cell carcinoma of the lung, may differ in clinical presentation, because the manifestations of a widely metastatic tumor (e.g., cachexia) may override the development of classic Cushing's syndrome. In such a patient, clinical features may be limited to muscle wasting and weakness, glucose intolerance, and hypokalemia. However, benign tumors and malignant tumors with slow growth rates may remain clinically silent for prolonged periods of time and thus allow the more typical clinical features of Cushing's syndrome to develop.

Diagnosis

The first step in diagnosing ectopic ACTH production by a neoplasm is the recognition of the features associated with hypercortisolism. An individual with the classic cushingoid habitus and other physical stigmata, hypertension, and glucose intolerance does not present a major clinical dilemma; on the other hand, those patients with widespread malignancy may have more subtle or atypical presentations. Once clinical suspicion is aroused, several tests for confirmation of hypercortisolism may be performed.

Serum cortisol levels above reference ranges at 0800 and 1600 h identify patients who should be evaluated further. Increased free urinary cortisol or 17-hydroxycorticosteroids in a 24-h urine specimen are indicative of adrenal hyperfunction. The overnight dexamethasone suppression test serves as a screening test, and failure of serum cortisol to fall below reference levels necessitates further investigation. Failure to suppress urinary free cortisol or 17-hydroxycorticosteroids with both low-dose (2 mg/d) and high-dose (8 mg/d) dexamethasone in conjunction with markedly elevated ACTH levels is most suggestive of an ectopic source of ACTH production. Pituitary adenomas are usually associated with lower levels of serum ACTH than are ectopic sources and usually show suppression with high-dose dexamethasone.

Metyrapone, an 11-hydroxylase inhibitor, prevents the conversion of 11-deoxycortisol to cortisol, and thus it would be expected to increase 11-deoxycortisol levels when ACTH elevation is due to pituitary adenoma.

$$11-\text{Deoxycortisol} \xrightarrow{\textit{11-Hydroxylase}} \text{Cortisol}$$

Metyrapone, however, has no appreciable effect on the levels of 11-deoxycortisol when ACTH production is ectopic. Corticotropin-releasing hormone (CRH) stimulates ACTH release from a pituitary adenoma and causes subsequent increase in glucocorticoid levels but is not expected to stimulate an ACTH-producing tumor. Marked hypokalemic alkalosis is also suggestive of ectopic production due to the very high cortisol levels seen in this condition.[1] High cortisol levels with attendant mineralocorticoid effect of the glucocorticoids lead to increased exchange of K^+ and H^+ for Na^+, thus leading to decreased potassium values and an increase in pH.

In some cases of ectopic ACTH production, especially from bronchial carcinoid tumors, high-dose dexamethasone causes significant suppression of urinary free cortisol levels, and metyrapone causes increased levels of 11-deoxycortisol, thus confusing the diagnostic picture since such a pattern is more consistent with ACTH from a pituitary adenoma than from an ectopic source. However, these findings may be due to production of CRH by the ectopic (tumor) source and subsequent stimulation of a normal pituitary to produce ACTH. Petrosal sinus sampling[5] is a test applicable to this diagnostic dilemma. A small catheter is threaded into each petrosal sinus in the head, blood samples are obtained, ACTH concentrations are determined, and sinus concentrations are compared with those in peripheral venous blood. A significant gradient between sinus and peripheral levels suggests pituitary adenoma; absence of a gradient is consistent with an ectopic source for ACTH. CRH stimulation can also be utilized to enhance the gradient. Detection of hormone gradients across other vascular beds may also be used to locate ectopic sources inaccessible to other diagnostic methods.

Once there is sufficient evidence from laboratory and clinical evaluation to establish ectopic ACTH production, radiology may be employed to locate the source. CT and magnetic resonance imaging (MRI) are invaluable for locating these tumors because they are quite small and not readily identified on routine X-rays. Marked symmetrical adrenal gland enlargement, to a degree detectable by CT scan, is more often associated with ectopic ACTH production than with pituitary or primary adrenal Cushing's syndrome, and this enlargement is felt to reflect the trophic stimulus of large amounts of ACTH released by tumors.

Elevation of 5-hydroxyindoleacetic acid (5-HIAA), a metabolic product of serotonin seen in carcinoid syndrome, is often not seen in bronchial carcinoids associated with ectopic ACTH production; bronchial carcinoids are foregut derivatives and may lack necessary enzymes to produce serotonin.

Treatment

The most logical and effective treatment for ectopic ACTH production, once the source has been located, is removal or destruction of the neoplastic source. After removal, laboratory and clinical parameters often return to the normal range, although signs and symptoms of Cushing's syndrome may require months to regress. In some cases, however, the source may not be found even after extensive workup; in cases of widespread malignancy, the tumor or tumors may be located, but resection may not be feasible. In these instances, drug therapy to interfere with hormone function or synthesis (ketoconazole or aminoglutethimide) or to destroy adrenal cortical parenchyma (mitotane) may be initiated. In other cases, adrenalectomy or adrenal gland infarction by selective embolization may be required.[6]

References

1. Leinung, M.C., Young, W.F., Whitaker, M.D., et al.: Diagnosis of corticotropin producing bronchial carcinoid tumors causing Cushing's syndrome. Mayo Clin. Proc., 65: 1314-1321, 1990.

2. Jex, R.K., van Heerden, J.A., Carpenter, P.C., and Grant, C.S.: Ectopic ACTH syndrome. Am. J. Surg., 149: 276-282, 1985.

3. White, A., Clark, A.J., and Stewart, M.F.: The synthesis of ACTH and related peptides by tumors. Baillieres Clin. Endocrinol. Metab., 4: 1-27, 1990.

4. Odell, W.D.: Bronchial and thymic carcinoids and the ectopic ACTH syndrome. Ann. Thorac. Surg., 50: 5-6, 1990.

5. Doppman, J.L., Nieman, L., Miller, D.L., et al.: Ectopic adrenocorticotropic hormone syndrome: Localization studies in 28 patients. Radiology, *172:* 115-124, 1989.

6. Del Gaudio, A.: Ectopic ACTH syndrome. Int. Surg., *73:* 44-49, 1988.

Additional Reading

Blunt, S.B., Sandler, L.M., Burrin, J.M., and Joplin, G.F.: An evaluation of the distinction of ectopic and pituitary ACTH dependent Cushing's syndrome by clinical features, biochemical tests, and radiological finds. Q. J. Med., *77:* 1113-1133, 1990.

Jung, T., and Sikora, K.: The ectopic ACTH syndrome. *In:* Endocrine Problems in Cancer. London, Heinemann Medical Books, 1984.

Murray, R.J., Criner, G.J., Andreus, G., and Valente, W.: Cushing's syndrome in a woman with left perihilar mass. Chest, *93:* 1249-1250, 1988.

Pass, H.I., Doppman, J.L., Nieman, L., et al.: Management of the ectopic ACTH syndrome due to thoracic carcinoids. Ann. Thorac. Surg., *50:* 52-71, 1990.

WEAKNESS, WEIGHT LOSS, AND HYPOTENSION

Emmanuel L. Bravo, Contributor
Michael J. Kelner, Reviewer

A 40-year-old single woman complained of increasing lassitude and fatigue over the past six months. For the past three months she had experienced recurrent upper respiratory tract infections and a poor appetite accompanied by abdominal cramps, diarrhea, and a weight loss of 25 lb (11 kg). The patient had given up aerobic exercise class because of joint pains, increasing muscle weakness, and dizzy spells following even mild exercise. She admitted to decline of libido and sexual performance but attributed the decline to her chronic illness. She denied recreational use of drugs and taking any medications. She noted amenorrhea for the past three months. Her history was negative for diabetes, tuberculosis, and malignancy.

Physical examination disclosed a well-developed woman, 64 inches (1.6 m) tall, weighing 102 lb (46 kg), and in no acute distress. Her supine blood pressure was 120/65 mm Hg and her heart rate was 86 BPM. After one minute of quiet standing, her blood pressure fell to 90/58 mm Hg, the heart rate increased to 120 BPM, and she complained of dizziness. Her skin had a soft texture; no abnormal pigmentations were noted, but patches of vitiligo were observed on the right leg. Neck examination revealed a diffusely enlarged thyroid without discrete masses; there were no cervical adenopathies. The heart displayed no abnormalities, and lungs were clear to auscultation and percussion. The abdomen was flat and diffusely tender with no rebound, no organomegaly, and no masses; hyperactive bowel sounds were heard. Extremities showed no edema; peripheral pulses were weak but bilaterally synchronous. External genitalia and distribution of pubic hair were those of a normal adult female. No central nervous system (CNS) abnormalities were observed.

Initial laboratory findings were as follows:

Analyte	Value, conventional units	Reference range, conventional units	Value, SI units	Reference range, SI units
Hemoglobin (B)	9.4 g/dL	11.7-15.5	5.83 mmol/L	7.26-9.62
Leukocyte count (B)	7.6 x 10^3/μL	4.8-10.8	7.6 x 10^9/L	4.8-10.8
Sodium (S)	126 mmol/L	136-145	Same	
Potassium (S)	5.8 mmol/L	3.5-5.1	Same	
Chloride (S)	98 mmol/L	98-107	Same	
CO$_2$, total (S)	20 mmol/L	23-29	Same	
Creatinine (S)	1.8 mg/dL	0.7-1.2	159 μmol/L	62-106
Calcium (S)	11.3 mg/dL	8.4-10.2	2.83 mmol/L	2.10-2.54
Phosphorus (S)	2.6 mg/dL	2.7-4.5	0.84 mmol/L	0.87-1.45
Urea nitrogen (S)	52 mg/dL	7-18	18.6 mmol urea/L	2.5-6.4
Urea nitrogen/creatinine ratio	29:1	12:1-20:1	117:1 (urea:creatinine mole ratio)	48.5:1-80.8:1
Urinalysis (U)	Within normal limits			

Chest X-ray examination showed a normal cardiac shadow. The electrocardiogram (ECG) was essentially normal except for peaked T waves.

Since the patient's presentation was suggestive of adrenal insufficiency, possibly Addison's disease, she was hospitalized, and hydration with isotonic saline was started. Blood specimens for ACTH, cortisol, aldosterone, FSH, and TSH were obtained. Results were as follows:

Analyte	Value, conventional units	Reference range, conventional units	Value, SI units	Reference range, SI units
ACTH (P)	100 pg/mL	10-50	22 pmol/L	2-11
Aldosterone (P)	7 ng/dL	7-24	194 pmol/L	194-666
Cortisol (S)	10 µg/dL	12-26	276 nmol/L	331-717
FSH (S)	40 mU/mL	≤18	40 U/L	≤18
TSH (S)	9.8 µU/mL	0.4-5.5	9.8 mU/L	0.4-5.5

Dexamethasone and fludrocortisone were initiated to forestall adrenal collapse during testing. On each of two successive days after baseline urine collections, 40 U of ACTH in 500 mL dextrose/saline were administered intravenously over an 8-h period. The results of the ACTH challenge test were

	17-OHCS, mg/d (µmol/d)	17-KS, mg/d (µmol/d)	Aldosterone, µg/d (nmol/d)
Day 1, baseline	2.2 (6.1)	3.8 (13.2)	2.3 (6.4)
Day 2, baseline	2.1 (5.8)	4.0 (13.9)	2.4 (6.7)
Day 3, ACTH	2.0 (5.5)	5.0 (17.3)	2.6 (7.2)
Day 4, ACTH	1.9 (5.2)	4.0 (13.9)	2.5 (6.9)
Day 5, post-ACTH	0.8 (2.2)	3.6 (12.5)	1.8 (5.0)

The results of the ACTH stimulation test clearly documented adrenal failure. Further, they pinpointed the problem as primary adrenal failure. Values after stimulation should rise at least to twice baseline and to absolute levels of >12 mg for urinary 17-hydroxycorticosteroids (17-OHCS) and 17-ketosteroids (17-KS) and of >15 µg for urinary aldosterone. Patients with primary adrenal failure show no increase in urinary metabolites with sustained ACTH stimulation. In secondary adrenal failure, a "stepladder" increase in the levels of urinary steroids is obtained with sustained ACTH stimulation. In addition, the elevated serum levels of pituitary hormones (ACTH, FSH, and TSH) provided additional evidence ruling out hypopituitarism as a cause of adrenal failure.

Additional tests and results included the following:

Tuberculosis serology	Negative
Histoplasmosis serology	Negative
Angiotensin-converting enzyme	Within reference range
Thyroid microsomal antibodies titer	1:50,000 (Normal, ≤ 1:100)

Differential Diagnosis

The symptom complex of weakness, anorexia, weight loss, easy fatigability, and postural hypotension is common to most forms of chronic illness. Chronic hypercalcemia from whatever cause can present with gastrointestinal manifestations (i.e., nausea, vomiting, abdominal cramps) and signs and symptoms indicative of volume depletion. This patient's hypercalcemia, however, was mild; symptoms do not usually occur until the serum calcium exceeds 13 mg/dL (3.24 mmol/L). Hypercalcemia can be associated with adrenal failure and may, in part, reflect the degree of dehydration or the lack of glucocorticoids that may enhance calcium reabsorption from the gut. Hyponatremia is common to both adrenocortical deficiency and syndrome of inappropriate antidiuretic hormone secretion (SIADH). Both may be associated with renal sodium wasting and decreased free water clearance. However, dehydration and hyperkalemia are present in adrenocortical deficiency, and hyponatremia in SIADH is not associated with hyperkalemia. Chronic renal failure may be present with fatigue, anorexia, lassitude, hyponatremia, hyperkalemia, and anemia. Furthermore, urea nitrogen and creatinine values in this patient are more indicative of prerenal azotemia than of renal failure.

A diagnosis of chronic adrenal insufficiency or of Addison's disease must always be considered when a patient presents with unexplained weakness, weight loss, hypotension, and anemia. Chronic adrenal insufficiency may result from primary adrenal failure (Addison's disease) or secondarily from decreased pituitary ACTH secretion (hypopituitarism). This patient's clinical picture is most consistent with Addison's disease. Her hyponatremia and hyperkalemia are indicative of the mineralocorticoid deficiency that is common in primary adrenal failure. Secondary adrenal failure is not usually associated with significant electrolyte changes because aldosterone production, being predominantly dependent on angiotensin II and potassium levels, remains within normal limits.

Changes in skin pigmentation, when present, may help in differentiating Addison's disease from secondary adrenal failure (hypopituitarism). Hyperpigmentation is a common finding in Addison's disease, because decreased feedback inhibition by cortisol increases synthesis of ACTH and related precursor peptides, both of which have melanocyte-stimulating activity. It is generally concentrated over palmar and other body creases, pressure points (i.e., knuckles, elbows), mucous membranes, scars, and areolas of the nipples. The actual color can vary from bronze to dark brown. The skin is soft in texture, and vitiligo may be present in 4-6% of these patients, especially when the cause is autoimmune in nature. In hypopituitarism, decreased pigmentation due to lack of β-lipoprotein may be observed. Lack of axillary and pubic hair is more common in female patients. Decreased libido more commonly occurs in patients with hypopituitarism but can also be seen in Addison's disease. Diminished sex drive is due, in part, to the debilitating chronic illness and, in part, to the associated primary gonadal failure.

Other associated laboratory abnormalities are hypoglycemia, eosinophilia, increased levels of circulating antidiuretic hormone (ADH), and metabolic acidosis. Hypoglycemia frequently occurs in patients who are fasted for prolonged periods and is due to defective gluconeogenesis. Increased circulating levels of ADH result primarily from hypovolemia, which serves as a potent stimulus to ADH release. Metabolic acidosis results from decreased secretion of ammonia and hydrogen ions due to mineralocorticoid deficiency.

The only specific diagnostic test for adrenal insufficiency is measurement of plasma cortisol or urinary 17-OHCS before and after administration of ACTH. The choice of diagnostic test depends on assessment of the patient's clinical status. If adrenal insufficiency has to be ruled out, the ACTH stimulation test can be helpful. Plasma cortisol is measured before the intravenous injection of 0.25 mg of ACTH and 30 minutes thereafter. Adrenocortical function is considered to be normal if resting plasma cortisol is greater than 20 µg/dL (552 nmol/L) and/or an increase of at least 11 µg/dL (304 nmol/L) is obtained.

Primary Adrenocortical Insufficiency

Primary adrenal insufficiency (Addison's disease) has two main causes. Granulomatous infections such as tuberculosis and histoplasmosis account for a minority of cases in the United States. In general, patients with tuberculous adrenalitis, especially if it is associated with active or miliary tuberculosis, tend to be more ill than are those with adrenalitis due to histoplasmosis. Addison's disease may occur years after "cure" of tuberculosis, and the patient's history will provide a clue to the possible cause. Histoplasmosis is an important cause of the disease in areas where it is endemic. Adrenal involvement occurs in as many as 50% of cases of disseminated histoplasmosis infection. Sarcoidosis can lead to adrenal failure since it may affect the hypothalamus, the pituitary, or the adrenals. The incidence of adrenal failure in sarcoidosis, however, is <2%.

A more common cause of Addison's disease is an autoimmune reaction in which lymphocytic and plasma cell invasion of the adrenal is accompanied by antiadrenal antibodies that can be detected in the plasma. The condition may occur alone or in association with other endocrine disorders. Association of autoimmune thyroiditis and autoimmune adrenal disease is well recognized. The combination of primary thyroid failure, primary adrenal failure, and diabetes mellitus represents autoimmune pluriglandular deficiency and has been termed Schmidt's syndrome. Primary gonadal failure of varying degrees may occur in patients with autoimmune adrenal failure. Another well-recognized combination is hypoparathyroidism, Addison's disease, and moniliasis with ovarian failure.

Other causes of adrenal insufficiency include a hereditary disorder marked by progressive myelin degeneration of the brain (adrenoleukodystrophy) and spinal cord (adrenomyelodystrophy). Adrenal insufficiency arising from infiltration of the adrenals by opportunistic pathogens or Kaposi's sarcoma may complicate the acquired immunodeficiency syndrome (AIDS). Etomidate (an anesthetic), ketoconazole (an antifungal drug), and the anticoagulant heparin may impair biosynthesis of corticosteroids and thus induce adrenal insufficiency.

The cause of this patient's Addison's disease is probably autoimmune adrenal destruction. After exclusion of tuberculosis, histoplasmosis, sarcoidosis, drugs, and metastatic disease, demonstration of coexistent autoimmune disease by laboratory evidence of Hashimoto's thyroiditis, occurrence of vitiligo, and ovarian failure seems to confirm this etiology.

Treatment

The patient's subsequent treatment consisted of prednisone (5.0 mg in a.m. and 2.5 mg in p.m., daily) and fludrocortisone (0.1 mg daily). Mineralocorticoid replacement is necessary in patients with primary adrenal failure. On the other hand, patients with secondary adrenal failure do not require mineralocorticoid replacement because their mineralocorticoid production is preserved. On this regimen, the patient's appetite improved, she gained weight, her electrolyte abnormalities resolved, and her cardiovascular homeostatic mechanisms were restored to normal. She was advised to wear an identification bracelet or carry a card at all times indicating the presence of adrenal failure and the need for increased steroid dosage during stressful situations such as surgery, infections, and physical injury.

Additional Reading

Aron, D. C.: Endocrine complications of the acquired immunodeficiency syndrome. Arch. Intern. Med., *149:* 330, 1989.

Leshin, M.: Southwestern Internal Medicine Conference: Polyglandular autoimmune syndromes. Am. J. Med. Sci., *290:* 77, 1985.

Moser, H. W., Moser, A. B., Kawamura, N., et al.: Adrenoleukodystrophy: Elevated C26 fatty acid in cultured skin fibroblasts. Ann. Neurol., *7:* 542, 1980.

Nerup, J.: Addison's disease — clinical studies. A report of 108 cases. Acta Endocrinol., *76:* 127, 1974.

Speckart, P. F., Nicoloff, J. T., and Bethune, J.E.: Screening for adrenocortical insufficiency with synthetic ACTH. Arch. Intern. Med., *128:* 761, 1971.

Tucker, W. S., Jr., Snell, B. B., Island, D. P., et al.: Reversible adrenal insufficiency induced by ketoconazole. JAMA, *253:* 2413, 1985.

Vita, J. A., Silverberg, S. J., Goland, R. S., et al.: Clinical clues to the cause of Addison's disease. Am. J. Med., *78:* 461, 1985.

Wagner, R. L., White, P. F., Kan, P. B., et al.: Inhibition of adrenal steroidogenesis by the anesthetic etomidate. N. Engl. J. Med., *310:* 1415, 1984.

BOY WITH THICK LIPS

Michael L. Cibull, Contributor
Ronald J. Whitley, Contributor
Michael J. Kelner, Reviewer

The patient, a 14-year-old male, presented for evaluation of hip pain that was the result of an accident while playing. Although the injury was found to be self-limited and the patient was otherwise asymptomatic, physical examination revealed several significant findings: the child had an unusual appearance; he was marfanoid with an elongated face and thickened "blubbery" lips; his tongue was quite "bumpy," and small nodules were noted to protrude bilaterally from the buccal mucosa; the conjunctiva contained several small nodules; he showed mild muscle wasting; and he had a kyphoscoliosis and mild pes cavus deformity. A firm, nontender nodule 2 cm in diameter was noted in the right midthyroid region; several enlarged, right cervical lymph nodes were also palpable. The remainder of the physical examination was unremarkable except for a mildly elevated blood pressure (145/90 mm Hg).

Requestioning the patient and his father elicited a family history of a maternal cousin with "thyroid cancer" and the demise of the patient's mother at age 35 because of a stroke. Further medical evaluation was advised, and several diagnostic procedures were subsequently performed. His electrocardiogram showed a heart rate of 72 BPM with normal sinus rhythm and left axis deviation consistent with ventricular hypertrophy; his chest film was clear. A technetium scan of his anterior neck demonstrated a cold (hypofunctioning) nodule in the right midthyroid. His thyroid function studies (total thyroxine, T_4; thyroid hormone-binding ratio, THBR; and free thyroxine index, FTI) were within normal limits.

At this point, the patient was referred to an endocrine clinic, where a fine-needle aspiration (FNA) biopsy of the thyroid nodule was performed. Cytological examination suggested medullary carcinoma, a tumor of the parafollicular cells (C cells) of the thyroid. Additional laboratory tests were requested to confirm the diagnosis and investigate the possibility of familial disease. The following results were obtained:

Analyte	Value, conventional units	Reference range, conventional units	Value, SI units	Reference range, SI units
Calcitonin, basal (S)	3850 pg/mL	3-26	3850 ng/L	3-26
Calcitonin, maximum response after calcium-pentagastrin stimulation* (S)	57,000 pg/mL	<350	57,000 ng/L	<350
PTH, intact (IRMA) (S)	35 pg/mL	10-65	3.8 pmol/L	1.1-7.0
Calcium, total (S)	9.2 mg/dL	8.4-10.0	2.30 mmol/L	2.10-2.50
Catecholamines, fractionated (U)				
Norepinephrine	180 μg/d	15-80	1064 nmol/d	89-473
Epinephrine	255 μg/d	0.5-20	1392 nmol/d	3-109
Dopamine	75 μg/d	65-400	490 nmol/d	424-2612
Vanillylmandelic acid (VMA) (U)	16.4 mg/d	<5	83 μmol/d	<25
Metanephrines, total (U)	5.1 mg/d	<1.3	25.9 μmol/d	<6.6

* Calcium (2 mg/kg) is infused over 1 min, followed by pentagastrin (0.5 μg/kg) infused over 5-10 s; serum calcitonin is measured before infusion and 2, 5, and 10 min thereafter.

On the basis of clinical and laboratory findings (elevated values of calcitonin and catecholamines, normal levels of PTH and calcium), the presence of a multiple endocrine neoplasia syndrome (MEN Type 3) was suspected, and the boy was referred to a surgeon.

The child was admitted to the hospital, where a computed axial tomographic (CAT) scan revealed a left adrenal mass. He underwent abdominal exploration with resection of both adrenals; a 3-cm pheochromocytoma was found in the left gland and a 0.5-cm pheo-chromocytoma in the right. Three weeks later he underwent a total thyroidectomy and modified right neck dissection. The right lobe of the thyroid contained a 2-cm tumor mass that was histologically diagnosed as medullary carcinoma; a smaller tumor measuring 3 mm in diameter was found in the left lower lobe of the thyroid. Several small foci of C-cell hyperplasia were observed in the tissue from both lobes. Twenty-seven nodes were found in the neck dissection; 13 contained metastatic medullary carcinoma.

The patient's postoperative recovery was uneventful except for an episode of tetany that responded to calcium replacement therapy. One month after surgery, the patient felt well and had no abnormalities on physical examination. His blood pressure was now 110/60 mm Hg, and his stimulated blood calcitonin level had dropped to 200 pg/mL (200 ng/L). The patient continued to be followed in the clinic at three-month intervals. Although he remained clinically well, his calcitonin levels after pentagastrin stimulation suggested the presence of progressive recurrent disease (Figure 1). Subsequent biochemical screening of his family led to a diagnosis of MEN 3 in one brother.

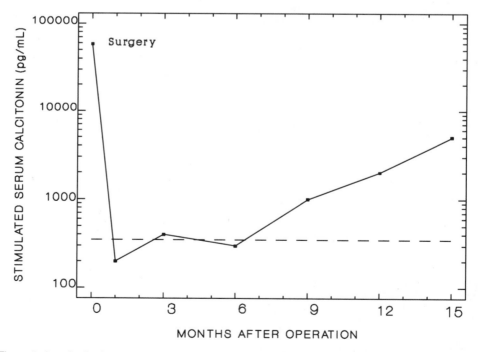

Figure 1. Longitudinal measurements of serum calcitonin in 14-year-old boy who underwent thyroidectomy for medullary thyroid carcinoma. Values shown are maximal serum calcitonin levels after provocative stimulation with calcium-pentagastrin immediately after surgery and after recurrence of tumor. The dashed line represents the upper limit of the reference range.

Definition of the Disease

Clinical Features. MEN 3 (also called MEN 2b) is a hereditary, multi-system disease characterized by a distinctive facial appearance and habitus that includes multiple mucosal neuromas and intestinal ganglioneuromas. Virtually all patients develop bilateral medullary thyroid carcinoma (MTC), often at an early age.[1] The tumor is more aggressive·in the setting of MEN 3 than when it is seen sporadically or as a part of other familial syndromes; many patients die of metastatic disease. Bilateral pheochromocytomas occur in about half of patients; signs and symptoms of these tumors include hypertension, palpitations, headache, and episodes of nervousness and sweating. Characteristic ophthalmological findings are also present and include enlarged corneal nerves seen on slit-lamp examination as well as conjunctival neuromas. MEN 3 patients frequently have intestinal motility problems with either diarrhea or constipation; parathyroid hyperfunction, however, does not occur.

Genetics. MEN 3 is inherited in an autosomal dominant pattern with variable expression in approximately one-half the cases. Although most affected persons develop MTC, the presence of the other manifestations of the syndrome is considerably less constant. It appears to be sporadic with no affected family members in the rest of the cases. Recently, the primary genetic defect in the MEN 3 syndrome has been localized to the centromeric region of chromosome 10.

Diagnosis

Syndromes of multiple endocrine neoplasia fall into three well-categorized patterns of endocrine and neuroendocrine lesions. Awareness of these patterns is crucial to early diagnosis and surgical cure. As shown in Table 1, the pattern of organ involvement is quite different between Type 1 and Types 2-3. For example, medullary thyroid carcinoma and pheochromocytoma occur in Types 2-3 but not in Type 1. Type 3 differs from Type 2 in a number of respects since the former is associated with abnormal physical appearance, lack of parathyroid disease, and a considerably more aggressive natural history for medullary carcinoma.

The diagnosis of MEN 3 should be suspected because of the unusual facies of affected individuals. Unfortunately, many patients are not recognized until they develop enlarged cervical lymph nodes or distant metastases, most commonly to the lung. Thin-needle biopsy of a "cold" thyroid nodule (i.e., one that fails to trap radioactive iodine) and cytological examination will usually lead to a correct identification of MTC. About 75% of these C-cell neoplasias produce abnormal amounts of calcitonin (CT), and increases of serum levels of this hormone may clarify the diagnosis in a patient in whom cytological study is suggestive but not diagnostic.[2] Unlike thyroid follicular cells, C cells do not produce thyroid hormones, nor do they respond to thyroid-stimulating hormone (TSH); patients with MEN-associated MTC are clinically euthyroid.

Medullary carcinomas comprise 7-10% of all thyroid tumors. Eighty percent of MTC cases occur sporadically; most are found in adults as a single nodule or mass in the lower portion of the thyroid gland. The remaining 20% of cases are familial and are often associated with other endocrine neoplasias in young individuals. Hereditary MTC is frequently bilateral and multifocal, and it is common to find areas of C-cell hyperplasia in areas distant from the primary tumor. Markedly increased serum CT levels can be seen in patients with widespread MTC; severe secretory diarrhea is relatively common, but some patients may be asymptomatic. Although acute administration of CT has a dramatic biological effect (i.e., hypocalcemia, inhibition of bone resorption), abnormalities in calcium or bone have not been consistently found in MTC. The physiological significance of CT in humans remains undefined.

Table 1. MULTIPLE ENDOCRINE NEOPLASIA SYNDROMES (MEN)

MEN SYNDROME

	1	2	3
Alternative name	Pluriglandular Wermer's	Sipple's	2b
Inheritance	Autosomal dominant	Autosomal dominant	Autosomal dominant
Organ involvement	Pituitary, 65%	Medullary carcinoma, 75-100%	Medullary carcinoma, 94%
	Parathyroid, 88%	Parathyroid, 45%	No parathyroid disease
	Adrenal cortex, 30%	Pheochromocytoma, 40-75%	Pheochromocytoma, 30-50%
	Pancreas, 81% (islet cell tumor)	Glioma	Ganglioneuromatosis, 100%; tongue, lips, alimentary tract, characteristic facies
	Thyroid (nonfunctional), 19%	Meningioma	
	Rare; lipoma, schwannoma, and carcinoid tumor	Glioblastoma	Skeletal anomalies, 81%; marfanoid habitus, pectus excavatum, pes cavus, scoliosis, slipped femoral epiphysis
			Corneal nerve hypertrophy

Modified from: Temple, W.J., Sugarbaker, E.V., and Ketcham, A.S.: The APUD system and its apudomas. Int. Adv. Surg. Oncol., *4:* 263, 1981. Reprinted by permission of Wiley-Liss, a division of John Wiley and Sons, Inc. Copyright © 1981, Wiley-Liss.

Elevated serum levels of CT are reliable markers of MTC as long as ectopic production can be excluded (i.e., some tumors of the lung, breast, or pancreas also produce CT). There is a positive correlation between tumor size and the basal serum concentration of CT. Occasionally, basal CT levels are borderline or normal, particularly early in the disease. In such cases, elevated serum levels of CT can be induced by stimulation with pentagastrin or calcium infusion. Both are potent secretagogues of CT. Within minutes after administration of these agents, there is a rise in the serum CT concentration in normal subjects and an exaggerated response in patients with MTC (or its premalignant form, C-cell hyperplasia). Most patients with MTC will respond to pentagastrin, but a few respond only to calcium. Combined calcium-pentagastrin stimulation provides a response of greater magnitude and is considered to be more effective and reliable than either agent alone. Provocative testing is an especially useful way to identify occult cancer, and asymptomatic family members of affected individuals should be screened every 6-12 months. Very mild elevations in CT or even the absence of the expected decrease in childhood levels should alert the physician to the possible presence of MTC.

Occasionally, medullary carcinomas secrete substances other than CT such as adrenocorticotropin (ACTH), serotonin, chromogranin A, or various prostaglandins; a confusing array of symptoms often results. For example, ectopic production of ACTH may cause Cushing's syndrome.

Pheochromocytomas are identified in about half of individuals with MEN 3. The elevated blood pressure and left ventricular hypertrophy reflected the effects of such a tumor in the case presented. Screening for these tumors usually involves evaluating urinary excretion of catecholamines, metanephrines, and VMA. MEN-associated pheochromocytomas have a predictable pattern of catecholamine secretion with a greater relative increase in epinephrine than in norepinephrine.[3] If urinary catecholamine values are high, CAT scans are usually obtained to localize the tumors preoperatively. In the context of MEN 3, these tumors are frequently bilateral, multicentric, or extra-adrenal. Pheochromocytomas can also be seen with other familial syndromes such as peripheral neurofibromatosis, von Hippel-Lindau syndrome, and McCune-Albright syndrome.[4]

Therapy

Surgery is the most effective treatment for both medullary carcinoma and pheochromocytoma. The pheochromocytoma is usually removed before thyroid surgery is performed in order to reduce the risk of a hypertensive crisis and fatal arrhythmia as a result of excessive catecholamine release. Total thyroidectomy is recommended for MTC since these tumors are frequently bilateral and multifocal. Cervical node dissections are usually a part of the surgical procedure, particularly in patients with palpable tumors. Radioiodine and X-ray therapies are not helpful in disseminated disease; chemotherapy is also of limited value. The preoperative stimulated level of CT has some prognostic significance. In patients with stimulated CT values <1000 pg/mL (<1000 ng/L), the surgical cure rate is about 96%. In patients with values >10,000 pg/mL (>10,000 ng/L), the cure rate is 40%; these patients also have a higher incidence of metastases and early death.[5]

Basal and stimulated CT determinations are very useful in evaluating patients postoperatively for recurrence and progression of disease. After successful surgery, basal CT levels should dramatically decrease and remain within the reference range. Increases in basal or stimulated CT levels, months to years after surgery, mark the presence of residual or metastatic disease. Measurement of carcinoembryonic antigen (CEA), an oncofetal antigen, also appears to be useful as a postoperative tumor marker; rising levels indicate a poor prognosis.[6]

References

1. Emmertsen, K.: Medullary thyroid carcinoma and calcitonin. Dan. Med. Bull., *32:* 1-28, 1985.

2. Stepanas, A., Samaan, N., Hill, C., and Hickey, R.: Medullary thyroid carcinoma. Cancer, *43:* 825-837, 1979.

3. Grauer, A., Raue, F., and Gagel, R.: Changing concepts in the management of hereditary and sporadic medullary thyroid carcinoma. Endocrinol. Metab. Clin. North Am., *19:* 613-635, 1990.

4. Schimke, R.: Multiple endocrine neoplasia: How many syndromes? Am. J. Med. Genet., *37:* 375-383, 1990.

5. Cance, W., and Wells, S.: Multiple endocrine neoplasia Type IIa. Curr. Probl. Surg., *22:* 1-56, 1985.

6. Saad, M., Ordonez, N., Rashid, R., et al.: Medullary carcinoma of the thyroid. Medicine, *63:* 319-342, 1984.

A WOMAN WITH PSYCHOSIS AND HYPERCALCEMIA

Susan A. Fuhrman, Contributor
Ronald J. Whitley, Reviewer

A 48-year-old female with a past history of mental illness was admitted to the hospital with new onset of bizarre psychotic behavior. She had been well for the past two years and had no significant history of medical problems. She denied any weakness, weight loss, abdominal pain, nausea, or vomiting. Physical examination revealed the following: weight 138 lb (62.7 kg), height 65 in (1.65 m), pulse 80 BPM and regular, blood pressure 130/75 mm Hg. The remainder of the examination was entirely normal except for the patient's mental status. She did not know where she was and was confused as to the current date and year.

The following laboratory results were obtained upon admission:

Analyte	Value, conventional units	Reference range, conventional units	Value, SI units	Reference range, SI units
Sodium (S)	141 mmol/L	136-146	Same	
Chloride (S)	107 mmol/L	99-108	Same	
Potassium (S)	3.9 mmol/L	3.7-5.2	Same	
Bicarbonate (S)	22 mmol/L	22-29	Same	
Glucose (S)	96 mg/dL	72-105	5.3 mmol/L	4.0-5.8
Urea nitrogen (S)	25 mg/dL	9-23	8.9 mmol urea/L	3.2-8.2
Creatinine (S)	0.9 mg/dL	0.3-1.0	80 µmol/L	27-88
Calcium (S)	13.8 mg/dL	8.4-10.1	3.44 mmol/L	2.10-2.52
Phosphorus (S)	2.8 mg/dL	2.5-4.5	0.90 mmol/L	0.81-1.45
Chloride/phosphorus ratio	38:1	<29:1	Same	
Magnesium (S)	2.2 mg/dL	1.7-2.7	0.91 mmol/L	0.70-1.11
Protein, total (S)	7.2 g/dL	6.4-8.3	72 g/L	64-83
Albumin (S)	4.2 g/dL	3.5-5.0	42 g/L	35-50
ALP (S)	64 U/L	50-120	1.1 µkat/L	0.8-2.0
AST (S)	25 U/L	0-50	0.42 µkat/L	0.00-0.83
ALT (S)	35 U/L	0-50	0.58 µkat/L	0.00-0.83
GGT (S)	29 U/L	10-40	0.48 µkat/L	0.17-0.67
LDH (S)	252 U/L	205-475	4.20 µkat/L	3.42-7.92

The physician's initial impression was recurrence of the patient's mental illness. However, review of the laboratory findings raised the distinct possibility of a central nervous system disorder due to hypercalcemia. The patient was treated to restore normocalcemia by administering intravenous fluids and oral furosemide to increase renal excretion of calcium. The etiology of the hypercalcemia was then investigated.

Although the differential diagnosis of hypercalcemia must consider a variety of causes (Table 1), the problem is somewhat simplified by first considering the most likely etiologies. The vast majority (>90%) of cases of sustained hypercalcemia have either primary hyperparathyroidism or malignancy. (Patients with primary hyperparathyroidism frequently have mild to moderate hypercalcemia, whereas patients with severe hypercalcemia [>13.0 mg/dL;

>3.25 mmol/L] usually have malignancy.) In unselected outpatients, hyperparathyroidism is more common; malignancy is more common in hospitalized ill patients.

Table 1. CAUSES OF HYPERCALCEMIA

Hyperparathyroidism	Physical immobilization
Malignancy	Adrenal insufficiency
Thiazide diuretics	Pheochromocytoma
Hypo- or hyperthyroidism	Acromegaly
Vitamin A or vitamin D intoxication	Lithium therapy
Sarcoidosis	Familial hypocalciuric hypercalcemia
Milk-alkali syndrome	Post renal transplant

In this patient, the low serum phosphorus and the high ratio of chloride to phosphorus (38:1) suggested hyperparathyroidism, but she had no history of bone pain, recent fractures, or kidney stones, all of which are associated with hyperparathyroidism. Use of diuretics, particularly of thiazide drugs, which decreases renal excretion of calcium and thus leads to hypercalcemia, was another possibility, but the patient denied their use. Physical examination had not indicated malignancy. Breast examination and mammography, as well as chest X-ray examination, were all negative for pathological changes. Additional studies were requested, and the following results were obtained:

Analyte	Value, conventional units	Reference range, conventional units	Value, SI units	Reference range, SI units
PTH, intact molecule (P)	56 pg/mL	9-51	6.0 pmol/L	1.0-5.5
Calcium, total (S)	13.6 mg/dL	8.4-10.1	3.39 mmol/L	2.10-2.52
Calcium, ionized (S)	6.9 mg/dL	4.4-5.5	1.72 mmol/L	1.10-1.37
Occult blood (F)	Negative	Negative		

The clinical impression was that the patient had hyperparathyroidism; this was confirmed by the laboratory data. Exploratory surgery of the patient's neck located and removed a large, solitary parathyroid adenoma. The patient's psychotic symptoms regressed as the serum calcium decreased, and she was discharged on the fifth postoperative day.

Definition of the Disease

Hyperparathyroidism as a clinical entity was first described in the mid-1920's. The condition is characterized by increased parathyroid hormone (parathormone) secretion, most often due to neoplasm. Initially thought to be rare and manifest clinically as the profound bone disease osteitis fibrosa cystica, the disease was soon discovered to include nephrolithiasis among its manifestations. Bone disease and kidney stones remain the most important clinical symptoms associated with the disorder.

Clinical Features.[1] The clinical presentation of hyperparathyroidism can be varied. The most common presentation is that of an asymptomatic patient with an increased serum calcium on a biochemical profile (serendipity syndrome). These patients present a management problem that will be discussed later. Other clinical manifestations that are seen in hyperparathyroid patients include bone pain, skeletal deformities, and pathological fractures, including compression fractures of the vertebrae. Renal manifestations of the disorder include episodes of flank pain and renal colic from nephrolithiasis. Central nervous system (CNS) involvement appears to be related to the degree of hypercalcemia; the symptoms include lethargy, confusion, and obtundation. These symptoms reverse with normalization of the serum calcium level. If the calcium is very high and remains untreated, coma and death may occur. The CNS findings in this patient represent a more unusual manifestation of the disease, specifically the psychoneurotic and psychiatric manifestations. These symptoms include depression, personality change, memory loss, or overtly psychotic behavior. In many cases in which patients present with these types of CNS manifestations, otherwise curative surgery does not result in resolution of these symptoms.

Other unusual presenting findings include neuromyopathic symptoms such as weakness, particularly of proximal muscles, fatigability, fine tongue fasciculations, hyperreflexia, and muscle atrophy. These neuromyopathic signs and symptoms are reversible following removal of the adenomatous or hyperplastic parathyroid tissue. Gastrointestinal symptoms have also been reported in conjunction with hyperparathyroidism; these include peptic ulcer disease with the associated symptoms of dyspepsia, pancreatitis, and diffuse nonspecific abdominal pain. Although frequently cited as a significant association, the relationship between peptic ulcer disease and hyperparathyroidism is under debate. Pancreatitis with associated severe abdominal pain is most likely directly related to the elevated calcium level. Diffuse abdominal pain unrelated to pancreatitis is seen in only a small percentage of patients, and the pain resolves following curative surgery. Nausea, vomiting, anorexia, constipation, and weight loss are all symptoms of hypercalcemia and are seen in 20-30% of cases of hyperparathyroidism. Hypertension is seen in a large percentage (20-50%) of patients with hyperparathyroidism, but because it is also seen frequently (20%) in the general population, one cannot be certain of a causative relationship in a given case. A radiographic profile of bone may show decreased density with widespread "punched-out" lesions. Joint pain and clubbing may also be observed.

Diagnosis

The diagnosis of primary hyperparathyroidism has traditionally been a difficult one to make with absolute certainty. This is because in the past, the assays for parathyroid hormone (PTH) were far from satisfactory. Parathyroid hormone circulates in a variety of active and inactive molecular forms. These have been categorized as C-terminal fragments, N-terminal fragments, mid-molecule fragments, and intact molecule. The half-lives of the intact molecule and the N-terminal fragments in the circulation are very short (5-6 min) so these species of PTH circulate in the lowest concentrations. Because the analytic sensitivity of previous assays was not adequate to accurately measure such low concentrations of hormone, earlier assays avoided measurement of the intact molecule or N-terminal fragment. C-terminal or mid-molecule assays were the test of choice because these fragments have a half-life of 30-40 min and therefore circulate in much higher concentrations than the intact molecule. In general mid-molecule fragments are more immunogenic than other PTH fragments, making mid-molecule assays technically very sensitive and easy to perform. Nevertheless, mid-molecule and C-terminal assays have several deficiencies: they do not measure the biologically active hormone; increased serum concentrations occur in patients with renal failure; and they show apparent cross-reactivity with other peptides found in normal sera. Bioassays for PTH, either direct (using cell cultures) or indirect (measuring urinary cyclic AMP), are seldom useful; moreover, these assays are difficult to perform.

More recently developed immunometric assays for intact PTH have analytical sensitivity adequate to distinguish hyperparathyroid patients from those with hypercalcemia of malignancy.[2] Results for the two groups, as determined with the older assays, often significantly overlap. Approximately 90% of patients with hyperparathyroidism will have absolute elevations of their PTH by these newer assays. The remaining 10% will have PTH values that are inappropriately elevated for the degree of hypercalcemia.[3] For this reason, it is important to obtain a concurrent ionized calcium whenever a PTH is ordered.

Concentrations of intact PTH are not always abnormal in patients with primary hyper-parathyroidism. Other laboratory tests helpful for diagnosis depend on the clinical circum-stances. Ionized calcium assay is the first choice of testing for the patient presenting with signs or symptoms of hyperparathyroidism. Ionized calcium, which is 45-50% of the total calcium, better indicates clinical state than does a value for total calcium and thus is a more sensitive marker for hyperparathyroidism than is PTH. If ionized and total calcium levels are persistently normal, then a diagnosis of hyperparathyroidism is essentially ruled out. If the calcium is elevated and the PTH is in the high normal range, hyperparathyroidism remains the most likely diagnosis.

Patients with hyperparathyroidism tend to have increased urine calcium excretion, low serum phosphorus, and increased urine phosphorus, as well as elevated 1α,25-dihydroxy-vitamin D levels. These abnormalities are the direct result of PTH action on renal tubular function. Even so, vitamin D levels are seldom needed for confirmation of a diagnosis of primary hyperparathyroidism; moreover, vitamin D assays are technically difficult to perform. These patients also tend to have high or high normal serum chloride, again the result of PTH effect on the renal tubule. The chloride/phosphorus ratio is another useful test for evaluating the probability of hyperparathyroidism. A value ≥29 is associated with almost all cases of hyperparathyroidism; a lower ratio makes the diagnosis unlikely.[4] In the hypercalcemic patient the ratio is particularly helpful for ruling out hyperparathyroidism and rapidly focusing attention on the possibility of hypercalcemia secondary to malignancy.

The calcium versus PTH diagram (Figure 1) can be very helpful in evaluating and interpreting PTH results and concurrent calcium values. Using this figure, there is clear-cut separation between the patients with hypercalcemia of malignancy and those with primary hyperparathyroidism.

It is sometimes difficult to distinguish hypercalcemia of malignancy from primary hyper-parathyroidism. Recently, immunometric assays for parathyroid hormone-related peptide (PTHrP) have been developed and may be of diagnostic help in these situations. PTHrP has many of the same biological effects as PTH. Unlike PTH, however, PTHrP concentrations are within reference limits in patients with primary hyperparathyroidism and in patients with chronic renal failure.[5,6]

Treatment

In cases of significant hypercalcemia, especially if symptomatic, serum calcium should be promptly decreased, even as an etiological cause is being sought. Intravenous fluids and furosemide (oral or intravenous) produce a decrease by increasing renal excretion of calcium. A very high serum calcium level or presence of life-threatening symptoms calls for more extreme measures, such as treatment with plicamycin or synthetic salmon calcitonin to achieve an acute drop in serum calcium level.[7]

Definitive therapy of the hyperparathyroid patient consists of removal of the adenoma-tous or hyperplastic tissue. In most instances, surgical exploration of the neck will identify the tissue and will lead to curative removal. When localization is difficult, venous catheter-ization studies and determination of afferent and efferent PTH levels may be necessary.

Asymptomatic hyperparathyroid patients present a particularly difficult management problem. Approximately 25% of those with a serum calcium level of <11 mg/dL (<2.74 mmol/L) will in the long run develop complications of hyperparathyroidism (nephro-lithiasis, decreased creatinine clearance, or hypertension) to a degree requiring consideration of surgery.[8] Since no one can predict which of these individuals will develop complications, surgery is recommended as a preventive measure.

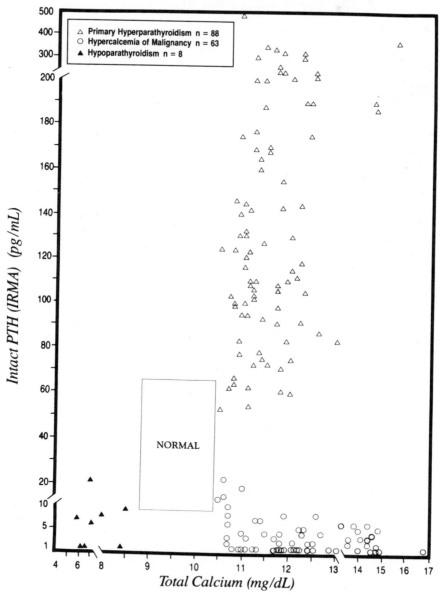

Figure 1. Intact PTH (IRMA) and total calcium in various disease states. (Reproduced with permission from: Pandian, M.R., Lavigne, J.R., Carlton, E.I., et al.: Immunoradiometric Assay for Intact PTH: A New Generation of PTH Assay for Assessment of Parathyroid Function. San Juan Capistrano, CA, Nichols Institute Reference Laboratories, 1989. Illustration courtesy of Nichols Institute Reference Laboratories.)

References

1.   Broadus, A.E.: Mineral metabolism. *In:* Endocrinology and Metabolism. P. Felig, J.D. Baxter, A.E. Broadus, and L.A. Frohman, Eds. New York, McGraw-Hill, 1981.

2.   Endres, D.B., Villanueva, R., Sharp, C.F., Jr., and Singer, F.R.: Immunochemilumino-metric and immunoradiometric determinations of intact and total immunoreactive parathyrin: Performance in the differential diagnosis of hypercalcemia and hypopara-thyroidism. Clin. Chem., *37:* 162-167, 1991.

3.   Howanitz, P.J., and Howanitz, J.H.: Calcium metabolism. *In:* Laboratory Medicine: Test Selection and Interpretation. J.H. Howanitz, P.J. Howanitz, et al., Eds. New York, Churchill Livingstone, Inc., 1991.

4.   Wong, E.T., and Frier, E.F.: The differential diagnosis of hypercalcemia: An algorithm for more effective use of laboratory tests. JAMA, *247:* 75-80, 1982.

5.   Bilezikian, J.P.: Parathyroid hormone-related peptide in sickness and health. N. Engl. J. Med., *332:* 1151-1153, 1990.

6.   Kao, P.C., Klee, G.G., Taylor, R.L., and Heath, H.: Parathyroid hormone-related peptide in plasma of patients with hypercalcemia and malignant lesions. Mayo Clin. Proc., *65:* 1399-1407, 1990.

7.   Garcia, J.C.: Mineral, parathyroid, and metabolic bone diseases. *In:* Manual of Medical Therapeutics, 26th ed. W.C. Dunagan and M.C. Ridner, Eds. St. Louis, Department of Medicine, Washington University, 1989.

8.   Scholz, D.A., and Purnell, D.C.: Asymptomatic primary hyperparathyroidism: 10-year prospective study. Mayo Clin. Proc., *56:* 473-478, 1981.

A CHILD WITH OSTEOPENIA AND RETARDED GROWTH

William H. Porter, Contributor
Richard A. Mc Pherson, Reviewer

Although normal at birth, this two-year-old white male had failed to grow and develop adequately. His appetite had been poor since birth, and he experienced vomiting and low weight gain. Measurement of sweat chloride had ruled out cystic fibrosis. When he was hospitalized at eight months of age, the following laboratory results had been obtained:

Analyte	Value, conventional units	Reference range, conventional units	Value, SI units	Reference range, SI units
Sodium (S)	148 mmol/L	139-146	Same	
Potassium (S)	7.6 mmol/L	4.1-5.3	Same	
Chloride (S)	114 mmol/L	98-108	Same	
CO_2, total (S)	15 mmol/L	20-28	Same	
Urea nitrogen (S)	105 mg/dL	5-18	37.5 mmol urea/L	1.8-6.4
Creatinine (S)	2.2 mg/dL	0.2-0.4	195 µmol/L	18-35
Calcium, total (S)	7.0 mg/dL	9-11	1.75 mmol/L	2.25-2.75
Phosphorus (S)	12.3 mg/dL	4.5-6.7	3.97 mmol/L	1.45-2.16
PTH, intact (S)	890 pg/mL	15-60	95.6 pmol/L	1.6-6.4
ALP (S)	480 U/L	124-255	8.0 µkat/L	2.1-4.3
Osteocalcin (S)	322 ng/mL	10-25	322 µg/L	10-25
1,25(OH)$_2$D (S)	6 pg/mL	15-60	14 pmol/L	36-144
25(OH)D (S)	34 ng/mL	9-52	85 nmol/L	23-130
pH (aB)	7.26	7.35-7.45	Same	
pCO_2 (aB)	27 mm Hg	27-41	3.6 kPa	3.6-5.5
pO_2 (aB)	93 mm Hg	83-108	12.4 kPa	11.1-14.4
Hematocrit (B)	22 %	30-40	0.22	0.30-0.40

Cystoscopy and retrograde pyelography at that time revealed evidence of aplasia of the right and hypoplasia of the left kidney. A clinical diagnosis of renal osteodystrophy was made.

His acidosis was corrected with sodium bicarbonate, and he was transfused for his anemia. Administration of 1,25-dihydroxyvitamin D [1,25(OH)$_2$D], calcium gluconate, and aluminum hydroxide-containing gel (Amphojel) was prescribed prior to discharge.

His current admission at age two was for respiratory difficulty and tremors of the extremities. He appeared malnourished and was extremely irritable. He had 10 teeth, but they lacked enamel. The following laboratory results were found:

Analyte	Value, conventional units	Reference range, conventional units	Value, SI units	Reference range, SI units
Sodium (S)	118 mmol/L	139-146	Same	
Potassium (S)	7.7 mmol/L	4.1-5.3	Same	
Chloride (S)	92 mmol/L	98-108	Same	
CO_2, total (S)	10 mmol/L	20-28	Same	

Analyte	Value, conventional units	Reference range, conventional units	Value, SI units	Reference range, SI units
Urea nitrogen (S)	250 mg/dL	5-18	89.3 mmol urea/L	1.8-6.4
Creatinine (S)	4.2 mg/dL	0.2-0.4	371 μmol/L	18-35
Calcium, total (S)	11.4 mg/dL	9-11	2.84 mmol/L	2.25-2.75
Phosphorus (S)	16.4 mg/dL	4.5-6.7	5.30 mmol/L	1.45-2.16
PTH, intact (S)	560 pg/mL	15-60	60.1 pmol/L	1.6-6.4
ALP (S)	320 U/L	124-255	5.3 μkat/L	2.1-4.3
pH (aB)	7.19	7.35-7.45	Same	
pCO_2 (aB)	28 mm Hg	27-41	3.7 kPa	3.6-5.5
pO_2 (aB)	72 mm Hg	83-108	9.6 kPa	11.1-14.4
Hematocrit (B)	18 %	30-40	0.18	0.30-0.40

X-ray studies showed flaring of the anterior edges of the ribs, marked irregularity and resorption of the femoral and humeral heads, generalized decrease in bone density, and calcification of peripheral arteries. There was marked subperiosteal bone resorption of the middle phalanges.

An attempt was made to place the patient on peritoneal dialysis in preparation for renal transplantation. His acidosis was very difficult to control, and administration of small amounts of fluid aggravated his respiratory difficulty and resulted in congestive heart failure. Following two respiratory arrests, he was placed on a respirator. He developed sepsis and died of cardiac arrest on the 10th hospital day.

Among the findings at autopsy were evidence of severe osteitis fibrosa, marked hyperplasia of the parathyroid glands, and the presence of modest amounts of stainable aluminum in bone. Aplasia of the right kidney and hypoplasia of the left kidney were confirmed. A diagnosis of renal osteodystrophy secondary to congenital kidney disease was made.

Etiology of Renal Osteodystrophy[1-3]

Renal osteodystrophy denotes metabolic bone disease associated with chronic renal failure. Its development is related to diminished conversion by the proximal tubular 1-α-hydroxylase enzyme of 25(OH)D (produced in the liver) to the many-times more active 1,25(OH)₂D.

The 1-α-hydroxylase enzyme is inhibited by increased levels of inorganic phosphorus. Thus, as renal disease progresses and glomerular filtration rate (GFR) declines and phosphate retention ensues, the formation of 1,25(OH)₂D is diminished. Furthermore, synthesis of 1,25(OH)₂D declines directly as a result of loss of functional nephrons.

With less 1,25(OH)₂D, intestinal absorption of dietary calcium is reduced, contributing to lower serum calcium. Moreover, the elevated serum phosphate complexes with calcium, thereby further depressing ionized calcium. This reduction of serum ionized calcium stimulates even greater release of parathyroid hormone (PTH) and development of secondary hyperparathyroidism. 1,25-Dihydroxyvitamin D normally inhibits PTH secretion, and thus reductions of this vitamin may contribute to the secondary hyperparathyroidism of renal failure.

PTH acts synergistically with 1,25(OH)₂D to stimulate bone turnover (bone formation and resorption). Thus, the low ionized calcium is initially compensated by the PTH-mediated release of calcium from bone. Additionally, the set-point for calcium-regulated PTH secretion may be elevated in renal failure; sustained PTH secretion may occur in normocalcemic or even hypercalcemic patients.[4] Reduced $1,25(OH)_2D$ may contribute to the altered calcium set-point.[5] The increased action of PTH on bone is evident histologically in about half the patients whose GFR has declined to 50% or less.

As renal disease progresses, the PTH responsiveness of bone is diminished, mediated at least in part by further decrements in $1,25(OH)_2D$ synthesis. The rate of bone resorption eventually is insufficient to offset the deficit in intestinal calcium absorption, and hypocalcemia develops along with further increases in serum PTH. Moreover, the decline in $1,25(OH)_2D$ contributes to the increased serum PTH by diminished feedback inhibition. Thus, the parathyroid glands may undergo marked hyperplasia.

In addition to acceleration of PTH-mediated resorption of bone, mineralization defects may also occur when the GFR falls below 40 mL/min. The mineralization defect (osteomalacia) presumably results from diminished $1,25(OH)_2D$ and lesser availability of calcium. Defective mineralization may also occur as a consequence of aluminum deposition in bone and of metabolic acidosis associated with end-stage renal disease. Patients with chronic renal failure are often treated with aluminum-containing phosphate-binding gels to inhibit intestinal phosphate absorption and thus lower serum phosphate concentrations. Such patients are therefore at increased risk of aluminum accumulation and deposition in bone.

Bone Pathology in Renal Osteodystrophy[1,2]

Based on histomorphometric indices, there are two major aspects to the bone disease in renal osteodystrophy, one that displays a high rate of bone turnover and another displaying low turnover.

A major determinant of *high-turnover renal osteodystrophy* is elevated PTH. Hyperparathyroid bone disease (osteitis fibrosa) is characterized by increased numbers of osteoclasts, osteoblasts, and osteocytes. Disorderly production of collagen may occur on the trabecular surface or in the marrow cavity and may cause peritrabecular and marrow fibrosis. Increased osteoclastic resorption leads to thinning of cortex and trabeculae. This bone loss may be evident on X-ray examination, especially the subperiosteal resorption occurring at the radial aspects of phalanges.

Low-turnover renal osteodystrophy is characterized by a marked decrease in the number of osteoblasts and osteoclasts and a diminished bone apposition rate. Often there is also accumulation of lamellar osteoid, a condition referred to as low-turnover osteomalacia. Some patients have low bone turnover and depressed mineralization but without accumulation of osteoid. This adynamic bone condition is referred to as "aplastic" bone.

Low-turnover osteomalacia differs from classic vitamin D-deficiency osteomalacia in that patients are refractory to the administration of $1,25(OH)_2D$, they have an increased incidence of bone fractures, and they are likely to experience debilitating bone pain. The associated biochemical features include normal or moderately elevated alkaline phosphatase and PTH and a tendency to hypercalcemia.

The etiological factors responsible for low-turnover osteomalacia or "aplastic" bone are not well understood. In a high proportion of such patients, marked deposition of aluminum in bone is evident.[6] The aluminum accumulates predominantly at the calcification front between the calcified matrix and osteoid. The principal source of the aluminum in patients with renal osteodystrophy is aluminum-containing phosphate-binding gels. Aluminum is known to inhibit bone formation (inhibit osteoblastic activity), to suppress PTH release from the parathyroid gland, and to interfere with bone mineralization. Such actions of aluminum might account for the low-turnover osteomalacia often associated with its deposition in bone.

Yet some patients with high-turnover osteodystrophy have increased bone aluminum, although generally not to the same degree as do those with low-turnover osteomalacia.

Metabolic bone disease in renal osteodystrophy is clearly complex. Patients with moderate to advanced renal failure who are on maintenance dialysis may have concurrent hyperparathyroid bone disease (osteitis fibrosa) and mineralization defects (osteomalacia). Occasionally there is even evidence of osteosclerosis. The bone disease in such patients has been referred to as mixed uremic osteodystrophy. However, in some patients the bone disease is almost entirely osteitis fibrosa, whereas others may have a marked predominance of low-turnover osteomalacia. The undefined role of aluminum in modifying the underlying bone disease and its association with low-turnover osteomalacia adds to the complexity. Some investigators consider aluminum-related bone disease a separate entity. Regardless, the distinction between hyperparathyroid bone disease and aluminum-related bone disease is important because therapeutic approaches in each condition are different.

The patient in this case had X-ray evidence of substantial bone resorption, marked parathyroid hyperplasia with elevated serum PTH, and severe osteitis fibrosa. There was modest stainable aluminum in bone. Thus, this child's bone disease was predominantly high-turnover hyperparathyroid renal osteodystrophy.

Hypercalcemia in Renal Osteodystrophy[7]

Although hypocalcemia is more common in renal osteodystrophy, some patients develop hypercalcemia from excessive therapy with $1,25(OH)_2D$ or calcium supplements or their combination. Marked hyperplasia of the parathyroid gland leading to "autonomous" secretion* of PTH ("tertiary" hyperparathyroidism) has also been suspected as a cause of hypercalcemia. Indeed parathyroidectomy may benefit some patients. Hypercalcemia may also be frequently associated with aluminum-related low-turnover osteomalacia presumably because deposits of aluminum at bone surfaces block normal mineralization with calcium from the blood.[8]

The patient in this case initially presented with hypocalcemia (age eight months) but then developed hypercalcemia by two years of age. The hypercalcemia occurred after administration of $1,25(OH)_2D$, calcium gluconate, and aluminum hydroxide. Children with renal osteodystrophy are especially prone to aluminum toxicity,[9] but aluminum-related bone disease was not evident in this child. Thus, the hypercalcemia in this patient was the result of "tertiary" hyperparathyroidism (the parathyroid glands were markedly hyperplastic) or vitamin D and calcium therapy, or a combination of these.

Laboratory Evaluation of Renal Osteodystrophy[1,2]

Useful biochemical parameters for the assessment of renal osteodystrophy include routine measurements of serum calcium, inorganic phosphorus, creatinine, urea nitrogen, and alkaline phosphatase. Additional important measurements include those for serum PTH, $1,25(OH)_2D$, osteocalcin, and aluminum.

Osteocalcin (bone Gla protein) is the major noncollagenous protein component of osteoid that, like alkaline phosphatase, is produced by osteoblasts. Increased serum levels of osteocalcin and alkaline phosphatase (in the absence of liver disease) are thus an indication of enhanced bone turnover. Osteocalcin, alkaline phosphatase, and PTH are all

---

* An altered set-point for calcium modulation of PTH secretion may be associated with the hyperplasia.

elevated to a more significant degree in patients with high-turnover osteodystrophy (osteitis fibrosa) than in those with low-turnover osteomalacia. However, biochemical parameters do not always distinguish between these two bone disorders, especially in hypercalcemic patients. The laboratory data for the patient in this case support the diagnosis of chronic renal failure and high-turnover osteodystrophy.

Newer methods for PTH determinations measure the intact molecule, compared with older and less specific methods that detected C-terminal and mid-molecule PTH fragments. These PTH degradation fragments are normally eliminated by the kidney but accumulate in the blood during renal failure. Thus, in patients with end-stage renal disease, disproportionate elevations in the PTH fragments occur in serum, and the preferred PTH measurement is for the intact molecule.

Although the measurement of serum aluminum is helpful to identify patients at risk for aluminum-related bone disease, such measurements cannot determine which patients actually have this disorder. A deferoxamine challenge test to detect aluminum overload has been proposed,[10] but its reliability is controversial.[2]

Bone biopsy, in association with tetracycline double labeling and aluminum staining, is the most reliable means to diagnose renal osteodystrophy and to distinguish among the various forms of the disorder.

Treatment for Renal Osteodystrophy[1,2]

The goal of therapy for renal osteodystrophy is to control the hyperphosphatemia and to alleviate the secondary hyperparathyroidism. Hyperphosphatemia may be treated by decreasing dietary intake of phosphate, by eliminating phosphate with dialysis, and by using phosphate-binding gels to decrease intestinal phosphate absorption. These gels often contain aluminum and thus place patients at increased risk of developing aluminum-related bone disease. If aluminum overload occurs, chelation therapy with deferoxamine to mobilize aluminum from tissues is required. Secondary hyperparathyroidism may be alleviated by the administration of 1-α-hydroxyvitamin D or 1,25(OH)$_2$D and calcium salts.

Parathyroidectomy may be necessary to control hypercalcemia in patients with mixed uremic osteodystrophy or those with predominantly osteitis fibrosa. On the other hand, hypercalcemic patients with aluminum-related low-turnover osteomalacia require chelation therapy and should not undergo parathyroidectomy, which may be detrimental.

References

1. Sherrard, D.J., and Andress, D.L.: Renal osteodystrophy. *In:* Diseases of the Kidney, 4th ed. R.W. Schrier and C.W. Gottschalk, Eds. Boston, Little, Brown and Co., 1988.

2. Malluche, H., and Faugere, M.-C.: Renal bone disease 1990: An unmet challenge for the nephrologist. Kidney Int., *38:* 193-211, 1990.

3. Llach, F., and Massry, S.G.: On the mechanism of secondary hyperparathyroidism in moderate renal insufficiency. J. Clin. Endocrinol. Metab., *61:* 601-606, 1985.

4. Brown, E.M., Wilson, R.E., Eastman, R.C., et al.: Abnormal regulation of parathyroid hormone release by calcium in secondary hyperparathyroidism due to chronic renal failure. J. Clin. Endocrinol. Metab., *54:* 172-179, 1982.

5. Delmez, J., Tindira, C., Grooms, P., et al.: Parathyroid hormone suppression by intravenous 1,25-dihydroxyvitamin D. J. Clin. Invest., *81:* 1349-1355, 1989.

6. Ott, S.M., Maloney, N.A., Coburn, J.W., et al.: The prevalence of bone aluminum deposition in renal osteodystrophy and its relation to the response to calcitriol therapy. N. Engl. J. Med., *307:* 709-713, 1982.

7. Piraino, B.M., Rault, R., Greenberg, A., et al.: Spontaneous hypercalcemia in patients undergoing dialysis. Am. J. Med., *80:* 607-615, 1986.

8. Piraino, B., Chen, T., and Puschett, J.B.: Elevated bone aluminum and suppressed parathyroid hormone levels in hypercalcemic dialysis patients. Am. J. Nephrol., *9:* 190-197, 1989.

9. Andreoli, S.P., Bergstein, J.M., and Sherrard, D.J.: Aluminum intoxication from aluminum-containing phosphate binders in children with azotemia not undergoing dialysis. N. Engl. J. Med., *310:* 1079-1084, 1984.

10. Millner, D.S., Nebeker, H.G., Ott, S.M., et al.: Use of the deferoxamine infusion test in the diagnosis of aluminum-related osteodystrophy. Ann. Intern. Med., *101:* 775-780, 1984.

EPISODIC HYPERTENSION

Gordon P. Guthrie, Jr., Contributor

A 35-year-old computer company executive was noted at his annual physical examination to have an elevated blood pressure. His blood pressure was 188/112 mm Hg in the left arm when seated. During each of his past two annual physical examinations, mild elevations in his blood pressure were also noted. These were, respectively, 160/94 mm Hg two years ago and 158/92 mm Hg one year ago. During the past two years, he had also noted occasional unusual episodes occurring approximately twice every month, characterized by a sensation of apprehension, moderately severe frontal headache, profuse perspiration, and rapid heart beat. These episodes seemed to have no clear precipitating factor, were abrupt in onset, and lasted approximately 10 to 15 minutes. During the episodes, his wife commented that his complexion appeared to become pale and his lips became blanched.

Physical examination, about 30 minutes after the above initial blood pressure reading, revealed his blood pressure again to be elevated at 178/110 mm Hg in the seated posture, with a pulse rate of 90 BPM. After three minutes of standing upright, his blood pressure was 152/94 mm Hg and his pulse rate 112 BPM. His optic fundi showed that his retinal arterioles were moderately narrowed; no hemorrhages or exudates were seen.

The following laboratory measurements were obtained during the initial appraisal of his hypertension:

Analyte	Value, conventional units	Reference range, conventional units	Value, SI units	Reference range, SI units
Sodium (S)	139 mmol/L	136-145	Same	
Potassium (S)	4.6 mmol/L	3.8-5.1	Same	
Chloride (S)	109 mmol/L	96-108	Same	
CO_2, total (S)	24 mmol/L	23-30	Same	
Urea nitrogen (S)	12 mg/dL	7-18	4.3 mmol urea/L	2.5-6.4
Creatinine (S)	1.0 mg/dL	0.7-1.3	88 µmol/L	62-115
Glucose (S)	99 mg/dL	75-105	5.5 mmol/L	4.2-5.8
Protein, total (S)	6.0 g/dL	6.0-7.8	60 g/L	60-78
Albumin (S)	3.9 g/dL	3.5-5.0	39 g/L	35-50
Urate (S)	6.0 mg/dL	4.5-8.0	357 µmol/L	268-476
Cholesterol (S)	210 mg/dL	140-220	5.43 mmol/L	3.62-5.69

A chest film showed his heart to be normal size, and an electrocardiogram showed minimal ST and T wave abnormalities in the lateral precordial leads, suggesting early left ventricular hypertrophy. Because of symptoms suggesting overactivity of the sympathetic nervous system, a random plasma specimen and 24-h urine were collected, and the following results were obtained:

Analyte	Value, conventional units	Reference range, conventional units	Value, SI units	Reference range, SI units
Vanillylmandelic acid (VMA) (U)	12.5 mg/d	2-7	63 µmol/d	10-35
Norepinephrine (U)	1800 µg/d	15-80	10,638 nmol/d	89-473

Analyte	Value, conventional units	Reference range, conventional units	Value, SI units	Reference range, SI units
Epinephrine (U)	100 µg/d	0-20	546 nmol/d	0-109
Metanephrines, total (U)	2.5 mg/d	<1.0	13 µmol/d	<5
Catecholamines (P)				
Norepinephrine	2500 pg/mL	174-624	14.78 nmol/L	1.03-3.69
Epinephrine	85 pg/mL	0-114	464 pmol/L	0-622

Because of his symptoms and abnormal laboratory values for catecholamines and catecholamine metabolites, a presumptive diagnosis of a pheochromocytoma was made. To localize the lesion, computed tomographic examination of the adrenals was performed; an 8-cm mass in the region of the left adrenal gland was seen. This mass was irregular in shape with a relatively radiolucent center. The patient was subsequently treated with a long-acting β-adrenergic blocker (nadolol) and an α-adrenergic blocker (phenoxybenzamine) for several weeks. During this interval, he had no further paroxysms, and his blood pressure remained consistently at approximately 110/78 mm Hg. He then underwent abdominal surgery, during which a 250-g pheochromocytoma was removed.

Definition of the Disease

A pheochromocytoma is a tumor of the adrenal gland or other catecholamine-secreting tissue that releases epinephrine or norepinephrine, or both. Clinical signs and symptoms are attributable to the release of these vasoactive hormones. Pheochromocytoma is a potentially fatal disorder because of the severe hypertension and cardiac arrhythmias caused by catecholamine surges. However, it is curable if detected in time.

Catecholamine biosynthesis usually occurs in sympathetic neurons, in so-called chromaffin tissue. Most chromaffin cells are in sympathetic nerve endings, including the paravertebral sympathetic chain. Almost all chromaffin tissue is capable of secreting norepinephrine, the major hormone produced by the sympathetic nervous system as both a neurotransmitter and circulating hormone. Specialized populations of chromaffin cells are further capable of producing epinephrine, predominantly a circulating hormone. The signs and symptoms of pheochromocytoma derive directly from the excessive norepinephrine or epinephrine or both secreted by these tumors.

Clinical Features. Pheochromocytoma often presents with dramatic clinical features; the triad of headache, diaphoresis, and palpitations is frequently present. Hypertension is quite common (90% of patients) and may be either sustained or intermittent. Many patients have "attacks" or paroxysms and episodic symptoms that suggest periodic release of large amounts of catecholamines. Seventy-five percent of patients with pheochromocytoma experience one or more symptomatic hypertensive attacks weekly; the attacks are often abrupt in onset and subside somewhat slowly. In most patients, they last less than one hour, but they may last a minute or as long as a week. Some attacks may be precipitated by pressure in the region of the tumor. The pressure may be initiated by bending over, by urination (some tumors occur in the wall of the urinary bladder), or by ingestion of foods or beverages (such as some cheeses or wines) that contain catecholamine-like substances capable of displacing norepinephrine or epinephrine from tumors.

Besides hypertension, headache is the most common symptom of pheochromocytoma, and it usually is quite severe and throbbing during a paroxysmal attack. Sweating, the next most common symptom, is usually generalized and often profuse. Other symptoms include anxiety, apprehension, palpitations, and a rapid heart beat, often with peak heart rates occurring during the paroxysmal attack; all are typical features of catecholamine release. Many patients lose weight, probably because of an increased metabolic rate caused by stimulation by the excess catecholamines.

A characteristic feature of these tumors is a marked fall in blood pressure when changing from the sitting or supine to the upright posture. In some patients, this fall in blood pressure is so remarkable that they develop syncope or near-syncope when they stand. This change in pressure occurs because of the profound vasoconstriction and depletion of the intracellular plasma volume as a result of sustained catecholamine exposure. Many patients develop constipation, even to the point of symptoms resembling intestinal obstruction. The pallor of the skin and lips during attacks is thought to be due to the vasoconstrictive action of catecholamines on the skin. Marked increases in both systolic and diastolic pressure occur in patients during paroxysmal attacks, although approximately one-half of all patients with pheochromocytoma have sustained increases in blood pressure without paroxysms.

Several pathological features of pheochromocytoma occur with a coincidental frequency of about 10%. For example, about 10% of such tumors are familial, in that they are part of an inherited pattern of endocrine tumors termed multiple endocrine neoplasia (MEN) 2 or 3. This is an autosomal dominant disorder having variable occurrence of pheochromocytoma, medullary thyroid cancer, mucosal neuroma, and thickened corneal nerves. Ten percent of pheochromocytomas occur outside the adrenal gland (along the chromaffin sympathetic chain), 10% are bilateral, and 10% are malignant.

Diagnosis

Any patient with a significantly elevated blood pressure might be a potential suspect for pheochromocytoma, although less than 1% of even severely hypertensive patients will prove to have this condition. Many clinicians believe that any patient with moderately severe or severe hypertension and any of the signs or symptoms of pheochromocytoma should be carefully scrutinized for the disease with an appropriate laboratory screening test. It is believed that a combination of clinical evaluation, laboratory studies, and imaging studies with high resolution scanners rarely fails to diagnose pheochromocytoma. In symptomatic hypertensives, a normal test for plasma or urinary catecholamines or vanillylmandelic acid (VMA) has a negative predictive value of >0.98.

The measurement of catecholamines and metabolites in a 24-h urine collection is the most reliable technique for screening for this disorder; 95% of the patients with pheochromocytoma have elevated urinary levels. VMA is a major metabolite of norepinephrine and epinephrine and is frequently elevated. Urinary metanephrines, which include metanephrine and normetanephrine, are metabolites proximal to VMA in the metabolic pathway and are also usually elevated. Finally, the catecholamines themselves, free norepinephrine and epinephrine, also appear in urine in excess in patients with pheochromocytoma (see Figure 1). VMA, metanephrines, free norepinephrine, and free epinephrine can all be determined on a single 24-h urine collection, to which hydrochloric acid is added as a preservative. Free urinary catecholamines and metanephrine seem to have an advantage (88% positive) over VMA (86% positive). Combination testing is recommended since some tumors will secrete only one or the other metabolite. Small tumors secrete more free catecholamines, whereas large tumors, having marked intratumor metabolism, excrete more metabolites. Laboratory values are increased more consistently and more significantly during hypertensive periods. On the other hand, there are 2-12% of patients with hypertension, without pheochromocytoma, who have increased catecholamine or metabolite values. In these cases, however, elevations are generally <50% above the upper limit of the reference range.

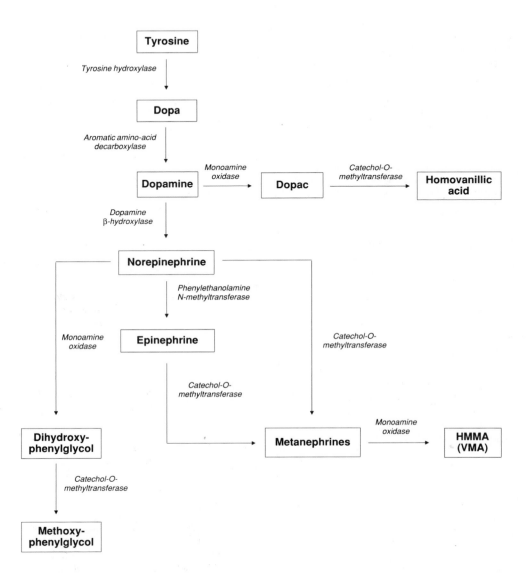

Figure 1. Simplified metabolic pathway of catecholamines.

Dopac = dihydroxyphenylacetic acid; HMMA = 4-hydroxy-3-methoxymandelic acid; VMA = vanillyl-mandelic acid. (Modified after Clauson, R.C., and Brown, M.J.: Ann. Clin. Biochem., *19:* 396, 1982, and Brown, M.J.: Eur. J. Clin. Invest., *14:* 67, 1984.)

Most recently, sensitive and specific techniques for measurement of plasma catecholamines have been added to the available diagnostic tests. Values <1000 pg/mL (<5.91 nmol/L) tend to exclude tumors, values between 1000 and 2000 pg/mL (5.91 and 11.82 nmol/L) are suspicious, and values ≥ 2000 pg/mL (≥11.82 nmol/L) are considered diagnostic (SI unit conversion factor based on molecular weight of norepinephrine of 169.18). Plasma catecholamine measurements are most discriminating when elevated levels are found at a time when levels are normally low, such as after administration of a drug like clonidine, which suppresses activity of the sympathetic nervous system. During periods of normotension, plasma values in patients with pheochromocytoma may be normal.

When a clinical and laboratory diagnosis of pheochromocytoma has been made, the task then is to localize the tumor. Computed tomography (CT) is extremely accurate in identifying lesions with a diameter of 1 cm or more in the adrenals or 2 cm or more in extra-adrenal locations. Magnetic resonance imaging (MRI) is equally sensitive. If a CT of the adrenals fails to reveal the presence of a tumor, CT scanning of other areas along the sympathetic chain is indicated; however, in extra-adrenal tumors, MRI is more reliable. These areas include the urinary bladder, the paravertebral sympathetic chain, and the neck. Some pheochromocytomas are very difficult to find, but these cases are rare. A new radiopharmaceutical agent, radioiodinated *m*-iodobenzylguanidine (MIBG), is taken up by pheochromocytomas, and thus nuclear scanning techniques may localize the agent and the tumor.

Treatment

Since the pathophysiological changes of pheochromocytoma are caused by the catecholamines produced by these tumors, blockade of the hormone effects relieves the signs and symptoms of the syndrome. α-Adrenergic blockers interfere with the vasoconstrictive actions of norepinephrine and epinephrine and are essential in the preoperative management of these patients. The preferable medication is phenoxybenzamine, a long-acting α-adrenergic blocker. Alternatives are prazosin, terazosin, or doxazosin, which are shorter acting agents. Many patients have β-adrenergic mediated symptoms, including tachycardia, which are usually most dramatic in epinephrine-secreting pheochromocytomas. For these patients, β-adrenergic blockade is essential, again with use of long-acting and potent agents such as nadolol or atenolol. Alternatively, labetalol, a combined α- and β-adrenergic blocker, may also be used. When the adrenergic effects of circulating catecholamines have been fully neutralized by drug therapy, a matter often of several weeks, the localized tumor is then removed by surgery.

Additional Reading

Bravo, E.L.: Diagnosis of pheochromocytoma. Hypertension, *17:* 742-744, 1991.

Grossman, G., Goldstein, D.S., Hoffman, A., and Keiser, H.: Glucagon and clonidine testing in the diagnosis of pheochromocytoma. Hypertension, *17:* 733-741, 1991.

Manger, W.M., and Gifford, R.W. Jr.: Hypertension secondary to pheochromocytoma. Bull. N.Y. Acad. Med., *58:* 139-158, 1982.

Stein, P.P., and Black, H.R.: A simplified diagnostic approach to pheochromocytoma. Medicine, *70:* 46-66, 1990.

Van Heerden, J.A., Sheps, S.G., and Hamberger, B.: Pheochromocytoma: Current status and changing trends. Surgery, *91:* 367-373, 1982.

DIARRHEA AND GASTROINTESTINAL HEMORRHAGE

A. Ralph Henderson, Contributor

A 54-year-old male office worker was admitted because of a one-year history of severe diarrhea and recurrent gastrointestinal hemorrhage; during this period he lost 44 lb (20 kg). The patient had evidence of malnutrition — paresthesias and altered sensation, angular stomatitis and cheilosis, and a pellagra-like dermatitis — and his clothes had clearly become too large for him. He commented that his belt had to be tightened three more inches than formerly. He was not jaundiced. He complained of epigastric pain that occurred 2-3 hours after meals, often awakened him at night, and was relieved by alkali and food. The troublesome diarrhea consisted of an increased frequency of bowel movements that were also more fluid than previously.

Blood pressure and pulse were normal. The abdomen was soft, and there was no guarding; on deep palpation, midline epigastric pain was elicited.

The following laboratory values were obtained:

Analyte	Value, conventional units	Reference range, conventional units	Value, SI units	Reference range, SI units
Sodium (S)	136 mmol/L	135-145	Same	
Potassium (S)	3.1 mmol/L	3.5-5.0	Same	
Chloride (S)	81 mmol/L	95-107	Same	
Bicarbonate (S)	35 mmol/L	24-32	Same	
Anion gap (S)	20 mmol/L	8-16	Same	
Creatinine (S)	0.5 mg/dL	0.8-1.6	44 µmol/L	70-140
Urea nitrogen (S)	5 mg/dL	7-18	1.8 mmol urea /L	3.0-6.5
Glucose (S)	60 mg/dL	61-126	3.3 mmol/L	3.4-7.0
Calcium (S)	7.52 mg/dL	8.4-10.2	1.88 mmol/L	2.10-2.55
Protein, total (S)	5.5 g/dL	6.0-8.0	55.0 g/L	60-80
Albumin (S)	1.6 g/dL	3.5-4.9	16.0 g/L	35-49
Urate (S)	3.6 mg/dL	4.5-8.0	214 µmol/L	270-480
Cholesterol (S)	120 mg/dL	154-268	3.10 mmol/L	3.98-6.95
Triglycerides (S)	203 mg/dL	44-320	2.3 mmol/L	0.5-3.6
Bilirubin, total (S)	0.6 mg/dL	0.4-1.3	10 µmol/L	7-22
ALT (S)	46 U/L	5-30	0.76 µkat/L	0.08-0.50
AST (S)	59 U/L	10-30	0.98 µkat/L	0.17-0.50
ALP (S)	97 U/L	18-113	1.6 µkat/L	0.3-1.9
Amylase, total (S)	150 U/L	30-220	2.50 µkat/L	0.50-3.69
Amylase, P-type (S)	71 U/L	16-115	1.18 µkat/L	0.27-1.92
% of total	47 %	45-50	0.47	0.45-0.50
Lipase (S)	131 U/L	30-190	2.18 µkat/L	0.50-3.17
pH (aB)	7.67	7.35-7.45	Same	
pCO2 (aB)	31 mm Hg	35-45	4.1 kPa	4.7-6.0
Hematocrit (B)	39 %	40-54	0.39	0.40-0.54
Hemoglobin (B)	10.1 g/dL	13.1-17.2	6.27 mmol/L	8.13-10.67
Urinalysis (U)	Within normal limits			

Analyte	Value, conventional units	Reference range, conventional units	Value, SI units	Reference range, SI units
Gastric residue after overnight fast	114 mL	<50	0.114 L	<0.50
Basal acid output (BAO)	38.3 mmol/h	<11	Same	
Peak acid output (PAO)	79.4 mmol/h	12-60	Same	
BAO/PAO ratio	0.48	<0.20	Same	
Gastrin (S)	340 ng/L	<100	Same	

A 72-h fecal fat determination was performed while the patient was on a 100-g fat diet. The result, by the titrimetric procedure, was 18 g/d (reference range, <6 g/d). A 25-g xylose absorption test showed a urinary xylose excretion in a 5-h period of 5.0 g (33.3 mmol/5 h); the reference range is >4 g/5 h (>26.6 mmol/5 h).

A jejunal biopsy showed no abnormality. A small ulcer was seen on endoscopy in the third portion of the duodenum; prominent gastric and duodenal mucosal folds were also observed.

Differential Diagnosis

The patient presented with four main complaints: recurrent gastrointestinal hemorrhages, loss of weight, malnutrition, and diarrhea. He had not been fully investigated for these complaints in the recent past, and he appeared to have been provided with only symptomatic treatment for these recurrent hemorrhages. Recurrent hemorrhages are often due to duodenal or gastric ulceration. About one-fifth of patients with these ulcers experience such hemorrhages, and about one-half of all hospital admissions for upper gastrointestinal hemorrhages are due to peptic ulcer disease. Other common causes of such hemorrhage include gastritis (often due to alcohol), esophageal tearing due to recurrent vomiting, and bleeding esophageal varices. These, and other causes, can usually be detected by endoscopy or barium studies. Indeed, as previously noted, endoscopy findings confirmed the classic duodenal ulcer history given by the patient. The gastric acid studies clearly suggested hypersecretion of gastric acid, which was supported by the elevated serum gastrin level.

The loss of weight and signs of malnutrition can reasonably be attributed to malabsorption;[1] hence the importance of establishing the existence of fat malabsorption (steatorrhea) and normal absorption of carbohydrate (xylose test). It appears likely that the paresthesia and altered sensation, angular stomatitis and cheilosis, and a pellagra-like dermatitis are due, respectively, to deficiencies of thiamine (vitamin B_1), riboflavin (vitamin B_2), and niacin (nicotinic acid; vitamin B_3) secondary to the malabsorption.

Diarrhea is present when there is an abnormal increase in stool weight, liquidity, or frequency.[2] In the present case, the patient noted both an increased fluidity and frequency of bowel movements. The osmolality of the stool was close to that of serum (about 294 mOsm/kg H_2O), and blood and pus were not detected in the stool; these findings suggest a type of secretory diarrhea.

Peptic Ulcer

The term *peptic ulcer* is used to describe a group of ulcerative disorders of the gastric and duodenal mucosa that are due to the combined action of pepsin and acid.[3] The common forms of peptic ulcer are chronic duodenal and gastric ulcers.

Duodenal ulcer is a recurring, chronic disease, and nearly all such ulcers occur in the first portion of the duodenum. They tend to be deep, sharply demarcated, and <1 cm in diameter. Disease prevalence is such that about 10% of the population have a duodenal ulcer sometime during their life. The disease tends to be slightly more common in males than in females, and it is about three times more common than gastric peptic ulcer. Duodenal ulcer patients secrete more gastric acid than normal, but the extent of the overlap in acid secretion between these populations is such that gastric acidity measurements are of limited usefulness as a diagnostic test for duodenal ulcer. Likewise, although fasting serum gastrin levels are often similar to those of the healthy population, more gastrin is secreted into the circulation on stimulation by a protein-containing meal. The same gastrin stimulus elicits a greater gastric acid response than in the healthy population. Several genetic traits have been associated with duodenal ulcer. Individuals with blood group O have a 30% increased risk of ulcer, nonsecretors of blood group antigens have a 50% increased risk, and a nonsecretor with blood group O has a 150% increase in ulcer risk. Also, several subtypes of ulcer disease have been delineated; rapid gastric emptying is one such subgroup. The duodenal ulcer patient usually complains of epigastric pain that occurs within 1-3 hours after eating and that can often awaken the patient at night. The pain is quickly relieved by antacids or by eating. The disease is characterized by remissions. Hemorrhage, ulcer perforation into the peritoneal cavity, and pyloric stenosis are complications that occur in 20%, 10%, and 5% of cases, respectively.

Gastric ulcers are less common than duodenal ulcers and tend to occur after age 60, which is about 10 years later than for duodenal ulcers. The ulcers usually occur in the gastric antrum, and their histological appearance is similar to that of duodenal ulcer. Although the pain of a gastric ulcer is similar to that of a duodenal ulcer, it is much less predictable in nature. Often, eating precipitates pain to the extent that weight loss is common owing to the resulting aversion to food. Patients with gastric ulcers commonly secrete less gastric acid than do normal, healthy persons, and gastric emptying may be delayed. The major complications are hemorrhage and perforation.

Zollinger-Ellison Syndrome

An uncommon cause of peptic ulcers is the Zollinger-Ellison syndrome. This syndrome is characterized by the clinical triad of gastric acid hypersecretion, severe peptic ulcer disease, and non-β islet cell tumors of the pancreas.[4] It occurs in about 1% of all patients with duodenal ulcer and is slightly more common in males than in females. Symptoms usually occur in the third to fifth decade of life. The gastrin-secreting tumor is usually found in the pancreas, most frequently in the head of the pancreas, and up to 15% of gastrinomas occur in the wall of the duodenum. These tumors vary in size from about 0.2 to over 20 cm in diameter, and about half of them are multiple. Sixty percent of these tumors are malignant and may metastasize to regional lymph nodes, liver, spleen, bone, mediastinum, peritoneum, and skin. About one-quarter of patients with gastrinomas have Type 1 multiple endocrine neoplasia syndrome (MEN 1), which consists of tumors of the parathyroid glands, pituitary, pancreatic islets, and thyroid.

The excessive secretion of gastrin increases the gastric parietal cell mass (due to the trophic effects of gastrin), increases gastric acid secretion, and is probably also responsible for the prominent gastric and duodenal mucosal folds that are often observed in this syndrome. Mucosal ulceration usually occurs in the first portion of the duodenum. However, 25% of such ulcers occur lower down in the duodenum, or even in the jejunum. The occurrence of an ulcer in these regions should immediately raise the suspicion of the Zollinger-Ellison syndrome. Characteristically, ulceration in the Zollinger-Ellison syndrome is recurrent and subject to the usual complications of duodenal ulcer. About one-third of patients with a gastrinoma will suffer from diarrhea because of the large amount of hydrochloric acid secreted into the gastrointestinal tract. Indeed, diarrhea may precede ulcer symptoms by many years, and in a few patients, diarrhea has occurred in the complete absence of clinical ulcer disease. Finally, steatorrhea may occur, although this is much less common than diarrhea. The low intraluminal pH inactivates pancreatic lipase and prevents the digestion of triglycerides. In addition, the acidity renders some bile acids insoluble, thus reducing the formation of micelles necessary for the absorption of fatty acids and monoglycerides.

Discussion

The case presents a series of symptoms that can be integrated into a single diagnostic entity — the Zollinger-Ellison syndrome. These symptoms are

Ulcer in third portion of duodenum or in jejunum
Marked prominence of mucosal folds in stomach and duodenum
Poor response to ulcer therapy
Recurring ulceration or a strong familial history of peptic ulcer
Evidence of diarrhea and steatorrhea
Parathyroid or pituitary tumors or a family history of such tumors
Gastric acid hypersecretion or hypergastrinemia

The possibility of gastrinoma should be considered when patients present with one or more of the above findings. However, patients may also present with a single symptom.

Because hypersecretion of gastrin is not a universal symptom in Zollinger-Ellison syndrome and may also occur in some cases of duodenal ulcer, the measurement of BAO and PAO may not be conclusive of the diagnosis of Zollinger-Ellison syndrome. However, values of BAO >20 mmol/h and PAO >60 mmol/h are highly suggestive of the syndrome. Therefore, barium contrast radiological examination of the gastric mucosa is often necessary as it will detect the prominent mucosal folds characteristic of this syndrome. Measurement of serum gastrin is an important diagnostic test; values >1000 ng/L, in the presence of high gastric acidity, are virtually diagnostic of Zollinger-Ellison syndrome. However, elevated levels of gastrin are also found in pernicious anemia, gastric atrophy, rheumatoid arthritis, diabetes mellitus, and renal insufficiency. In pernicious anemia, gastrin levels may be up to 1000 ng/L, which is in the same range as many patients with a gastrinoma. Thus, an elevated level of gastrin alone may not be specific for a gastrinoma, although many cases do have fasting gastrin levels >500 ng/L. In fact, hypergastrinemia may not always be a feature in Zollinger-Ellison syndrome, and provocative tests for gastrin secretion may be necessary. Such stimulation of gastric secretion is produced by secretin injection, by calcium infusion, or by ingestion of a standard test meal.[4] Once the diagnosis is established, the tumor must be located, but this is often difficult or impossible. It is estimated that in nearly 50% of cases with unequivocal evidence of gastrinoma, the tumor cannot be identified at surgery.

Treatment

Treatment options[4] will be mandated by the location of the tumor (if known), its multiplicity, and whether or not it is malignant. The characteristics of this case, outlined in the Discussion above, clearly suggest a diagnosis of the Zollinger-Ellison syndrome. Thus, although no tumor could be found, a not uncommon circumstance in this syndrome, the patient was placed on the potent H_2-receptor blocker famotidine, which reduced the gastric acid secretion, healed the ulcer, completely arrested the diarrhea, and permitted the patient's return to his previous weight.

References

1. Tietz, N.W., Rinker, A.D., and Henderson, A.R.: Gastric, pancreatic, and intestinal function. *In:* Textbook of Clinical Chemistry. N.W. Tietz, Ed. Philadelphia, W.B. Saunders Co., 1986.

2. Fine, K.D., Kreijs, G.J., and Fordtran, J.S.: Diarrhoea. *In:* Gastrointestinal Disease: Pathophysiology, Diagnosis, and Management, 4th ed., vol. 1. M.H. Sleisenger and J.S. Fordtran, Eds. Philadelphia, W.B. Saunders Co., 1989.

3. McGuigan, J.E.: Peptic ulcer. *In:* Harrison's Principles of Internal Medicine, 11th ed. E. Braunwald, K.J. Isselbacher, R.G. Petersdorf, et al., Eds. New York, McGraw-Hill, 1987.

4. McGuigan, J.E.: The Zollinger-Ellison syndrome. *In:* Gastrointestinal Disease: Pathophysiology, Diagnosis, and Management, 4th ed., vol. 1. M.H. Sleisenger and J.S. Fordtran, Eds. Philadelphia, W.B. Saunders Co., 1989.

WOMAN WITH FACIAL FLUSHING

Jerome M. Feldman, Contributor

The patient, a 46-year-old female, had developed easy fatigability and weakness seven months prior to admission to a local hospital. Her physician had told her she must be under stress and that her symptoms were probably due to "nerves." In the following two months, however, she experienced spells of intermittent diarrhea with 2-3 semisolid bowel movements per day. She also noted bouts of facial warmth, "as if the blood were rushing to my face." These episodes were also marked by facial reddening; they would last 2-4 minutes and then fade. The flushing could be consistently provoked by drinking wine or beer. Although the patient's menstrual cycle was normal, her physician told her that her flushing might be due to early menopause.

In the two months prior to admission to the local hospital, the patient had developed a "choking sensation" when she tried to eat. Her appetite had decreased, and she had lost 10 lb (4.5 kg). She was complaining of almost continuous frontal headaches. A month prior to this admission, her physician had palpated left cervical and supraclavicular lymph nodes that were hard in texture and had suspected malignant lymphoma. The pathology report on a scalene lymph node removed at the time of this admission read as follows:

> The tissue contains sections of fibroadipose tissue containing numerous nests of tumor characterized by anaplastic, pleomorphic cells with large hyperchromic and occasionally bizarre nuclei. The tumor nests frequently contain central areas of necrosis. Several mitotic figures per high power field are seen. The tumor nests are separated by bands of dense fibrous tissue.
>
> *Interpretation:* This scalene node biopsy contains poorly differentiated carcinoma, probably squamous cell.

The diagnosis of a rapidly progressing, highly malignant tumor brought about the transfer of the patient to the University Medical Center. Physical examination at admission revealed a woman who appeared relatively healthy and complained of severe headache. The most striking features were telangiectasia on the patient's cheeks and the mass of hard lymph nodes, some 2 cm in diameter, in the left supraclavicular area. Hepatosplenomegaly was not found. Laboratory studies (complete blood count and liver and kidney function tests) were all normal.

Chest X-ray examination revealed large bilateral hilar masses with several nodules in both lung fields. Abdominal computed tomography (CT) showed numerous space-occupying lesions in the liver that were compatible with malignant tumor. Brain CT scan gave evidence of metastases in the brain stem. Liver-spleen scan with ^{99m}Tc sulfur colloid revealed multiple photopenic areas in the liver. ^{131}I-*m*-iodobenzylguanidine (^{131}I-MIBG) scan of the head, chest, and abdomen indicated uptake of ^{131}I-MIBG in the hilar nodes as well as in the suspected tumor nodules in the liver.

Medical Center pathologists re-examined the slides from the scalene node removed earlier. Although they agreed with the original description of the tissue, they noted also areas of cytological uniformity with some focal rosette formations, a finding that suggested tumor with some neuroendocrine differentiation. Immunoperoxidase stains were then performed on fixed and paraffin-mounted sections from the original biopsy. These stains were positive for neuron-specific enolase and negative for chromogranin A. The tumor was now thought more likely to be adenocarcinoma than squamous cell carcinoma. Possible diagnoses for this type of adenocarcinoma included metastatic ductular breast carcinoma or neuroendocrine tumor.

In consideration of a diagnosis of neuroendocrine tumor, serum, plasma, platelets, and 24-h urine specimens were analyzed for serotonin; urine was also assayed for serotonin metabolite (5-hydroxyindoleacetic acid, 5-HIAA). The following results were obtained:

Analyte	Value	Reference range
5-HIAA (U)	83 μmol/d	10-41
Serotonin (U)	8272 nmol/d	284-1250
Serotonin (S)	3239 nmol/L	100-1500
Serotonin (Plt)	2546 nmol/g	300-2200
Serotonin (P)	78 nmol/L	5-100

These findings, together with imaging information, suggested that the patient had carcinoid tumor of unknown origin that was metastatic to cervical nodes, liver, and brain. The presence of bilateral hilar nodes and urine excretion of serotonin much greater than that of 5-HIAA caused the patient's physicians to think the tumor was most likely a histologically and biochemically atypical bronchial carcinoid tumor.

After the patient was given a large dose of dexamethasone to prevent brain edema, she was treated with external radiation to the head and then started on a five-day course of combination therapy with the antineoplastic drugs streptozocin and 5-fluorouracil. The therapeutic plan was for 5-8 cycles of these chemotherapeutic agents at one-month intervals. Two weeks after the first cycle was started, the patient already showed a fall in serotonin and 5-HIAA levels (Table 1). Four weeks after starting therapy, serotonin and 5-HIAA levels had returned to normal, and the patient had had a parallel reduction in all of her symptoms.

Table 1. RESPONSE OF 5-HIAA AND SEROTONIN TO ANTINEOPLASTIC THERAPY

Analyte	Reference range	Therapy (weeks) 0	2	4
5-HIAA (U), μmol/d	10-41	83	67	36
Serotonin (U), nmol/d	28-1250	8272	3381	1034
Serotonin (S), nmol/L	100-1500	3239	1604	768
Serotonin (Plt), nmol/g	300-2200	2546	1474	1137
Serotonin (P), nmol/L	5-100	78	65	13

Definition of Carcinoid Tumors

Carcinoid tumors are a subgroup of neuroendocrine tumors that arise from neural crest cells. Other neuroendocrine tumors that are thought to arise from neural crest cells include pheochromocytoma, medullary carcinoma of the thyroid, islet cell carcinoma, and malignant melanoma. During embryological life, the neural crest cells migrate from the neural crest area to distant organs throughout the body. If these cells should become neoplastic during later life, they give rise to neuroendocrine tumors such as carcinoid tumors. Thus, carcinoid tumors have been described in almost every organ in the body. The term *Karzenoide* (carcinoid) was first used to describe tumors of the small intestine that histologically resembled adenocarcinomas but were not as aggressive. The majority of carcinoid tumors synthesize and secrete serotonin. Some, but not all, patients who harbor serotonin-secreting carcinoid tumors may develop flushing, diarrhea, and cardiac valvular disease — a constellation of symptoms called the carcinoid syndrome.

One of the more helpful ways to classify carcinoid tumors has been to group them according to the division of the gut from which they arise — foregut, midgut, and hindgut tumors. If tumors contain enough serotonin to reduce silver salts to elemental silver, the tumors are called argentaffin positive. *Foregut carcinoid tumors* (bronchus, stomach, duodenum, and pancreas) are argentaffin negative, have a low serotonin 5-hydroxytryptamine (5-HT) content, sometimes secrete 5-hydroxytryptophan (5-HTP) or adrenocorticotropic hormone (ACTH), and may metastasize to bone. Like the present patient, patients with foregut carcinoid tumors may have an unusually large amount of serotonin in their urine. *Midgut carcinoid tumors* (jejunum, ileum, and right colon) are argentaffin positive, have a high serotonin content, rarely secrete 5-HTP or ACTH, and rarely metastasize to bone. *Hindgut carcinoid tumors* (transverse colon, left colon, and rectum) are argentaffin negative, rarely contain serotonin, rarely secrete 5-HTP or ACTH, and may metastasize to bone.

Diagnosis

Histological Tests. The diagnosis of a carcinoid tumor is usually first suggested by the appearance of the tumor in tissue sections stained with hematoxylin and eosin. The small polygonal or round cells have uniform-appearing basophilic nuclei with only rare mitotic figures. The cells are organized into clusters, nests, rosettes, or pseudoacinar patterns.

With light microscopy, carcinoid tumors are frequently difficult to distinguish histologically from other neuroendocrine tumors since many present as atypical variants from the classic carcinoid picture. As in the present case, they may be mistaken for undifferentiated carcinoma or adenocarcinoma. In other patients they may be mistaken for small-cell (oat cell) carcinoma. Rarely, as in this case, they are confused with squamous cell carcinoma.

Histochemical tests have been useful to distinguish neuroendocrine tumors from other types of tumors. Stains for argentaffin, serotonin, neuron-specific enolase, and chromogranin A have particular application to carcinoid detection. However, the immunological stain for serotonin is limited in usefulness because it is only semiquantitative, and small amounts of serotonin may occur in some noncarcinoid tumors. Staining for neuron-specific enolase may not be highly specific for neuroendocrine tumors. As in this case, a number of atypical bronchial carcinoid tumors were found to be positive for neuron-specific enolase and negative for chromogranin A.

More useful is demonstration of neurosecretory granules by transmission electron microscopy to differentiate neuroendocrine tumors, such as carcinoid, from non-neuroendocrine tumors. The highest quality electron micrographs are obtained when tissue has been properly fixed in glutaraldehyde. However, for purposes of diagnosis, the neurosecretory granules are adequately preserved even in tissues initially fixed in formalin or in sections from paraffin blocks. Electron microscopy was not performed in this case.

Diagnostic Laboratory Tests. Measurement of histamine, dopamine, or substance P in plasma and urine is helpful for diagnosis in some patients. However, since the most specific marker of carcinoid tumors is serotonin, the measurement of serotonin and its metabolites in urine and blood fractions remains the mainstay of diagnosis. Quantitative determination of urinary 5-HIAA excretion is important for both diagnosis and judging the stability of the patient's tumor mass. Although circulating levels of serotonin in serum, platelets, and plasma are not as important in judging stability, they are valuable for establishing the diagnosis. Some data indicate that 9% of the patients with proven carcinoid tumors had normal 5-HIAA excretion but increased serum serotonin concentration.

The measurement of urinary excretion of serotonin is particularly helpful in the evaluation of patients with suspected carcinoid tumors of foregut origin. Some foregut carcinoid tumors are biochemically "atypical" because they are deficient in the enzyme aromatic amino acid (AAA) decarboxylase. Because this enzyme is required for the conversion of 5-hydroxy-tryptophan (5-HTP) to serotonin, deficient tumors secrete 5-HTP rather than serotonin. As in the present patient, when the 5-HTP is converted to serotonin by the AAA decarboxylase in normal kidney tissue, serotonin excretion dominates 5-HIAA excretion.

Imaging techniques that are helpful in diagnosing the presence and estimating the spread of carcinoid tumors include ultrasonography, CT, ^{99m}Tc liver-spleen scans, magnetic resonance imaging (MRI), and ^{131}I-MIBG scans. ^{131}I-MIBG, an isotopically labeled analogue of norepinephrine, is concentrated by the cells of many carcinoid tumors, by pheochromo-cytomas, and by occasional medullary carcinomas of the thyroid and islet cell carcinomas. The present patient concentrated ^{131}I-MIBG in her tumor.

Treatment

Many patients with carcinoid tumors do well for years without specific antineoplastic therapy, whereas other patients with aggressive tumors rapidly deteriorate. For patients with an indolent tumor and no diarrhea or facial flushing, initial therapy is not needed. The patient should have periodic tests of serotonin production and imaging procedures to monitor stability of the tumor mass.

If the patient has troublesome diarrhea, the serotonin-receptor antagonist cyprohepta-dine or methysergide is administered orally. If the diarrhea is not controlled with these measures or if bouts of facial flushing or hypotension are a problem, octreotide (Sandostatin) may be given subcutaneously. Octreotide is an analogue of the naturally occurring polypep-tide somatostatin; it apparently inhibits the secretion of serotonin and other neurohumors from the carcinoid tumor and thus reduces the severity of the flushing and the diarrhea. Finally, if the tumor is growing rapidly, antineoplastic therapy is required. For a carcinoid tumor of midgut origin, interferon alfa-2b (Intron A) is given. For a tumor of foregut origin, a combina-tion of streptozocin (Zanosar) and 5-fluorouracil is used. Because the clinical and biochem-ical features suggested that the carcinoid tumor of the present patient arose in the bronchus, this combination was selected in the present case. Combination therapy of cisplatin (Platinol) or etoposide (VP-16) has been found effective in the patient with either a rapidly growing carcinoid tumor of foregut or midgut origin or a tumor that has failed to respond to the above-described therapy.

Additional Reading

Feldman, J.M., and Lee, E.M.: Serotonin content of foods: Effect on urinary excretion of 5-hydroxyindoleacetic acid. Am. J. Clin. Nutr., *42:* 639-643, 1985.

Feldman, J.M.: Urinary serotonin in the diagnosis of carcinoid tumors. Clin. Chem., *32:* 840-844, 1986.

Feldman, J.M.: Carcinoid tumors and the carcinoid syndrome. Curr. Probl. Surg., *12:* 830-885, 1989.

Hanson, M.W., Feldman, J.M., Blender, R.A., et al.: ^{131}I-MIBG imaging in patients with carcinoid tumors. Radiology, *172:* 699-703, 1989.

Kvols, L.K.: The carcinoid syndrome: A treatable malignant disease. Oncology, *2:* 33-39, 1988.

Moertel, C.G.: Treatment of the carcinoid tumor and the malignant carcinoid syndrome. J. Clin. Oncol., *1:* 727-740, 1983.

PREGNANCY COMPLICATED BY ABDOMINAL PAIN

Lisa A. Sprague, Contributor
Susan Cox, Contributor

A 23-year-old black female with sickle cell disease and 33 weeks pregnant was admitted to the delivery suite complaining of four hours of crampy abdominal pain. No other gastrointestinal or genitourinary symptoms were present, and the patient denied vaginal bleeding. She had been closely followed since early in the pregnancy, and the prenatal course had been unremarkable. On physical examination, the oral temperature was 100 °F (37.8 °C), and the abdomen was gravid (fundal height 33 cm) with mild tenderness localized to the uterus. A vaginal examination was performed, and the cervix was found to be dilated 3 cm instead of closed as would be expected at this stage of pregnancy. Monitoring with an external tocometer and a fetal monitor showed regular uterine contractions and a reassuring fetal heart tracing.

The following laboratory data were obtained upon arrival:

Analyte	Value, conventional units	Reference range, conventional units	Value, SI units	Reference range, SI units
Sodium (S)	137 mmol/L	136-145	Same	
Potassium (S)	4.5 mmol/L	3.8-5.1	Same	
Chloride (S)	110 mmol/L	96-104	Same	
CO_2, total (S)	24 mmol/L	23-29	Same	
Urea nitrogen (S)	11 mg/dL	7-18	3.9 mmol urea/L	2.5-6.4
Creatinine (S)	0.6 mg/dL	0.6-1.1	53 μmol/L	53-97
Bilirubin, total (S)	1.9 mg/dL	0.2-1.0	32 mmol/L	3-17
Hematocrit (B)	21 %	37-47	0.21	0.37-0.47
Leukocyte count (B)	$15 \times 10^3/\mu L$	4.8-10.8	$15 \times 10^9/L$	4.8-10.8
Platelet count (B)	$250 \times 10^3/\mu L$	150-450	$250 \times 10^9/L$	150-450
Differential count (B)				
Segmented neutrophils	65 %	41-71	0.65	0.41-0.71
Band forms	20 %	5-10	0.20	0.05-0.10
Lymphocytes	25 %	24-44	0.25	0.24-0.44
Reticulocyte count, corrected (B)	10 %	1-2	0.10	0.01-0.02
Urinalysis (U)	Within normal limits			

The resident physician considered a variety of diagnostic possibilities that included sickle cell abdominal crisis, infectious processes possibly of the amniotic fluid or membranes, preterm labor, or urinary tract infection such as pyelonephritis. Magnesium sulfate, a medication often effective in arresting early labor by decreasing smooth muscle activity, was started intravenously.

The elevation of leukocyte count and hematocrit was attributed to labor, and the elevation of reticulocytes and bilirubin to sickle cell crisis. During a four-hour period of observation, the patient developed progressively worse abdominal pain, and her temperature increased to 101.2 °F (38.4 °C). Because the resident physician became more concerned about the possibility of an intra-amniotic infection or chorioamnionitis, the magnesium sulfate infusion, contraindicated in intrauterine infections, was stopped. An amniocentesis was performed to obtain fluid for Gram stain, anaerobic and aerobic cultures, and fetal lung maturity studies. The following results were obtained on the amniotic fluid:

	Patient value	Reference range
Gram stain, uncentrifuged fluid	Few gram-positive organisms seen	No organisms
Lecithin/sphingomyelin (L/S) ratio	2.0	≥2 indicates fetal lung maturity
Phosphatidylglycerol (PG)	3 mg/L	>2 mg/L indicates fetal lung maturity
Foam stability index	50	48-50 indicates fetal lung maturity

The amniotic fluid studies indicated that chorioamnionitis was present and that fetal lung maturity was likely. Empiric antibiotic therapy was started, labor was allowed to progress, and the patient delivered a 4-lb (1816-g) male infant.

Discussion and Definition of Disease

Sickle Cell Disease. Sickle cell disease is the homozygous state of a hemoglobinopathy caused by an amino acid substitution on both β-chains of the hemoglobin molecule. Affected individuals develop a hemolytic anemia and recurrent episodes of sickle crisis characterized by vaso-occlusive events and subsequent microinfarctions of involved organs. Common laboratory abnormalities during sickle crisis include low hematocrit and hemoglobin, a high reticulocyte count, a high leukocyte count, hyperbilirubinemia, and hematuria. Abdominal pain as a result of the vaso-occlusive phenomenon in abdominal organs is a common presentation for sicklers in crisis; however, sicklers are also particularly susceptible to certain infections and may develop appendicitis, cholelithiasis, pancreatitis, and the usual diseases of the reproductive tract. It is often difficult to make a definitive diagnosis in a sickle cell patient presenting with abdominal pain. Pregnancy in patients with sickle cell anemia remains a substantial clinical problem. Statistically there is an increase in maternal morbidity and mortality as well as fetal mortality. The most common pregnancy complications include sickle cell crisis, chest syndrome, urinary tract infections, and rarely strokes, hepatitis, and septicemia. Undesired fetal and perinatal outcomes include spontaneous abortion, low birth weight, stillbirth, and preterm delivery. A tenfold reduction in perinatal mortality, however, has been reported in women given prophylactic transfusions.

Chorioamnionitis. Infections of the placental membranes, the chorion and the amnion, can be caused by aerobic and anaerobic bacteria as well as *Mycoplasma*, *Chlamydia*, and viruses. Infection is frequently implicated as a factor in premature onset of labor. The biochemical basis for the pathway to amnionitis-induced premature labor is believed to result from phospholipase A_2 cleaving arachidonic acid, which is then converted to prostaglandin. An alternative explanation is that bacterial endotoxin from gram-negative organisms stimulates the decidual cells to produce cytokines and prostaglandins, which then initiate labor. The diagnosis of chorioamnionitis is made by a constellation of symptoms including maternal fever, uterine tenderness, fetal or maternal tachycardia, and a foul smell to the amniotic fluid. Confirmatory evidence may be provided by Gram stain and cultures of amniotic fluid obtained by a transabdominal amniocentesis. Amniocentesis is done by introducing a needle through the mother's abdominal wall into a pocket of amniotic fluid localized by ultrasonography. A positive Gram stain of organisms in a noncentrifuged specimen is highly indicative of infection as long as membranes are not ruptured. Both mother and fetus can develop catastrophic sepsis if amnionitis goes untreated for a period of time usually quoted as 12 hours.

Premature Onset of Labor. Prematurity is one of the major health hazards of our time. Eight percent of infants are delivered at less than 37 weeks' gestation; yet, they account for 75% of neonatal mortality (death during the first 28 days of life) and 50% of neurological morbidity including cerebral palsy and minimal cerebral dysfunction. The cause of premature labor is unknown, and researchers have been unable to identify characteristic biochemical markers in these women. In fact, the changes in progesterone, estrogen, and prostaglandin levels identified in term pregnancies do not occur in any consistent pattern in pregnancies that terminate prematurely. There are, however, strong clinical correlates that allow identification of pregnancies at risk for preterm delivery. These correlates include (1) previous preterm delivery; (2) medical complications of pregnancy, namely, hypertension, diabetes, renal disease, heart disease, anemia, and systemic infections; (3) obstetrical complications such as abruptio placentae, placenta previa, multiple gestation, and polyhydramnios; (4) genital tract abnormalities; and (5) infection. Much of the research to date links infection (chorioamnionitis) to a very large percentage of pregnancies that terminate prematurely. In particular, analyses of amniotic fluid for bacteria or markers of inflammation (i.e., lipopolysaccharide, interleukin-1B, interleukin-6, tumor necrosis factor, and interleukin-8) suggest that 30-40% have infection.

Fetal Lung Maturity Studies. The fetal lung is generally considered to be well developed with respect to gas exchange by 25 weeks' gestation. Despite this fact, premature infants are often unable to maintain oxygenation adequately because the lungs do not produce sufficient surfactants, which are substances that decrease the surface tension at the air-fluid interface in the respiratory acinus, thereby preventing alveolar collapse. Inadequate surfactant causes a disorder known as respiratory distress syndrome (RDS) or hyaline membrane disease. Surfactant is produced by the Type II pneumocytes and consists of three phospholipids: dipalmitoyl lecithin phosphatidylcholine, phosphatidylinositol, and phosphatidylglycerol. Surfactant enters the amniotic fluid, and its level in the fluid can be used as an assessment of fetal lung maturity. The lecithin/sphingomyelin (L/S) ratio, quantitative phosphatidylglycerol, and the foam stability test are the common studies used to determine the presence of adequate quantities of these phospholipids and thus indicate lung maturity.

Lecithin and sphingomyelin are present in amniotic fluid in equal concentration until 34 weeks' gestation, at which time the fetal lung's production of lecithin markedly increases. The L/S ratio is calculated from the relative concentrations of the two substances, which are usually determined by densitometry of a thin layer chromatogram. Respiratory distress syndrome of the newborn is very unlikely when the ratio is ≥ 2. False high L/S ratios are, however, possible if blood or meconium — common contaminants of amniotic fluid — is present. The L/S ratio may be a misleading indicator of fetal lung maturity in mothers with diabetes, probably because of the isolated underproduction of phosphatidylglycerol, a phospholipid not measured in the L/S ratio determination. In such cases, phosphatidylglycerol should be assayed by two-dimensional chromatography. This assay is not invalidated by presence of blood or meconium in the amniotic fluid sample. Phosphatidylglycerol levels have been shown to correlate better than L/S ratios with lung maturity in diabetic mothers.

The surfactant property of the phospholipids can be used as an indicator for fetal lung maturity in the "shake test" or foam stability index. In this procedure, agitation of amniotic fluid diluted with ethanol produces a ring of bubbles at the air-fluid interface. Persistence of the ring for 15 minutes or more predicts that the risk for neonatal RDS is low. The shake test, like the L/S ratio, may be invalidated by contamination with blood or meconium and also by other substances such as vaginal secretions, oils used for lubrication of plastic syringes, and obstetrical creams.

A new test that uses the technique of fluorescence polarization to measure the concentration of phospholipid in amniotic fluid has been introduced recently.[1] The automated test provides a rapid estimate of the relative concentrations of surfactant and albumin (surfactant/albumin ratio). Preliminary studies suggest this test may be a more accurate predictor of fetal lung maturity than is the L/S ratio.

Treatment

Sickle Cell Disease. Current methods of management of sickle cell disease include prophylactic red blood cell transfusions at mid-pregnancy with a goal to maintain the hematocrit greater than 25% and the hemoglobin S less than 60%. The drawbacks to transfusion therapy are obvious and include risk for hepatitis, alloimmunization, and AIDS (HIV infection).

Chorioamnionitis. The management of chorioamnionitis depends on the expected time of delivery. If the infant and placenta are removed expeditiously, antibiotics may be withheld. Obviously the infant is better off the sooner it is delivered from this hostile environment. The question then remains how best to effect delivery. At the present time, if delivery is not expected to occur within 1-2 hours, broad-spectrum antibiotics are begun. All attempts are made to allow vaginal delivery since cesarean section is associated with a high incidence of postpartum endometritis.

Antibiotics should be selected to cover the major pathogens — *Escherichia coli, Streptococcus agalactiae*, and *Peptostreptococcus*. To maximize amniotic fluid and fetal levels, antibiotics that readily cross the placenta should be selected. Ideal agents are ampicillin or ampicillin-gentamicin. A point to remember is that if chorioamnionitis is the cause of preterm labor, tocolytic agents to inhibit uterine contractions are *absolutely* contraindicated (see Table 1).

Table 1. CONTRAINDICATIONS TO TOCOLYSIS

Absolute Contraindications
Severe pregnancy-induced hypertension
Severe abruptio placentae
Chorioamnionitis
Fetal demise
Fetal anomaly
Fetal distress
Fetal growth retardation
Undiagnosed bleeding

Relative Contraindications
Hypertension — maternal
Diabetes (poorly controlled)
Hyperthyroidism
Maternal heart disease
Multiple gestation

Adapted from: Main, D.M., and Main, E.K.: Management of preterm labor and delivery. *In:* Obstetrics: Normal and Problem Pregnancies. S.G. Gabbe, J.R. Niebyl, and J.L. Simpson, Eds. New York, Churchill Livingstone, 1986.

Preterm Labor. Treatment of preterm labor consists of bed rest, adequate hydration, and pharmacological suppression of smooth muscle activity. None of these interventions have been proved to prevent preterm delivery, but often several additional days *in utero* can be gained. Three major classes of drugs are currently used to arrest labor, namely, magnesium sulfate, β-adrenergic agents, and prostaglandin inhibitors. All three work through their indirect effects on myosin light chain kinase, the enzyme responsible for contractions because of its effect on myosin light chain phosphorylation. Magnesium sulfate is believed to competitively inhibit free intracellular calcium, which is required for activation of myosin light chain kinase. β-Adrenergic drugs, e.g., terbutaline and ritodrine, work via the adenylate cyclase pathway to increase intracellular concentrations of *c*AMP, which directly inhibits myosin light chain kinase by phosphorylation of the enzyme. Antiprostaglandins, e.g., indomethacin, inhibit prostaglandin production, and prostaglandins are thought to be responsible for uterine contractions.

Fetal Lung Immaturity. It is currently possible to accelerate fetal lung maturation by using glucocorticosteroids in high risk patients. Perinatal mortality and morbidity are decreased in the treatment group if the baby is delivered between one and seven days after treatment. Importantly, the effect of therapy is more marked in infants between 30 and 32 weeks of gestation, and less so in infants of less than 30 and between 32 and 34 weeks of gestation. Effective steroids include betamethasone or dexamethasone (Decadron). Steroids should not be used if chorioamnionitis is suspected.

Reference

1. Russell, J.D., Cooper, C.M., Ketchum, C.H., et al.: Multicenter evaluation of TDx test for assessing fetal lung maturity. Clin. Chem., *35:* 1005-1010, 1989.

Additional Reading

Chapman, J.F., and Herbert, W.N.P.: Current methods of evaluating fetal lung maturity. Lab. Med., *17:* 597-602, 1986.

Klein, V.R., and Cunningham, F.G.: Amniotic fluid. A source for fetal evaluation. Semin. Perinatol., *10:* 125-135, 1986.

WOMAN WITH AMENORRHEA

Holly Gallion, Contributor
Larry E. Puls, Reviewer

A 30-year-old, gravida 2 para 2, white female was referred for evaluation of amenorrhea and an elevated level of serum hCG (human chorionic gonadotropin*). She reported that her menses had become irregular over the last two years and that she had not had any menstrual bleeding for nine months prior to referral. Over the last few months she had experienced mild frontal headaches and nausea. The patient was concerned that she might be pregnant. Indeed, she was found to have a positive pregnancy test by her local physician. However, diagnostic laparoscopy and dilation and curettage prior to referral to the University Hospital failed to demonstrate evidence of an intrauterine or ectopic pregnancy.

The patient's physical examination on admission was unremarkable. Her past medical history was significant in that she had undergone a tubal ligation after the birth of her last child six years ago. Laboratory results included the following:

Analyte	Value, conventional units	Reference range, conventional units	Value, SI units	Reference range, SI units
Chorionic gonadotropin, β-subunit (β-hCG) (S)	3800 mU/mL	0-3.1	3800 U/L	0-3.1
Prolactin (S)	8 ng/mL	0-27	8 μg/L	0-27
Thyroid-stimulating hormone (TSH) (S)	4.7 μU/mL	0.7-7	4.7 mU/L	0.7-7

Four days after her admission, her serum β-hCG had risen to 6200 mU/mL (6200 U/L). Ultrasonography of the pelvis demonstrated a slightly prominent uterus without evidence of intrauterine contents or adnexal masses. A mass in the left lung was present on chest X-ray examination. Further radiological evaluation including computed tomographic (CT) images of the head, chest, and abdomen revealed a 3 by 4-cm loculated mass in the left lower lobe of the lung, a 1-cm lesion in the right frontal lobe, and a 2 by 2.5-cm lesion in the left parietal lobe. Based on the findings of metastases and an elevated hCG, a presumptive diagnosis of choriocarcinoma was made. Stereotactic biopsy of the lung lesion confirmed the diagnosis.

---

* Human chorionic gonadotropin is a glycoprotein selectively produced by trophoblastic cells. It is composed of an α- and a β-chain. The α-subunit of hCG is similar to that of thyroid-stimulating hormone (TSH), luteinizing hormone (LH), and follicle-stimulating hormone (FSH), which are produced by the pituitary gland. It is the β-subunit that gives hCG its unique biological and immunological specificity. hCG can be measured as an intact molecule (intact hCG) only or as the combination of intact hCG and free β-subunits of hCG (total β-hCG). Research methods can also measure the free α- or β-subunits without detection of the intact hCG. Since most tumors may secrete either the intact hCG or the free β-subunit, or a combination of both, the measurement of total β-hCG is indicated for use as a tumor marker. In contrast, pregnant individuals produce mainly intact hCG, and thus either test would be satisfactory to detect normal pregnancy. In the patient in this report, the rise in β-hCG that heralded the presence of recurrent tumor was not associated with detectable levels of intact hCG.

The patient was initially treated with whole-brain radiation and modified Bagshawe chemotherapy (doxorubicin, cyclophosphamide, hydroxyurea, actinomycin D, vincristine, and methotrexate). After three courses of chemotherapy, β-hCG was undetectable, and one additional course of chemotherapy was given. Three months later, despite undectable intact hCG, β-hCG rose to 14 mU/mL (14 U/L), thus indicating tumor recurrence. Repeat physical and radiological examination failed to demonstrate the site of metastatic disease. Six months later, despite four additional courses of chemotherapy (cisplatin and etoposide) and hysterectomy, her β-hCG rose to 36 mU/mL (36 U/L). At this time, CT scan evaluation revealed an isolated metastasis in the upper lobe of the right lung. Following surgical resection of the lung metastasis and four courses of salvage chemotherapy (etoposide, methotrexate, dactinomycin, vincristine, and cyclophosphamide), her β-hCG levels fell to <5.0 mU/mL (<5.0 U/L). Following completion of therapy, the patient has remained in complete clinical and laboratory remission for the past 48 months.

CORRELATION OF SELECTED β-hCG AND INTACT hCG VALUES WITH TREATMENT REGIMEN

Treatment Regimen	β-hCG, mU/mL (U/L)	Intact hCG, mU/mL (U/L)
Admitted with metastasis in lung and brain	3800 (3800)	
First course of chemotherapy	6200 (6200)	
Second course of chemotherapy	138 (138)	
Third course of chemotherapy	5.4 (5.4)	
Fourth course of chemotherapy	<5.0 (<5.0)	
Tumor recurrence	14 (14)	<5.0 (<5.0)
Following hysterectomy and four additional courses of chemotherapy	36 (36)	<5.0 (<5.0)
One week following resection of lung metastases	7.7 (7.7)	<5.0 (<5.0)
Salvage chemotherapy instituted	15 (15)	<5.0 (<5.0)
Completion of salvage chemotherapy	<5.0 (<5.0)	<5.0 (<5.0)
48 months following completion of therapy	<5.0 (<5.0)	<5.0 (<5.0)

Gestational Trophoblastic Neoplasia

The term *gestational trophoblastic neoplasm* (GTN) collectively refers to a group of human malignant tumors that arise from the fetal placenta. These tumors — hydatidiform mole, invasive mole, and choriocarcinoma — have several unusual features that make them especially interesting. First, although they arise from fetal tissues, they almost exclusively invade and metastasize to maternal structures. Second, these tumors characteristically produce large amounts of the glycoprotein hormone, human chorionic gonadotropin (hCG). The amount of hCG produced is directly related to the number of viable tumor cells present and has proved to be a sensitive tumor marker for this disease. Finally, GTN is exquisitely sensitive to chemotherapeutic agents. Choriocarcinoma, which was almost uniformly fatal prior to the mid 1950's, is now one of the most curable disseminated gynecological malignancies.

Clinical Features

In the United States, hydatidiform mole occurs in approximately 1 in 1200 pregnancies. This tumor is characterized histologically by hydropic degeneration of the chorionic villi, absent fetal vessels, and trophoblastic proliferation. When invasion of the uterine myome-trium by molar villi is present, this form of GTN is called an invasive mole, but because hysterectomy and histological examination are not usual for patients with GTN, this diagnosis is rarely made. *Choriocarcinoma* is a rare, highly malignant form of GTN with a propensity to spread hematogenously to the lung, brain, liver, and kidney. This form of GTN is seen in 3-7% of patients with hydatidiform mole. Although most cases of choriocarcinoma follow a molar pregnancy, the antecedent pregnancy may also have been a miscarriage, an ectopic pregnancy, or even a term pregnancy as was the case in the patient reported here.

Hydatidiform mole is most common in women over the age of 40 and women who have had one previous molar pregnancy. These patients usually present with suspected preg-nancy and vaginal bleeding or the passage of molar tissue. Pre-eclampsia, hyperemesis gravidarum, and hyperthyroidism are also frequently present. Patients with choriocarcinoma usually present with signs or symptoms from metastatic lesions in the lung or brain. However, because of high gonadotropin production, choriocarcinoma may also present with amenor-rhea followed by vaginal bleeding.

Treatment

The diagnosis of a molar pregnancy is usually based on an ultrasonographic examination that reveals multiple intrauterine echoes and absence of a fetus or gestational sac. Because uterine curettage rarely reveals the presence of choriocarcinoma, this diagnosis is frequently not made until the patient develops symptoms from metastatic disease. Once the diagnosis of a molar pregnancy is established, curettage to remove the molar tissue is performed. Following evacuation of the uterus, serial serum β-hCG determinations are performed. Since quantitative serum β-hCG concentrations correlate with tumor burden, therapeutic decisions are made on the basis of this marker for GTN. In the majority of patients with a molar pregnancy, the fall of β-hCG level to normal within 8-12 weeks indicates the complete resolution of all trophoblastic disease. However, in approximately 20% of patients, hCG levels remain elevated or rise and thus indicate the presence of persistent trophoblastic disease. In these cases, as well as in patients with histologically confirmed choriocarcinoma, treatment is required after radiological evaluation of the lung, liver, and brain has been completed.

If the β-hCG is <40,000 mU/mL (<40,000 U/L) and there are no brain or liver metastases, single agent chemotherapy (methotrexate or actinomycin) is begun. However, if the β-hCG is >40,000 mU/mL (>40,000 U/L), the patient has a poor prognosis, and intensive multiple agent chemotherapy is necessary. During treatment, serial measurements of β-hCG are performed to monitor disease status. The absence of detectable β-hCG in the serum for three consecutive weeks indicates complete laboratory remission. Treatment is discontinued after one to three additional courses of chemotherapy. Patients are subsequently followed with serum hCG determinations for at least one year after completion of therapy.

Additional Reading

Goldstein, D.P., and Berkowitz, R.S.: Advances in gestational trophoblastic disease — An invitational symposium. J. Reprod. Med., *29:* 783-812, 1984.

Morrow, C.P., and Townsend, D.E.: Tumors of the placental trophoblast. *In:* Synopsis of Gynecologic Oncology. C.P. Morrow and D.E. Townsend, Eds. New York, John Wiley and Sons, 1987.

A HEALTHY MULTIPAROUS WOMAN WHOSE BABIES BECAME JAUNDICED

Douglas W. Huestis, Contributor

A 30-year-old woman, about 34 weeks pregnant, came to her obstetrician for late prenatal care and eventual delivery. She herself was in good health. Her family consisted of a boy of 10, a girl of 9, and another girl of 7 years of age. All the children were in good health, born of the same husband in another country. When questioned further, the patient volunteered the information that she had some sort of blood problem and that both the girls had "yellow jaundice" at birth. The younger girl had been severely jaundiced and had been given two blood transfusions. The mother had never had transfusions herself.

The obstetrician obtained routine prenatal laboratory tests, including blood counts, serological test for syphilis (STS), blood typing, and a blood group antibody screen. The results indicated no anemia or other blood abnormality; the STS was nonreactive; and the patient was found to be type O, Rh-negative. The antibody screen, however, was positive, and the laboratory identified the presence of anti-Rh$_0$ (D), the most common type of Rh antibody seen in persons immunized by pregnancy or transfusion. Her husband's blood type was O, Rh-positive.

The laboratory reported the Rh antibody titer to be 32, i.e., the serum reacted with Rh-positive test erythrocytes at a dilution of 1:32. This result indicated that the mother was producing significant amounts of antibody.

At this point the obstetrician did not know whether the fetus was Rh-positive or whether it was seriously affected by maternal antibody. The extent of the hemolytic process can be determined by sampling the amniotic fluid and measuring the bilirubinoid pigments that would result from excessive fetal blood breakdown. The physician can then correlate this observation with the history, physical findings, and ultrasonographic image.

To accomplish this, the obstetrician collected amniotic fluid by transabdominal puncture (amniocentesis) and sent it to the laboratory (see Figures 1 and 2). The results indicated a severely involved fetus. The obstetrician judged that by 36 weeks the fetus was mature enough for preterm delivery. This impression was confirmed by a lecithin/sphingomyelin (L/S) ratio of 2.5:1.

A boy weighing 5 lb 15 oz (2.7 kg) was delivered. He breathed spontaneously. On physical examination, the near-term baby seemed to be in fairly good clinical condition but was pale and had an enlarged liver. He quickly became jaundiced. Tests on the cord blood gave the following results:

Analyte	Value, conventional units	Reference range, conventional units	Value, SI units	Reference range, SI units
Blood type	O, Rh-positive		Same	
Direct antiglobulin (Coombs) test	Strongly positive	Negative	Same	
Hemoglobin (B)	10.5 g/dL	14-19	6.52 mmol/L	8.69-11.79
Reticulocytes (B)	17 %	3-5	0.17	0.03-0.05
Bilirubin (S)	4.1 mg/dL	0.2-2.5	70 µmol/L	3-43

The test results showed that the baby was Rh-positive and had abundant antibody adsorbed onto the erythrocytes (presumably maternal anti-Rh), along with moderate-to-severe anemia, marked reticulocytosis, and severe hyperbilirubinemia. On the stained blood smear, one could see numerous nucleated erythrocytes, with polychromasia and macrocytosis of the erythrocytes. Six hours after birth, the baby's condition had worsened, and the bilirubin had risen to 13.3 mg/dL (227 μmol/L), a dangerous rate of rise of over 1.5 mg/dL (26 μmol/L) per hour. The only applicable treatment at this stage was exchange transfusion.

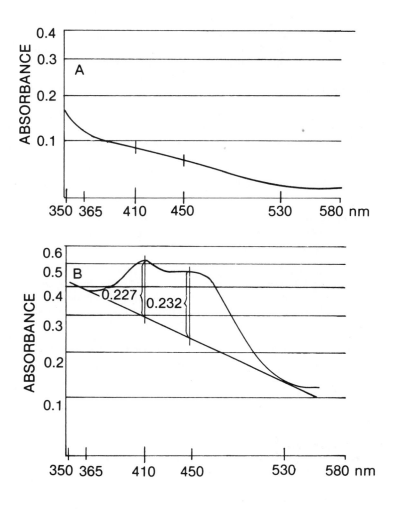

Figure 1. A. Normal amniotic fluid. Note near linearity of the curve. B. Amniotic fluid showing bilirubin peak at 450 nm and oxyhemoglobin peak at approximately 410 nm. Note baseline drawn between linear parts of the curve, from 550 to 365 nm. (Reproduced with permission from: Greene, M.F., Montserrat, DeM. F., and Tulchinsky, D.: Biochemical aspects of pregnancy. In: Textbook of Clinical Chemistry. N.W. Tietz, Ed. Philadelphia, W.B. Saunders Co., 1986.)

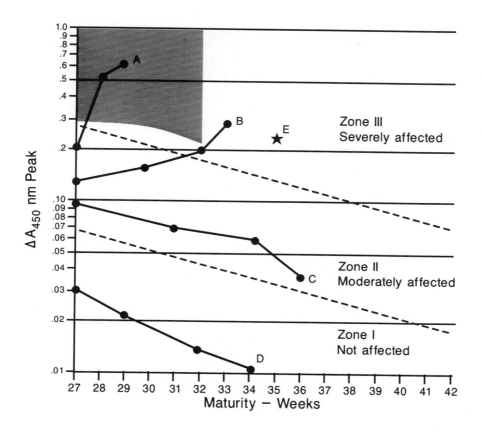

Figure 2. Chart of amniotic fluid absorbance at 450 nm related to fetal gestational age. The dashed lines separate three zones: the top zone indicates severe fetal hemolytic disease; the middle one, moderate involvement; and the bottom, mild disease or an unaffected fetus. The shaded zone indicates where intrauterine transfusion is usually necessary. The solid lines show readings on individual patients in the following circumstances: (A) intrauterine fetal death, (B) severe hemolytic disease with survival, (C) mild hemolytic disease, (D) Rh-negative fetus, and (E) the star shows the single reading in this case presentation. (Modified from: Huestis, D.W., Bove, J.R., and Case, J.: Practical Blood Transfusion, 4th ed. Boston, Little, Brown and Co., 1988.)

The neonatologist carried out this procedure via an umbilical catheter, using fresh O Rh-negative whole blood adjusted to a hematocrit of 55% to correct the baby's anemia while removing the jaundiced plasma and antibody-coated erythrocytes. Exchange transfusion was accomplished using a three-way stopcock, removing the baby's blood with a 20-mL syringe and substituting 20 mL of donor blood at a time. A single unit of blood (about 450 mL, or twice the baby's blood volume of 90 mL/kg) usually accomplishes an exchange of about 85%. The Rh-negative donor blood will not be affected by residual maternal antibody in the baby's body. (More than one exchange is sometimes necessary, depending on the level and rate of rise of the serum bilirubin.) After this treatment, the baby's jaundice subsided, and he was sent home at 10 days of age.

This case illustrates the classic blood type incompatibility that leads to Rh hemolytic disease of the newborn (*erythroblastosis fetalis*). The Rh-negative mother had an Rh-positive husband; the first child was unaffected, subsequent ones suffered progressively more severe jaundice, and the last baby required blood transfusions (presumably an exchange). Nevertheless, these findings are referable to the effects of previous pregnancies. To find out about the present pregnancy requires a direct test of that fetus, such as amniocentesis.

Pathogenesis

A mother can be immunized by leakage of fetal erythrocytes across the placenta into her circulation. Whether immunization occurs depends on the presence of an immunogenic fetal erythrocyte antigen, its absence in the mother, the mother's capacity for producing antibodies, and the ability of the antibody to reach the fetus (i.e., the antibody must be of type IgG).

Erythroblastosis can be caused by antibodies to any erythrocyte antigen, but in most severe cases the major Rh antigen Rh_O (D) is involved. Rh and most other erythrocyte antigens are clearly detectable at early stages of fetal development and can therefore be affected by maternal antibody throughout pregnancy. A more common but less severe form of hemolytic disease is associated with fetomaternal ABO incompatibility.

To induce immunization, fetal erythrocytes must enter the mother's circulation and remain there long enough to stimulate antibody production. Fetal ABO incompatibility with the mother protects against this to some extent (but not fully), probably because maternal anti-A or anti-B antibodies destroy incoming fetal ABO-incompatible, Rh-positive erythrocytes before they can cause antibody formation. There are also quantitative aspects. Immunization is more likely to take place in response to a relatively large influx of fetal cells (e.g., 1-5 mL), such as may occur with fetomaternal hemorrhage or at the time of delivery. Other important considerations include the following:

> Some persons make antibody readily; others do not. About 30% of Rh-negative subjects fail to become immunized even to repeated injections of Rh-positive erythrocytes.

> If the father is heterozygous for the gene controlling the principal Rh factor, he has an even chance of fathering Rh-negative babies. An Rh-negative fetus would not cause formation of Rh antibody, nor would it be affected by existing Rh antibody.

> Serological methods are available to estimate whether a person is homozygous or heterozygous for Rh_O (D). Other observations may make this obvious. For example, an Rh-negative child in the family indicates that the father, if Rh-positive, is heterozygous.

> Placental permeability to fetal erythrocytes may be important in the formation of IgG-type antibody.

> The greater the number of Rh-positive pregnancies, the more likely is immunization.

Discussion

The Rh antibody titer indicates only that the mother is immunized to Rh_O (D). Specifically, it does not indicate that the fetus is Rh-positive or that it is seriously affected by Rh hemolytic disease. Although a rising titer usually means an Rh-positive fetus, many immunized women maintain a fixed titer. Failure of the titer to rise does not mean the fetus is Rh-negative.

In serial titration, a difference of two dilutions (i.e., from 2 to 8 or from 64 to 256) is the borderline of significance. Quantitative or automatic titration techniques add little, if anything. The titration procedure must measure IgG-type antibody by a carefully standardized method to ensure comparability from one sample to the next. Because small differences in technique can affect results, the titers obtained in one laboratory should not be directly compared with those obtained in another.

Figure 1 shows the absorption spectrum of a normal amniotic fluid specimen and that of one with a marked elevation of bilirubin and hemoglobin. (The critical measurement is the ΔA_{450}, shown by the vertical line between the peak and baseline at 450 nm.) Figure 2 shows plots of sequential measurements of ΔA_{450} from several patients with fetal involvement ranging from none to severe. Our patient's value appears as a star (E) on Figure 2, since she was tested only once. Generally, serial determinations are preferred, but in this case of advanced pregnancy, the obstetrician judged, on the basis of ultrasonographic imaging, that the fetus was mature enough for preterm delivery at 36 weeks.

Alternatives

What if the fetus had been allowed to go to term? Continued exposure to maternal antibody would have resulted in increasing destruction of fetal erythrocytes with compensatory hematopoietic hyperplasia, which involves not only the bone marrow but also the liver and spleen, with production of massive hepatosplenomegaly. Overproduction cannot keep pace with erythrocyte destruction, and anoxia damages the heart, liver, and brain. Heart failure combined with liver failure and decreased production of albumin bring about generalized edema (anasarca). The extreme form of this sequence is called *hydrops fetalis* and usually results in intrauterine death. Such stillborns are pale and bloated but not jaundiced, because the excess bilirubin is cleared through the placenta.

What if the fetus is too immature to survive delivery? With amniocentesis or percutaneous umbilical blood sampling, hemolytic disease may be diagnosed too early in fetal life for delivery to be considered. If the involvement seems so severe that it would not be possible to keep the fetus alive until it could be delivered (30 to 32 weeks), there is the option of intrauterine transfusion of Rh-negative erythrocytes. These are injected percutaneously into the fetal abdominal cavity, from which they are absorbed into the fetal blood stream via the subdiaphragmatic lymphatics. There is a reasonable likelihood of success, although several such transfusions may be needed. A newer technique involves actual intravascular transfusions of the fetus, using an umbilical vessel observed by ultrasonographic imaging.

What if the baby had not had an exchange transfusion after delivery? The live-born baby no longer has access to its mother's placental waste-disposal system. It is possible to correct the anemia by a simple transfusion (not exchange). However, the antibody, diffused throughout the body, continues to destroy the baby's remaining Rh-positive erythrocytes. This process causes rapidly increasing anemia and also jaundice, since excess bilirubin is no longer disposed of through the placenta. The hyperbilirubinemia (mostly indirect or unconjugated bilirubin) is toxic to the immature brain, causing edema and yellow staining (*kernicterus*), particularly of the basal ganglia. The result can be death, a form of cerebral palsy, or other forms of brain damage.

Can Rh hemolytic disease be effectively prevented? It has already been seen that ABO incompatibility offers some protection against Rh immunization, presumably by hemolyzing incompatible erythrocytes before they can effectively stimulate the mother's immune mechanisms. Experimentally, Rh-negative volunteers given Rh-positive erythrocytes are less likely to make Rh antibody if the erythrocytes are first coated with Rh antibody. Passively administered Rh antibody possibly blocks Rh epitopes on Rh-positive erythrocytes, thus suppressing antibody response by host lymphocytes. Because the main influx of fetal erythrocytes takes place at the time of delivery, a single dose of Rh immune globulin (RhIg) following delivery prevents immunization in about 90% of cases. The few failures are caused either by immunization *during* pregnancy, including spontaneous or unrecognized miscarriages, or occasionally by an unusually large influx of fetal cells at delivery. Immunization during pregnancy can usually be prevented by a small dose of RhIg at 28 weeks' gestation. The effect of a larger-than-usual hemorrhage at delivery, when detected, can be prevented by a larger dose of RhIg after delivery.

Additional Reading

Allen, F.H., Jr., and Diamond, L.K.: Erythroblastosis Fetalis. Boston, Little, Brown, and Co., 1957.

Mollison, P.L., Engelfriet, C.P., and Contreras, M.: Blood Transfusion in Clinical Medicine, 8th ed. Oxford, Blackwell, 1987, pp. 637-677.

Queenan, J.T.: Erythroblastosis fetalis: Closing the circle. N. Engl. J. Med., *314:* 1448-1449, 1986.

Thaler, M.M.: Perinatal bilirubin metabolism. Adv. Pediatr., *19:* 215-235, 1972.

Zimmerman, D.R.: Rh. The Intimate History of a Disease and Its Conquest. New York, Macmillan Publishing Co., 1973.

WOMAN WITH A FAMILY HISTORY OF BREAST CANCER

Deborah E. Powell, Contributor

The patient, a 40-year-old married nurse, was seen by her gynecologist for her annual examination, which included breast examination and cervical/vaginal (Papanicolaou) smear. No breast masses were detected by palpation, but because of her age, a routine screening mammogram was performed. It was interpreted as showing fibrocystic changes. Because of a history of breast cancer in her maternal grandmother and an aunt, she was advised to have annual screening mammograms. She chose, however, not to do so.

Four years later, the patient again saw her gynecologist, complaining of a small thickening in the upper outer quadrant of the left breast. A mammogram was again obtained; it showed a focal area of small clusters of irregular calcifications in the left upper outer quadrant. Biopsy was suggested, and because the area was difficult to palpate, a wire-localization procedure was performed to localize the mass prior to surgery. When the mass was excised, a specimen mammogram confirmed the presence of small microcalcifications. All of the tissue was submitted for histological examination. The tissue diagnosis was infiltrating ductal adenocarcinoma, Grade II, 1.2 cm in greatest dimension, with identifiable lymph- vascular invasion. Since no tissue had been saved frozen for estrogen and progesterone receptor assay, immunohistochemistry and flow cytometry were performed on the formalin-fixed, paraffin-embedded tissue. Immunohistochemical examination revealed small numbers of cells (<10% of total) positive for estrogen and progesterone receptors (i.e., staining of nucleus equal to or greater than that seen in normal duct epithelial cells with a negative control slide). Flow cytometry showed a small aneuploid peak. The patient was advised of the need for further therapy and was given the options of lumpectomy and radiation therapy with axillary sampling or mastectomy with axillary node dissection. She chose mastectomy; histological examination of this specimen revealed no evidence of residual tumor, and no metastases were found in the 23 axillary lymph nodes removed. There was no recommendation for further therapy.

Eighteen months after surgery, a small nodule was found by X-ray examination in the upper lobe of the right lung; no other abnormalities were noted. A repeat chest film three months later showed no enlargement of the mass, but another X-ray film six months later showed an increase in its size. Bronchoscopy washings and brushings were obtained and interpreted as highly suspicious for malignancy. Because the patient was a 60 pack-year-smoker,* thoracotomy was expected to discover a primary lung tumor. However, the tumor removed at surgery was interpreted as metastatic adenocarcinoma consistent with breast as primary site. This tumor was 2 by 1 cm in size. Half of the specimen was snap-frozen for estrogen and progesterone receptor assays and other studies. A part was taken for flow cytometry. The estrogen-receptor binding was 12 fmol/mg cytosol protein; progesterone-receptor binding was 22 fmol/mg cytosol protein. Flow cytometry showed a large aneuploid peak in addition to the normal cell population.

The patient was started on chemotherapy. Within six months she had developed back pain, and a bone scan revealed lytic lesions in T10, L4, L5, and several ribs. She became

---

* Pack-year = packs smoked per day × number of years of smoking.

jaundiced and developed a pathological fracture of the left hip. Despite supportive therapy, she died three years after the initial diagnosis of adenocarcinoma.

Discussion

Carcinoma of the breast is the second leading cause of cancer deaths in women in the United States. Only lung cancer kills more women annually. One in ten women in the United States will develop breast cancer, and over 50% will die of their disease. Known risk factors include a family history of premenopausal breast cancer in maternal relatives, a personal history of atypical proliferative fibrocystic breast disease, and nulliparity or late age of first childbearing. Women who have had cancer in one breast have an increased risk of developing cancer in the second breast. Dietary factors, such as diets high in animal fats, are also important factors of added risk. Dietary involvement is supported by the unusual geographical distribution of breast cancer, with high rates in Western populations and relatively low rates in Far Eastern populations, e.g., indigenous Japanese women. Nevertheless, Japanese women born in the United States and consuming Western diets develop a risk of breast cancer similar to that of American women. Whether the use of exogenous estrogens or alcohol creates risk remains controversial.

Despite the known risks for developing breast cancer, most women who have developed breast cancer are not at high risk for nonsurvival. The best "treatment" of the disease is early detection, usually by physical examination (including regular self-examination) and mammography. The American Cancer Society recommends first or baseline screening mammography for women between the ages of 35 and 40, with regular repeats every two years until age 50, and annually after 50. For women subject to known risk factors, annual screening mammograms should start prior to age 50.

Several features of a detected, excised, and diagnosed tumor are useful for prognosis. Histopathological features include tumor size, presence or absence of metastasis to axillary lymph nodes, tumor type and grade, and presence or absence of lymph-vascular invasion in the primary tumor. Larger tumors carry a more serious prognosis. Tumors with >4 positive axillary lymph nodes have the worst prognosis; a count of 1-4 positive nodes is better; and a count of zero positive nodes is best. Identifiable lymph-vascular invasion by tumor cells within the breast tissue worsens the prognosis, even if no lymph nodes are positive. Histological grade of the tumor may be recorded as I, II, or III, with Grade III tumor having the worst prognosis. Some types of invasive carcinoma, e.g., tubular carcinomas, medullary carcinomas, and colloid or mucinous carcinomas, are less likely than others to metastasize and hence have a somewhat better prognosis.

Certain biochemical features of tumor tissue are important for determining the prognosis of breast cancer and, in addition, are helpful for planning treatment after surgery. Detection and *quantitation of estrogen receptors* (ER) and *progesterone receptors* (PR) — binding proteins for the steroid hormones estrogen and progesterone — are well established as an adjunct to prognosis and therapy. These receptors are present in both cytoplasm and the nucleus of cells in normal and tumor tissue. They occur within normal duct epithelium and perilobular stroma of the human breast as well as in tissues in multiple other sites. The receptor proteins in the cytoplasm bind estrogen and progesterone and translocate the hormones into the nucleus, where they exert their action.

The most commonly used quantitative biochemical procedure for ER and PR involves in vitro saturation of receptor binding sites with radiolabeled estrogen or progesterone, removal of free label with dextran-coated charcoal, and counting of bound radioactivity. Scatchard analysis is then applied to the binding data to determine binding capacity and affinity of receptors. Results are reported as femtomole (fmol) hormone bound per milligram of cytosol protein isolated from the specimen. In the past, at least 500 mg of tumor tissue have been required for the assays, but recently, micromethods have been developed. The routine approach is to test both estrogen and progesterone binding on the same specimen. The specimen must be snap-frozen within 15 minutes or less after acquisition and kept frozen at -70 °C or lower until assayed. Usually a mirror image slice of tumor is evaluated histologically in order to ensure that the tissue tested for ER and PR is representative of the tumor.

Tumors with undetectable or very low binding of the hormone, i.e., ≤3 fmol/mg protein, are considered receptor-negative and usually do not respond to antisteroid hormone therapy. Receptor hormone binding of 3-20 fmol/mg protein is an indeterminate range, and binding >20 fmol/mg protein is considered to be positive. Receptor-positive tumors, especially those that are strongly positive, i.e., >100 fmol/mg protein, often respond to hormonal therapy, e.g., with the anti-estrogen tamoxifen.

Immunohistochemical methods for ER and PR utilize non-isotopically labeled antibodies directed against the receptor proteins. Once the labeled antibody has reacted with the receptor protein in the cells in the thin section on a microscope slide, a histochemical reaction versus the label localizes and visualizes the receptor material. The immunoperoxidase methodology is typical of these methods. With staining of receptors *in situ* and quantitation by image analysis, these assays have proved to be highly sensitive and able to provide results closely comparable to the biochemical procedures. They have the advantages of requiring less sample than the isotopic method and of applicability to both fresh, unfixed and formalin-fixed, paraffin-embedded tissue. They are, as well, unlikely to give receptor-negative results in the initial cancer of postmenopausal women on estrogen (Premarin) or in a recurrent cancer in women being treated with anti-estrogen.

In this patient's case, it is interesting that immunochemically receptor-positive cells were seen in the original tumor, but the metastatic tumor removed several months later did not show significant levels of ER or PR by biochemical methods. Possibly the metastatic cells were less differentiated than their precursors and consequently less able to synthesize receptor proteins. As a result of these findings, chemotherapy rather than antihormone therapy was indicated.

Recently *flow cytometry*, used to measure the DNA content of proliferating cells, has become an important tool for prognosis of carcinoma of the breast. The procedure can be performed on fresh tumor tissue removed at surgery or on formalin-fixed, paraffin-embedded tissue. The primary tumor of this patient was evaluated as fixed tissue, whereas the metastatic tumor was examined as fresh tissue. Breast tumors with totally diploid DNA content have been found to have better prognosis than tumors containing an aneuploid cell population. Furthermore, tumors with large numbers of actively proliferating cells (high S-phase fraction) imply a worse prognosis than do those with small numbers of cells in S-phase. Aneuploid peaks in both the original and metastatic tumor implied unfavorable prognosis for the patient presented in this case history.

Other studies[1-4] are currently investigating various biochemical markers and their prognostic utility for patients with breast cancer. These markers include cathepsin D, *neu* oncogene (c-erb B-2), and epidermal growth factor receptors. *Cathepsin D* is a protease; its synthesis is stimulated by estrogens, and its secretion occurs in some estrogen receptor-positive breast cancer cells. However, recent studies have shown somewhat contradictory data regarding the role of cathepsin D as a prognostic predictor in breast cancer. Whereas one large study[1] suggested that cathepsin D could be an independent indicator of poor prognosis in patients with node-negative breast cancer, another showed it to be associated with favorable outcomes in patients with positive lymph node metastases, but not in node-negative patients.[2] *neu Oncogene* is a gene that codes for *neu* oncoprotein; in breast cancer, expression of this gene is associated with increased levels of *neu* oncoprotein. In a study of patients with axillary lymph node-positive breast cancer, amplification of the *neu* oncogene was related to earlier recurrence of disease and shorter survival times.[3] *Epidermal growth factor receptors (EGFR)* are glycoproteins that are present on cell membranes in many human tissues. These receptors have been shown to be present on membranes prepared from human breast cancers and lymph node metastases. Recurrence of disease is higher in patients with EGFR-positive tumors than with EGFR-negative tumors.[4] Increased levels of EGFR significantly correlate with poor prognosis and may predict poor response to endocrine therapy in patients with breast cancer.

Principles of Treatment

Today multiple modalities of therapy are available for the patient with breast cancer. Surgery, radiation therapy, hormonal therapy, and chemotherapy all have roles in treatment. Breast-conserving surgery is widely utilized, and newer strategies for treatment of metastatic disease are utilizing autologous bone marrow transplantation. In short, treatment may be individualized for each patient and requires consultation with the patient and physicians familiar with the various treatment strategies.

References

1. Tandon, A.K., Clark, G.M., Chamness, G.C., et al.: Cathepsin D and prognosis in breast cancer. N. Engl. J. Med., *322:* 297-302, 1990.

2. Henry, J.A., McCarthy, A.L., Angus, B., et al.: Prognostic significance of the estrogen-regulated protein, cathepsin D, in breast cancer. Cancer, *65:* 265-271, 1990.

3. Slamon, D.J., Clark, G.M., Wong, S.G., et al.: Human breast cancer: Correlation of relapse and survival with amplification of the Her-2/*neu* oncogene. Science, *235:* 177-182, 1987.

4. Sainsbury, J.R.C., Farndon, J.R., Needham, G.K., et al.: Epidermal growth factor receptor status as a predictor of early recurrence and death from breast cancer. Lancet, *1:* 1398-1402, 1987.

Additional Reading

McGuire, W.L., Tandon, A.K., Allred, D.C., et al.: How to use prognostic factors in axillary node-negative breast cancer patients. J. Natl. Cancer Inst., *82:* 1006-1015, 1990.

WOMAN WITH ABDOMINAL DISTENTION

Paul D. DePriest, Contributor
J. R. van Nagell, Jr., Reviewer

The patient was a 51-year-old white female referred to the University Hospital for evaluation of increasing abdominal girth. Two months prior, the patient had developed a sensation of abdominal bloating and early satiety. She also complained of recent onset of constipation and urinary frequency. The patient had experienced increasing fatigue and a 25-lb weight loss over the preceding six months. She had shortness of breath when sitting and when exercising. She had been married for 31 years but had never had children and had never used contraception. She had not had menses in over one year.

The patient's past medical history was significant for hypertension and a previous myocardial infarction. She had no prior surgery and had taken no medications in over one year. However, she gave a history of smoking two packs of cigarettes per day for over 20 years and admitted to a daily intake of at least two 12-oz cans of beer.

Physical examination revealed a blood pressure of 180/100 mm Hg. There were decreased breath sounds at both lung bases; the sounds were particularly pronounced on the right side. Heart rate and rhythm were regular, but a Grade III/VI systolic ejection murmur was noted. The abdomen was markedly distended with a positive fluid wave. The liver margin was not palpable. Pelvic examination revealed a fullness in the right adnexal region and a bulging of the cul-de-sac. There was 1+ pitting edema of both lower extremities.

Based on the above findings, the admitting diagnosis was congestive heart failure with subsequent fatigue, shortness of breath, ascites, and edema. A chest X-ray examination and electrocardiogram (ECG) were ordered. The chest film revealed bilateral pleural effusions with the right-sided effusion twice as large as the left. There was no pulmonary edema noted, but the heart was slightly enlarged. The ECG showed signs of an old anterolateral myocardial infarction and left ventricular strain pattern. An echocardiogram was performed to evaluate the ventricular wall motion and to examine the valvular anatomy. Echocardiogram results showed concentric left ventricular wall thickening, mildly thickened aortic valve leaflets, and normal wall motion.

Because of the signs of pelvic fullness on clinical examination, an abdominopelvic ultrasonographic examination was ordered. This scan showed a large amount of fluid in the abdomen and a normal-sized liver and spleen. There was a cystic mass approximately 10 cm in diameter noted on the right side of the pelvis, which was confluent with the uterus. This mass was felt to be consistent with a multiloculated, complex ovarian neoplasm.

On admission, the following laboratory results were obtained:

Analyte	Value, conventional units	Reference range, conventional units	Value, SI units	Reference range, SI units
Leukocyte count (B)	5.5 x 10³/μL	4.8-10.8	5.5 x 10⁹/L	4.8-10.8
Hematocrit (B)	30 %	37-47	0.30	0.37-0.47
Hemoglobin (B)	10.9 g/dL	12-16	6.76 mmol/L	7.45-9.93

Analyte	Value, conventional units	Reference range, conventional units	Value, SI units	Reference range, SI units
MCV (B)	70 fL	81-99	Same	
MCH (B)	25 pg	27-31	Same	
MCHC (BErcs)	29 g Hb/dL	31-36	18 mmol Hb/L	19-22
Platelet count (B)	525 x 10^3/μL	150-450	525 x 10^9/L	150-450
Differential count (B)				
Neutrophils	84 %	41-71	0.84	0.41-0.71
Lymphocytes	10 %	24-44	0.10	0.24-0.44
Monocytes	3 %	3-7	0.03	0.03-0.07
Eosinophils	3 %	0-1	0.03	0-0.01
Partial thromboplastin time (PTT) (P)	28 s (patient) 29 s (control)	23.1-33.3	Same	
Prothrombin time (PT) (P)	14.5 s (patient) 12 s (control)	11.5-13.5	Same	
Sodium (S)	138 mmol/L	136-145	Same	
Potassium (S)	4.0 mmol/L	3.8-5.1	Same	
Chloride (S)	105 mmol/L	98-108	Same	
CO_2, total (S)	25 mmol/L	23-29	Same	
Urea nitrogen (S)	11 mg/dL	7-18	3.9 mmol urea/L	2.5-6.4
Creatinine (S)	0.8 mg/dL	0.7-1.2	71 μmol/L	62-106
Glucose (S)	86 mg/dL	75-105	4.8 mmol/L	4.2-5.8
Protein, total (S)	5.8 g/dL	6.0-7.8	58 g/L	60-78
Albumin (S)	2.9 g/dL	3.4-4.8	29 g/L	34-48
Urate (S)	5.8 mg/dL	2.5-6.2	345 μmol/L	149-369
Cholesterol (S)	95 mg/dL	120-210	2.46 mmol/L	3.10-5.43
Bilirubin, total (S)	0.3 mg/dL	0.2-1.1	5 μmol/L	3-19
AST (S)	32 U/L	13-35	0.53 μkat/L	0.22-0.58
ALT (S)	31 U/L	7-35	0.52 μkat/L	0.12-0.58
LDH (S)	175 U/L	100-190	2.92 μkat/L	1.67-3.17
ALP (S)	82 U/L	30-100	1.4 μkat/L	0.5-1.7
GGT (S)	27 U/L	10-50	0.45 μkat/L	0.17-0.83
Calcium, total (S)	6.8 mg/dL	8.4-10.2	1.70 mmol/L	2.10-2.54
Calcium, ionized (S)	4.70 mg/dL	4.60-5.08	1.17 mmol/L	1.15-1.27

Since ultrasonographic examination had shown a pelvic mass, a primary or metastatic ovarian lesion was suspected. Assays for carcinoembryonic antigen (CEA) and cancer antigen 125 (CA 125) gave the following results:

Analyte	Value, conventional units	Reference range, conventional units	Value, SI units	Reference range, SI units
CEA (S)	2.5 ng/mL	0-5.0	2.5 μg/L	0-5.0
CA 125 (S)	378 U/mL	<35	378 kU/L	<35

A barium enema revealed extrinsic sigmoid colon compression secondary to the pelvic mass. An intravenous pyelogram (IVP) showed right hydronephrosis but otherwise normal renal architecture.

Thoracentesis was performed to document the type of effusion. One liter of clear, straw-colored fluid was removed from the right pleural space. The following results of assays on the fluid were obtained:

Analyte	Value, conventional units	Value, SI units
Cytology	No malignant cells	Same
Cell count	Rare leukocyte; rare erythrocyte	Same
LDH	78 U/L	1.30 μkat/L
Protein	2.3 g/dL	23 g/L
Glucose	67 mg/dL	3.7 mmol/L

The physician felt these results were compatible with a transudative* effusion. Total parenteral nutrition was begun, and the patient was taken to the operating room seven days later. At the time of laparotomy, a large right ovarian tumor was removed that was a serous cystadenocarcinoma. The tumor was 25 by 30 cm in size. The right ovary was replaced with tumor, and the left ovary had small metastatic implants on its surface. The omental specimen revealed multiple microscopic metastases. Multiple biopsies of the peritoneal cavity were negative for tumor. Samples of the ascitic fluid taken from four abdominal quadrants were negative for malignant cells. The pathology report indicated that the patient had Stage IIIA epithelial ovarian cancer.

Definition of the Disease

Incidence of Ovarian Cancer. In 1991, it was anticipated that there would be over 21,000 new cases of ovarian carcinoma diagnosed in the United States and that over 12,000 women would die of the disease.[1] Seventy-five percent of patients will have advanced stage disease (Stage III or IV) at the time they first consult a physician, and their five-year survival will be only 15-20%. Ovarian cancers of epithelial origin and serous cystadenocarcinomas account for about 70% of all cases.

Risk Factors. Predisposing risk factors include nulliparity, a positive family history of ovarian carcinoma in primary relatives, and age. It is postulated that in the absence of pregnancy there is incessant ovulation, which places the germinal epithelium of the ovary at risk for neoplastic transformation. Lynch has reported three familial syndromes associated with an increased risk for ovarian cancer.[2] These include site-specific familial ovarian cancer in which a woman's mother, grandmother, or sister has ovarian cancer. In this situation, predisposition to ovarian cancer may be inherited as an autosomal dominant trait. Therefore, the risk of ovarian cancer in a woman with two or more primary relatives who have the disease may be as high as 50%. The two other familial syndromes associated with an increased predisposition for ovarian cancer are the breast cancer-ovarian cancer syndrome and the Lynch Type II syndrome. In the latter, non-polyposis–related colon cancer is associated with ovarian cancer. Although ovarian cancer occurs most commonly in the fifth and sixth decades (mean age, 59 years), familial ovarian neoplasia occurs approximately 10 years earlier.

Differential Diagnosis

In a patient with ascites and pleural effusion, the diagnostic possibilities include congestive heart failure, liver disease, infectious disease, and malignancy. When there is a pelvic mass, ascites, and a pleural effusion, the differential diagnosis is more limited and includes only primary ovarian neoplasms (benign and malignant) and metastatic lesions to the ovary. Cancers that frequently spread to involve the ovaries include breast, gastric, colon, and uterine carcinomas.

---

* The fluid in transudative effusions has LDH values <200 U/L, pleural fluid LDH/serum LDH = <0.6, and pleural fluid protein/serum protein = <0.5. Values in exudates are above these limits.

Diagnosis

This patient's symptoms were initially attributed to a presumptive diagnosis of congestive heart failure (CHF). CHF is a generalized dysfunction of the cardiac muscle. When the heart is unable to pump blood effectively, the pressure in the right side of the heart (atrium and ventricle) increases. This increased pressure manifests as an enlarged heart, pulmonary congestion (edema), and liver congestion. The liver congestion eventually results in a rise in the portal circulation pressure. This portal hypertension leads to ascites. Other primary hepatic disorders such as cirrhosis will cause a similar accumulation of ascites.

Symptoms and signs of ovarian cancer appear late in the course of the disease. Therefore, diagnosis is usually not made until the disease has spread beyond the pelvis. The most common presenting symptoms include abdominal swelling, pelvic pressure, constipation, urinary frequency, fatigue, and early satiety. The most common sign is a firm, fixed pelvic mass, and the diagnosis of an ovarian tumor is usually made by pelvic examination. Pelvic imaging with ultrasonography and computed tomography (CT) is effective in delineating pelvic masses. However, in very large masses, accurate measurement may be precluded by areas of the cyst wall being pushed against the parietal peritoneum. As in this patient, the ultrasonogram can overestimate ascites volume and underestimate actual ovarian neoplasm size. Recently, several investigators have reported that transvaginal sonography (TVS) is an effective screening method for ovarian cancer.[3,4] In a study of 1300 asymptomatic postmenopausal women with no known pelvic abnormality, two primary ovarian cancers were detected by TVS. Both patients had early Stage I disease, and both were cured by conventional therapy. At the present time, TVS is an experimental diagnostic method that is undergoing evaluation in carefully controlled national trials.

In the patient with ascites from ovarian cancer, the laboratory evaluation can be exceedingly helpful. Ovarian cancer rarely metastasizes into the liver; therefore, the liver function tests are normal. By contrast, in CHF and cirrhosis there can be varying degrees of liver function test abnormalities in the patient with advanced ovarian carcinoma. The laboratory examination will usually detect poor nutrition (decreased albumin, decreased total protein, decreased cholesterol) and anemia. Recently, serum from ovarian cancer patients has been found to contain a distinct antigen called CA 125. Bast and colleagues[5,6] reported that CA 125 is overexpressed in ovarian cancer patients. CA 125 is an antigenic determinant on a high-molecular-weight glycoprotein[5] that is elevated (>35 U/mL; >35 kU/L) in the serum of approximately 80% of patients with nonmucinous epithelial ovarian cancer. The frequency of CA 125 elevation is related directly to the stage of disease; it varies from 50% in patients with Stage I disease to 90% in patients with Stage III or Stage IV lesions. The relatively low clinical sensitivity (50-83%, depending on the stage of the disease) of the CA 125 test precludes its use as a reliable screening test for ovarian cancer; however, the test has been used effectively to monitor disease status after chemotherapy and to detect recurrence.[6]

Clinical Features

Ovarian cancer spreads directly over peritoneal surfaces and less commonly metastasizes via lymphatic or hematogenous routes. The presence of ascites is frequent in advanced stage ovarian cancer. The cause of the ascites is increased production of fluid and decreased clearance by the efferent lymphatics of the omentum and right hemidiaphragm.

The patient described herein had vague symptoms and an ill-defined pelvic abnormality. Other worrisome findings included a right-sided pleural effusion and ascites. Evaluation of the pleural effusion was mandatory to rule out malignant or infectious causes. Even when ascites or pleural effusion is due to underlying ovarian carcinoma, only 25% of samples will reveal malignant cells.[7] Most of the time, the ascitic fluid meets the criteria of a transudate (pleural fluid LDH/serum LDH <0.6, pleural fluid protein/serum protein <0.5, and pleural fluid LDH <200 U/L).[8,9] Paracentesis is not recommended in a woman with a suspected ovarian neoplasm because of the possibility of tumor rupture by the paracentesis needle. If a localized, encapsulated ovarian tumor is ruptured, then seeding of the abdominal cavity is probable, with subsequent advancement of the stage of disease.

In the patient with ascites and a pleural effusion, the physician must be concerned about underlying congestive heart failure. In this patient, the echocardiogram was normal, and the heart was not massively enlarged. Primary cirrhosis can also cause ascites. Primary liver dysfunction, either acute or chronic, is associated with increased ALT, AST, GGT, and ALP. This patient had normal liver function tests. The decreased serum albumin and slight increase in prothrombin time were due to malnutrition and not to primary liver failure.

Treatment

Ovarian cancer is optimally treated by a combination of surgery and chemotherapy. Prognosis is related directly to the amount of tumor remaining after surgical debulking, so every effort should be made to remove all visible and palpable areas of disease. Following surgery, patients with epithelial ovarian cancer should be treated with cisplatin-based chemotherapy, one treatment per month for six months. If, after completion of chemotherapy, the patient has a normal serum CA 125 level and no clinical evidence of disease, a second-look laparotomy should be performed. Patients with no histopathological or cytological evidence of persistent ovarian cancer at second-look surgery can have their treatment stopped. If a microscopic or visible tumor is present at second-look laparotomy, chemotherapy should be continued for an additional six months.

References

1. Boring, C., Squires, T., and Tong, T.: Cancer statistics 1991. CA, *41:* 19-36, 1991.

2. Lynch, H.T., Watson, P., Bewtra, T.A., et al.: Hereditary ovarian cancer: Heterogeneity in age at diagnosis. Cancer, *67:* 1460-1466, 1991.

3. Higgins, R.V., van Nagell, J.R., Donaldson, E.S., et al.: Transvaginal sonography as a screening method for ovarian cancer. Gynecol. Oncol., *34:* 402-406, 1989.

4. van Nagell, J.R., Higgins, R.V., Donaldson, E.S., et al.: Transvaginal sonography as a screening method for ovarian cancer: A report of the first 1000 cases screened. Cancer, *65:* 573-577, 1990.

5. Davis, H.M., Zurawski, V.R., Jr., Bast, R.C., Jr., and Klug, T.L.: Characterization of the CA 125 antigen associated with human epithelial ovarian carcinomas. Cancer Res., *46:* 6143, 1986.

6. Bast, R.C., Jr., Klug, T.L., St. John, E., et al.: A radioimmunoassay using a monoclonal antibody to monitor the course of epithelial ovarian cancer. N. Engl. J. Med., *309:* 883, 1983.

7. Berek, J.S., and Hacker, N.F.: Staging and second-look operations in ovarian cancer. *In:* Ovarian Malignancies. M.S. Piver, Ed. Edinburgh, Churchill Livingstone, Inc., 1987.

8.   Sahn, S.A.: Malignant pleural effusions. *In:* Pulmonary Diseases and Disorders, 2nd ed. A.P. Fishman, Ed. New York, McGraw-Hill, 1988.

9.   Winterbauer, R.H.: Non-neoplastic pleural effusions. *In:* Pulmonary Diseases and Disorders, 2nd ed. A.P. Fishman, Ed. New York, McGraw-Hill, 1988.

POLYDIPSIA, POLYURIA, AND A PERISELLAR MASS

Deborah E. Powell, Contributor

The patient, a 14-year-old female, had been seen a year earlier by her pediatrician with a complaint of frequent headaches and a history of increased water intake and urinary output over 2-3 years. During the previous several months, these symptoms had intensified. She had been seen by several physicians, and repeated diagnostic tests did not lead to a definitive diagnosis. Finally a computed tomographic (CT) scan was performed, and a lesion was noted in the area of the pituitary gland. During exploratory surgery, a perisellar mass was found that, on biopsy, was interpreted as dysgerminoma. Radiation therapy of 7000 rads (7000 cGy) to the primary tumor and 5000 rads (5000 cGy) to the whole brain was administered.

At completion of the radiation program, the patient was complaining of nausea and vomiting. Chest X-ray examination at this time revealed several lesions in both lung fields, most prominent on the right side. A needle biopsy was performed with CT-directed guidance on one of the right lung nodules. The biopsy showed tumor cells with areas of necrosis. Some cells had single, extremely large, vesicular nuclei. Some multinucleated tumor giant cells were seen that stained positive for chorionic gonadotropin (hCG) by immunohistochemical techniques. Stains for α-fetoprotein (AFP) were negative. Serum levels of AFP and hCG were determined; AFP was undetectable, and hCG determined by a total β-hCG assay was 425,000 mU/mL (425,000 U/L; reference range, <3.1). The patient was then given radiation therapy to the right lung while the left lung was shielded.

Five months after cranial surgery, the chest lesions had enlarged, and the patient was severely short of breath. The serum hCG level was 1,140,000 mU/mL (1,140,000 U/L). Chemotherapy with cisplatin, vinblastine, and bleomycin was started. After four courses on this regimen, the tumor size determined by X-ray study was reduced by 50%. The patient suffered moderate hematotoxicity. The serum hCG level fell initially to 1550 mU/mL (1550 U/L) but then started to rise again. Three months after start of chemotherapy, the hCG level was 2950 mU/mL (2950 U/L). Treatment was changed to vinblastine twice monthly, but about a month later the patient experienced increasing nausea and vomiting, numbness of the right cheek, and seizure activity. Seizures were well controlled with phenytoin, but repeat CT scan showed several small metastases to the central nervous system. Serum hCG levels had risen to 230,000 mU/mL (230,000 U/L).

The patient was readmitted to the hospital for radiation and chemotherapy. Upon admission she was found to have paralysis of the right third and seventh nerves and a left Babinski reflex with 2-3 beats of clonus at the left ankle. Chest X-ray examination revealed significant increase in the size of the pulmonary lesions. One week later, a repeat chest film showed continued enlargement of the tumor nodules with consolidation in the right upper lobe. The patient became increasingly short of breath and developed rales in the left upper lobe posteriorly. A clinical diagnosis of pneumonia was made (the patient was unable to produce sputum for confirmation by culture), and gentamicin and penicillin were started. Nine days after admission a sudden episode of apnea with hypotension and dilation of the left pupil ended in death. The final diagnosis was widely metastatic mixed germ cell tumor, presumably originating in the perisellar area.

Discussion

Germ Cell Tumors. These tumors are neoplasms that affect primarily children and young adults. Although the most common sites of both benign and malignant germ cell tumors are the ovaries and testes, these tumors can arise in extragonadal tissues. The most common locations for such extragonadal germ cell neoplasms are the retroperitoneum, the anterior mediastinum, and the area of the pineal gland and perisellar areas of the brain. In the central nervous system the pineal gland is the most common site of germ cell tumors. In this patient, however, the pineal gland was grossly and microscopically normal.

Germ cell tumors account for 50% of the tumors of the pineal gland. In any location, a germ cell tumor can be pure, consisting of only one identifiable cell type, or mixed, consisting of several different types of neoplastic germ cells. Because the pineal gland was not involved in this child, the origin of the tumor was believed to be in the suprasellar area. Similar cases have been reported.

Germ cell tumors can be classified according to the following scheme. The most primitive of these tumors are the *dysgerminoma/seminoma*. These neoplasms, composed of large, undifferentiated cells frequently embedded in lymphocyte-rich stroma, are extremely radio-sensitive. Although they have been associated occasionally with the presence of multi-nucleated syncytiotrophoblast-like giant cells, serum levels of chorionic gonadotropin in these patients are usually not markedly elevated. *Germ cell tumors* may show evidence of embryonic or extraembryonic differentiation. Extraembryonic differentiation is manifested in the endodermal sinus tumor and the choriocarcinoma. Embryonic differentiation is manifested as different types of teratoma (benign or malignant) and embryonal carcinoma. Both of these groups of neoplasms are much more common in ovary and testes than elsewhere, although they have been seen in extragonadal locations. All of the other types of germ cell neoplasms are less radiosensitive than is the dysgerminoma/seminoma group, and early and aggressive chemotherapy is usually required to control the disease when other tumor types are present. Any of the different types of germ cell tumors can occur alone (pure germ cell tumors) or as a mixture of two or more types (mixed germ cell tumors), as mentioned previously.

One of the important features of germ cell tumors is their association with production of tumor markers or oncofetal antigens by the tumor cells. Germ cell tumors produce several of these substances, including α-fetoprotein (AFP), human chorionic gonadotropin (hCG), human placental lactogen (hPL), and α_1-antitrypsin (AAT). Endodermal sinus tumors are associated with production of AFP, choriocarcinomas with the production of hCG and hPL, and embryonal carcinomas with the production of AAT, AFP, and hCG.

This case illustrates the inadequacy of a small biopsy specimen for diagnosis of mixed germ cell tumors. Although the original biopsy showed only dysgerminoma, clearly the rapid progress of this patient's disease indicated other elements had been present, most likely choriocarcinoma, a highly malignant cell type less sensitive to radiation therapy. A small biopsy obtained at craniotomy cannot reasonably be expected to provide a complete picture of the different histological types of tumor. Therefore, an important adjunct in classifying such tumors is the determination of the presence and level of abnormal tumor-produced substances, i.e., tumor markers or oncofetal antigens. The probability of choriocarcinoma cells in this patient's tumor was enhanced by the elevation of hCG level found early on in the disease. Effect of therapy on tumor burden could be and was followed with measurement of serum levels of hCG. Tumor markers generally can be used to good purpose for monitoring the course of disease and the response to therapeutic measures.

Human chorionic gonadotropin is a glycoprotein hormone produced normally by the syncytiotrophoblast of the developing placenta. In a normal pregnancy its level rises dramatically in the first trimester to fall again after approximately 60 days of gestation to low levels that are maintained throughout the pregnancy. It is also produced by certain neoplasms, including germ cell tumors (most notably choriocarcinoma and embryonal carcinoma), hydatidiform moles and other types of trophoblastic disease, and tumors of other sites such as large cell undifferentiated carcinoma of the lung. The intact hCG molecule consists of two noncovalently bound dissimilar subunits designated α and β. The α-subunit of hCG has a high degree of structural homology with the α-subunits of luteinizing hormone (LH), follicle-stimulating hormone (FSH), and thyroid-stimulating hormone (TSH), all produced by the anterior pituitary. However, the β-subunits, which determine the biological activity, are structurally and immunologically different for these hormones, allowing them to be measured without interference from each other in radio- and enzyme immunoassays. Both whole (intact) hCG and hCG β-subunit assays are available. However, the intact hCG assays do not measure *free* β-hCG subunits that may be present to a significant degree in specimens from some patients with tumors. In contrast, a *total* β-hCG assay measures β-subunits present as free β-subunits as well as those that are part of the intact hCG molecule. Although assays for intact hCG are adequate for detecting and monitoring pregnancies, they may not be satisfactory for tumor diagnosis. Certain tumors may produce only the β-subunit, and in these particular neoplasms, assays for the intact molecule are unsatisfactory since they will not detect the β-subunits being secreted.[1,2]

High levels of chorionic gonadotropin such as those seen with multiple gestations and certain tumors can be associated with important clinical symptoms. Probably the most common of these is the presence of excessive nausea and vomiting, which is seen as the typical "morning sickness" of a normal first trimester pregnancy. In addition, other symptoms may be associated with the TSH-like effect of chorionic gonadotropin. These include rapid heart rate and sometimes frank congestive heart failure.

Summary

The importance of correct classification of germ cell tumors into mixed and pure categories cannot be overstated. Approximately 6% of germ cell tumors of the ovary are mixed cell types; as many as 35% of intracranial germ cell tumors fall into this category.[3] The patient's course will be determined by the most malignant cell type present because it will be the type most likely to metastasize. Germ cell neoplasms are common tumors in children and young adults. Their production of tumor markers is always a help to the astute clinician who, upon observing detectable tumor in the gonads, retroperitoneum, mediastinum, or suprasellar area of children, is then faced with classifying and treating it.

Treatment

Germ cell tumors, both gonadal and extragonadal, are treated with a combination of surgery and multi-drug chemotherapy. The pure dysgerminomas or seminomas can be treated successfully with radiation therapy because of their extreme radiosensitivity.

References

1. Odell, W.W.: Humoral manifestations of cancer. *In:* Williams Textbook of Endocrinology, 7th ed. J.D. Wilson and D.W. Foster, Eds. Philadelphia, W.B. Saunders Co., 1985.

2. Rinker, A.D., and Tietz, N.W.: β-hCG vs. intact hCG assays in the detection of trophoblastic disease. Clin. Chem., *35:* 1799-1806, 1989.

3. Kurman, R.J., and Norris, H.J.: Malignant mixed germ cell tumors of the ovary: A clinical and pathologic analysis of 30 cases. Obstet. Gynecol., *48:* 579-589, 1976.

WOMAN WITH ANEMIA AND HYPERTENSION

John A. Koepke, Contributor
Richard A. Mc Pherson, Reviewer

This 47-year-old woman had several pregnancies complicated by bouts of urinary frequency and urgency. The diagnosis of recurrent urinary tract infections had been made and several courses of treatment with sulfonamides had been given during and following her pregnancies.

About two years ago, the patient complained of increasing weakness and fatigue, with occasional episodes of dizziness and headache. At that time, she was seen by her family practitioner. Physical examination showed a pale, chronically ill woman who appeared to be somewhat short of breath. Significant positive physical findings included the lung fields, which were dull at both bases with a few rales in the lower lung fields. There was a pitting edema of the feet and ankles. Examination of the abdomen was unremarkable. Her blood pressure was 155/97 mm Hg.

A urinalysis, a blood count, and a panel of chemistry tests were performed, and the following results were obtained:

Analyte	Value, conventional units	Reference range, conventional units	Value, SI units	Reference range, SI units
Sodium (S)	146 mmol/L	138-145	Same	
Potassium (S)	5.9 mmol/L	4.1-5.3	Same	
Chloride (S)	110 mmol/L	98-107	Same	
CO_2, total (S)	20 mmol/L	22-30	Same	
Urea nitrogen (S)	60 mg/dL	8-18	21 mmol urea/L	2.9-6.4
Creatinine (S)	4.0 mg/dL	0.6-1.1	353 µmol/L	53-97
Glucose (S)	96 mg/dL	70-105	5.3 mmol/L	3.9-5.8
Protein, total (S)	5.6 g/dL	6.2-8.0	56 g/L	62-80
Albumin (S)	3.0 g/dL	3.8-5.4	30 g/L	38-54
Iron (S)	220 µg/dL	70-180	39 µmol/L	13-32
Iron-binding capacity (S)	295 µg/dL	250-400	53 µmol/L	45-72
Ferritin (S)	80 µg/L	20-90	Same	
Creatinine clearance (S, U)	25 mL/min	85-125	0.42 mL/s	1.42-2.08
Hemoglobin (B)	9.0 g/dL	12.0-16.0	5.59 mmol/L	7.45-9.93
MCV (B)	87 fL	80-100	Same	
MCH (B)	29 pg	27-33	Same	
Reticulocyte count (B)	$20 \times 10^3/\mu L$	10-75	$20 \times 10^9/L$	10-75
Leukocyte count (B)	$3.7 \times 10^3/\mu L$	3.2-9.8	$3.7 \times 10^9/L$	3.2-9.8
Specific gravity (U)	1.007	1.010-1.035	Same	
pH (U)	5.0	4.5-8.0	Same	
Protein (U)	2+	Negative		
Glucose (U)	Negative	Negative		
Microscopic (U)				
Leukocytes	Few	<10/hpf		
Erythrocytes	Occasional	<3/hpf		

Analyte	Value, conventional units	Reference range, conventional units	Value, SI units	Reference range, SI units
Microscopic (U), cont.				
Casts	10-15; broad, waxy	<3/hpf		
Bacteria	None	None		

A diagnosis of renal disease was made based upon the clinical history, evidence of fluid retention, and hypertension. The laboratory data were consistent with chronic renal disease and early renal failure. Therefore, the patient was advised to have a renal biopsy, to which she consented. The percutaneous renal biopsy showed loss of renal tissue, interstitial fibrosis, and infiltration with lymphocytes and other inflammatory cells; these histological findings were consistent with chronic pyelonephritis.

The patient was placed on a program of chronic renal dialysis (twice each week). Although she improved symptomatically while under this treatment regimen, her anemia continued to require the transfusion of a unit of packed red blood cells about every six weeks.

Differential Diagnosis

Additional elements of a patient's medical history and physical examination may be relevant to the diagnosis of anemia and to establishing its etiological origin. Anemia causes paleness of the skin; particularly useful for clinical evaluation is the color of the nail beds and mucous membranes in patients with pigmented skin. (In renal failure a sallow complexion may indicate severe azotemia.) Clubbing of the fingers, an unusual finding, may result from poor oxygenation due to anemia. Examination of the heart can reveal dramatic flow murmurs due solely to the decreased blood viscosity of severe anemia. Other abnormal heart sounds may suggest hemolysis from mechanical trauma during closure of calcified or artificial valves.

The presence of organomegaly of liver or spleen may suggest hemolysis or other causes of anemia such as malaria. Malnutrition or malabsorption can be suspected if there is a history of diarrhea or constipation (e.g., bacterial overgrowth). A neurological examination may reveal changes in mentation, vibratory sensation, and reflexes that suggest a vitamin deficiency (e.g., B_{12}) that may also be responsible for anemia. Endocrine abnormalities can cause anemia so that thyroid studies as well as an evaluation of the pituitary and adrenal glands may ultimately be necessary. Both stool and urine should be examined for evidence of occult or frank hemorrhage to rule out an ulcer or malignancy. Women should be asked about excess menstrual blood loss. Urinalysis may suggest hemolysis if the urobilinogen is elevated.

Careful examination of the peripheral blood film is particularly useful in delineating many forms of anemia. The MCV clearly distinguishes microcytic (e.g., iron deficiency or thalassemia) from macrocytic (e.g., folate or vitamin B_{12} deficiency) anemia. Abnormal erythrocyte morphological features can suggest hemolysis (fragmented cells, microspherocytes), hemoglobinopathy (sickled cells, target cells), and membrane protein or enzyme defects that result in poikilocytosis and anisocytosis.

Mild to moderate anemia in middle-aged female patients requires a fairly complete laboratory study. Although chronic renal disease is probably the cause of anemia in this patient, iron deficiency, chronic blood loss, hemolytic disorders, and other less frequent causes must also be considered or ruled out. Therefore, serum iron, transferrin (or total iron-binding capacity, TIBC), and ferritin levels are commonly measured, as well as the reticulocyte count and occult blood in feces. Bone marrow aspiration and biopsy may be indicated in some cases.

In this case, iron deficiency was ruled out with the evidence of a normal serum iron and iron-binding capacity. In iron deficiency states, the serum iron is characteristically very low but the iron-binding capacity is increased, and the percentage of transferrin saturation with iron is usually <15%. (Alternatively, total iron and serum transferrin, the protein that transports iron in blood, can be determined and the percent saturation calculated.) In this patient, the percent saturation was greater than normal, the opposite of what would have been seen in iron deficiency.

In iron deficiency states, one would also expect a deficiency or absence of storage iron in the bone marrow. In the past, a bone marrow biopsy or aspirate for cytochemical staining with Prussian blue would have been required to assess the iron stores. Although this procedure is most reliable, it can be rather traumatic for the patient. Now, a surrogate test, serum ferritin, is available. Ferritin levels in normal individuals are a reliable guide for tissue iron stores, and levels above 20 µg/L indicate adequate stores. However, since ferritin is a so-called acute phase protein (i.e., the serum level increases in a wide variety of acute infections and reactions), it may be increased in patients with either acute or chronic disease. In patients with chronic disease, only ferritin levels above 60 µg/L should be considered as evidence for ruling out iron deficiency.

Other causes of anemia include a wide variety of hemolytic anemias as well as blood loss. For example, sickle cell disease can be complicated by renal papillary necrosis with urinary tract infection leading to chronic renal failure and subsequent anemia of chronic disease. A normal reticulocyte count ruled out hemolytic processes as the basis for this patient's anemia. Elevated counts are characteristic of chronic hemolytic processes that stimulate premature release of erythrocytes from the bone marrow. Blood loss, in this case, was not a serious consideration since the clinical history and tests for fecal blood were negative, and iron studies had ruled out the probability of iron deficiency anemia characteristic of chronic blood loss.

Whereas in the past the anemia of chronic disease has been frequently a diagnosis of exclusion, this entity is now more widely recognized and diagnosed primarily rather than by exclusion.[1] The diagnosis of chronic renal disease is well documented in this case by the findings of renal biopsy. Although the patient responded quite well to renal dialysis, the anemia remained a significant problem.

In chronic renal disease, the destruction of renal parenchyma is associated with the decreased synthesis of the hematopoietic growth factor erythropoietin. This hormone normally stimulates maturation of the bone marrow erythroblasts and causes the release of red cells from the marrow in order to maintain a normal peripheral erythrocyte level. The decrease or absence of erythropoietin that occurs in renal disease thus results in anemia.[2]

The anemia of chronic disease is characteristically normocytic and normochromic. Hemoglobin concentrations are 7.0-11.0 g/dL (4.34-6.83 mmol/L), and the absolute reticulocyte count is normal or low. Although bone marrow examination was not done in this case, the expected picture would be a normal or low cellularity with an increase in storage iron. These patients fail to incorporate iron into developing erythrocytes, hence the iron stores are overfilled. This picture could be modified, of course, if there were supervening complicating factors such as gastrointestinal bleeding or hemolytic processes.[3]

Treatment

A patient with a chronic disease (in this case, chronic renal disease) and an associated anemia may be a difficult problem for long-term care. Patients with chronic renal disease are frequently placed on long-term dialysis programs while awaiting a renal transplant. While being chronically dialyzed, they may require frequent erythrocyte transfusions. Problems associated with chronic transfusions include the development of erythrocyte antibodies, the accumulation of excess storage iron, and the risk of infection with hepatitis viruses, cytomegalovirus (CMV), or human immunodeficiency virus (HIV).

Patients sometimes treat themselves with iron since they know that iron deficiency is a common cause of anemia. Iron therapy for anemia of chronic disease carries an important risk. In most kinds of anemia, there is an increased absorption of dietary iron (the expected physiological response) whether or not the anemia is due to iron deficiency. Normally about 10% of dietary iron is absorbed, but in the hemolytic anemias such as sickle cell disease or thalassemia, the amount of iron absorbed increases markedly. The phenomenon occurs because there is an increased synthesis of apoferritin in the intestinal mucosal cells, and increased amounts of apoprotein increase the absorptive capability for iron. When more iron is administered orally or when blood transfusions are used in long-term treatment of anemia, the body's normal storage capacity for iron is exceeded. The excess iron is taken up by hepatocytes, in which it is toxic and can result in cirrhosis. If there is significant hepatic fibrosis, this type of iron storage disease is termed hemochromatosis. Excess iron also irreversibly affects the myocardium and the cardiac conduction system; it may also affect the pancreas and lead to diabetes. Increased melanin deposition in the skin and testicular atrophy, probably secondary to hypothalamic-pituitary malfunction, may also be noted.

Recently the use of recombinant human erythropoietin (r-HuEPO) has been successful to treat anemia in patients on chronic renal dialysis, although some patients with chronic renal disease appear to respond more promptly and completely than do others. The treatment has allowed a marked reduction in transfusion requirements for these patients and thus diminishes the risks associated with transfusions.[4]

References

1. Erslev, A.J.: Anemia of chronic disorders. Glenside, PA, Toltzis Communications, Inc., 1987.

2. Paganini, E.P.: Overview of anemia associated with chronic renal disease: Primary and secondary mechanisms. Semin. Nephrol., 9: 3, 1989.

3. Lewis, J.P., and Meyers, F.J.: The anemia of renal insufficiency. In: Laboratory Hematology. J.A. Koepke, Ed. New York, Churchill Livingstone, Inc., 1984.

4. Lundin, A.P.: Recombinant erythropoietin and chronic renal failure. Hosp. Prac., pp. 45-53, 15 April 1991.

Additional Reading

Erslev, A.J., Adamson, J.W., Eschbach, J.W., and Winearls, C.G., Eds.: Erythropoietin: Molecular, Cellular, and Clinical Biology. Baltimore, Johns Hopkins University Press, 1991.

CHILD WITH PNEUMONIA

John A. Koepke, Contributor
Richard A. Mc Pherson, Reviewer

A 12-year-old Afro-American male child was admitted to the hospital through the emergency room because of severe illness marked by high fever, 103 °F (39.6 °C), and rapid, shallow breathing.

Physical examination indicated consolidation of the left lower lung fields where no breath sounds could be auscultated. The heart appeared to be somewhat enlarged on X-ray film, but this judgment was difficult to make because of the changes in adjacent lung regions. Examination of the abdomen revealed that the liver was enlarged, but the spleen could not be palpated. The patient had several healed scars and open sores on his ankles.

A blood sample drawn in the emergency room provided the following results:

Analyte	Value, conventional units	Reference range, conventional units	Value, SI units	Reference range, SI units
Hemoglobin (B)	11.0 g/dL	13.6-17.2	6.83 mmol/L	8.44-10.67
MCV (B)	82 fL	80-110	Same	
MCH (B)	28 pg	27-33	Same	
Leukocyte count (B)	28 x 10^3/μL	3.2-9.8	28 x 10^9/L	3.2-9.8

Review of the peripheral blood film showed poikilocytosis with crescent-shaped erythrocytes. There was a granulocytosis with a marked left shift, i.e., many immature granulocytes in the circulation. Many granulocytes contained toxic granulations and had Döhle bodies. Chemical urinalysis showed proteinuria, but screening tests for urinary tract infection, i.e., nitrite and leukocyte esterase, were negative. Examination of stained sputum showed many gram-positive cocci in pairs and short chains, sometimes within granulocytes. Sputum culture grew *Streptococcus pneumoniae*, which was consistent with the initial Gram stain of the sputum. Portable X-ray examination of the chest showed consolidation of the left lower lobe of the lung. Based on these laboratory and radiological findings, the patient was treated with penicillin for bacterial (pneumococcal) pneumonia. He did well and was discharged from the hospital in five days.

Differential Diagnosis

The combination of anemia and pneumococcal pneumonia in an Afro-American child directs attention to consideration of another underlying disorder possibly involving a hemoglobinopathy. The findings of proteinuria and mild hepatomegaly without apparent splenomegaly or lymphadenopathy also provide the clinician with leads that can be pursued with appropriate laboratory examination.

Laboratory investigation of anemia begins with an automated complete blood count (CBC) that differentiates anemias into normocytic (MCV, 80-100 fL), microcytic (MCV,

<80 fL), or macrocytic (MCV, >100 fL) types. Normocytic anemia, such as this case showed, mandates examination of the peripheral blood smear for unusual or abnormal erythrocytes that demonstrate microcytosis, hypochromia, spherocytosis, anisocytosis, poikilocytosis, or presence of target or sickle cells. Howell-Jolly bodies in some erythrocytes indicate a nonfunctioning spleen that can result from sickle cell disease. Multiple episodes of crisis cause splenic ischemia and infarction, finally culminating in splenic fibrosis and atrophy (i.e., autosplenectomy).

A reticulocyte count is very useful in differentiating hemolytic anemias with normal erythropoiesis from nonhemolytic anemias in which erythrocyte production is diminished. The reticulocyte count is elevated in most hemolytic anemias (in this case, the reticulocyte count was $310 \times 10^3/\mu L$ [$310 \times 10^9/L$], reference range 24-84), although a normal or low count may occur in aplastic crises.

The diagnosis of hemolytic anemia was made on the basis of a moderate anemia coupled with an elevated reticulocyte count. Because the patient was Afro-American, sickle cell disease (with a prevalence of 1 in 600 Afro-Americans) was at the top of the list of possible diagnoses. In this patient, the sickle cell screening test was positive. This test checks for the decreased solubility of sickle hemoglobin (Hb S) in a specially constituted buffer solution.

Glucose-6-phosphate dehydrogenase (G-6-PD) deficiency should also be considered in the differential diagnosis. The gene for G-6-PD is carried on the X chromosome, and consequently G-6-PD deficiency is a sex-linked disorder. Its incidence in Afro-American males is roughly 1 in 8. Erythrocytes of these individuals contain levels of G-6-PD that, although low, are usually adequate to sustain cell maintenance. However, exposure to oxidizing substances (e.g., primaquine for prophylaxis of malaria, nitrofurantoin for urinary tract infection, or fava beans) or an acute febrile illness may overwhelm the fragile system operating with marginal levels of G-6-PD and lead to acute hemolysis. In interim periods, the erythrocytes of patients deficient in G-6-PD survive normally. G-6-PD deficiency is detected with a screening procedure followed by quantitative assay for specific enzyme activity. The G-6-PD screening test was negative in this patient, indicating normal G-6-PD activity.

Afro-American patients may be afflicted with thalassemia or thalassemia-sickle cell disease, and therefore the possibility of these conditions must not be ignored. Hemoglobin electrophoresis plus measurement of the concentrations of fetal hemoglobin and hemoglobin A_2 are necessary to make these diagnoses. The exact delineation of the various kinds of thalassemia can at times be quite difficult, and family studies as well as more sophisticated laboratory studies (e.g., α- and β-hemoglobin chain synthetic ratios; globin gene deletion by DNA analysis) may be required in certain cases.[1]

Additional studies such as assays for total and conjugated bilirubin, urine urobilinogen, haptoglobin, and other analytes are usually abnormal in cases of accelerated hemolysis, regardless of cause. These determinations may be useful for following the severity and progression of a hemolytic process, but they do not add more to establishing a specific diagnosis.

On the basis of the positive sickle cell screening test, hemoglobin electrophoresis was performed to confirm the diagnosis because false positive or false negative results may be obtained with the hemoglobin solubility screening test. Hemoglobin electrophoresis uses cellulose acetate or agarose gels at pH 8.6 for convenient resolution of hemoglobins A, F, C, and S. A second supplemental electrophoretic procedure to separate some of the abnormal hemoglobins, e.g., hemoglobins D and G, is performed at acid pH (6.0) in agar gels.

In the electrophoretic procedure, the relative proportions of normal as well as abnormal hemoglobins can be quantitated. In this case the proportion of hemoglobin S (Hb S) was 82%, fetal hemoglobin (Hb F) 14%, and hemoglobin A_2 (Hb A_2) 4%. The patient had not received any erythrocyte transfusions in the previous several weeks, and therefore there was no contamination of the specimen with normal adult hemoglobin A (Hb A) from transfused blood. When ordering hemoglobin electrophoresis in suspected cases of sickle cell disease, the physician must take recent transfusions into account. A mistaken diagnosis of sickle cell *trait* could be made in a patient with sickle cell disease who had recently been transfused with red cells containing normal Hb A.

Whereas diagnostic electrophoresis should be restricted to a time long after transfusion, effectiveness of a transfusion can be monitored by hemoglobin electrophoresis afterwards. By measuring amounts of Hb A and Hb S periodically, the proportion of Hb S can be monitored and new transfusions invoked to maintain Hb S at <30% and thus avert sickle cell crises.

Other conditions in which Hb S may be present include sickle cell trait (Hb S plus normal Hb A; prevalence 1 in 12), SC hemoglobinopathy (Hb S plus Hb C; prevalence 1 in 800), and SD hemoglobinopathy (Hb S plus Hb D). All of these conditions are usually less severe clinically than sickle cell disease (Hb SS). Most of these hemoglobinopathies can be accurately diagnosed in the laboratory by standard hemoglobin electrophoresis or by more specialized means such as isoelectric focusing or even by direct sequencing of the amino acids in an abnormal hemoglobin molecule.[2] Prenatal diagnosis of a hemoglobinopathy is best done by DNA analysis of fetal cells obtained by sampling the chorionic villi.

Treatment

The standard treatment for sickle cell disease has not changed a great deal in the last decade. Chronic transfusions are usually required to maintain a patient's hemoglobin near 10.5 g/dL (6.52 mmol/L). The many transfusions these patients receive raise the risk of developing various antibodies to donor erythrocytes. About one-quarter of sickle cell patients will develop antibodies, and procuring compatible blood becomes more difficult. The use of designated, related donors whose erythrocyte antigen phenotypes match those of the recipient lessens the rate of immunization and also improves the chances of finding compatible blood.[3]

Another problem associated with chronic transfusions is transfusion hemosiderosis, the buildup of stored iron in the patient's body. Each unit of transfused erythrocytes contains from 150 to 250 mg of elemental iron. When the transfused cells finally are cleared, the iron from their hemoglobin is stored in the reticuloendothelial cells. By this means the body naturally conserves iron. In addition, intestinal absorption of dietary iron increases in patients with chronic hemolytic anemia. Both of these mechanisms cause massive storage of iron, which can lead to parenchymal organ (liver, heart) and endocrine gland (especially pancreas) dysfunction. The risk of iron overload may be lessened by use of partial exchange transfusions.

Infection is the major cause of death in children with sickle cell disease because, after loss of splenic function, susceptibility increases for infections with encapsulated organisms, e.g., *Streptococcus pneumoniae, Haemophilus influenzae*. Osteomyelitis with *Salmonella* is also common in patients with sickle cell disease. General preventive measures include immunization with a polyvalent pneumococcal vaccine or even chemoprophylaxis with antibiotics. Folate supplementation should also be administered to prevent depletion in the presence of life-long brisk hematopoiesis.

Painful, acute sickle cell crises are treated with oral or parenteral fluid replacement and with analgesia, e.g., narcotics. Sickle cell crises are especially severe when they follow diseases such as pneumonia in which there is impaired oxygenation of the blood and subsequent intravascular sickling and vaso-occlusion. A vicious cycle of deoxygenation leading to polymerizaton of Hb S and erythrocyte sickling results in sludging of blood in the small vessels with capillary obstruction and subsequent organ injury. This ischemia and necrosis causes acidosis, which in turn causes further sickling and worsening of the crisis state. In such cases oxygen therapy is indicated.[4]

The complications of vaso-occlusive crises involve many organs including lung, liver, brain (cerebrovascular accidents), penis (priapism), bone (aseptic necrosis), retina, kidney, spleen, and skin (leg ulcers). Congestive heart failure is common. Erythrocyte exchange transfusion can lead to visible improvement of skin ulcers such as this patient displayed. The necrosis and periosteitis of metacarpal and metatarsal bones causes a painful deformation termed the hand-foot syndrome. Aplastic crisis (acute failure to produce erythrocytes) may result from infection with human parvovirus that selectively affects erythroid precursors in bone marrow. A further complication of any hereditary hemolytic disorder is formation of bilirubin gallstones to a degree that may require cholecystectomy.

A number of innovative therapeutic initiatives are currently under active investigation; they include trials of new drugs and bone marrow transplantation. New drugs are designed to inhibit Hb S polymerization. The most promising of them is the chemotherapeutic agent hydroxyurea; its use has been associated with significant increases in the proportion of Hb F in the patient's cells.[5] Increased concentrations of Hb F increase the minimum gelling concentration of deoxygenated Hb S solutions. Some medical centers are now performing bone marrow transplant for hemoglobinopathies, primarily for treatment of thalassemia, but there exists a potential for application to sickle cell disease in the future.

References

1. Steinberg, M.H.: The interactions of α-thalassemia with hemoglobinopathies. Hematol. Oncol. Clin. North Am., 5: 453-473, 1991.

2. Kaufman, R.E.: Analysis of abnormal hemoglobins. In: Practical Laboratory Hematology. J.A. Koepke, Ed. New York, Churchill Livingstone, Inc, 1991.

3. Kanter, M.H., and Hodge, S. E.: The probability of obtaining compatible blood from related directed donors. Arch. Pathol. Lab. Med., 114: 1013-1016, 1990.

4. Fabry, M.E., and Kaul, D.K.: Sickle cell vaso-occlusion. Hematol. Oncol. Clin. North Am., 5: 375-398, 1991.

5. Rodgers, G.P.: Recent approaches to the treatment of sickle cell anemia. JAMA, 265: 2097-2101, 1991.

Additional Reading

Mentzer, W.C., and Wagner, G.M., Eds.: The Hereditary Hemolytic Anemias. New York, Churchill Livingstone, Inc., 1989.

A WOMAN WITH FATIGUE AND PALLOR

Naif Z. Abraham, Jr., Contributor
Douglas A. Nelson, Contributor
Susan A. Fuhrman, Reviewer

A 59-year-old secretary was observed by her employer to show fatigue and weakness that had developed insidiously over a period of seven months. Recently she had become very pale and exhibited irritability, forgetfulness, personality change, and mood swings. Her work had deteriorated so greatly that her employer demanded that she seek medical attention. Upon physical examination, she appeared very pale with slightly icteric skin and sclerae. Her pulse was rapid, and auscultation revealed a systolic flow murmur. Her tongue was not sore, but it appeared smooth and beefy red (atrophic glossitis) on inspection. In addition, she described the recent onset of tingling and prickling sensations (paresthesias) localized symmetrically in her hands and feet. The neurological examination was remarkable for diminished vibration and position sense as well as for impaired cutaneous touch and pain sensation in the lower extremities. Although the patient admitted to having episodes of weakness and lightheadedness, she denied hallucinations or other disturbances of mentation.

Initial laboratory results were as follows:

Analyte	Value, conventional units	Reference range, conventional units	Value, SI units	Reference range, SI units
Leukocyte count (B)	$3.8 \times 10^3/\mu L$	4.5-11.0	$3.8 \times 10^9/L$	4.5-11.0
Erythrocyte count (B)	$1.36 \times 10^6/\mu L$	3.8-5.3	$1.36 \times 10^{12}/L$	3.8-5.3
Hemoglobin (B)	6.1 g/dL	11.7-16.0	3.79 mmol/L	7.26-9.93
Hematocrit (B)	18 %	35-47	0.18	0.35-0.47
MCV (B)	131 fL	81-101	Same	
MCH (B)	44.9 pg	27-34	Same	
MCHC (BErcs)	34.3 g Hb/dL	31-36	21 mmol Hb/L	19-22
Platelet count (B)	$83 \times 10^3/\mu L$	150-450	$83 \times 10^9/L$	150-450
Reticulocyte count (B)	0.2 %	0.5-1.5	0.002	0.005-0.015
Albumin (S)	4.2 g/dL	3.5-5.0	42 g/L	35-50
ALP (S)	78 U/L	25-100	1.3 μkat/L	0.4-1.7
ALT (S)	38 U/L	8-20	0.63 μkat/L	0.13-0.33
AST (S)	73 U/L	8-20	1.22 μkat/L	0.13-0.33
LDH (S)	1535 U/L	140-280	25.59 μkat/L	2.33-4.67
Bilirubin, total (S)	2.1 mg/dL	0.2-1.0	36 μmol/L	3-17
Urea nitrogen (S)	8 mg/dL	7-18	2.9 mmol urea/L	2.5-6.4
Creatinine (S)	0.6 mg/dL	0.6-1.1	53 μmol/L	53-97
Cholesterol (S)	131 mg/dL	172-300	3.39 mmol/L	4.45-7.76
Peripheral blood leukocyte differential count				
Neutrophils	$2.1 \times 10^3/\mu L$ (56%)	1.5-6.7	$2.1 \times 10^9/L$ (0.56)	1.5-6.7
Eosinophils	$0.04 \times 10^3/\mu L$ (1%)	0.0-0.7	$0.04 \times 10^9/L$ (0.01)	0.0-0.7
Basophils	$0.0 \times 10^3/\mu L$ (0%)	0.0-0.15	$0.0 \times 10^9/L$ (0)	0.0-0.15
Lymphocytes	$1.5 \times 10^3/\mu L$ (39%)	1.5-4.0	$1.5 \times 10^9/L$ (0.39)	1.5-4.0
Monocytes	$0.15 \times 10^3/\mu L$ (4%)	0.2-0.95	$0.15 \times 10^9/L$ (0.04)	0.2-0.95

Erythrocyte morphology: Marked anisocytosis; moderate poikilocytosis; moderate polychromasia; moderate macrocytosis, including oval macrocytes.

Leukocyte morphology: Occasional hypersegmented neutrophils present; nucleated erythrocytes present (3 per 100 leukocytes counted).

Results from the patient's complete blood count indicated a macrocytic anemia. The differential diagnosis of macrocytic anemia includes megaloblastic anemia, myelofibrosis with myeloid metaplasia, alcohol abuse, liver disease, and the myelodysplastic syndromes.[1] Presence of numerous oval macrocytes, combined with the presence of hypersegmented neutrophils, favored megaloblastic anemia as the most likely diagnosis. In addition, the neurological findings raised the question of megaloblastic anemia due to cobalamin (vitamin B_{12}) deficiency, and additional laboratory tests were requested and are given below.

Analyte	Value, conventional units	Reference range, conventional units	Value, SI units	Reference range, SI units
Cobalamin (S)	114 pg/mL	200-900	84 pmol/L	148-664
Folate (S)	3.1 ng/mL	3-16	7.2 nmol/L	7-36
Folate (Erc)	100 ng/mL	130-628	227 nmol/L	294-1422

The low serum cobalamin and the normal serum folate supported a diagnosis of cobalamin deficiency as the cause of the macrocytic anemia. In the United States, cobalamin deficiency is virtually always due to malabsorption, and thus a Schilling test* was performed in order to distinguish lack of intrinsic factor (IF), which binds to cobalamin in the stomach, from disease of the terminal ileum (the site for IF-facilitated absorption of cobalamin).

	Value, conventional units	Reference range, conventional units	Value, SI units	Reference range, SI units
Schilling Test (% of labeled cobalamin excreted in urine)				
Stage I	3 %	>9 %	0.03	>0.09
Stage II	15 %	>9 %	0.15	>0.09

The patient had impaired absorption of cobalamin (Stage I) that was corrected in the presence of exogenously administered intrinsic factor (Stage II). In the absence of evidence of gastric disease or of previous gastric surgery (gastrectomy), the Schilling test provided strong evidence for the diagnosis of pernicious anemia.

The patient was treated with administration of hydroxycobalamin (1000 µg/d, intramuscularly, for two weeks). The patient began to feel better within the first few days after therapy was begun. After two weeks, the following laboratory results were obtained:

---

* **Schilling test:** *Stage I.* The fasting patient is given an oral dose of radiolabeled (tracer) cobalamin, followed two hours later by a large, parenteral dose of unlabeled cobalamin in order to saturate the tissue-binding sites; saturation allows the absorbed labeled cobalamin to be excreted in the urine. Radioactivity is then measured in the urine collected over the next 24 hours. Normal levels of radioactivity in the urine indicate normal absorption of cobalamin. An abnormally low level of radioactivity in the urine indicates poor absorption of cobalamin and necessitates further testing. *Stage II.* The test is repeated, and this time the oral dose of labeled cobalamin is given together with hog intrinsic factor. Normal radioactivity in the 24-h urine specimen indicates that a lack of intrinsic factor in the patient is the cause of cobalamin deficiency, whereas abnormally low radioactivity in the Stage II sample indicates intestinal malabsorption.

Analyte	Value, conventional units	Reference range, conventional units	Value, SI units	Reference range, SI units
Leukocyte count (B)	$15.5 \times 10^3/\mu L$	4.5-11.0	$15.5 \times 10^9/L$	4.5-11.0
Erythrocyte count (B)	$3.28 \times 10^6/\mu L$	3.8-5.3	$3.28 \times 10^{12}/L$	3.8-5.3
Hemoglobin (B)	11.3 g/dL	11.7-16.0	7.01 mmol/L	7.26-9.93
Hematocrit (B)	34 %	35-47	0.34	0.35-0.47
MCV (B)	104.7 fL	81-101	Same	
MCH (B)	34.5 pg	27-34	Same	
MCHC (BErcs)	32.9 g Hb/dL	31-36	20 mmol Hb/L	19-22
Platelet count (B)	$460 \times 10^3/\mu L$	150-450	$460 \times 10^9/L$	150-450
Reticulocyte count (B)	5.1 %	0.5-1.5	0.051	0.005-0.015
Cobalamin (S)	1037 pg/mL	200-900	765 pmol/L	148-664

Despite marked improvement in hematological status, the patient's neurological manifestations were not entirely reversed. She showed a persistent deficit in vibration sense, and her paresthesias showed minimal change. However, the prognosis for improvement of her neurological manifestations was good, because of the relatively short duration of the neurological symptoms before treatment. The longer the duration of neurological symptoms, the less likely that neurological changes will be reversed by therapy.[2]

Definition of the Disease

Pernicious anemia (PA) is megaloblastic anemia caused by cobalamin deficiency attributable to atrophy of the gastric oxyntic (parietal) cell mucosa. This condition results in deficient secretion of hydrochloric acid and of intrinsic factor (IF) into the gastric fluid. IF is a glycoprotein with a high affinity for cobalamin; the IF-cobalamin complex eventually attaches to IF receptors in the ileum and thus facilitates absorption of cobalamin. In the absence of IF, malabsorption of cobalamin occurs and leads to frank cobalamin deficiency. The deficiency becomes apparent only after three to four years because the stores of the vitamin in normal liver tissue are sufficient for that length of time.

The gastric antral mucosa remains unaffected, and consequently serum gastrin levels may be elevated as a result of loss of feedback inhibition by hydrochloric acid on gastrin secretion. The serum gastrin assay is an ancillary test and may be useful in assessing the significance of a low serum cobalamin level.[3] However, definitive diagnosis of PA is obtained with a Schilling test, which, unlike serum tests, assesses the actual absorption of cobalamin.[4]

An autoimmune process may be the etiology responsible for failure of the parietal cell mucosa in PA. Patients affected by PA frequently suffer from other autoimmune diseases such as Graves' disease, Hashimoto's thyroiditis, and vitiligo. Three types of autoantibodies have been identified in many (but not all) patients with PA: blocking antibodies that bind IF and prevent its binding with cobalamin; binding antibodies that react with IF-cobalamin complexes; and parietal canalicular antibodies directed against the microvilli of the gastric parietal cell itself. These autoantibodies may be the agent producing the atrophic fundal gastritis, rather than a result of the atrophy, but the relationship is not proved. Even so, an autoimmune process is believed to underlie development of Type A (fundal or oxyntic) gastritis, which in about 10% of patients progresses to overt PA.[5]

Either cobalamin deficiency or folate deficiency can impair DNA synthesis throughout the body by interfering with the utilization of tetrahydrofolate and its derivatives.[1,6] Consequently, the tissues most seriously affected are those in which rapid cell division occurs, namely, the bone marrow and the lining of the gastrointestinal tract. In the bone marrow, impaired DNA synthesis leads to characteristic megaloblastic hematopoiesis. Nuclear maturation is retarded compared with cytoplasmic maturation, i.e., nuclear-cytoplasmic asynchrony occurs; the result is larger cell size with immature-appearing nuclei. These changes occur in erythroid, granulocytic, and megakaryocytic cell lineages.

Folate deficiency can produce a hematological picture of megaloblastic anemia identical to that of cobalamin deficiency. However, the two deficiencies must be distinguished. Folate deficiency can be identified primarily by low serum and erythrocyte folate levels, elevation of urinary formiminoglutamic acid after a histidine load, and full therapeutic response to physiological (not pharmacological) doses of folate.[6,7] The neurological sequelae of cobalamin deficiency are believed to be unrelated to the block of DNA synthesis. Impairment of DNA synthesis is not believed to be responsible for the neurological sequelae of cobalamin deficiency, but myelin formation may be impaired by some as yet unknown mechanism.[1]

Clinical Features

PA is insidious in its onset; the disease progresses slowly. Classically, as in this case, the patient presents with nonspecific signs and symptoms of anemia and with characteristic neurological abnormalities. In some patients, however, involvement may be selective, affecting either bone marrow or nervous system and having little or no effect on other organ systems.[2] PA usually occurs after age 40 and is seen particularly in persons of Northern European origin. Afro-American and South African women who develop PA do so at an earlier age.[8]

Weakness, fatigue, syncope, angina, lightheadedness, palpitations, pallor, dyspnea, and cardiac flow murmurs — if present — are due to the anemia *per se*. A minimal fever may occur; slight jaundice and scleral icterus may develop as a result of increased heme breakdown associated with rapid turnover in bone marrow. Purpura due to severe thrombocytopenia occurs rarely. Gastrointestinal signs and symptoms include a smooth, beefy red tongue (atrophic glossitis), anorexia, weight loss, and constipation or diarrhea.

Demyelination, axonal degeneration, and eventual neuronal death produce neurological manifestations typical of cobalamin deficiency, but these changes are not seen with folate deficiency. Classic signs and symptoms include (1) symmetrical tingling and numbness in the feet and fingers and diminished vibratory and position sense (*posterior* column degeneration) and (2) weakness, spasticity, and hyperactive deep reflexes (*lateral* column degeneration). Irritability, forgetfulness, or other disturbances in mentation, as well as peripheral nerve involvement that produces distal symmetrical impairment of superficial sensation, may also be present.[6] Neurological sequelae of cobalamin deficiency may occur in the absence of anemia. Thus, neurological complaints may be the initial, presenting symptoms in patients with deficiency.[2]

Diagnosis

Patients with PA usually have an anemia with significant macrocytosis. Ineffective erythropoiesis produces the characteristic morphological changes in peripheral blood and bone marrow cells. The peripheral blood film shows poikilocytosis and anisocytosis as well as large, fully hemoglobinized, oval macrocytes. Small teardrop erythrocytes may also be seen. If megaloblastic anemia develops in an individual with iron deficiency or with thalassemia minor (disorders that are characterized by microcytosis), the MCV may be in the normal range. Mild thrombocytopenia is common, as is mild leukopenia. The presence of large neutrophils with hypersegmented nuclei (>5 lobes per nucleus) is a distinctive feature of megaloblastic anemia. Bone marrow examination characteristically shows megaloblastic hematopoiesis: marked erythroid hyperplasia with typical megaloblasts, giant band neutrophils, giant metamyelocytes with immature chromatin, and large megakaryocytes with nuclear separation and nuclear fragments. Iron stores are increased.[9] However, bone marrow examination is not necessary when peripheral blood films show morphological changes consistent with megaloblastic anemia and noninvasive tests yield clear results.[10] Bone marrow examination is indicated in a patient with macrocytic anemia that has not resolved despite therapy with folate and cobalamin.

A number of laboratory tests reflect effects of the ineffective hematopoiesis of megaloblastic anemia. *Serum lactate dehydrogenase (LDH)* is markedly elevated because of the increased intramedullary destruction of cells. *Serum iron* is increased because of decreased erythropoiesis and iron utilization. A mild increase in *serum unconjugated bilirubin* results from both ineffective erythropoiesis and hemolysis of abnormal erythrocytes.

Once megaloblastic anemia is identified, serum cobalamin as well as erythrocyte and serum folate assays should be performed.[6,7,10] Although the erythrocyte folate level may be decreased in cobalamin deficiency, the serum folate level is usually normal or high (see Table 1). This is in contrast to folate deficiency, in which serum and erythrocyte folate levels are both decreased. The serum cobalamin assay is the primary diagnostic test for cobalamin deficiency, and values usually are diagnostically low when deficiency is present. Although clinical signs generally appear when serum cobalamin levels fall below 150 pg/mL (111 pmol/L), serum levels may not always be true indicators of tissue levels. A better indicator of low tissue levels is elevation of serum and urine methylmalonate because their concentrations increase before a decrease in serum cobalamin levels occurs. Methylmalonate concentrations remain at normal (trace) levels in folate deficiency. Serum homocysteine is elevated in both cobalamin and folate deficiencies and, like methylmalonate, appears to be a more sensitive indicator of intracellular cobalamin depletion. However, assays for methylmalonate and homocysteine are difficult and not readily available.[6,7,11] Differentiation of cobalamin deficiency from folate deficiency can be made by administering a physiological dose of cobalamin and observing the reticulocyte response in 5-7 days; a response will occur in PA but not in megaloblastic anemia due to folate deficiency.[1,6] This test is, however, contraindicated for diagnosis of a critically ill patient for whom optimal therapy should not be delayed.[1]

Table 1. SERUM COBALAMIN, SERUM FOLATE, AND ERYTHROCYTE FOLATE LEVELS IN MEGALOBLASTIC ANEMIA[10]

Disorder	Cobalamin (S)	Folate (S) *	Folate (Erc)
Cobalamin deficiency	Decreased	Normal or increased	Decreased
Folate deficiency	Normal	Decreased	Decreased
Cobalamin and folate deficiency	Decreased	Decreased	Decreased

* Fluctuates with changes in dietary folate.

The Schilling test allows differentiation of cobalamin deficiency due to a small intestinal malabsorption defect from PA due to lack of IF. The result of Stage I testing indicates ability or inability to absorb cobalamin in the small intestine. If inability is demonstrated, the result of Stage II testing indicates whether malabsorption is due to lack of IF from the gastric mucosa or to an absorption defect in the small intestine. Normal absorption of labeled cobalamin provided with exogenous IF in the Stage II test is strong evidence for a diagnosis of PA (provided that the patient has not had a gastrectomy).

Treatment

The mainstay of treatment of PA is replacement therapy with cobalamin by intramuscular injection of synthetic vitamin (cyanocobalamin or hydroxycobalamin). Sufficient doses should be given to replace daily losses and to replenish storage pools. Parenteral maintenance therapy must be continued for the rest of the patient's life; oral therapy is unreliable.[12] Because patients with PA have an increased incidence of gastric cancer, long-term follow-up should include routine periodic examinations for occult blood in stool.[9]

During the early treatment of patients with severe PA, hypokalemia may suddenly develop. Potassium depletion is due to the immediate return of normal hematopoiesis and the potassium requirements of so many young erythrocytes. To prevent the possibility of cardiac arrhythmia and sudden death secondary to hypokalemia, oral potassium supplements can be started at the same time as the cobalamin therapy and continued during the first 10 days of treatment. Cobalamin deficiency should never be treated with folic acid alone. Although the hematological abnormalities may respond partially to folic acid therapy, the neurological lesions do not respond and may progress and become irreversible.[6]

Response to replacement therapy occurs within 1-2 days; the patient experiences increased strength and an increased sense of well-being. Megaloblastic features of the marrow revert to normal within 2-3 days, and reticulocytosis peaks within 10 days. Normal hemoglobin levels are usually achieved within 1-2 months.[12] Marked improvement occurs in neurological symptoms of recent onset;[2] however, a lesser degree of improvement can be expected for longstanding neurological symptoms.

References

1. Rappaport, S.I.: Megaloblastic anemias. *In:* Introduction to Hematology, 2nd ed. S.I. Rappaport, Ed. Philadelphia, J.B. Lippincott Co., 1987.

2. Healton, E.B., Savage, D.G., Brust, J.C.M., et al.: Neurologic aspects of cobalamin deficiency. Medicine, *70:* 229-245, 1991.

3. Miller, A., Slingerland, D.W., Cardarelli, J., et al.: Further studies on the use of serum gastrin levels in assessing the significance of low serum B_{12} levels. Am. J. Hematol., *31:* 194-198, 1989.

4. Nickoloff, E.: Schilling test: Physiologic basis for and use as a diagnostic test. Crit. Rev. Clin. Lab. Sci., *26:* 263-276, 1988.

5. Green, L.K., and Graham, D.Y.: Gastritis in the elderly. Gastroenterol. Clin. North Am., *19:* 273-292, 1990.

6. Beck, W.S.: Megaloblastic anemias. *In:* Hematology, 5th ed. W.S. Beck, Ed. Cambridge, The MIT Press, 1991.

7. Beck, W.S.: Diagnosis of megaloblastic anemia. Ann. Rev. Med., *42:* 311-322, 1991.

8. Beck, W.S.: Megaloblastic anemias. *In:* Cecil Textbook of Medicine, 18th ed. J.B. Wyngaarden and L.H. Smith, Eds. Philadelphia, W.B. Saunders Co., 1988.

9. Babior, B.M., and Bunn, H.F.: Megaloblastic anemia. *In:* Harrison's Principles of Internal Medicine, 12th ed. E. Braunwald, K.J. Isselbacher, R.G. Petersdorf, et al., Eds. New York, McGraw-Hill Co., 1991.

10. Kjeldsberg, C., Beutler, E., Bell, C., et al.: Practical Diagnosis of Hematologic Disorders. Chicago, American Society of Clinical Pathologists, 1989.

11. Allen, R.H., Stabler, S.P., Savage, D.G., et al.: Diagnosis of cobalamin deficiency I: Usefulness of serum methylmalonic acid and total homocysteine concentrations. Am. J. Hematol., *34:* 90-98, 1990.

12. Babior, B.M.: Erythrocyte disorders: Anemias related to the disturbance of DNA synthesis (megaloblastic anemia). *In:* Hematology, 4th ed. W.J. Williams, E. Beutler, A.J. Erslev, and M.A. Lichtman, Eds. New York, McGraw-Hill Co., 1990.

Additional Reading

Carmel, R.: Subtle and atypical cobalamin deficiency states. Am. J. Hematol., *34:* 108-114, 1990.

Stabler, S.P., Allen, R.H., Savage, D.G., et al.: Clinical spectrum and diagnosis of cobalamin deficiency. Blood, *76:* 871-881, 1990.

PNEUMONIA, LEUKOPENIA, AND ECCHYMOSES

Marcel E. Conrad, Contributor
Susan A. Fuhrman, Reviewer

The patient, a 15-year-old white male, presented to the Emergency Department of the University Hospital because of weakness and a fever of 102 °F (38.9 °C). There was no prior history of illness. At the time of admission, the patient appeared pale and had tenderness over the sternum. There were ecchymoses over the anterior abdominal wall and right buttock. Blood pressure was 110/65 mm Hg and pulse 105 BPM. Examination of the chest showed dullness over the right posterior lung fields. Breath sounds were bronchial in this area with rales. The liver was palpable at the costal margin, but the spleen was not palpated. A chest X-ray was normal except for linear streaks in the region of the right lower lobe.

The following laboratory values were reported on admission:

Analyte	Value, conventional units	Reference range, conventional units	Value, SI units	Reference range, SI units
Leukocyte count (B)	$3.4 \times 10^3/\mu L$	4.5-13.0	$3.4 \times 10^9/L$	4.5-13.0
Platelet count (B)	$31 \times 10^3/\mu L$	150-450	$31 \times 10^9/L$	150-450
Hemoglobin (B)	10.4 g/dL	12.3-16.6	6.45 mmol/L	7.63-10.30
MCV (B)	98.7 fL	83-97	Same	
Peripheral blood smear				
Neutrophils	18 %	40-80	0.18	0.40-0.80
Bands	8 %	0-6	0.08	0.00-0.06
Lymphocytes	50 %	15-50	0.50	0.15-0.50
Monocytes	24 %	2-11	0.24	0.02-0.11
Sodium (S)	141 mmol/L	138-145	Same	
Potassium (S)	4.5 mmol/L	4.0-5.3	Same	
Chloride (S)	105 mmol/L	98-108	Same	
CO_2, total (S)	21 mmol/L	22-29	Same	
Urea nitrogen (S)	15 mg/dL	7-18	5.4 mmol urea/L	2.5-6.4
Creatinine (S)	0.8 mg/dL	0.2-1.0	71 µmol/L	18-88
Glucose (S)	100 mg/dL	70-115	5.6 mmol/L	3.9-6.4
Protein, total (S)	6.0 g/dL	6.0-8.0	60 g/L	60-80
Albumin (S)	3.6 g/dL	3.5-5.5	36 g/L	35-55
Urate (S)	8.8 mg/dL	2.0-6.0	523 µmol/L	119-357
Cholesterol (S)	86 mg/dL	70-200	2.22 mmol/L	1.81-5.17
Bilirubin, total (S)	0.7 mg/dL	0.2-1.0	12 µmol/L	3-17
AST (S)	55 U/L	15-35	0.92 µkat/L	0.25-0.58
ALT (S)	35 U/L	10-30	0.58 µkat/L	0.17-0.50
LDH (S)	320 U/L	150-250	5.33 µkat/L	2.50-4.17
Prothrombin time (PT) (P)	16.5 s	10.2-13.5	Same	
Partial thromboplastin time (PTT) (P)	45 s	28-35	Same	

To evaluate the abnormal coagulation studies, measurement of fibrinogen and fibrin split products was ordered and the following values were obtained:

Analyte	Value, conventional units	Reference range, conventional units	Value, SI units	Reference range, SI units
Fibrinogen (P)	110 mg/dL	210-400	1.1 g/L	.2.1-4.0
Fibrin split products (P)	1:80	<1:20		
D-dimer test (P)	2 µg/mL	<0.5		

Thrombocytopenia, abnormal PT and PTT, decreased fibrinogen and increased fibrin split products, in conjunction with peripheral ecchymoses, suggested a diagnosis of disseminated intravascular coagulation (DIC). In the presence of leukopenia and a possible pneumonia, blood, sputum, and urine cultures were obtained, and the patient was started on piperacillin and amikacin. Cultures grew no organisms.

A bone marrow biopsy and aspirate were obtained from the posterior iliac crest. The aspirate was scanty and obtained with difficulty. The bone marrow biopsy core was white rather than pink in gross appearance. The bone marrow aspirate specimen was dilute and contained fat but no spicules. No megakaryocytes were seen. Fifty-eight percent of cells were mononuclear and contained azurophilic granules. The cells varied considerably in size and shape, and some cells were reniform whereas others were bilobular. The biopsy specimen was markedly hypercellular and contained few fat globules. There were few megakaryocytes and erythroid precursors. The cells had a uniform, monotonous appearance; many contained nucleoli, and most contained azurophilic granules.

Portions of the aspirate were sent for cytogenetic studies and immunological marker determination. Cytogenetic analysis revealed occasional aneuploidy, and many cells showed a t(15:17) translocation; no Philadelphia (Ph[1]) chromosome was seen. Cell surface markers showed many cells were positive for CD13, CD15, CD32, and CD33; T-cell and B-cell markers were nonreactive.

Discussion

The patient presented with pancytopenia and pneumonia with sternal tenderness. The sternal tenderness suggested that the pancytopenia was caused by a hypercellular marrow rather than an aplastic marrow. The pneumonia was associated with neutropenia. The physical evidence of pneumonia predominated over the radiological findings because marked neutropenia precluded granulocytic infiltration. Hence roentgenographic changes in the affected area of the lung were delayed and less prominent than in a patient with normal granulocytes. The ecchymoses were explained by the laboratory studies showing evidence of DIC.

Diagnosis

The patient had pancytopenia with a markedly hyperplastic marrow containing a predominance of immature cells. This picture was compatible with a diagnosis of leukemia. In childhood, the most common acute leukemia is lymphoblastic, whereas in adults, it is myeloblastic. An adolescent is in the age interface where both types are relatively commonplace. The peripheral blood findings were not diagnostic because the patient was leukopenic without blasts in the peripheral smear. However, the bone marrow was hyperplastic, and most of the cells were promyelocytes. The presence of DIC in a patient with a hyperplastic bone marrow and cells that contain azurophilic granules strongly suggests that the patient has acute promyelocytic leukemia (M3 in FAB classification). Results of cell surface marker studies were typical of those found in granulocytic cell lines and were compatible with a myeloid leukemia. The finding of t(15:17) chromosomal translocation was characteristic of a progranulocytic leukemia.

Initially this patient presented with pancytopenia. A bone marrow biopsy and aspirate showing a marrow that was hyperplastic and contained hematopoietic cells excluded aplastic anemia and infiltration of the bone marrow with solid tumor cells or myelofibrosis as an etiology for the pancytopenia. The presence of more than 50% progranulocytes excluded the myelodysplastic syndromes from consideration. Occasionally, bone marrow biopsy specimens obtained from children or adolescents following an aregenerative crisis contain a large percentage of early myeloid precursors at a single stage of development. These bone marrow biopsy specimens are usually not markedly hypercellular and usually contain proportionate numbers of repopulating erythroid precursors and megakaryocytes in addition to early granulocytes. Whenever there is doubt about the differential between acute promyelocytic leukemia and a recovering bone marrow, chromosomal studies should be performed and a bone marrow biopsy should be repeated after several days' wait to ascertain whether there has been further maturation of the granulocytic precursors. The finding of Auer rods in the cytoplasm of the immature granulocytes would provide assurance of a diagnosis of leukemia. Although Auer rods were not reported in this patient's bone marrow, they are commonly present in acute promyelocytic leukemia. In the present case, the t(15:17) chromosomal translocation assured the diagnosis of leukemia of a progranulocytic type. Special stains (Sudan black, peroxidase, PAS) and cell surface marker studies would not be helpful in the differential diagnosis of acute promyelocytic leukemia and a recovering bone marrow because they would merely identify the cells as granulocytes.

Definition of the Disease

Acute myelogenous leukemia (AML) has a low incidence in childhood (<1 case in 100,000 per year). Among adults, the incidence rises increasingly rapidly with age, from approximately 1/100,000 in the fourth decade of life to approximately 10/100,000 in those over 70 years of age. The natural course of AML can range from a slowly progressive disease to one of acute virulence with the slower clinical course being more commonplace in the elderly. In 1976 a collaborating group of French, American, and British hematologists (FAB group) classified the leukemias based upon the morphology of the cells in the bone marrow and the percentage of each type of cell present. The acute myeloid leukemias include the granulocytic leukemias (M1-M3), myelomonocytic (M4), monocytic leukemia (M5), erythroleukemia (M6), and acute megakaryocytic leukemia (M7). The clinical manifestations are similar in all forms of acute myelogenous leukemia; patients usually seek medical attention because of symptoms and complications associated with decreased production of normal blood cells. Other than the more pronounced bleeding and bruising from disseminated intravascular coagulation (DIC), there are no clinical findings that separate myelogenous leukemia from other acute leukemias. However, it needs to be pointed out that other types of acute leukemia may be complicated by DIC. Progranulocytic leukemia is usually acute in onset and most common in young adults, whereas M1, M2, and M4 occur more commonly with increasing age. Usually the total blood leukocyte count is near normal or low rather than increased. A specific karyotypic abnormality, the t(15:17) translocation, is commonly found in this form of leukemia. Unlike other forms of acute myelogenous leukemia, patients enter a remission following treatment with retinoids. This phenomenon indicates that progranulocytic leukemia is a distinct clinical entity with an etiology different from other leukemias.

Treatment

Hemorrhagic complications may be averted by platelet transfusion and administration of fresh-frozen plasma. Low-dose heparin therapy is generally recommended in combination with platelets and clotting factors. Unlike other acute leukemias, APL is responsive to therapy with all-*trans* retinoic acid, and remissions will occur without producing bone marrow aplasia or exacerbation of coagulopathy. Retinoid therapy was discovered because the patients usually have a t(15:17) translocation and the breakpoints on chromosome 17 in APL cells are clustered in the first intron of the retinoic acid receptor (RAR-α) gene. Retinoic acid receptors are ligand-inducible transcription factors that seem to regulate the expression of genes that are important in determining myeloid maturation. In most cases, APL appears to be characterized by abnormal retinoic acid receptors; the abnormality is responsible for the maturation arrest of granulocytic precursors at the progranulocytic stage of development. The patient was simultaneously administered platelets and fresh-frozen plasma and was heparinized in order to treat the disseminated coagulopathy associated with progranulocytic leukemia. Allopurinol was administered. The preferred treatment options of chemotherapy were either cytosine arabinoside and daunomycin or all-*trans* retinoic acid (all-TRA). All-TRA was chosen, and after four weeks of therapy, the patient entered complete remission without developing severe pancytopenia.

Additional Reading

Bioudi, A., Ramkaldi, A., Alcalau, M., et al.: RAR-α gene rearrangements as a genetic marker for diagnosis and monitoring in acute promyelocytic leukemia. Blood, *77:* 1418-1422, 1991.

Borrow, J., Goddard, A.D., Sheer, D., et al.: Molecular analysis of acute promyelocytic leukemia breakpoint chister region on chromosome 17. Science, *249:* 1577-1590, 1990.

Huang, M., Le, H.C., Chen, S.R., et al.: Use of all-*trans* retinoic acid in the treatment of acute promyelocytic leukemia. Blood, *72:* 567-572, 1988.

Stone, R.M., and Mayer, R.J.: The unique aspects of acute promyelocytic leukemia. J. Clin. Oncol., *8:* 1913-1921, 1990.

A MAN WITH SPLENOMEGALY

Douglas A. Nelson, Contributor
Richard A. Mc Pherson, Reviewer

A 52-year-old man went to see his physician because of increased frequency of feeling fatigued. He had had to stop jogging, one of his favorite recreational activities. His appetite was poorer, and he had lost weight. In addition, he often noted a sense of fullness in the left upper quadrant of his abdomen.

On physical examination, his spleen was palpable about 5 cm below the left costal margin, and his liver was questionably palpable at the right costal margin. He appeared slightly pale but not jaundiced, and no other significant physical findings were noted.

Laboratory results were as follows:

Analyte	Value, conventional units	Reference range, conventional units	Value, SI units	Reference range, SI units
AST (S)	16 U/L	8-20	0.27 µkat/L	0.13-0.33
Bilirubin (S)	0.9 mg/dL	0.2-1.0	15 µmol/L	3-17
Cholesterol (S)	220 mg/dL	158-227	5.69 mmol/L	4.09-5.87
Creatinine (S)	1.1 mg/dL	0.7-1.3	97 µmol/L	62-115
Protein, total (S)	6.9 g/dL	6.0-8.0	69 g/L	60-80
Albumin (S)	3.6 g/dL	3.5-5.0	36 g/L	35-50
Leukocyte count (B)	170 x 10^3/µL	4.5-11.0	170 x 10^9/L	4.5-11.0
Erythrocyte count (B)	3.23 x 10^6/µL	4.2-5.6	3.23 x 10^{12}/L	4.2-5.6
Hemoglobin (B)	10 g/dL	13.1-17.2	6.21 mmol/L	8.13-10.67
Hematocrit (B)	30 %	39-50	0.30	0.39-0.50
MCV (B)	92.9 fL	81-101	Same	
MCH (B)	31 pg	27-35	Same	
MCHC (BErcs)	33.3 g Hb/dL	32-36	21 mmol Hb/L	20-22
Platelet count (B)	825 x 10^3/µL	150-450	825 x 10^9/L	150-450
Reticulocytes	1.5 %	0.5-1.5	0.015	0.005-0.015
Leukocyte differential count (B)				
Blast cells	1.7 x 10^3/µL (1%)	0	1.7 x 10^9/L (0.01)	0
Promyelocytes	8.5 x 10^3/µL (5%)	0	8.5 x 10^9/L (0.05)	0
Neutrophil myelocytes	35.7 x 10^3/µL (21%)	0	35.7 x 10^9/L (0.21)	0
Neutrophil metamyelocytes	15.3 x 10^3/µL (9%)	0	15.3 x 10^9/L (0.09)	0
Neutrophil band cells	23.8 x 10^3/µL (14%)	0.2-2.1	23.8 x 10^9/L (0.14)	0.2-2.1
Neutrophils	61.2 x 10^3/µL (36%)	1.5-6.7	61.2 x 10^9/L (0.36)	1.5-6.7
Eosinophils	6.8 x 10^3/µL (4%)	0-0.7	6.8 x 10^9/L (0.04)	0-0.7
Basophils	10.2 x 10^3/µL (6%)	0-0.15	10.2 x 10^9/L (0.06)	0-0.15
Monocytes	3.4 x 10^3/µL (2%)	0.2-0.95	3.4 x 10^9/L (0.02)	0.2-0.95
Lymphocytes	3.4 x 10^3/µL (2%)	1.5-4.0	3.4 x 10^9/L (0.02)	1.5-4.0
Normoblasts (nucleated erythrocytes)	One per 100 leuko-cytes			

The laboratory data provided no evidence of liver disease. Because of the leukocytosis with immature granulocytes and nucleated erythroid precursors circulating in the blood (leukoerythroblastosis) and the thrombocytosis, a primary myeloproliferative disorder was suspected.* Therefore, bone marrow aspiration and biopsy with cytogenetic studies on the aspirated cells, as well as additional chemical studies, were performed.

Bone marrow aspiration and biopsy: Increased cellularity, increase particularly in the granulocytic cell lines but also in megakaryocytes and erythroid cells; morphologically the cells appeared to have normal maturation.

Cytogenetic analysis of bone marrow myeloid cells: 26/26 karyotypes showed a small chromosome #22; it was determined to be the result of t(9;22). This shortened chromosome #22 is known as the Philadelphia (Ph[1]) chromosome.

Analyte	Value, conventional units	Reference range, conventional units	Value, SI units	Reference range, SI units
Urate (S)	11 mg/dL	4.5-8.2	654 μmol/L	268-488
Cobalamin (S)	1100 pg/mL	100-700	812 pmol/L	74-516
Neutrophil ALP score [†]	6	40-130	Same	

The peripheral blood differential cell count, the bone marrow cellular picture, the low score for neutrophil ALP, and the characteristic translocation of chromosomes 9 and 22 were judged diagnostic of chronic myelogenous leukemia.

The patient was treated with hydroxyurea, a drug that inhibits DNA synthesis, and this brought his leukocyte and differential counts back within normal limits. The patient improved clinically, regained a sense of well-being, and resumed full activity. The bone marrow, however, remained hypercellular, and the Philadelphia (Ph[1]) chromosome persisted; this picture is typical of response to treatment at this stage.

After four years, the hydroxyurea no longer controlled the leukocyte count. Despite increasing dosages, the count gradually increased as did numbers of blast cells in the peripheral blood. Flow cytometry determined the immunophenotype of the blast cells; they were positive for CD10 (CALLA[‡]) and the B-cell antigens CD19 and CD20. Terminal deoxynucleotidyl transferase (TdT[§]) was also positive. These findings indicated that the blast "crisis," a new phase of the patient's disease, was a lymphoblastic transformation. The patient responded briefly to chemotherapy for lymphoblastic leukemia but died of hemorrhage.

---

* The myeloproliferative disorders include essential (idiopathic) thrombocythemia, polycythemia vera, myelofibrosis with myeloid metaplasia, and chronic myelogenous leukemia.[1]

[†] Neutrophil ALP (alkaline phosphatase) is a cytoplasmic enzyme of blood neutrophilic leukocytes. Typically it is measured (or "scored") cytochemically.

[‡] CD10 or CALLA (common acute lymphoblastic leukemia-associated antigen) is a membrane antigen present in immature B-lymphoid cells in normal individuals and in the blast cells of acute lymphoblastic leukemia of early B-lineage phenotype.

[§] TdT (terminal deoxynucleotidyl transferase) is a nuclear enzyme that is present in immature lymphoid cells in normal individuals and in the blast cells of acute lymphoblastic leukemia.

Differential Diagnosis

Enlargement of the spleen (splenomegaly) in nontropical countries is usually due to malignant lymphoma, leukemia, myeloproliferative disease, hemolytic anemia, or portal hypertension. The chemical tests performed for this patient (serum AST, bilirubin, albumin, and protein) are quite normal and do not provide evidence for liver disease that might cause portal hypertension. The normocytic anemia was very unlikely to be hemolytic, i.e., due to increased destruction of erythrocytes, because the reticulocyte count is not elevated and the bilirubin is normal. Therefore, the last two of the listed causes of splenomegaly were unlikely.

Leukoerythroblastosis (or leukoerythroblastotic reaction) is present when both nucleated erythrocytes (normoblasts) and immature granulocytes (at the myelocyte stage or younger) circulate in the blood; these are detected by examining the peripheral blood film. Leuko-erythroblastosis can be caused by hemolysis, acute blood loss, severe infection, or massive trauma. A very important cause is involvement of the bone marrow by a neoplastic process such as metastatic carcinoma or sarcoma, malignant lymphoma, leukemia, multiple my-eloma, or a myeloproliferative disorder. If one of the conditions in the first group is not present, then examination of the bone marrow by aspiration and biopsy is clearly indicated.[2]

The type of leukocytosis, as determined by the distribution of cells in the leukocyte differential count, is helpful in pointing to the nature of the underlying condition. In infection, for example, usually only one type of cell is increased in number: neutrophils in the case of acute bacterial infection; monocytes in chronic infection; lymphocytes or atypical lymphocytes in viral infections; or eosinophils in allergic reactions. In this patient, there was an increase in the absolute counts of neutrophils, eosinophils, basophils, and monocytes. These findings implied a disorder involving a precursor cell common to these cell lines, i.e., the hematopoietic stem cell. In addition, there was a bimodal distribution in the neutrophilic series: a peak in the number of neutrophils and in the number of neutrophilic myelocytes. This differential cell count strongly suggested a diagnosis of chronic myelogenous leukemia (CML).[3]

The increase in serum urate can be attributed to increased purine degradation associ-ated with augmented production and destruction of myeloid cells. Serum cobalamin (vitamin B_{12}) rises because transcobalamin I, a cobalamin-binding protein and a normal constituent of the specific granules of neutrophils,[4] is released from dying neutrophils. Increased serum cobalamin may also be seen in monocytic proliferation. Neutrophil ALP is present in a membrane fraction or novel granule in the cytoplasm of neutrophils.[4] In CML its activity is typically very low, whereas it is elevated in neutrophilia due to infections, in polycythemia vera, and in myelofibrosis with myeloid metaplasia. The low value seen in this patient is further support for the diagnosis of CML.

Bone marrow examination is necessary to demonstrate that the hypercellularity is due to an increase in the number of proliferating cells of the myeloid lines, primarily in the number of granulocytes. Increase in megakaryocyte numbers is usual, and increase in erythroid cells sometimes occurs.

Diagnosis

The diagnosis of CML requires the presence of the typical hematological findings discussed previously: neutrophilia with bimodal distribution of myelocytes and mature cells; basophilia; usually eosinophilia; hypercellular bone marrow with increase in all myeloid cells; and low neutrophil alkaline phosphatase. In addition, the diagnosis must be confirmed by demonstration of the Philadelphia (Ph[1]) chromosome (or the bcr/abl fusion gene) in the proliferating myeloid cells.

Discussion

Chronic myelogenous leukemia is an acquired disease. Some of the evidence for this statement is that CML very rarely is found in both identical twins and that an increased incidence of CML has been found in survivors of the atomic bombs in Hiroshima and Nagasaki. This acquired genetic abnormality occurs at the pluripotential stem cell level.

Cytogenetic study of the blood or bone marrow reveals a typical small abnormal chromosome 22, the Ph[1] chromosome, in almost all cases of CML.[5] This is a result of a reciprocal translocation of the long arms of chromosomes 9 and 22 that is designated t(9;22). The Ph[1] chromosome is present in granulocytes, monocytes, erythrocytes, platelets, and usually in some B lymphocytes, but it is not present in fibroblasts of the bone marrow or skin.

The presence of the Ph[1] chromosome in all of these bone marrow cells suggests that they constitute a clonal population. Monoclonality has been demonstrated by studies in women who happen to have a heterozygosity for the X-linked gene for glucose-6-phosphate dehydrogenase (G-6-PD). In these women, both the A and B isoenzymes of G-6-PD can be distinguished by electrophoresis. Both isoenzymes occur in all the somatic tissues, including skin, lymphocytes, and other hematopoietic cells. But in those heterozygous females who develop CML, only one or the other (A or B) isoenzyme is to be found in their erythrocytes, granulocytes, platelets, and some B lymphocytes. This distinctive distribution indicates that cells with only one isoenzyme are monoclonal and that CML involves not only granulocytes but also erythroid cells, megakaryocytes and platelets, and in some cases B lymphocytes. The common hematopoietic stem cell is consequently identified as the point of origin for the disease.[6]

In some patients with typical CML who lack the Ph[1] chromosome, molecular probe analysis will reveal the presence of the fusion gene bcr/abl.[2] The genetic abnormality that is essential for the genesis of CML is the fusion of the bcr gene on chromosome 22q with the abl oncogene translocated from chromosome 9q. The resultant bcr/abl fusion gene transcribes an mRNA molecule of 8.5 kb, resulting in a protein product of a molecular weight of 210, 000 with strong tyrosine kinase activity. There is experimental evidence that this bcr/abl protein can induce CML.[7] The few patients with CML who lack the Ph[1] chromosome and bcr/abl have a worse prognosis than do those who have t(9;22) and the fusion gene.

The Ph[1]-positive clone of cells is genetically unstable, as indicated by the high risk of development of additional cytogenetic abnormalities coinciding with the onset of either an accelerated phase of the disease or a blast crisis. The additional karyotypic changes usually include yet another Ph[1] chromosome, an extra chromosome #8 (+8), or an isochromosome #17 (i{17q}).[8]

Malignant transformation inevitably occurs in CML and may do so at any time during the course of the disease; the median time is three to four years after diagnosis. The manifestations of this transformation are variable — from an *aggressive phase* in which there is a loss of control of leukocyte counts by the drugs to a *blast phase*. This blast phase (acute leukemia) is preceded by one of the additional cytogenetic abnormalities referred to above and often is heralded by progressive immaturity of blood granulocytes and an increase in basophils. The blast cells eventually prevail; the patient develops intractable infections or hemorrhages and subsequently dies. The blast cells may be lymphoblasts, as in this patient, but more often they are myeloblasts, megakaryoblasts, or blasts that display the cytochemical or immune phenotype of more than one lineage.

Treatment

After the diagnosis of CML has been established, the first objective of treatment is to bring the leukocyte count under control; success generally relieves the symptoms. Either busulfan, an alkylating agent, or hydroxyurea, a cycle-specific inhibitor of DNA synthesis, may be used. Usually, however, even though the cell counts become normal and the bone marrow may *appear* normal, the Ph[1]-positive clone remains present in the bone marrow. α-Interferon has been used successfully to control the leukocyte counts with loss of the Ph[1]-positive clone in some patients. None of these drugs prevents eventual transformation of the disease to the acute phase.

Once control of the cell counts has been achieved, the next treatment of choice is allogeneic bone marrow transplantation from an HLA-identical sibling donor, if one is available. If such a donor is not available, marrow from an HLA-matched unrelated donor may be used, although the success rate is lower in this event. Bone marrow transplantation with marrow from a normal donor is the only curative therapy currently available for CML. The option of bone marrow transplantation is usually not attempted, however, if the patient is over 50 years of age because of the excessively high morbidity and much lower success rate in older individuals.

References

1. Munker, R., and Koeffler, H.P.: Pathobiology of the myeloproliferative disorders. *In:* Hematology: Basic Principles and Practice. R. Hoffman, E.J. Benz, Jr., S.J. Shattil, et al., Eds. New York, Churchill Livingstone, inc., 1991.

2. Bagby, G.C., Jr.: Leukocytosis and leukemoid reactions. *In:* Cecil Textbook of Medicine. J.B. Wyngaarden and L.H. Smith, Jr., Eds. Philadelphia, W.B. Saunders Co., 1988.

3. Spiers, A.S.D., Bain, B.J., and Turner, J.E.: The peripheral blood in chronic granulocytic leukaemia: Study of 50 untreated Philadelphia-positive cases. Scand. J. Haematol., *18:* 25-38, 1977.

4. Boxer, L.A., and Smolen, J.E.: Neutrophil granule constituents and their release in health and disease. Hematol. Oncol. Clin. North Am., *2:* 101, 1988.

5. Kurzrock, R., Gutterman, J.U., and Talpaz, M.: The molecular genetics of Philadelphia chromosome-positive leukemias. N. Engl. J. Med., *319:* 990-998, 1988.

6. Fialkow, P.J., Jacobson, R.J., and Papayannopoulou, T.: Chronic myelocytic leukemia: Clonal origin in a stem cell common to the granulocyte, erythrocyte, platelet and monocyte/macrophage. Am. J. Med., *63:* 125-130, 1977.

7. Goldman, J.M., Grosveld, G., Baltimore, D., and Gale, R.P.: Chronic myelogenous leukemia — The unfolding saga. Leukemia, *4:* 163-167, 1990.

8. Alimena, G., Dallapiccola, B., Gastaldi, R., et al.: Chromosomal, morphological and clinical correlations in blastic crisis of chronic myeloid leukaemia: A study of 69 cases. Scand. J. Haematol., *28:* 103-117, 1982.

A CASE OF IMPOTENCE AND PROGRESSIVE FATIGUE

John C. Spinosa, Contributor
Richard A. Mc Pherson, Contributor
Dennis Ross, Reviewer

A 44-year-old man, previously in good health, sought medical evaluation because of impotence and increasing fatigue. He had a past history of sporadic impotence that had increased in frequency over the last 18 months. Attendant with the impotence was a history of progressive fatigue, primarily manifested as exercise intolerance accompanied by painful leg cramps. The patient denied any chest pain, respiratory difficulties, or episodes of vertigo or syncope. The patient also denied fevers, night sweats, or additional constitutional symptoms. His past medical history was significant for mild hypertension that had been amenable to dietary restrictions. At this time he was not taking medications and denied smoking, significant alcohol consumption, or recreational drug use. His father had died from hairy-cell leukemia; his mother and siblings were in good health.

On physical examination, the patient was afebrile and vigorous. His blood pressure was 140/90 mm Hg, pulse 72 BPM, and respiratory rate 16/min. Abnormal physical findings were limited to the abdomen in which a splenic tip was palpable 4 cm below the costal margin at the midclavicular line. The liver was normal-sized, and there was no lymphadenopathy. Neither ecchymoses nor purpura was present. Laboratory findings were as follows:

Analyte	Value, conventional units	Reference range, conventional units	Value, SI units	Reference range, SI units
Sodium (S)	144 mmol/L	135-145	Same	
Potassium (S)	4.3 mmol/L	3.9-5.4	Same	
Chloride (S)	108 mmol/L	97-106	Same	
CO_2, total (S)	27 mmol/L	23-30	Same	
Urea nitrogen (S)	21 mg/dL	7-18	7.5 mmol urea/L	2.4-6.4
Creatinine (S)	1.3 mg/dL	0.5-1.2	115 μmol/L	44-106
Glucose (S)	85 mg/dL	70-105	4.7 mmol/L	3.9-5.8
Protein, total (S)	7.7 g/dL	6.1-8.0	77 g/L	61-80
Albumin (S)	4.5 g/dL	3.3-4.8	45 g/L	33-48
Urate (S)	3.2 mg/dL	3.7-8.1	190 μmol/L	220-482
Cholesterol (S)	133 mg/dL	150-220	3.44 mmol/L	3.88-5.69
Triglycerides (S)	58 mg/dL	55-160	0.65 mmol/L	0.62-1.80
Calcium (S)	9.7 mg/dL	8.4-10.2	2.42 mmol/L	2.10-2.54
Phosphorus (S)	3.7 mg/dL	2.5-4.5	1.19 mmol/L	0.81-1.45
Iron (S)	93 μg/dL	30-180	17 μmol/L	5-32
Bilirubin, total (S)	0.6 mg/dL	0-1.5	10 μmol/L	0-26
ALT (S)	32 U/L	2-40	0.53 μkat/L	0.03-0.67
AST (S)	24 U/L	2-40	0.40 μkat/L	0.03-0.67
LDH (S)	175 U/L	94-190	2.92 μkat/L	1.57-3.17
ALP (S)	66 U/L	30-120	1.1 μkat/L	0.5-2.0
GGT (S)	42 U/L	4-51	0.70 μkat/L	0.07-0.85
Leukocyte count (B)	$1.1 \times 10^3/\mu L$	4.5-11.0	$1.1 \times 10^9/L$	4.5-11.0
Erythrocyte count (B)	$2.8 \times 10^6/\mu L$	4.3-5.9	$2.8 \times 10^{12}/L$	4.3-5.9

Analyte	Value, conventional units	Reference range, conventional units	Value, SI units	Reference range, SI units
Hemoglobin (B)	9.0 g/dL	13.9-18.0	5.59 mmol/L	8.63-11.17
MCV (B)	92.3 fL	80-97	Same	
MCH (B)	32.5 pg	26-34	Same	
MCHC (BErcs)	35.2 g Hb/dL	31-37	22 mmol Hb/L	19-23
Platelet count (B)	$23 \times 10^3/\mu L$	130-400	$23 \times 10^9 L$	130-400
Leukocyte differential count (B)				
Segmented neutrophils	$0.07 \times 10^3/\mu L$(6%)	1.6-7.3(36-66)	$0.07 \times 10^9/L$(0.06)	1.6-7.3(0.36-0.66)
Band neutrophils	$0.03 \times 10^3/\mu L$(3%)	0.0-1.2(0-11)	$0.03 \times 10^9/L$(0.03)	0.0-1.2(0.00-0.11)
Lymphocytes	$1.0 \times 10^3/\mu L$(90%)	1.1-4.8(24-44)	$1.0 \times 10^9/L$(0.90)	1.1-4.8(0.24-0.44)
Monocytes	$0.0 \times 10^3/\mu L$(0%)	0.0-1.2(0-10.7)	$0.0 \times 10^9/L$(0.00)	0.0-1.2(0.00-0.11)
Eosinophils	$0.01 \times 10^3/\mu L$(1%)	0.0-0.7(0-6.1)	$0.01 \times 10^9/L$(0.01)	0.0-0.7(0.00-0.06)
Basophils	$0.0 \times 10^3/\mu L$(0%)	0.0-0.3(0-2.5)	$0.0 \times 10^9/L$(0.00)	0.0-0.3(0.00-0.03)
Serum-soluble IL-2 receptor (sIL-2R)	60,500 U/mL	<800	60.5×10^6 U/L	<0.8

The peripheral smear demonstrated atypical mononuclear cells characterized by intermediate size, moderate amounts of pale cytoplasm with frequent frayed cytoplasmic borders showing hairlike projections, and oval to reniform nuclei containing evenly dispersed reticular chromatin and inconspicuous nucleoli. Many of these atypical mononuclear cells contained granules positive for tartrate-resistant acid phosphatase (TRAP).

The clinical history, laboratory evaluation, and peripheral smear findings were highly suspicious for hairy-cell leukemia, and a confirmatory bone marrow aspiration was performed. The aspiration was a "dry tap" that yielded no cells. The core biopsy contained a patchy infiltrate of abnormal mononuclear cells with morphological features of hairy cells. Hematopoiesis was diminished but otherwise unremarkable.

Based on these findings, a diagnosis of hairy-cell leukemia was made, and the patient was begun on a 5-day course of treatment with 2-chlorodeoxyadenosine (2-CDA). He showed rapid improvement with resolution of his splenomegaly and normalization of his hematological parameters. A repeat bone marrow aspirate contained only normal hematopoietic elements; typical hairy-cell infiltrates were absent. There was no TRAP activity in mononuclear cells from a buffy coat preparation made after treatment. The patient's fatigue improved rapidly following therapy. Although he sought medical attention for his impotence, this problem remained and was felt to predate development of his malignancy. The patient is alive and well without further evidence of disease.

Definition of the Disease

Hairy-cell leukemia (HCL) is a rare, indolent malignancy of B lymphocytes that primarily affects older individuals. The mean age at diagnosis is 50 years, although individuals as young as 18 years and as old as 88 years have presented with HCL. A 4:1 male to female predominance exists. Rare familial clustering of HCL has been reported (as in this case), but no accepted genetic or environmental risk factors are recognized for the disease.[1]

Clinical Findings. The clinical presentation of HCL is usually vague and nonspecific. Patient complaints of fatigue and general malaise or abdominal fullness are common. Most of the symptoms can be related to either the underlying pancytopenias or the splenomegaly or both. Pancytopenia of mild to moderate degree typically occurs. Occasionally, absolute lymphocyte counts are normal; if absolute lymphocyte counts are elevated because of hairy cells in the circulation, absolute counts of other leukocytes will be diminished. Splenomegaly is invariably present and often massive enough to cause significant abdominal symptoms. Lymphadenopathy, when present, is typically isolated to small clusters of lymph nodes and can be found in up to 20% of patients.[1] Nodal enlargement as a prominent feature of the disease is unusual.

The natural history of HCL shows slow progression with gradually worsening cytopenias and increasing splenomegaly. If the disease is left untreated, the average life expectancy is 5-7 years from the time of diagnosis. Death is usually a result of infection, because of worsening leukopenia. A bleeding diathesis due to thrombocytopenia is an occasional cause of death. Splenic rupture due to massive splenomegaly is a less frequent cause of death. Several very effective treatment options now exist for patients with HCL (see *Treatment*).

Diagnosis of HCL

The diagnosis of HCL is based on cytological and morphological features in bone marrow or, occasionally, in splenectomy specimens.[2] Several additional laboratory studies including immunophenotyping studies, immunoglobulin gene rearrangement analysis, and soluble interleukin-2 receptor measurements provide useful diagnostic and prognostic information for the clinician.

Morphological Features. In the peripheral smear, hairy cells are recognized by their characteristic fine cytoplasmic projections of "hairs." This can be seen best by phase contrast examination of a fresh wet preparation of blood, although hairy cells are also seen on fresh blood smears stained with Wright-Giemsa stain. Artifacts caused by incorrect sample storage can diminish these projections in true hairy cells or even induce the formation of atypical projections in otherwise normal cells. The definition of true hairy projections may require electron microscopy of carefully preserved cells to prevent artifactual distortion.

The hairy cells are intermediate in size and have moderate amounts of pale cytoplasm. Nuclei are centrally located and are oval to reniform, occasionally angulated, and contain evenly dispersed reticular chromatin. Nucleoli are inconspicuous or absent. Hairy-cell infiltrates in the bone marrow are typically patchy with some interstitial infiltration; tumor can represent 5-95% of the marrow elements. The abnormal cells have a background of reticulin fibrosis, which accounts for the frequency with which bone marrow aspirates prove inade-quate for diagnosis ("dry taps"). In biopsy material, the hairy cells are characterized by moderate amounts of amphophilic cytoplasm and have centrally placed oval to angulated nuclei. Cytoplasmic borders are indistinct. Mitoses are exceedingly rare and, if present, cast doubt on a diagnosis of HCL. Bone marrow aspirate smears, when successful, yield abnormal mononuclear cells with cytological features similar to those seen in the peripheral smear. Touch preparations of a bone marrow core biopsy are useful when the aspiration has produced no material. However, the number of cells containing "hair-like" cytoplasmic projections is diminished in air-dried bone marrow smears.

The differential diagnosis of HCL in the bone marrow includes distinction of other low grade lymphocytic malignancies such as small lymphocytic lymphoma or leukemia, plas-macytoid lymphocytic lymphoma, and small cleaved follicular center cell lymphoma.[2-4] Distinction among these possibilities is hindered when the biopsy specimen is not properly fixed and processed. Fixation with B-5 (a mercuric-based fixative) yields results superior to formalin fixation. Systemic mastocytosis will mimic the spindle cell pattern of HCL and should be suspected when there are associated skin changes. Giemsa stain readily identifies the mast cells within the bone marrow specimen.

At least two rare variants of HCL are seen, the prolymphocytic variant of HCL[3] and splenic lymphoma with circulating villous lymphocytes (SLVL).[4] The former entity has circulating cells showing a composite morphological pattern of hairy cells and lymphocytes; they possess abundant pale cytoplasm with villous projections and round nuclei containing coarse reticular chromatin and prominent central nucleoli. The SLVL condition has cells with polar villous projections and shows more involvement of splenic white pulp.

Rarely, the diagnosis of HCL cannot be rendered on the basis of bone marrow findings alone, and a splenectomy may be necessary. HCL distends and infiltrates the red pulp of the spleen in a characteristic fashion.[2] Red pulp distention is also associated with the generation of red cell lakes. Other lymphomas and leukemias that can be confused with HCL do not typically involve the red pulp in such a dramatic fashion and mainly involve the white pulp.

Histochemical demonstration of tartrate-resistant acid phosphatase (TRAP) activity in the abnormal mononuclear cells of bone marrow or peripheral blood is a well established criterion for confirming the presence of hairy cells.[5] TRAP granules in HCL are abundant and easily detectable. Oftentimes, the number of granules will obscure the nuclear features of the cell. Although intimately associated with HCL, mildly TRAP-positive cells can be seen in plasmacytoid lymphocytic lymphomas, large granular lymphocytes, and activated macrophages.[5] Osteoclasts are also TRAP positive. Several other histochemical stains have been tried in HCL but are not diagnostically helpful.

Laboratory Features. Ancillary laboratory studies can aid immensely in the diagnosis of HCL and appear to have prognostic significance. Immunoglobulin gene rearrangement studies and immunophenotyping by flow cytometry have firmly established that HCL is a clonal proliferation of B lymphocytes even though aberrantly they express a T-cell surface marker.[1,6,7] The cell of origin in HCL is not known, but there is suggestive evidence that hairy cells derive from a preplasmacytic precursor.[1]

In nearly every case of HCL, immunoglobulin gene rearrangements can be demonstrated by Southern blot analysis.[6] This technique includes extraction of DNA, enzymatic digestion, DNA fragment electrophoresis, transfer to a membrane, probing with a gene of interest, and exposure by autoradiography or other means. Most times, both light and heavy chain rearrangements are found, but occasional clones will demonstrate rearrangement of only one chain. These gene rearrangement studies confirm the clonal origin and lineage (i.e., B cell versus T cell) of lymphocytic proliferations and thus can help establish the diagnosis of HCL. When successful treatment and remission of HCL have significantly reduced the number of abnormal cells in peripheral blood and in bone marrow aspirates, molecular studies are useful for monitoring their recurrence. Hairy cells express a characteristic immunophenotype when analyzed by flow cytometry.[7,8] The abnormal cells express pan-B cell antigens CD19, CD20, and CD22 as well as the activation antigen, CD11c (Leu-M5), and IL-2 receptor, CD25 (TAC), usually found on T cells. Surface immunoglobulin is invariably detected and shows light chain restriction. The intensity of surface immunoglobulin staining may be variable. Recently, a new antibody, B-ly7, has been described that appears to have improved sensitivity in distinguishing the hairy-cell phenotype.[8] The threshold for detecting hairy cells is 2% or less of total lymphocytes with use of two-color flow cytometric analysis.

Hairy cells express extremely high levels of CD25, the IL-2 receptor that is normally cleaved proteolytically, resulting in a soluble fragment of IL-2R (termed sIL-2R) to be shed into the blood. This phenomenon is the basis for a recently introduced assay to estimate hairy-cell leukemic mass by measuring the serum concentration of sIL-2R.[9] Patients with inflammatory conditions show a mild increase in detectable receptor, and patients with T-cell malignancies can have up to a 10-fold increase in sIL-2R over normal controls. By contrast, patients with HCL generally have serum levels of IL-2R 50-100 times those seen in normal controls. Serial measurements of sIL-2R appear to be reliable evaluators of disease progression and activity in T-cell malignancies and HCL. The sIL-2R test has received approval from the Food and Drug Administration (FDA) for these applications.

Treatment

Three recently released drugs have shown efficacy in the treatment of HCL. The first drug is the biological response modifier α-interferon. Pharmacological doses of recombinant α-interferon cause partial or complete remission of HCL in more than 75% of patients.[10] The remissions appear to be durable but require continued administration of the drug. Once the administration of the drug stops, proliferation of hairy cells may occur.

More recently, two nucleoside-based agents have shown utility in HCL — deoxycoformycin (DCF) and 2-chlorodeoxyadenosine (2-CDA). Both agents are directed against adenosine deaminase and were initially studied in patients with severe combined immunodeficiency. These drugs increase intracellular concentrations of adenosine in lymphocytes and appear to cause cell death by apoptosis. They are not cell-cycle specific agents. More than 90% of patients treated with either DCF or 2-CDA have partial or complete remissions that appear to be durable.[11,12] DCF may require several months of therapy,[12] whereas 2-CDA appears efficacious with only a single 5-day course of intravenous administration.[11]

Summary

Initial diagnosis of HCL and subsequent monitoring for residual disease and recurrence requires bone marrow biopsy and examination of buffy coat preparations from peripheral blood. Demonstration of TRAP-positive mononuclear cells and immunophenotyping of circulating mononuclear cells has utility in detecting minimal residual disease. Advances in molecular biology, particularly the immunoglobulin gene rearrangement and sIL-2R tests, have substantially improved our ability to diagnose HCL and to monitor therapy. Novel therapies, based on natural and pharmacological modification of cellular biological responses, have been developed for elimination or control of HCL.

References

1. Dalal, D.I., and Fitzpatrick, L.A.: Hairy-cell leukemia: An update. Lab. Med., *22:* 31-36, 1991.

2. Burke, J.S., and Rappaport, H.: The diagnosis and differential diagnosis of hairy-cell leukemia in bone marrow and spleen. Semin. Oncol., *11:* 334-346, 1984.

3. Catovsky, D., O'Brien, M., Melo, J.V., et al.: Hairy-cell leukemia (HCL) variant: An intermediate disease between HCL and B prolymphocytic leukemia. Semin. Oncol., *11:* 362-369, 1984.

4. Melo, J.V., Robinson, D.S., Gregory, C., et al.: Splenic B cell lymphoma with "villous" lymphocytes in the peripheral blood: A disorder distinct from hairy-cell leukemia. Leukemia, *1:* 294-298, 1987.

5. Yam, L.T., Janckila, A.J., Li, C.Y., et al.: Cytochemistry of tartrate-resistant acid phosphatase: 15 years' experience. Leukemia, *1:* 285-288, 1987.

6. Foroni, L., Catovsky, D., and Luzzatto, L.: Immunoglobulin gene rearrangements in hairy-cell leukemia and other B cell lymphoproliferative disorders. Leukemia, *1:* 389-392, 1987.

7. Melo, J.V., San Miguel, J.F., Moss, V.E., et al.: The membrane phenotype of hairy-cell leukemia: A study with monoclonal antibodies. Semin. Oncol., *11:* 381-385, 1984.

8. Thaler, J., Dietze, O., Faber, V., et al.: Monoclonal antibody B-ly7: A sensitive marker for detection of minimal residual disease in hairy-cell leukemia. Leukemia, *4:* 170-176, 1990.

9. Pizzolo, G., Ambrosetti, F., Vinante, M., et al.: Serum interleukin-2 receptor as index of tumor burden in hairy-cell leukemia. Blood, *77:* 2540-2542, 1991.

10. Quesada, J.R., Lepe-Zuniga, J.L., and Gutterman, J.U.: Mid-term observations on the efficacy of α-interferon in hairy-cell leukemia and status of the interferon system of patients in remission. Leukemia, *1:* 317-319, 1987.

11. Piro, L.D., Carrera, C.J., Carson, D.A., et al.: Lasting remissions in hairy-cell leukemia induced by a single infusion of 2-chlorodeoxyadenosine. N. Engl. J. Med., *322:* 1117-1121, 1990.

12. Bournocle, B.A., Grever, M.R., and Kraut, E.H.: Treatment of hairy-cell leukemia: The Ohio State University experience with deoxycoformycin. Leukemia, *1:* 350-354, 1987.

PATIENT WITH PLEURITIC PAIN AND HYPERGAMMAGLOBULINEMIA

Philip R. Greipp, Contributor
David N. Bailey, Reviewer

A 60-year-old optometrist developed acute onset of fever, productive cough, and left-side pleural pleuritic pain. In addition, he had malaise, chills, and diaphoresis. Other recurrent problems included mild, stable angina pectoris.

Physical examination revealed an acutely ill, but alert, oriented man; height, 67.5 inches (1.71 m); weight, 171 lb (78 kg); blood pressure, 137/60 mm Hg; pulse rate, 72 BPM and regular. The left chest was splinted, restricting movement of that side of the chest during inspiration. Dullness and decreased breath sounds were noted in the left chest. The physical examination was otherwise unremarkable.

The initial clinical impression was probable pneumococcal pneumonia and left pleural effusion. The following laboratory test results were reported:

Analyte	Value, conventional units	Reference range, conventional units	Value, SI units	Reference range, SI units
Hemoglobin (B)	8.5 g/dL	12.9-16.6	5.28 mmol/L	8.01-10.30
Leukocyte count (B)	$9.8 \times 10^3/\mu L$	4.1-10.9	$9.8 \times 10^9/L$	4.1-10.9
Platelet count (B)	$217 \times 10^3/\mu L$	184-370	$217 \times 10^9/L$	184-370
Creatinine (S)	0.9 mg/dL	0.7-1.1	80 μmol/L	62-97
Calcium, total (S)	9.1 mg/dL	8.4-10.1	2.27 mmol/L	2.10-2.52
Protein, total (S)	10.2 g/dL	6.0-7.8	102 g/L	60-78
Protein electrophoresis (S)				
Albumin	3.0 g/dL	3.1-4.3	30 g/L	31-43
α_1-globulin	0.2 g/dL	0.1-0.3	2 g/L	1-3
α_2-globulin	0.7 g/dL	0.6-1.0	7 g/L	6-10
β-globulin	1.1 g/dL	0.7-1.4	11 g/L	7-14
γ-globulin	4.2 g/dL	0.7-1.6	42 g/L	7-16

The chest film showed a left, lower lobe infiltrate and a left pleural effusion. Sputum showed polymorphonuclear leukocytes containing gram-positive diplococci.

Differential diagnostic considerations included causes for pneumonia with hypergamma-globulinemia such as tuberculosis or advanced liver disease with pneumonia, which are associated with polyclonal gammopathy, or multiple myeloma with pneumonia, which is associated with monoclonal gammopathy.

Review of the serum protein electrophoretic pattern showed a sharp monoclonal band within the γ-globulin fraction. Immunoelectrophoresis of the same serum revealed an IgA κ monoclonal protein. It is generally important to detect and quantitate Bence Jones protein-uria in patients suspected of having multiple myeloma. A value >500 mg in 24 hours suggests active disease requiring treatment. A metastatic bone survey, including X-ray study of the skull, axial skeleton, and proximal long bones, was negative. A bone marrow aspirate showed 40% plasma cells. Normal hematopoiesis was slightly diminished. A 24-h urine protein electrophoresis was not performed. In this patient the diagnosis of multiple myeloma was made based on the marrow findings and results of serum electrophoretic and immuno-electrophoretic findings. Following successful antibiotic treatment of his pneumonia, the patient was advised to consider chemotherapy, but he decided to defer treatment.

The patient was re-evaluated five months later. His hemoglobin had increased to 10.8 g/dL (6.70 mmol/L), and the bone marrow aspirate still showed 45% plasma cells. The plasma cell labeling index, a measure of the number of plasma cells in S-phase of the cell cycle, was 0.2%. A monoclonal β-γ spike, on electrophoresis, measured 2.31 g/dL (23 g/L), and the total γ-globulin 4.1 g/dL (41 g/L). Serum creatinine and calcium were normal. Urine showed a small amount of monoclonal κ protein. β_2-Microglobulin was normal, and C-reactive protein was normal. There were no circulating plasma cells detected by immunofluorescence on a mononuclear cell preparation that had been depleted of T cells. The physician elected to continue observation of the patient.

Two months later, the patient's monoclonal immunoglobulin spike was unchanged; the hemoglobin concentration had increased to 11.7 g/dL (7.26 mmol/L), and creatinine and calcium were still normal. The diagnosis was smoldering multiple myeloma. Continued follow-up was advised. Influenza and pneumococcal vaccination were given.

The patient was observed without chemotherapy for four uneventful years. Then his hemoglobin concentration decreased, and there was an increase in the myeloma spike, lytic lesions on bone survey, and an increase in bone marrow plasma cells with an increased plasma cell labeling index. β_2-Microglobulin remained low. Circulating plasma cells were observed in the immunofluorescent preparation of T cell-depleted mononuclear cells from peripheral blood.

Definition of the Disease

Multiple myeloma is characterized by the production in 75% of cases of a monoclonal protein in the serum (IgG, IgA, IgD, or IgE) and the presence in 80% of cases of κ or λ monoclonal light chain in the urine (Bence Jones proteinuria). Immunoelectrophoresis is necessary to define the specific monoclonal protein in the serum and urine. Immunofixation is more sensitive and may be used when the monoclonal protein is small in amount. Bone lesions are absent in one-third of cases, and anemia may be mild. One must be suspicious of the diagnosis of multiple myeloma in older individuals who present with only anemia, hypercalcemia, or renal insufficiency but have no bone lesions. Diagnostic criteria include a monoclonal protein in the serum or urine, lytic bone lesions with >10% plasma cells in the bone marrow, or biopsy-proven plasmacytoma. Patients with no bone lesions who have only a small amount of myeloma protein in the urine and negative ancillary tests (β_2-microglobulin, C-reactive protein, plasma cell labeling index of the bone marrow plasma cells, and tests for circulating myeloma cells) may have stable disease that does not require treatment. When bone radiographs are negative or show only osteoporosis, a criterion of 30% plasma cells is used.

The β_2-microglobulin, C-reactive protein, bone marrow plasma cell labeling index, and tests of the blood for circulating plasma cells using immunofluorescence examination of the T cell-depleted specimen are used as ancillary diagnostic tests.[1] It is best to obtain the bone marrow plasma cell labeling index at the time of the initial diagnostic marrow to avoid the unnecessary pain and expense of an additional marrow biopsy. The information gained may be used to help assess prognosis in patients who require treatment.

Patients with smoldering multiple myeloma have no bone lesions. They have >10% plasma cells in the bone marrow, and the plasma cell labeling index is very low — usually 0.0-0.2%. They remain stable without treatment for one year or more.

Presentation of Multiple Myeloma

About two-thirds of patients present with bone pain or bone lesions detected by x-ray, and most remaining patients have anemia. One-fourth of patients present with renal insufficiency and one-fifth of patients have hypercalcemia at diagnosis. Two-thirds of patients have a monoclonal spike in the serum, and 50% of patients have a monoclonal spike in the urine. Ten percent of patients will have a nondiagnostic serum and urine protein electrophoresis. Immunoelectrophoresis and immunofixation must be done to define the myeloma protein on such patients.

Bone marrow plasma cell labeling index is elevated in most patients with multiple myeloma.[2] β_2-Microglobulin and C-reactive protein may be elevated. Two-thirds of patients with multiple myeloma have circulating plasma cells detectable by immunofluorescence examination of a mononuclear cell preparation that has been depleted of T cells.[3] Although pneumonia caused by *Diplococcus pneumoniae* is a "classic" presentation of patients with multiple myeloma, its occurrence is uncommon, and recurrent infections with this organism are unusual. Even when pneumococcal vaccine is utilized, it may be ineffective because of the patient's lack of a primary antibody response.

Treatment

Standard chemotherapy for multiple myeloma utilizes melphalan and prednisone. Combination chemotherapies result in a higher response rate and more rapid response, but overall survival is not changed. Survival is best predicted by measuring the plasma cell labeling index and β_2-microglobulin concentrations.[4] Allogeneic or autologous bone marrow transplant may be used in younger patients who satisfy criteria for various transplant programs investigating the efficacy of this approach.

This patient had multiple myeloma that smoldered for four years, later necessitating treatment. Earlier treatment may have resulted in unnecessary expense and complications including acute leukemia.

Multiple Myeloma and Acute Leukemia

Acute leukemia occurs in about 10% of patients alive ten years after a diagnosis of multiple myeloma. Most patients with multiple myeloma who require treatment die within 30-36 months of initiation of treatment. Those who survive are at continuous risk of development of acute leukemia or relapse of myeloma. Rarely is treatment of acute leukemia effective. Deferral of treatment in patients with smoldering multiple myeloma avoids this unnecessary complication. On the other hand, one must avoid deferring treatment unnecessarily.

It has been said that no single test distinguishes the patient with overt multiple myeloma from the patient who will remain stable. Only close follow-up with serial measurement of serum protein electrophoresis can conclusively demonstrate stability and the absence of need for treatment. Newer tests such as the plasma cell labeling index and tests for circulating plasma cells may identify groups who require chemotherapy within six months.

References

1. Greipp, P. R.: Monoclonal gammopathies: New approaches to clinical problems in diagnosis and prognosis. Blood Rev., 3: 222-236, 1989.

2. Greipp, P. R., Witzig, T. E., and Gonchoroff, N. J.: Immunofluorescence labeling indices in myeloma and related monoclonal gammopathies. Mayo Clin. Proc., 62: 969-977, 1987.

3. Witzig, T. E., Gonchoroff, N. J., and Katzmann, J. A.: Peripheral blood B cell labeling indices are a measure of disease activity in patients with monoclonal gammopathies. J. Clin. Oncol., 6: 1041-1046, 1988.

4. Greipp, P. R., Katzmann, J. A., O'Fallon, W. M., et al.: Value of beta2-microglobulin level and plasma cell labeling indices as prognostic factors in patients with newly diagnosed myeloma. Blood, 72: 219-223, 1988.

Additional Reading

Kyle, R. A., and Greipp, P. R.: Multiple myeloma and other plasma cell disorders. *In:* Current Diagnosis, 8th ed. R.B. Conn, Ed. Philadelphia, W.B. Saunders Co., 1991.

PREGNANCY WITH ELEVATED MATERNAL SERUM α-FETOPROTEIN

Anjana Lal Pettigrew, Contributor

A 25-year-old white female was seen by her obstetrician for her second pregnancy. Her last normal menstrual period had begun 10 weeks prior to the visit. She was sure of this date but had a history of irregular menstrual cycles. Other than mild nausea in the morning and a tired feeling, she had had no illness or fever in the past two months. She was taking carbamazepine daily for a seizure disorder that was well controlled, her last seizure having occurred one year before. She admitted to drinking several glasses of wine each weekend. Her first pregnancy had produced a healthy daughter now two years old. Her cousin had had an anencephalic male child who died at birth. Her husband's sister had had a single miscarriage. There was no known family history of chromosome abnormalities, other birth defects, or known genetic disorders.

Physical examination was normal. The uterine size was consistent with a pregnancy of 9-10 weeks' gestation. Laboratory results were as follows:

Analyte	Value, conventional units	Reference range, conventional units	Value, SI units	Reference range, SI units
Hemoglobin (B)	13.5 g/dL	12-16	8.38 mmol/L	7.45-9.93
Hematocrit (B)	39 %	37-47	0.39	0.37-0.47
MCV (B)	91 fL	81-99	Same	
Carbamazepine (S)	7.5 μg/mL	Therap.: 4-12	32 μmol/L	17-51
Blood group and type	A, Rh$_O$ positive			
Antibody screen	Negative			
Rubella antibody	Immune			
Syphilis serology	Negative			
Urinalysis (U)	Negative for protein, glucose, and ketones; microscopical examination within normal limits			
Cervical/vaginal smear (Pap test)	Within normal limits			

At the time of her 16th week visit, the patient reported that her morning nausea had resolved; she had had no intercurrent illness or problem with the pregnancy. Physical examination showed the uterine size was consistent with 17 weeks' gestation. Doppler ultrasonographic examination indicated normal fetal heart tones. At this visit, she, like all obstetric patients visiting at 16 weeks, was given a pamphlet describing screening available for detection of a fetal neural tube defect (NTD) and Down syndrome. Her physician explained to her that these are two common disorders affecting infants and that a "positive" screening result would lead to recommendation for further testing to confirm or identify a problem. The patient elected to have the blood test performed.

The laboratory was provided with the following information that is required for interpretation of the laboratory tests, since levels of the analytes tested (especially α-fetoprotein) vary with the phase of gestation, with single versus multiple gestation, and with maternal age, race, weight, and diabetes.

Weeks of gestation	16.9 (estimate from LMP*)
Patient age, expected at delivery	25.5 y
Weight	130 lb (59.9 kg)
Race	Caucasian
Insulin-dependent diabetes	No
History of NTD	Anencephaly in second cousin of patient

The laboratory results of the screening tests were as follows:

Maternal serum

α-Fetoprotein (AFP)	110.4 ng/mL (3.18 MoM[†])
Estriol, unconjugated (uE$_3$)	0.83 ng/mL (0.92 MoM)
Human chorionic gonadotropin (hCG)	69.6 U/mL (2.71 MoM)

Interpretation

Open NTD risk: This serum AFP value, adjusted for maternal weight, is *elevated* for a singleton pregnancy at this gestational age. An ultrasonographic examination to date the pregnancy accurately and a repeat serum AFP test are recommended.

Down syndrome risk: The risk for fetal Down syndrome, based on the maternal serum AFP, uE$_3$, and hCG, is less than 1 in 200.[‡]

The patient was asked to return to discuss the abnormal results and was very upset. She was told that her fetus was not found to be at high risk for Down syndrome, but that an elevated AFP indicated increased risk for certain types of birth defects. She was also told that most women with elevated serum AFP levels are carrying a normal fetus, but that elevation could indicate an open spine or abdominal wall defect in the fetus. Additional testing was recommended, specifically an ultrasonographic examination to determine fetal age more accurately and a repeat test for maternal serum AFP. Fetal age was determined by ultrasonography to be 17.3 weeks. The laboratory results for maternal serum AFP were as follows:

Maternal serum	142.3 ng/mL (4.1 MoM)

This serum AFP value, adjusted for maternal weight, is *elevated* for a pregnancy at this gestational age. Further testing is recommended.

---

* LMP, last menstrual period.

† MoM, multiples of median value as defined by maternal age, weight, race, diabetic status, and weeks of gestation. A "positive" test is usually defined as ≥2.5 MoM. A positive result occurs in about 3% of all tests but is not of itself diagnostic of an open fetal defect.

‡ The risk for Down syndrome is calculated from maternal age and the AFP, uE$_3$, and hCG values. A risk calculated to be ≥1:200 is usually defined as a "positive" screen result for Down syndrome. A positive screening test occurs in about 5% of pregnant women.

The patient was asked to return to discuss the latest findings. The obstetrician explained that the elevation of AFP indicated that the fetus was at increased risk of having a neural tube or abdominal wall defect. He recommended that she consider further tests that consisted of a high resolution ("genetic") ultrasonographic examination and an amniocentesis for determination of amniotic fluid AFP, presence of acetylcholinesterase (AChE), and chromosome analysis.

The sonogram showed a 3-cm neural tube defect in the thoracic spine, but no other abnormalities were detected. The amniotic fluid AFP value was elevated at 48.6 µg/mL (4.5 MoM), and an acetylcholinesterase band was detected. Chromosome analysis showed a 46,XY normal male chromosome pattern. After telling the patient that the results were consistent with an isolated open spine defect, the obstetrician referred her to a medical geneticist. Genetic counseling included explanation of the cause of NTD's, description of therapy and prognosis of cases with NTD, and discussion of options for current and future pregnancies.

Definition of the Disease

Neural tube defects (NTD's) are among the most common major congenital abnormalities. In the United States, the incidence is 1-2 per 1000 live births. The two most frequent forms of NTD's are anencephaly and the various types of spina bifida. Both result from a failure of the neural tube to close completely in the fourth week of fetal development. Anencephaly is characterized by absence of the cerebral hemispheres and cranial vault and is lethal soon after birth. Spina bifida lesions are either meningoceles or myeloceles or a combination of the two. Meningoceles involve herniation of the meninges through an open defect with the spinal cord remaining intact and in its normal position. Myeloceles involve the spinal cord, and even small lesions are associated with significant neurological impairment below the level of the lesion (weakness, paralysis, bowel and bladder incontinence).

The cause of NTD's is heterogeneous. The majority (about 80%) are due to multifactorial inheritance with the interaction of several genes and environmental factors. In the remaining cases, the NTD may be attributed to a specific cause such as mendelian inheritance (e.g., autosomal dominant inheritance), certain genetic syndromes, or chromosome abnormalities (e.g., trisomy 13). A few of the "maternal" environmental factors that have been implicated as a cause of NTD's are diabetes mellitus, hyperthermia, folic acid deficiency, alcohol ingestion, and fetal exposure to valproic acid, aminopterin, or carbamazepine.[1,2] About 95% of infants with an NTD are born to a couple with no prior family history of spina bifida.

Down syndrome is the most frequently observed chromosome abnormality present in liveborn infants and has an incidence of 1 in 800. It is the most common chromosomal cause of mental retardation. The majority of cases are sporadic and are due to nondisjunction at meiosis (trisomy 21). Although the risk for Down syndrome increases with advancing maternal age, there is a small risk of having a child with Down syndrome at any maternal age. Because younger women have a proportionately larger number of pregnancies, a substantial number of Down syndrome infants are born to younger women. Although specific prenatal testing for Down syndrome by amniocentesis or chorionic villus sampling in the pregnancies of older women is routinely recommended, many cases of Down syndrome in younger women are not detected. Familial Down syndrome due to inheritance of a robertsonian translocation involving chromosome 21 accounts for 1% or less of all cases of Down syndrome.

Screening for NTD's and Down Syndrome

The AFP profile is a group of tests performed on a single maternal serum sample; it screens for open fetal defects (mainly neural tube defects) and for Down syndrome. Down syndrome and NTD's are common and usually sporadic, occurring in families without any prior history. Thus, a screening test to identify affected pregnancies is desirable. AFP testing of maternal serum was originally developed to screen for the *elevation* of AFP associated with fetal open NTD's. Subsequently, *low* levels of AFP were seen to be associated with fetuses with Down syndrome. Recently, studies have shown that use of maternal serum unconjugated estriol and human chorionic gonadotropin measurements along with AFP levels improves the sensitivity of the AFP test for identifying Down syndrome pregnancies.

α-Fetoprotein, Unconjugated Estriol, and Human Chorionic Gonadotropin. AFP is a glycoprotein that is synthesized mainly by the fetal liver. It is excreted through the fetal kidneys into fetal urine, which is the major source of amniotic fluid in the second trimester. AFP enters the maternal circulation from the amniotic fluid. The levels of AFP in fetal blood, amniotic fluid, and maternal serum vary with gestational age. The optimal time for measuring maternal serum AFP is 16-18 weeks (range, 15-20 weeks). With an open defect in the fetal skin, such as an NTD, AFP in the fetal circulation leaks out and is found in higher than normal levels in the amniotic fluid and maternal blood. Elevated AFP levels are also associated with other open defects such as omphalocele and gastroschisis, both ventral wall defects.[1] Because AFP levels are influenced by factors such as singleton versus multiple gestation, race, maternal weight, and maternal diabetes mellitus, this information must be supplied to the laboratory so that accurate risk information can be calculated.

Abnormally low levels of AFP are associated with an increased risk for Down syndrome.[3] The low levels of AFP and uE_3 associated with Down syndrome pregnancies are thought to be due to decreased AFP and uE_3 synthesis by an immature fetal liver. The concentration of hCG in maternal serum declines between 10 and 20 weeks of pregnancy. The abnormally high level of hCG seen in Down syndrome pregnancies is thought to be due to an immature placenta and a delayed decrease in hCG during pregnancy.

Recommended Screening Protocol. Overall, 1 in 12 pregnant women (8%) will have a positive screen indicating an increased risk for either a fetal open defect or Down syndrome. The most frequent cause for a false positive screen is an error in dating the pregnancy. Therefore, an ultrasonographic examination to measure the fetus and date the pregnancy accurately is indicated if the original test interpretation was based on a gestational age derived from the LMP date. A recommended protocol for follow-up of the initial abnormal AFP profile is outlined in Figure 1.

If the repeat maternal serum AFP is elevated or if the triple profile of AFP, uE_3, and hCG is still abnormal, specific testing is recommended. An amniocentesis is performed for determining the amniotic fluid AFP and acetylcholinesterase. Amniotic fluid AFP levels are elevated in the majority of open neural tube and abdominal wall defects. Acetylcholinesterase, which is synthesized by nerve cells, will be present in the amniotic fluid in almost all cases of an open spine defect and is used to help differentiate between these and abdominal wall defects. A chromosome analysis is also performed. A high resolution ("genetic") ultrasonographic examination, which is a detailed anatomical study of the fetus, is performed to try to identify any structural abnormalities. In cases of an abnormal AFP profile and increased Down syndrome risk, an amniocentesis for chromosome analysis is performed.

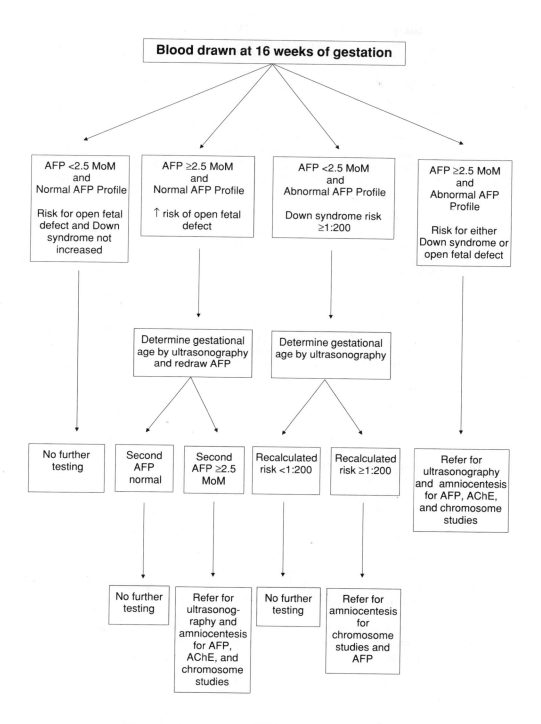

Figure 1. Recommended AFP Profile Screening Protocol.

Sensitivity of AFP Profile Screen in Detecting NTD's and Down Syndrome. In general, the odds of a fetus being affected with an NTD, after an elevated maternal serum AFP is first found, are about 1 in 50. The higher the AFP value, the greater the likelihood of an anatomical lesion. The odds of a fetus being affected with Down syndrome after a positive screen are approximately 1 in 55. In those cases in which a specific fetal anomaly is not present, an elevated maternal serum AFP may be associated with various complications of pregnancy that warrant closer monitoring during the remainder of the pregnancy.[4,5] These include poor fetal growth, fetal distress, threatened miscarriage, and fetal death. If the recommended protocol (Figure 1) is followed, antenatal diagnosis is possible for 95% of cases of anencephaly, 80% of all cases of spina bifida, and 60% of cases of Down syndrome.[6] Referral to a medical geneticist to discuss the fetal condition, etiology, treatment, pregnancy options, recurrence risks, and future pregnancy diagnostic options is warranted.

Some of the known causes of NTD's — which include hyperthermia, folic acid deficiency, maternal diabetes, and chromosome abnormality — can be excluded in the present case since there was no history of high fever or prolonged exposure in a sauna and no evidence of megaloblastic anemia. With multifactorial disorders, a family history of an affected first or second degree relative is considered significant and would place the fetus at increased risk. However, the anencephalic child in this family is a distant relative, and the occurrence is most likely coincidental. Two potential teratogens, alcohol and carbamazepine, must be considered as a possible cause of the NTD. Recent studies indicate that with first trimester exposure to carbamazepine there is an increased risk for an NTD.[2] NTD's are an occasional finding in infants exposed to alcohol in the first trimester. The NTD in the present case could have been caused by either agent or by both agents acting together. A genetic syndrome involving an NTD and other malformations not detectable by ultrasonography cannot be excluded prenatally.

References

1. Milunsky, A.: The prenatal diagnosis of neural tube and other congenital defects. *In:* Genetic Disorders in the Fetus: Diagnosis, Prevention, and Treatment. A. Milunsky, Ed. New York, Plenum Press, 1987.

2. Rosa, F.W.: Spina bifida in infants of women treated with carbamazepine during pregnancy. N. Engl. J. Med., *324:*674-677, 1991.

3. Knight, G.J., Palomaki, G.E., and Haddow, J.E.: Use of maternal serum α-fetoprotein measurements to screen for Down's syndrome. Clin. Obstet. Gynecol., *31:* 306-327, 1988.

4. Burton, B.K.: Outcome in infants born to mothers with unexplained elevations in maternal serum α-fetoprotein. Pediatrics, *77:* 582-586, 1986.

5. Milunsky, A., Jick, S.S., and Bruell, C.L.: Predictive values, relative risks, and overall benefits of high and low maternal serum α-fetoprotein screening in singleton pregnancies: New epidemiologic data. Am. J. Obstet. Gynecol., *161:* 291-297, 1989.

6. Wald, N.J., Cuckle, H.S., Densem, J.W., et al.: Maternal serum screening for Down's syndrome in early pregnancy. Br. Med. J., *297:* 883-887, 1988.

ACUTE HEMIPARESIS

Kevin R. Nelson, Contributor
Steven L. Hoover, Contributor

A 37-year-old woman presented to the Emergency Department because of progressive left arm and leg weakness. Difficulty was first noted three days earlier when she arose from bed and her leg felt "heavy." Weakness in the leg worsened over the next five days and extended to the left arm as well. She had also noted that "electric shocks go down my arms" when she flexed her neck (Lhermitte's phenomenon).

Neurological examination disclosed 6 mm pupils briskly reactive to light. With the swinging flashlight test, her left pupil dilated when the light was swung to that eye (Marcus Gunn pupil). Corrected visual acuity was 20/20 O.D. (oculus dexter; right eye) and 20/30 O.S. (oculus sinister; left eye). On gaze to the left, her right eye would incompletely adduct, and horizontal nystagmus was present in the left eye. Ocular movements were otherwise normal, including convergence. Examination of the facial and other cranial nerves was unremarkable. Sensation was preserved. The patient had no voluntary movement of her left leg. She was able to raise her left arm off the bed and flex her elbow but had no other motion. Deep tendon reflexes in the left arm and leg were exaggerated, with sustained ankle clonus and a positive Babinski's sign.

Hemiparesis with facial sparing raised the concern for an acute spinal cord lesion and prompted cervical magnetic resonance imaging (MRI). No tumor or herniated intervertebral disk was found, but T_2 weighted images disclosed an increase of the signal within the spinal cord at the C3 level. Consequently, the following cerebrospinal fluid (CSF) analyses were performed:

Analyte	Value, conventional units	Reference range, conventional units	Value, SI units	Reference range, SI units
Erythrocyte count (CSF)	0/µL	0		
Leukocyte count (CSF)	11/µL; 100% lymphocytes	≤5; 100% lymphocytes	11×10^6/L	≤5
Protein (CSF)	51 mg/dL	15-45	0.51 g/L	0.15-0.45
Glucose (CSF)	68 mg/dL	40-70	3.8 mmol/L	2.2-3.9
Oligoclonal IgG bands (CSF)	Present	Absent		
IgG index	1.1	0.3-0.7	Same	
IgG synthesis rate	+ 13.5 mg/d	−9.9 to + 3.3		
Myelin basic protein (CSF)	9 ng/mL	≤4	9 µg/L	≤4

Further inquiry disclosed that three years previously the patient had experienced a loss of vision in her left eye lasting several weeks, from which she recovered. She has had momentary diplopia, which was more prominent when she was fatigued or feverish.

Clinical and laboratory findings established the diagnosis of multiple sclerosis (MS) in this patient. Within days her weakness spontaneously stabilized. Over the following six weeks, strength in the arm and leg improved, leaving the patient with mild residual weakness.

Definition of the Disease

Multiple sclerosis is an autoimmune disorder of unknown cause. The immune response is directed largely against oligodendrocytes that form myelin sheaths around axons. The specific antigen(s) have yet to be identified, and both humoral as well as cell-mediated limbs of the immune system appear involved. MS is pathologically characterized by discrete multifocal inflammatory demyelinating plaques of varying age. Most plaques are concentrated in the white matter, often with a perivenular and periventricular distribution. Lymphocytes and macrophages predominate within the plaque. Also common is scattered demyelination of small axonal groups with few signs of active inflammation. Immunoglobulin is produced by B lymphocytes in or near the plaque.

Acute clinical manifestations of MS are caused by a combination of incidental axonal injury and demyelination. Myelin is critical for propagation of the axonal action potential because it maintains proper membrane characteristics. Acute demyelination blocks propagation of the action potential between cell body and nerve terminal. The specific clinical effects depend upon which neurons are affected.

Regardless of what causes demyelination, remyelination and resumption of saltatory conduction occurs to a far less extent in the central nervous system (CNS) than in the peripheral nervous system. Clinical improvement in MS is thought to occur primarily by overcoming conduction block with continuous, nonsaltatory conduction of the action potential through the demyelinated region. Patients with MS typically have exacerbations when they are hot. Elevated temperature may increase sodium channel inactivation and aggravate conduction block by limiting the amount of depolarizing sodium current. The degree of remission depends heavily upon the extent of axonal injury.

Clinical Features. Multiple sclerosis is often clinically evident before the age of 40. Some patients may be asymptomatic lifelong, and others suffer premature death from disseminated demyelination. The disease course is characterized by exacerbations and remissions, or it can be steadily progressive at a slow or rapid rate.

Signs and symptoms produced by MS reflect areas of pathological predilection. Demyelination within the posterior columns results in paresthesia ("pins and needles") and perhaps sensory loss. The initial symptoms of MS are commonly sensory; they are often of an unusual nature without objective confirmation and thus may prompt consultation with a psychiatrist. Involvement of the cerebellum and its interconnections causes ataxia, and impairment of central vestibular tracts produces vertigo. Neuropsychiatric manifestations include depression, dementia, and emotional lability.

Diagnosis

To diagnose MS it is necessary to establish CNS impairment, which varies in time and location. In many instances, this criterion is satisfied by history and neurological examination alone. However, MS may not be confirmed on this basis when the disease is early or otherwise restricted. In such cases, laboratory evaluation is of great value,[1] but it may be more important to exclude other treatable neurological conditions than to confirm a diagnosis of MS.

Cerebrospinal fluid (CSF) analysis aids in the diagnosis of MS by providing evidence of inflammation within the CNS. During an exacerbation, the CSF usually contains less than 20 leukocytes/μL (20 x 10^6/L), nearly all of which are lymphocytes. Inflammation disrupts the blood-brain barrier and mildly elevates CSF protein up to 60 mg/dL (0.60 g/L).

CSF IgM, IgA, and IgG (including IgG_1 and κ light chains) are increased during MS exacerbation. Therefore, the demonstration of CNS immunoglobulin synthesis is useful for supporting the diagnosis of MS. Production of CNS IgG must be differentiated from serum IgG transudation when the blood-brain barrier is disrupted by inflammation. CSF albumin can be used as a permeability reference because it is not synthesized in the CNS. By expressing CSF and serum IgG as a ratio to CSF and serum albumin, a converted relative measure of IgG synthesis in CSF can be obtained. Mathematically, this is expressed as

$$\text{IgG Index} = \frac{\text{CSF IgG/serum IgG}}{\text{CSF albumin/serum albumin}}$$

Investigators have calculated CSF IgG synthesis rates using many formulas.[2] Like the IgG index, the IgG synthesis rate corrects for blood-brain barrier disruption by using serum and CSF values for albumin and IgG. Either the IgG index or synthesis rate is abnormal in over 90% of patients with MS. However, 30-60% of patients with other inflammatory CNS disorders may show similar abnormalities. Also, the magnitude of CNS IgG synthesis rate correlates poorly with disease severity.

High resolution electrophoresis of CSF (sometimes enhanced with isoelectric focusing or immunofixation) yields IgG oligoclonal bands (OCB) in 80% of patients with MS[3] (Figure 1). However, 40% of patients with other causes of CNS inflammation will also have OCB. OCB appear early in the course of MS and retain their pattern regardless of disease activity. A recent study has suggested that IgM OCB may be an indicator of recent exacerbation.[4]

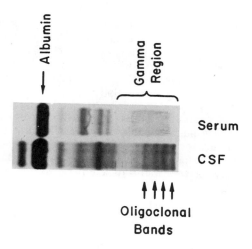

Figure 1. Cerebrospinal fluid electrophoresis in a patient with multiple sclerosis. IgG oligoclonal bands are present (arrows) and directed against currently unknown antigen(s). In some cases, results of OCB patterns require subjective interpretation.

Myelin basic protein (MBP) constitutes 30% of CNS myelin. Elevated CSF levels of MBP are found up to 14 days after CNS injury. In MS, elevated CSF MBP can be used as an objective measure of recent demyelination.[5]

Sensory evoked potentials can be recorded over cerebral cortex and spinal cord. These waveforms reflect neural conduction in optic tracts, brain stem auditory pathways, or somatosensory tracts between spinal cord and cortex. Both conduction block and continuous conduction will produce abnormal evoked potentials. After recovery from acute demyelination, the velocity of continuous action potential conduction is slower than saltatory conduction. This slowing is of little functional consequence but is important in the physiological evaluation for MS by producing delayed waveforms. Either absent or delayed waveforms can provide evidence of previously undetected lesions.

MRI of the CNS may contribute greatly to the diagnosis of MS by revealing clinically discernible and indiscernible plaques.[6] The exclusion of other neurological disorders is also important. The MRI is abnormal in most cases of MS. However, the MRI findings of MS can be seen in many other disease states and in some healthy individuals as well. Like all laboratory studies in MS, MRI must be interpreted in the proper clinical context.

In this patient, history and neurological examination detected CNS lesions separated in time and space. Acute demyelination of the pyramidal tracts led to weakness, hyperreflexia, and a positive Babinski's sign. Lhermitte's phenomenon presumably arose from mechanical stimulation of irritable posterior columns as the spinal cord stretched during neck flexion. Previous demyelination of the optic nerve caused mild residual visual loss. Impairment of the medial longitudinal fasciculus led to internuclear ophthalmoplegia and diplopia. The detection of MBP in the CSF implied injury to neural elements containing myelin. CNS inflammation was substantiated by CSF pleocytosis, intrathecal IgG production, and the presence of CSF oligoclonal bands.

Treatment

Treating an autoimmune disorder with immunosuppression possesses a certain logic. However, immunosuppression for MS has remained controversial for many years. It is difficult to establish the efficacy of therapy in an illness with highly variable clinical manifestations and whose natural history is often unpredictable and characterized by remission. Furthermore, the use of drugs with potentially serious complications must be undertaken with caution in a disorder in which up to 30% of untreated patients have minimal lifetime disability.

It is generally accepted that corticosteroids increase the rate of recovery from an acute exacerbation,[7] but there is little support that such therapy favorably alters the long-term course of MS. Azathioprine has been used for patients with progressive disease.[8] Treatment with the alkylating agent cyclophosphamide has been advocated by some,[9] but it is perhaps best reserved for ambulatory patients with a rapidly progressing course. Other forms of immunotherapy are experimental at this time.

References

1. Poser, C.M., Paty, D.W., Scheinberg, L., et al.: New diagnostic criteria for multiple sclerosis: Guidelines for research protocols. Ann. Neurol., *13:* 227-231, 1983.

2. Tourtellotte, W.W., Staugaitis, S.M., Walsh, M.J., et al.: The basis of intra-blood-brain-barrier IgG synthesis. Ann. Neurol., *17:* 21-27, 1985.

3. Farrell, M.A., Kaufmann, J.C.E., Gilbert, J.J., et al.: Oligoclonal bands in multiple sclerosis: Clinical-pathologic correlation. Neurology, *35:* 212-218, 1985.

4. Sharief, M.K., and Thompson, E.J.: The predictive value of intrathecal immunoglobulin synthesis and magnetic resonance imaging in acute isolated syndromes for subsequent development of multiple sclerosis. Ann. Neurol., *29:* 147-151, 1991.

5. Whitaker, J.N., and Synder, D.S.: Myelin components in the cerebrospinal fluid in diseases affecting central nervous system myelin. Clin. Allergy Immunol., *2:* 469-482, 1982.

6. Paty, D.W., Oger, J.J.F., Kastrukoff, L.F., et al.: MRI in the diagnosis of MS: A prospective study with comparison of clinical evaluation, evoked potentials, oligoclonal banding, and CT. Neurology, *38:* 180-185, 1988.

7. Thompson, A.J., Kennard, C., Swash, M., et al.: Relative efficacy of intravenous methylprednisolone and ACTH in the treatment of acute relapse in MS. Neurology, *39:* 969-971, 1989.

8. Goodkin, D.E., Bailly, R.C., Teetzen, M.L., et al.: The efficacy of azathioprine in relapsing-remitting multiple sclerosis. Neurology, *41:* 20-25, 1991.

9. Weiner, H.L., and Hafler, D.A.: Immunotherapy of multiple sclerosis. Ann. Neurol., *23:* 211-222, 1988.

YOUNG MAN WITH CHEST PAIN

Evan A. Stein, Contributor

A 42-year-old male executive presented to the Emergency Department with severe substernal chest pain of 45 minutes' duration. The pain radiated into his left upper and lower arm and was associated with severe dyspnea, diaphoresis, and nausea. The pain had started while he was hurrying through the airport. An electrocardiogram (ECG) in the Emergency Department demonstrated marked ST segment depression and deep Q waves, consistent with acute myocardial infarction. The patient was immediately started on intravenous streptokinase therapy and morphine; his pain rapidly subsided. Coronary angiography demonstrated a totally occluded proximal, left anterior descending (LAD) coronary artery that gradually opened on thrombolytic therapy to reveal a fixed 70% stenosis. Two other lesions of 60% and 40% stenosis were seen on the distal part of the right coronary and the left main coronary arteries, respectively.

Past history revealed occasional brief episodes, lasting one to three minutes, of chest discomfort or heaviness and associated numbness of the left hand. The episodes were associated with vigorous effort and had occurred over the past two years. Otherwise, the patient had enjoyed excellent health. He was taking no regular medications. His personal habits included using 100 mL of alcohol equivalents per week, smoking a pack of cigarettes daily, following a modified low fat diet, and maintaining a regular exercise program two to three times per week.

His family history indicated that his father was alive and well. His mother had died at age 59 from ischemic heart disease after having had coronary artery bypass surgery at age 57. Her father had died suddenly from myocardial infarction at age 48, as had her brother at age 39. The patient had two sisters, aged 36 and 34, and a brother aged 32. All were in good health, as were his three children, two girls and a boy, ages 2, 7, and 12, respectively.

His weight of 178 lb (81 kg) was appropriate for his height of 68 inches (1.74 m). Blood pressure was 110/70 mm Hg. Faint white deposits were noted on the lower lateral aspects of both corneas. Examination of the head and neck was noncontributory. Heart sounds were normal; no murmurs were heard. There was a faint bruit, Grade I/VI, heard over the left carotid artery. The rest of the pulses were present and equal, and no bruits were detected over either the abdominal aorta or femoral arteries. There were no masses in the abdomen, and the lungs were clear. Careful examination revealed that his left Achilles tendon was enlarged and nodular. The rest of the examination was unremarkable.

On the first day of admission, laboratory investigations included a routine biochemical profile, complete blood count, and urinalysis. The results were the following:

Analyte	Value, conventional units	Reference range, conventional units	Value, SI units	Reference range, SI units
Chemistry profile (S)				
Glucose	126 mg/dL	54-108	7 mmol/L	3-6
Triglycerides	319 mg/dL	53-266	3.6 mmol/L	0.6-3.0
Cholesterol	282 mg/dL	154-200	7.3 mmol/L	4.0-5.2

Analyte	Value, conventional units	Reference range, conventional units	Value, SI units	Reference range, SI units
CK, AST, LDH	All mildly elevated			
CK-MB	~18% of total	<5%	~0.18 of total	<0.05
Other analytes	Within normal limits			
Complete blood count (B)				
Leukocyte count	Mildly elevated			
	Other findings within normal limits			
Urinalysis (U)	Within normal limits			

The patient remained stable in the coronary care unit. After three days, he was placed in the step-down unit. His enzyme levels returned to normal, and he was discharged after seven days with a plan for a follow-up for either coronary artery bypass surgery or possibly angioplasty, depending on noninvasive cardiovascular evaluation to be carried out one month after discharge. In addition, the patient was referred to the local lipid clinic for further evaluation of the lipid disorder.

Follow-up of the patient at the lipid clinic took place three months later. The corneal arcus and tendon xanthoma were confirmed, and the following laboratory results were obtained with the patient in a fasting state:

Analyte	Value, conventional units	Reference range, conventional units	Value, SI units	Reference range, SI units
Cholesterol (S)	347 mg/dL	154-200	9 mmol/L	4.0-5.2
Triglycerides (S)	133 mg/dL	53-266	1.5 mmol/L	0.6-3.0
HDL-cholesterol (S)	39 mg/dL	35-65	1.0 mmol/L	0.9-1.7
LDL-cholesterol (S)	282 mg/dL	80-160	7.3 mmol/L	2.0-4.2
Apolipoprotein A-I (S)	105 mg/dL	125-155	1.05 g/L	1.25-1.55
Apolipoprotein B (S)	213 mg/dL	70-120	2.13 g/L	0.7-1.2
Lipoprotein little A antigen [Lp(a)]	86 mg/dL	<30	0.86 g/L	<0.3

Results were confirmed at a second visit two weeks later, also in a fasting state. The patient was found to have normal thyroid function, liver function, renal function, and glucose homeostasis.

With additional dietary therapy by a trained nutritionist, the patient maintained good compliance and, in effect, achieved Step 2 in the guidelines of the National Institutes of Health's National Cholesterol Education Program (NCEP). However, his lipid levels failed to decrease. A diagnosis of probable heterozygous familial hypercholesterolemia (FH) was made, and the lipid profiles of the patient's siblings and three children were tested. One sister of the patient had a marked elevation of LDL-cholesterol and apolipoprotein B. The children's results were as follows:

Serum Lipid	Reference range	Daughter, 2 y	Daughter, 7 y	Son, 12 y
Cholesterol	<4.40 mmol/L	7.36	4.04	6.27
Triglyceride	<1.14 mmol/L	0.98	0.68	1.14
HDL-cholesterol	>1.04 mmol/L	1.04	1.42	0.91
LDL-cholesterol	<2.85 mmol/L	5.88	2.31	4.84
Apolipoprotein A-I	1.25-1.55 g/L	1.15	1.38	1.08
Apolipoprotein B	<1.0 g/L	1.96	0.61	1.51
Lp(a)	<0.20 g/L	0.03	0.41	0.62

Definition of the Disease

The patient and his family have confirmed heterozygous familial hypercholesterolemia (FH), a dominant non-sex-linked genetic disorder that was described more than 50 years ago. The probable cause, a defect in the LDL-receptor, was discovered and described by Goldstein and Brown.[1] The gene frequency in the North American population is now estimated to be one in 300-500. In certain groups, particularly Lebanese, French-speaking Canadians, and the white Afrikaner population of South Africa, the gene frequency is substantially higher, in some cases documented as one in 66. A number of specific defects affecting the LDL-receptor mechanism have now been described. These have been shown to affect any one of a number of stages in receptor synthesis and post-synthetic modification.

The disorder manifests at birth and can be diagnosed by detection of elevated cord blood LDL-cholesterol and apolipoprotein B levels. The defective LDL-receptor causes an inability to catabolize and remove LDL from the circulation. The increased circulating LDL-cholesterol is postulated to be more readily taken up by macrophage scavenger cells. The macrophage becomes a foam cell, enters into the arterial wall, undergoes lysis, and releases both the lipid and a number of chemotactic factors; the eventual result is an atherosclerotic plaque. The inability to deliver cholesterol via the LDL pathway to hepatic cells also causes increased 3-hydroxy-3-methylglutaryl-CoA (HMG-CoA) reductase activity and enhanced cholesterol biosynthesis.

The homozygous condition is extremely rare, being found in less than one in one million persons in the United States. It is more common in the populations listed above in which the heterozygous gene is also more frequent. Homozygous FH is, in fact, usually a combination of two different gene defects (i.e., compound heterozygosity) in the United States. Although homozygous FH is a very serious condition leading invariably to atherosclerosis before age 20, there are two main clinical subtypes that vary in severity. The first subtype is receptor negative, with LDL-receptor activity <2% of normal. In these subjects, coronary atherosclerosis appears to manifest earlier and is more often lethal. The second subgroup is receptor defective, with LDL-receptor activity <20% of normal. Although this second disorder produces atherosclerosis at a very early age, it is generally not as strongly associated with premature death.

Clinical Features. The heterozygous disorder is often marked by a family history of early atherosclerosis. In individuals with the disorder, the risks of coronary artery disease manifesting clinically[2,3] are

Age (y)	Males (%)	Females (%)
<30	5.4	---
<50	51.1	12.2
<65	85.4	57.7

Clinical features are usually detectable by the mid- to late-20's and include extensor tendon xanthomas, mainly of the ring and middle fingers, nodular and thickened Achilles tendon xanthomas, and corneal arcus. Occasionally, xanthelasma and xanthomas over the elbows may be found. In the homozygote, xanthomas are seen usually before the age of two and are present interdigitally, in the cleft of the buttocks, over the knees, behind the knees, over the elbows, and around the ankles; they lead to the biochemical confirmation and diagnosis.

Diagnosis

The diagnosis is based on family history of early atherosclerosis, presence of xanthomas, and a marked increase in LDL-cholesterol. Although LDL-cholesterol is usually greater than 232 mg/dL (6 mmol/L), it can be as low as 154 mg/dL (4 mmol/L). Two- or three-generation transmission is generally necessary to confirm the diagnosis, since there is no specific test for LDL-receptors at this time. The LDL-receptor defect, if known, as in specific populations in which gene frequency is high and a gene founder effect is known to have occurred, may be diagnosed by use of specific gene probes. However, gene probes are not as yet recommended for routine clinical testing. Other disorders known to produce secondary hyperlipidemia — hypothyroidism, diabetes, renal disease such as nephrotic syndrome, or hepatic dysfunction — should be excluded.

Lipid levels are affected acutely by serious illness such as acute myocardial infarction, as in the patient described, and an erroneous diagnosis may be made or the diagnosis missed if the lipid assessment is carried out under unstable conditions. Wait three months after myocardial infarction, bypass surgery, or any major illness or operation to confirm the diagnosis.

The disorder seldom responds to dietary manipulation. Other possible disorders include familial defective apolipoprotein B. In this disorder, a defect in the apolipoprotein B, known as B-3500, can produce moderate elevations of LDL and a familial pattern. The defect is not associated with LDL-receptor abnormalities; instead, the defective apolipoprotein B does not bind adequately to the LDL-receptor.

Diagnosis of the homozygous condition is made clinically but can be confirmed by fibroblast culture and detailed LDL-receptor genetic analysis.

Lp(a) is useful not only as an independent risk factor for atherosclerosis when other lipid levels are "normal" but also as an important factor in subjects with heterozygous FH; if it is elevated, subjects have an even greater risk of earlier coronary artery disease.[4] Elevated Lp(a) may also dictate drug therapy because the bile acid sequestrants (BAS) and the HMGCoA reductase inhibitors (RI) do not alter Lp(a), whereas nicotinic acid (NA) does.

Treatment

As for all subjects at risk for atherosclerosis, other factors such as smoking, obesity, and exercise should receive attention if lipid reduction is to be beneficial in reducing atherosclerosis. There is now unequivocal evidence that long-term reduction in blood cholesterol, specifically in LDL-cholesterol, results in a reduced risk of coronary atherosclerotic related morbidity and mortality.[5] This reduction in risk of ischemic heart disease is ~2% for every 1% reduction in total cholesterol over a seven-year period. More recent studies using coronary angiography have clearly demonstrated that it is possible not only to stop the atherosclerotic process but also to reverse it.[6] Reversal is, however, a slow process, probably requiring substantial reductions in LDL-cholesterol to levels below 97 mg/dL (2.5 mmol/L) and occurring at about 1% per year of therapy. However, even in the most severely affected heterozygous familial hypercholesterolemic subjects, regression of coronary atherosclerosis has been shown to occur.[7]

The first step in treatment is dietary and should be instituted in all subjects with primary or familial hypercholesterolemia as soon as the diagnosis is confirmed. In children, this step is recommended after age two. Detailed dietary guidelines are available from either the

American Heart Association (AHA) or the National Institutes of Health's National Cholesterol Education Program (NCEP). There are two steps in the NCEP. Step 1 reduces total fat to <30% of calories, saturated fats to <10%, and mono- and polyunsaturated fats to <10% of calories. Dietary cholesterol should be <300 mg/d. The total energy intake should be reduced, if necessary for the subject to achieve ideal body weight. In the Step 2 diet, dietary cholesterol is reduced further to <200 mg/d and saturated fat to <7% of calories, with total fat making up <25% of total daily energy requirements. Any caloric replacement should be made with complex carbohydrates.

The effects of diet on cholesterol reduction are usually modest (5-15%) in FH subjects. The low fat, low saturated fat diet often reduces both LDL- and HDL-cholesterol. The full impact of diet often takes 8-12 weeks to occur.

Drug Therapy. Drug therapy centers around three therapeutic classes: the bile acid sequestrants (BAS), nicotinic acid (NA), and the HMG-CoA reductase inhibitors (RI). The *bile acid sequestrants* are nonabsorbable agents that work by binding and removing bile acids, a major breakdown product of cholesterol, and preventing their recycling through the enterohepatic circulation. The resultant depletion of hepatic intracellular cholesterol that occurs with conversion of cholesterol to replace these bile acids is, in turn, replaced either by *de novo* cholesterol biosynthesis or by increased LDL-receptor activity and uptake of circulating LDL-cholesterol into the cell. Increased cellular uptake of LDL-cholesterol causes marked decreases in plasma total and LDL-cholesterol; the degree of decrease is somewhat proportional to the dose of BAS consumed. The currently marketed resins, cholestyramine (Questran) and colestipol (Colestid), are administered as loose powders mixed in a liquid vehicle in doses ranging from 4-30 g/d with meals. Although inconvenient and slightly unpalatable, they have an excellent safety record and have even been used for more than 20 years in children with FH. LDL-cholesterol reduction ranges from 10% at small doses to 25% at very large doses. Side effects are unpalatability, abdominal distention, and constipation.

Nicotinic acid (niacin; Nicolar; Niacor) is the oldest lipid-lowering agent, having been used for over 35 years. Its mechanism of action has not been clearly elucidated, probably because it is used as a vitamin in very small amounts and thus has no patent protection. It exerts its major lipid-lowering effect by reducing hepatic synthesis of both lipid and protein components of lipoproteins. The protein effect may be part of a generalized effect on hepatic protein synthesis, and often the "window" between the lipid-lowering effect and generalized hepatotoxicity is small. This makes therapy with niacin potentially toxic, more so than with any other lipid-lowering agent. The effect on LDL and VLDL is often substantial, and niacin is the most potent elevator of HDL-cholesterol and apolipoprotein A-I currently available. It is also the only drug shown to have a consistent lowering effect on Lp(a) and may be used in conjunction with the BAS or RI or both.

The 3-hydroxy-3-methylglutaryl-CoA reductase inhibitors (lovastatin, simvastatin, and pravastatin) have over the last few years become the most widely used agents for lowering LDL-cholesterol both in the United States and the rest of the world. They specifically inhibit the rate-limiting step in *de novo* cholesterol biosynthesis, thereby stimulating cell surface LDL-receptor activity and increasing LDL removal with resultant reductions in plasma LDL-cholesterol. Their major advantages over BAS and NA are excellent patient tolerance and extremely uniform and predictable large reductions in LDL-cholesterol. At the largest dose, maximum LDL reductions of 35-40% are attainable. Potentially serious side effects are increased levels of aminotransferases and CK. Elevation of CK is usually rare; elevations of liver enzymes occur at a rate of one in 100-1000, depending on dose. Regular monitoring of these serum enzymes is necessary. The first generation fermentation products will soon be joined by a number of second generation synthetic RI currently in clinical trials.

In order to achieve desirable LDL-cholesterol levels, especially in FH subjects such as the family described here, the physician must use combination therapy with either two or three of the agents described above. Again, the optimal combination of agents and their respective dosages is an "art" and each patient a "clinical trial of one." Since these three drug groups are the only effective agents available and FH is a lifelong disorder, the clinician should proceed slowly and systematically assess efficacy, side effects, patient compliance, and cost-effectiveness at each step of therapy.

In very severe heterozygous familial hypercholesterolemics and in homozygotes, more extensive efforts to lower LDL are required. These include repetitive plasmapheresis or LDL-apheresis in addition to drug therapy and, in homozygotes, even hepatic transplantation to provide LDL-receptors absent in the patient.

References

1.   Goldstein, J.L., and Brown, M.S.: Familial hypercholesterolemia. *In:* The Metabolic Basis of Inherited Disease. C. Scriver, A.L. Beaudet, W.S. Sly, and D. Valle, Eds. New York, McGraw-Hill, 1989.

2.   Stone, N.J., Levy, R.I., Fredrickson, D., et al.: Coronary artery disease in 116 kindred with familial type II hyperlipoproteinemia. Circulation, *49:* 476-488, 1974.

3.   Slack, J.: Risks of ischemic heart disease in familial hyperlipoproteinemic states. Lancet, *2:* 1380-1382, 1969.

4.   Seed, M., Hoppichler, F., Reaveley, D., et al.: Relation of serum lipoprotein(a) concentration and apolipoprotein(a) phenotype to coronary heart disease in patients with familial hypercholesterolemia. N. Engl. J. Med., *322:* 1494-1499, 1990.

5.   Lipid Research Clinic Program: The Lipid Research Clinics Coronary Primary Prevention Trial results. II. The relationship of reduction in incidence of coronary heart disease to cholesterol lowering. JAMA, *251:* 365-374, 1984.

6.   Brown, G., Albers, J.J., Fisher, L.D., et al.: Regression of coronary artery disease as a result of intensive lipid-lowering therapy in men with high levels of apolipoprotein B. N. Engl. J. Med., *323:* 1289-1298, 1990.

7.   Kane, J.P., Malloy, M.J., Ports, T.A., et al.: Regression of coronary atherosclerosis during treatment of familial hypercholesterolemia with combined drug regimens. JAMA, *264:* 3007-3012, 1990.

MIDDLE-AGED WOMAN WITH RECURRENT ABDOMINAL PAIN

Evan A. Stein, Contributor

A 56-year-old woman was seen by a gastroenterologist after her internist had been unable to find the cause of her abdominal pain. The pain was intermittent and had first started in her late 40's. It appeared to coincide with a gain in weight from 132 to 150 lb (60 to 68 kg) following menopause and was aggravated by postmenopausal estrogen therapy. Although not directly related to food intake, this most recent and most severe bout of pain had occurred after her 30th wedding anniversary dinner party, during which time she had had a fat-rich meal and about four glasses of wine. At that time, the pain radiated into her back, was associated with nausea and vomiting, and was relieved somewhat if she leaned forward on her hands and knees.

Previous history indicated that cholecystectomy had not stopped the pain. An upper and lower gastrointestinal series had led to the presumptive diagnosis of functional bowel disease ("spastic colitis"), but neither alteration in diet nor inhibition of gastric acid secretion with cimetidine had improved symptoms.

The patient smoked 30 cigarettes daily and had done so for 40 years. She did minimal exercise and consumed moderate amounts of alcohol (280 mL equivalent or about ten drinks per week). She followed no particular diet restriction but did admit her pain was less pronounced when she tried to restrict her intake of fatty foods.

Family history revealed no other family member with similar problems. Her mother had developed noninsulin-dependent diabetes mellitus (NIDDM) at age 62 and died of a stroke at age 73. Her brother, aged 47, was healthy and was a long-distance runner. Her two children, both female, aged 28 and 26, were both apparently healthy.

Examination revealed a very tender abdomen with guarding and rigidity of the abdominal wall, especially over the epigastric area. Her temperature was 101.3 °F (38.5 °C).

The patient was admitted to the medical unit because she was dehydrated and was in increasing pain. A routine admission blood specimen was drawn for a battery of laboratory tests in hematology and biochemistry. The phlebotomist noted that the blood looked like "a strawberry milkshake," and the clinical chemistry laboratory reported a very lipemic serum that appeared to interfere with a number of analyses. (The lipemic appearance was due to the presence of high amounts of chylomicrons.) Results were reported as follows:

Analyte	Value, conventional units	Reference range, conventional units	Value, SI units	Reference range, SI units
Sodium (S)*	124 mmol/L	133-145	Same	
Potassium (S)*	3.3 mmol/L	3.5-5.0	Same	
Glucose (S)	132 mg/dL	70-105	7.3 mmol/L	3.9-5.8
Creatinine (S)	1.4 mg/dL	0.7-1.4	124 µmol/L	62-124
ALT (S)	30 U/L	5-25	0.50 µkat/L	0.08-0.42

* Measured by indirect ion selective electrode method.

Analyte	Value, conventional units	Reference range, conventional units	Value, SI units	Reference range, SI units
AST (S)	34 U/L	8-22	0.57 μkat/L	0.13-0.37
Bilirubin (S)	1.8 mg/dL	0.1-1.1	31 μmol/L	2-19
Albumin (S)	2.1 g/dL	3.5-5.0	21 g/L	35-50
Protein, total (S)	5.0 g/dL	6.0-8.0	50 g/L	60-80
Urate (S)	8.1 mg/dL	3.0-6.0	482 μmol/L	178-357
Triglycerides (S)	6823 mg/dL	35-135	77.03 mmol/L	0.40-1.53
Cholesterol (S)	418 mg/dL	<240	10.81 mmol/L	<6.21
HDL-cholesterol (S)	12 mg/dL	30-85	0.31 mmol/L	0.78-2.20

The complete blood count was within the reference ranges except for mild leukocytosis. Serum and urine amylase tests were then ordered. The initial laboratory report showed a normal to low serum amylase value. Upon repeat of the amylase test on a serial dilution, the activity increased considerably (a phenomenon frequently seen in hyperlipemic serum) and was eventually confirmed as being six times the upper limit of the reference range. The urinary amylase was three times the upper limit of the reference range. Thus, a diagnosis of acute pancreatitis was made. A computed tomographic (CT) scan confirmed an enlarged, edematous pancreas.

The patient was placed on intravenous fluids, rehydrated, and given sufficient analgesics to keep her pain-free. Only sips of water and ice were allowed to keep her mouth moist. After 24 hours, the pain decreased, and it was virtually gone after 72 hours.

Repeat laboratory evaluations were done on a daily basis. Within 24 hours of intravenous fluids, the lipemia was diminished, the triglyceride and cholesterol levels decreased, and the HDL-cholesterol concentration increased as follows:

Analyte	Day 1	Day 2	Day 3
Cholesterol (S)	365 mg/dL (9.45 mmol/L)	302 mg/dL (7.82 mmol/L)	268 mg/dL (6.94 mmol/L)
Triglycerides (S)	4010 mg/dL (45.27 mmol/L)	2166 mg/dL (24.45 mmol/L)	964 mg/dL (10.89 mmol/L)
HDL-cholesterol (S)	14 mg/dL (0.36 mmol/L)	18 mg/dL (0.47 mmol/L)	20 mg/dL (0.52 mmol/L)

The patient's estrogen therapy was discontinued, and she was started on a very low fat diet rich in complex carbohydrates. She lost 10 lb in the seven days prior to discharge. At the time of discharge, her cholesterol was 256 mg/dL (6.62 mmol/L), triglycerides 596 mg/dL (6.73 mmol/L), and HDL-cholesterol 23 mg/dL (0.60 mmol/L).

The patient was seen every two weeks at the lipid center. Her weight loss was maintained, and she was started on a program of aerobic exercise of 40-min periods at least three days per week. Alcohol was strictly forbidden. Despite emphasis placed on the need to stop smoking, the patient continued, although at a slightly reduced rate of 20 cigarettes per day.

Her lipids on this improved life style remained moderately elevated with a cholesterol of 242 mg/dL (6.27 mmol/L), triglycerides of 474 mg/dL (5.36 mmol/L), and HDL-cholesterol of 26 mg/dL (0.67 mmol/L). Her brother and two daughters were assessed in the fasting state to determine their lipids, and the following results were obtained:

Serum lipid	Brother, age 47 (Recommended range)	Daughter, age 28 (Recommended range)	Daughter, age 26 (Recommended range)
Cholesterol	196 mg/dL (<240)	184 mg/dL (<220)	220 mg/dL (<200)
Triglycerides	212 mg/dL (40-160)	95 mg/dL (35-135)	308 mg/dL (35-135)
HDL-cholesterol	33 mg/dL (30-70)	54 mg/dL (30-75)	35 mg/dL (30-75)
LDL-cholesterol	121 mg/dL (<130)	111 mg/dL (<130)	124 mg/dL (<130)

Metabolic Defect

This patient fulfills the criteria for familial hypertriglyceridemia (FHTG), namely, severe triglyceridemia with high triglyceride-rich lipoprotein (TRL) that is not secondary to another metabolic disorder, that does not normalize when diet and life style are modified, and that is similarly manifested in other family members. The patient obviously has a defect in TRL metabolism. This defect appears to have a familial basis, given the residual lipid abnormality in the patient despite removal of potential underlying causes of hypertriglyceridemia (e.g., excess weight, alcohol, high fat diet, and estrogen). In addition, there was a similar, although less severe, finding in other family members.

The most likely defect causing the lipid disorder is in lipoprotein lipase (LPL), the endothelial/adipose tissue-bound enzyme responsible for triglyceride removal from the two major triglyceride-rich lipoproteins, chylomicrons and very low-density lipoprotein (VLDL). LPL activity is difficult to quantitate, although there are now assays for both LPL activity and LPL mass available. Defects in LPL structure associated with impaired function have been described.[1] The other possible genetic defect could be in apolipoprotein CII, which is a cofactor needed for the activation of LPL.[1,2] Apolipoprotein CII is synthesized in the liver and is a major component of both chylomicrons and VLDL.

Definition of the Disease

FHTG is an autosomal recessive condition that may become manifest only when associated with other metabolic conditions such as smoking, obesity (usually truncal), alcohol intake, diabetes, or estrogens. Although smoking and obesity may further impair LPL activity, alcohol, estrogens, and diabetes may increase TRL synthesis sufficiently to fully saturate an already impaired LPL system. This heterozygote condition is usually not manifest in children, although low HDL-cholesterol levels and slightly higher than average triglyceride levels may be a "marker" for the condition in childhood and early adulthood. A more severe and rare disorder of triglyceride metabolism, familial hyperchylomicronemia, is manifest in children and probably reflects a "compound heterozygote" rather than a true homozygote disorder affecting LPL or apolipoprotein CII.

Clinical Features

The disorder is often totally asymptomatic, although in many patients, upon close questioning, a history of recurrent abdominal pain, gastrointestinal procedures, or multiple surgeries to the gastrointestinal tract can be found.

In some patients, episodes of severe hypertriglyceridemia may be associated with eruptive xanthomas over the shoulders, back, buttocks, elbows, or knees. This "rash," which looks like coarse sandpaper, may be the presenting feature to a dermatologist or primary care physician. Other clinical features include corneal arcus and xanthelasma (yellow-colored flat areas on the eyelids or under the eyes).

Associated metabolic abnormalities include impaired glucose tolerance, noninsulin-dependent diabetes mellitus (NIDDM), and hyperuricemia or gout. The patients often have central obesity ("pear shape") and hypertension. Atherosclerosis may not be a feature, although its occurrence is highly variable in families and may depend on other associated factors, such as smoking, NIDDM, and enhanced synthesis of Apo B lipoproteins. If atherosclerosis does develop, it often affects peripheral vessels (e.g., femoral or carotid arteries or the abdominal aorta) before it affects the coronary arteries.

Diagnosis

The diagnosis is based on finding severe hypertriglyceridemia that is not associated with disorders known to produce secondary hypertriglyceridemia, that does not normalize with modification of life style and diet, and that occurs in similar form in another family member. Demonstration of defects in LPL activity, mass, or structure is possible, as is demonstration of apolipoprotein CII deficiency, but tests are available in only a few research laboratories worldwide. In reaching a diagnosis, exclusion of lipid "phenocopies" is advisable; among these are familial combined hyperlipidemia and familial dysbetalipoproteinemia. Familial combined hyperlipidemia is a dominant disorder usually associated with increase in Apo B100 level; by contrast, FHTG usually shows decreased Apo B100 concentrations. Familial dysbetalipoproteinemia is a defect in the processing of intermediate-density lipoprotein (IDL). This disorder is characterized by an increased cholesterol/triglyceride ratio (>0.35) in the density fraction <1.006, a distinct lipoprotein electrophoretic pattern known as "floating B" in the density fraction <1.006, and an Apo E isoform phenotype known as E2/E2.[3]

Treatment

The most effective therapy is an extremely strict, low fat diet; fat must be <10% of total caloric intake. Such limitation is extremely difficult to achieve in our society and even more difficult to sustain for an indefinite period. The primary restriction should be in saturated fatty acids. Medium-chain triglycerides (MCT) can be used for cooking or to add fat for taste or calories, since MCT are transported directly to the liver by the portal system without prior incorporation into chylomicrons. Simple sugars should also be restricted since they tend to stimulate endogenous triglyceride and VLDL synthesis. Because many patients are overweight, total calorie restriction is usually necessary. Alcohol is also prohibited. The difficulty of the dietary regimen cannot be overemphasized, and the assistance of a trained, experienced nutritionist is considered essential if any success is to be achieved.

Other factors that tend to aggravate the condition and that may precipitate acute pancreatitis should be individually evaluated and treated appropriately. These factors include diabetes, hypothyroidism, estrogen therapy, and administration of thiazide diuretics.

Pharmacological therapy may prove helpful but is usually only supplemental to diet. The most effective agents are the fibric acid derivatives. These include the first generation fibrate, clofibrate (Atromid-S), second generation gemfibrozil (Lopid), and third generation products such as fenofibrate and bezafibrate. The third generation drugs, which have been used in Europe for nearly a decade, should be available in the United States soon. The fibrates are generally well tolerated but may cause gastrointestinal discomfort, some reduction in libido in men, and significant increase in the long-term risk of gallstones.

Should a fibrate prove ineffective, very large doses of omega-3 fatty acids (fish oil) may be used in dosages of 4-8 g/d. The omega-3 fatty acids appear to inhibit hepatic triglyceride synthesis. However, there are potential side effects that include disturbance of glucose homeostasis.

The third alternative is large doses of nicotinic acid, which can be very effective but may adversely affect glucose control. The use of nicotinic acid is described in greater detail in *Case 53*. With caution, these drug therapies may be used in combination.

References

1. Sprecher, D.L., Knauer, S.L., Black, D.M., et al.: Chylomicron-retinyl palmitate clearance in Type I hyperlipidemic families. J. Clin. Invest., *88:* 985-994, 1991.

2. Kashyap, M.L., Srivastava, L.S., Tsang, R.C., et al.: Apolipoprotein CII in Type I hyperlipoproteinemia: A study in three cases. J. Lab. Clin. Med., *95:* 180-187, 1980.

3. Gregg, R.E., and Brewer, H.B.: The role of apolipoprotein E and lipoprotein receptors in modulating the *in vivo* metabolism of apolipoprotein B-containing lipoproteins in humans. Clin. Chem., *34:* B28-B32, 1988.

CHILD WITH RECURRENT VOMITING

Ronald J. Whitley, Contributor
Michael W. Stelling, Reviewer

The patient is a 17-month-old white female admitted to the University Hospital because of intractable vomiting of four months' duration. Emesis occurred 2-4 times a day, usually after meals. It often began with ataxia and was accompanied by some abdominal cramping. Several diet changes were tried, but none was helpful. Two months ago the patient was admitted to a community hospital because of vomiting, lethargy, dehydration, and irritability. An intestinal tract infection was suspected clinically, even though diarrhea and fever were not prominent manifestations. She was also mildly alkalotic. This finding was somewhat puzzling since children with gastroenteritis are likely to be acidotic. She responded quickly to intravenous fluids, but vomiting recurred soon after she returned home.

At the time of her current admission, the patient again had persistent vomiting and was lethargic without evidence of volume depletion. On physical examination, her liver was substantially enlarged to 4 cm below the right costal margin, but jaundice or cataracts were not noted. Her parents denied any history of severe diarrhea or rash, but they noticed that she was more clumsy when walking and that she was talking less than before. Her physicians now suspected an encephalopathy secondary to meningoencephalitis or to increased intracranial pressure. A radiographic computed axial tomogram (CT scan) of the head demonstrated cortical atrophy; there was no evidence of inflammation, cerebral edema, or an intracranial mass.

On admission, the following serum levels were reported:

Analyte	Value, conventional units	Reference range, conventional units	Value, SI units	Reference range, SI units
Sodium (S)	138 mmol/L	138-145	Same	
Potassium (S)	4.5 mmol/L	4.1-5.3	Same	
Chloride (S)	109 mmol/L	98-107	Same	
CO_2, total (S)	22 mmol/L	20-28	Same	
Urea nitrogen (S)	11 mg/dL	5-18	3.9 mmol urea/L	1.8-6.4
Creatinine (S)	0.4 mg/dL	0.2-0.4	35 µmol/L	18-35
Glucose (S)	99 mg/dL	60-100	5.5 mmol/L	3.3-5.6
Protein, total (S)	6.1 g/dL	6.2-8.0	61 g/L	62-80
Albumin (S)	3.6 g/dL	3.8-5.4	36 g/L	38-54
Urate (S)	3.4 mg/dL	2.0-5.5	202 µmol/L	119-327
Cholesterol (S)	86 mg/dL	70-175	2.22 mmol/L	1.81-4.53
Bilirubin, total (S)	0.3 mg/dL	0.2-1.0	5 µmol/L	3-17
AST (S)	880 U/L	9-80	14.67 µkat/L	0.15-1.33
ALT (S)	1070 U/L	10-28	17.84 µkat/L	0.17-0.47
LDH (S)	792 U/L	180-430	13.2 µkat/L	3.00-7.17
ALP (S)	271 U/L	124-255	4.52 µkat/L	2.07-4.25
Lactate (S)	1.4 mmol/L	0.5-2.2	Same	
Ammonia (P)	208 µmol/L	40-80	Same	

The patient's plasma ammonia level was significantly increased; however, her physicians initially thought that her hyperammonemia reflected venous stasis at the time of a difficult venipuncture. Her affect and clinical appearance again improved after standard intravenous therapy, and cautious low protein oral intake was started. Within 12 hours she had a severe episode of vomiting and appeared encephalopathic. Her ammonia level at that time was 440 μmol/L (reference range, 40-80). On the basis of her clinical presentation and laboratory results, an inborn metabolic defect was suspected, and assays for plasma amino acids and urinary organic acids were requested. The following results were obtained:

		μmol/L	Reference Mean
Urine:	Increased orotic acid		
Plasma:	Arginine	10	78
	Citrulline	12	22
	Glutamine	1123	518
	Alanine	686	386

The combination of clinical findings, hyperammonemia, orotic aciduria, and low plasma levels of citrulline and arginine suggested a defect in one of the urea cycle enzymes, namely, ornithine transcarbamylase (ornithine carbamoyltransferase, EC 2.1.3.3).

Enzyme and Genetic Defect

In the human body, protein catabolism produces ammonia, a compound that is highly toxic if allowed to accumulate. The majority of ammonia is removed from cells and from blood by way of the synthesis and excretion of urea. Ornithine transcarbamylase (OTC) is one of the enzymes governing this disposal process, and an inherited defect in its biosynthesis leads to a disease known as ornithine transcarbamylase deficiency.

The gene for OTC is located on the X chromosome, and the disease is expressed as X-linked.[1,2] Partial or total deficiencies of OTC lead to hyperammonemia of varying degree. In most hemizygous males, OTC activity is very low or absent (<2% of normal), and lethal neonatal hyperammonemia is the usual outcome. A few of these males have a late onset form of the disease as a result of a partial enzyme defect. In affected heterozygous females, residual OTC activity (4-25% of normal) accounts for a variable clinical presentation. Normal levels of enzyme activity may be expressed in asymptomatic carriers (females).

Clinical Features[3]

In *males* with neonatal disease, conversion of ammonia to urea is severely impaired, and ammonia accumulating in large amounts rapidly produces a fatal toxic encephalopathy. Symptoms of hyperammonemia appear soon after birth, within hours to a few days after protein intake; the symptoms include vomiting, seizures, hyperventilation, lethargy, and coma progressing to early death. Plasma ammonia levels are extremely high, often over 600 μmol/L.

In *females*, the clinical picture is more variable; symptoms of hyperammonemia may start in infancy or as late as 9 years of age. Many females remain asymptomatic until attacks are precipitated by an increase in protein intake, acute infection, surgery, or vaccination. These episodic attacks are often accompanied by vomiting, feeding difficulties, irritability, intense headaches, and seizures. Hepatomegaly is also noted in some patients. In general, the severity of these symptoms correlates with plasma ammonia levels. Motor and intellectual retardation may progress with each recurrent episode. Although the clinical course is generally less malignant in females than in males, hyperammonemic coma and death may occur even after a number of symptom-free years.

Diagnosis

The greatest problem in the diagnosis of this disorder is considering the possibility of its presence, since the incidence of the disease is only 1:70,000-100,000. Recurrent vomiting, lethargy, and coma are not pathognomonic for OTC deficiency, and other conditions such as neonatal sepsis and intracranial hemorrhage may present with similar physical findings. Hyperammonemia is the major biochemical finding, and early detection is essential for a favorable prognosis. Concentrations of postprandial blood ammonia are regularly increased in clinically affected individuals, but normal levels may be found in patients with episodic symptoms, particularly if these persons are on a low protein diet.

Urea cycle enzyme defects are the major cause (70%) of hyperammonemia in children, but inherited disorders of organic acid metabolism (such as methylmalonic aciduria and propionic aciduria) as well as severe liver disease and Reye's syndrome also induce high ammonia levels.[4] Differentiation cannot be based solely on clinical grounds or on plasma ammonia concentrations. In some cases, abnormalities in acid-base balance will point to the correct diagnosis. For example, the presence of a respiratory alkalosis may suggest a urea cycle defect, whereas metabolic acidosis with a high anion gap is consistent with an organic aciduria.

A specific diagnosis of OTC deficiency, however, will require measurement of amino acids in blood and organic acids in urine.[1,3] These assays should be run in parallel, and results should be available within 24 hours in order to facilitate appropriate treatment. As shown in Figure 1, ornithine transcarbamylase catalyzes the synthesis of citrulline from ornithine and carbamylphosphate.

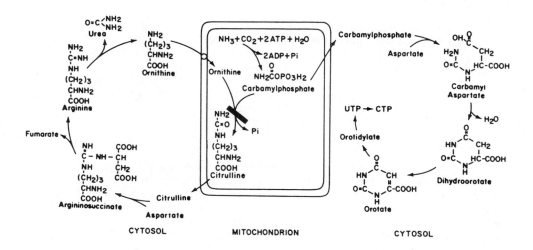

Figure 1. Principal reactions of the urea cycle and related reactions. The site of the defect in ornithine transcarbamylase deficiency is indicated. (Reprinted with permission from: Nyhan, W.L.: Abnormalities in Amino Acid Metabolism in Clinical Medicine. Norwalk, CT, Appleton-Century-Crofts, 1984.)

A deficiency of this enzyme may result in decreased amounts of citrulline, argininosuccinic acid, and arginine in blood, depending on the residual enzyme activity. Increased levels of these urea cycle intermediates, on the other hand, effectively rule out OTC deficiency as a cause of the hyperammonemia. In this disorder precursors of urea, principally glutamine and alanine, accumulate, thus confirming the high plasma levels of ammonia but not identifying the underlying defect.

The most characteristic biochemical finding in OTC deficiency is severe orotic aciduria. Carbamylphosphate, in the absence of ornithine transcarbamylase, is diverted from the urea cycle and flows into the path of pyrimidine synthesis. The result is increased urinary output of orotic acid, as well as of uracil and uridine (see Figure 1).

The definitive diagnosis of OTC deficiency is established by assaying ornithine transcarbamylase in liver tissue. Specimens obtained by duodenal or rectal biopsy may also be used for this purpose. Prenatal diagnosis of OTC deficiency can be made by assaying the enzyme in the fetal liver.[5] Asymptomatic carriers can be detected by measuring orotic acid after allopurinol challenge. Heterozygote detection and prenatal diagnosis can also be made by analysis of DNA restriction fragment length polymorphisms (RFLPs) using amniocytes or chorionic villus biopsy tissue. Newborn screening does not appear to be practical for detecting acute neonatal forms of the disease.

Treatment

Treatment aims at reducing the nitrogen load and increasing waste nitrogen removal.[1,4] Dietary protein is restricted while covering the demand for essential amino acids, vitamins, minerals, and carnitine; arginine (or citrulline) supplementation is required to promote normal growth. Patients with residual enzyme activity respond favorably, as a rule, to low protein diets aimed at preventing episodic hyperammonemia. Regrettably, most patients with complete OTC deficiency fail to respond to protein restriction or therapeutic measures aimed at removing ammonia and other urea precursors (e.g., peritoneal dialysis, hemodialysis, exchange transfusion).

Acute ammonia intoxication must be vigorously treated. For comatose patients, prompt and repeated hemodialysis may be required. In milder cases, therapy with pharmacological agents can provide an alternative pathway for getting rid of nitrogen that cannot be removed as urea. For example, sodium benzoate can be conjugated with glycine and phenylacetate can be combined with glutamine and thus allow urinary excretion of waste nitrogen as hippurate and phenylacetylglutamine. Frequent monitoring of blood ammonia and plasma glutamine may be required to guide effective therapy.

Helpful Notes

At physiological pH, almost all plasma ammonia is present in the ionized (NH_4^+) form. Although the use of the term *ammonium* is justified, by tradition most laboratories report results as ammonia (or ammonia nitrogen). Reliable estimates of plasma ammonia can be difficult to obtain unless preanalytical sources of error are carefully controlled. For example, ammonia concentrations increase rapidly as a result of amino acid deamination once a specimen is drawn. Atmospheric contamination or poor venipuncture technique may also result in increased ammonia levels. Therefore, free flowing venous blood should be collected without a tourniquet in pre-chilled anticoagulated tubes. The sample should be immediately placed on ice and promptly centrifuged at 4 °C. The plasma should then be stored at 4 °C until analysis. If the ammonia assay cannot be performed within an hour, the sample can be stored at -20 °C for 24 hours.

Some investigators have found that healthy infants and children have higher plasma ammonia levels than do adults (<40 µmol/L); others have found insignificant intergroup differences.[6,7] Reasons for these discrepancies may relate, in part, to the control of pre-analytical sources of error described in the preceding.

References

1. Brusilow, S., and Horwich, A.: Urea cycle enzymes. *In:* The Metabolic Basis of Disease. C. Scriver, A.L. Beaudet, W.S. Sly, et al., Eds. New York, McGraw-Hill, 1989.

2. Ampola, M.: Metabolic Disease in Pediatric Practice. Boston, Little, Brown and Co., 1982, pp. 141-147.

3. Nyhan, W., and Sakati, N.: Diagnostic Recognition of Genetic Disease. Philadelphia, Lea and Febiger, 1987, pp. 150-159.

4. Bachmann, C.: Urea cycle disorders. *In:* Inborn Metabolic Diseases: Diagnosis and Treatment. J. Fernandes, J.M. Saundubray, and K. Tada, Eds. Berlin, Springer-Verlag, 1990.

5. Rodeck, C., Patrick, A., Pembrey, M., et al.: Fetal liver biopsy for prenatal diagnosis of ornithine carbamyltransferase deficiency. Lancet, *2:* 297-300, 1982.

6. Green, A.: When and how should we measure plasma ammonia. Ann. Clin. Biochem., *25:* 199-209, 1988.

7. Batshaw, M., and Brusilow, S.: Asymptomatic hyperammonemia in low birth weight infants. Pediatr. Res., *12:* 221-224, 1978.

HYPERACTIVE BOY WITH INFANTILE SPEECH

Ronald J. Whitley, Contributor

A six-year-old white male was referred to the University Hospital for evaluation of hyperactivity and delayed language development. Speech and behavioral problems were first noticed when the boy was two years of age. At that time he could phonate, but his language was very difficult to understand. A local physician attributed his dysphasia to deafness, but subsequent hearing tests were normal. At age five the patient was enrolled in kindergarten, where it was soon appreciated that he was not comparable, developmentally or intellectually, to his peers. His attention span was very short, and he made little progress in school. His hyperkinetic behavior and unpredictable temper tantrums eventually prompted his transfer to a special education classroom. His IQ was estimated to be 50 to 60. The patient was the product of a full-term pregnancy of a 34-year-old mother (gravida 5, para 3). No perinatal problems were encountered at birth, and he walked at 13 months. Both parents were high-school graduates, and there was no family history of mental retardation or consanguinity.

Physical examination revealed a well-nourished, very active, prepubertal boy with fair complexion, blond hair, and blue eyes. No dysmorphic features were demonstrated, and his head circumference, height, and weight were appropriate for his age. Examinations of neck, chest, and abdomen were also unremarkable, and no unusual body odors or skin rashes were apparent. On neurological examination, his gross motor movements were found to be clumsy and more appropriate for a two-year-old. Although his gait was normal, he could not walk on his toes, stand on one foot, or jump with direction. Phonically, he could use simple words like "dog," "car," and "truck," but he was only able to put together rudimentary sentences such as "mommy store."

At first the patient's medical problems were attributed to an "attention deficit hyperactive disorder," and methylphenidate was prescribed to reduce his restlessness, distractibility, and impulsive behavior. Although no stigmata of metabolic disease were apparent, a urine metabolic screen was also requested to rule out the possibility of a genetic basis for his neurological problems. The following results were obtained: ferric chloride test, 4+; dinitrophenylhydrazine test, 4+; ketones, glucose, reducing substances, protein, cystine, homocystine, methylmalonic acid and mucopolysaccharides, all negative; phenylalanine (by thin layer chromatography, TLC), strongly positive. The urine sample was also noted to have a peculiar musty odor. To confirm these unexpected findings, a blood phenylalanine determination was subsequently performed; the result was 30.6 mg/dL (1851 µmol/L; reference range, 0.8-1.8; 48-109).

An inborn error of phenylalanine metabolism was now suspected, and additional laboratory tests were requested to document the disease and identify the specific phenotype. The following results were obtained:

Analyte	Value, conventional units	Reference range, conventional units	Value, SI units	Reference range, SI units
Phenylalanine (P)	25.5 mg/dL	0.8-1.8	1544 µmol/L	48-109
Tyrosine (P)	0.5 mg/dL	0.56-1.29	28 µmol/L	31-71

Analyte	Value, conventional units	Reference range, conventional units	Value, SI units	Reference range, SI units
Dihydropteridine reductase (DHPR) (B)	2.1 nmol/min/mg Hb	1.4-5.0	135.5 kU/mol Hb	90.3-322.5
Biopterin (U)	21.2 % of total pterins	20-42	0.212	0.20-0.42

The combination of clinical findings, hyperphenylalaninemia, hypotyrosinemia, and normal levels of DHPR and percent biopterin pointed to an inherited defect in phenylalanine hydroxylation, namely, phenylketonuria (PKU). A low phenylalanine diet was started in order to reduce the patient's phenylalanine levels and to improve his behavioral problems. Within four days his blood phenylalanine diminished to only trace levels. A month later his parents filed a legal action against the local hospital for failing to test their son properly for PKU at birth.

Definition of the Disease

Enzyme and Genetic Defect. Phenylalanine is an essential amino acid for protein synthesis. During early growth, about 50% of dietary phenylalanine is utilized for this purpose; most of the remainder is normally converted to tyrosine. Inability to carry out this hydroxylation reaction results in an accumulation of phenylalanine in blood, urine, and cerebrospinal fluid (CSF). Depending on its pathogenesis and degree, this disturbance in phenylalanine metabolism can have serious clinical consequences. Associated diseases are collectively known as the hyperphenylalaninemias, with classic phenylketonuria being the most common (see Table 1).

Table 1. **THE SPECTRUM OF INHERITED HYPERPHENYLALANINEMIAS**

Phenotype	Defect	Blood Phenylalanine
Phenylketonuria (classic PKU)	Phenylalanine hydroxylase absent (<1% of normal activity)	>20 mg/dL (>1211 μmol/L)
Non-PKU hyperphenylalaninemia (benign variant)	Phenylalanine hydroxylase deficiency (1-35% of normal activity)	2-20 mg/dL (121-1211 μmol/L)
BH$_4$-deficient hyperphenylalaninemias (cofactor variants)	Dihydropteridine reductase (DHPR) deficiency	>2 mg/dL (>121 μmol/L)
	Guanosine triphosphate cyclohydrolase (GTP-CH) deficiency	
	6-Pyruvoyltetrahydropterin synthase (6-PTS) deficiency	

As shown in Figure 1, parahydroxylation of phenylalanine requires oxygen, phenylalanine hydroxylase (PAH), tetrahydrobiopterin (BH$_4$), and dihydropteridine reductase (DHPR). DHPR is needed to keep the pterin cofactor in an active, reduced state. BH$_4$ is an obligatory component in this catalytic system.

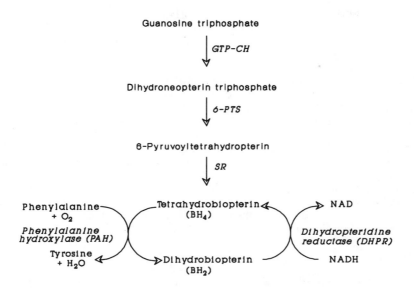

Figure 1. Phenylalanine hyroxylation and cofactor transformations. The principal biosynthetic pathway to BH$_4$ begins with GTP. SR = sepiapterin reductase; for additional abbreviations see Table 1. (Modified and used with permission from: Cotran, R.S., Kumar, V., and Robbins, S.L.: Diseases of infancy and childhood. *In:* Robbins Pathologic Basis of Disease, 4th ed. Philadelphia, W.B. Saunders Co., 1989.)

Most of the hyperphenylalaninemias are due to primary deficiencies of PAH (i.e., PKU and non-PKU hyperphenylalaninemias).[1] Some 1-2% of cases, however, are not the result of PAH deficiency but are disorders of DHPR activity or BH$_4$ synthesis. PKU and other genetic forms of hyperphenylalaninemia are transmitted as autosomal recessive traits. As a group, the hyperphenylalaninemias have an incidence of about 1:10,000 live births; rates are as high as 1:4500 in Ireland and as low as 1:100,000 in Finland. Classic PKU accounts for nearly half of these and is widely distributed among Caucasian ethnic groups and Orientals; it is rare in blacks.

In classic phenylketonuria, hepatic PAH activity is almost or completely absent. As a result, untreated persons on normal diets have sustained and markedly elevated levels of phenylalanine in tissues and blood; progressive impairment of cognitive development is the principal clinical concern. The non-PKU phenotype, on the other hand, is less severe clinically; PAH activity is higher (1-35% of normal), blood phenylalanine values are lower, and the associated risk of mental retardation in probands is smaller. Genetic studies have revealed the identity of several distinct mutations in the PAH gene that are responsible for the PKU phenotype;[1,2] other mutant alleles at the PAH locus confer the less severe, non-PKU form of hyperphenylalaninemia.

Clinical Symptoms[3]

Affected children appear normal at birth, and retarded intellectual development may not be evident for several months. The earliest symptoms are usually nonspecific — eczema, irritability, feeding difficulties, and vomiting. The vomiting can be of such severity that operations for pyloric stenosis are performed. The skin, hair, or urine of some children may also have the unusual but characteristic musty odor of phenylacetic acid. PKU patients are often good-looking children; over 90% of patients are fair-haired, fair-skinned, and blue-eyed. This hypopigmentation is related to phenylalanine inhibition of tyrosinase, a key enzyme in the pathway of melanin synthesis.

Without proper dietary control, retardation progresses relentlessly; 50 IQ points may be lost in the first year of life alone. Older children may also show hyperactivity, agitated and aggressive behavior, failure to talk or walk, seizures, abnormal electroencephalographic findings, and muscular hypertoxicity. General physical development and nutritional state, however, are remarkably good. Nevertheless, fewer than 4% of untreated cases will achieve an IQ of more than 60; most will have IQ values below 20. Irreversible brain injury appears to be related to phenylalanine accumulation and to its effects on reducing the synthesis of myelin, norepinephrine, and serotonin. Injury to brain tissue begins within the second or third week of life and becomes maximal at eight or nine months.[4] However, children whose defect is detected at birth and treated promptly show none of these abnormalities. Moreover, children with non-PKU hyperphenylalaninemia are usually not at risk for the clinical consequences seen in untreated PKU patients.

Diagnosis

In view of the disastrous effects of PKU, great emphasis is placed on early diagnosis and initiation of dietary treatment. Routine screening of all newborns for elevated blood phenylalanine is now a mandatory practice throughout the United States and Europe. In North America, the Guthrie bacterial inhibition assay is the most widely used screening method. This semiquantitative test should be carried out several days after the infant has been on an adequate dietary protein challenge. About 1% of babies screened each year will have a blood phenylalanine >2 mg/dL (>121 μmol/L).[5] Abnormal results should be confirmed with a quantitative chromatographic or fluorometric assay.

Only 1% of infants with a positive screening test will prove to have an inherited form of hyperphenylalaninemia. In fact, the most common cause of an elevated phenylalanine level in neonates is transient tyrosinemia of the newborn, a temporary disorder caused by delayed hepatic maturation of the tyrosine oxidizing system. Often seen in low birth weight and premature infants, this condition is not a genetic defect, and blood levels of phenylalanine (and tyrosine) decline toward normal as the neonate matures.

Two-thirds of patients with persistent hyperphenylalaninemia will have classic PKU; phenylalanine values >20 mg/dL (>1211 μmol/L) and tyrosine levels <2 mg/dL (<121 μmol/L) are typical. In contrast, the non-PKU form of PAH deficiency will manifest a persistent elevation of phenylalanine in the range of 2 to 20 mg/dL (121-1211 μmol/L). For some children, distinction of classic PKU from non-PKU hyperphenylalaninemia will depend on following serial phenylalanine concentrations as a function of age and diet. Diagnosis in some cases may also require the use of a phenylalanine loading study or a PAH enzyme assay. Patients with a non-PKU variant will usually have a rise in plasma phenylalanine to levels <20 mg/dL when challenged with 180 mg/kg of phenylalanine per day for 72 hours. Unfortunately, these loading tests cannot be used in the newborn, i.e., at the time they are most needed.

Ideally, PAH activity should be measured. Patients with classic PKU are readily distinguished from those with the non-PKU phenotype, since partial enzyme activity is the rule in the latter. Unfortunately, PAH is normally present only in liver cells, and a liver biopsy is not accepted by many parents.

Every infant who has hyperphenylalaninemia must be investigated for an underlying defect in the synthesis or regeneration of tetrahydrobiopterin. These "malignant" forms of hyperphenylalaninemia require early identification, since dietary restriction in phenylalaninemia fails to arrest progressive neurological damage. As shown in Table 1, three enzyme deficiencies have been recognized. In addition to their role in phenylalanine metabolism, these enzymes are also involved in the hydroxylation of tyrosine and tryptophan, an essential step in the synthesis of serotonin and the catecholamines. A lack of these neurotransmitters contributes to the neurological deterioration. Measurement of blood phenylalanine alone is inadequate to detect these malignant variants, and additional diagnostic methods must be used to identify and classify them. These usually include direct assay of DHPR (in dried blood spots on filter paper) and measurement of urinary pterins such as neopterin and biopterin; levels of neurotransmitters and their metabolites can also be assayed in plasma, urine, or CSF.

Prenatal diagnosis is possible in all forms of hyperphenylalaninemia by various combinations of DNA analyses, enzyme assays, and pterin measurements in amniotic fluid.[1] Reliable classification of PKU heterozygotes is also important in reproduction counseling, particularly since 2% of the Caucasian population are carriers of the defective gene. In PKU, heterozygotes can be detected by use of the phenylalanine tolerance test; DNA analysis also identifies PKU heterozygotes in about 75% of families.

Treatment and Prognosis

The classic treatment of PKU consists of dietary restriction of phenylalanine initiated before the onset of brain damage. This diet is based on special formulas (e.g., Lofenalac or Phenylfree) in which the bulk of the protein is replaced by an amino acid mixture low in phenylalanine. These formulas are supplemented with small amounts of natural foods to provide the phenylalanine necessary for normal growth. Blood phenylalanine levels are frequently checked and diet-managed to maintain them at 2-8 mg/dL (121-484 µmol/L). Phenylalanine-containing foods are tolerated as long as blood phenylalanine levels remain acceptable. Unfortunately, dietary restriction will not reverse mental retardation once it has developed; however, diet control will usually decrease the rate of further central nervous system damage and may lead to improved behavioral control.

Dietary treatment of PKU is unquestioned in children with phenylalanine levels of >20 mg/dL (>1211 µmol/L). Children who have some variant of PKU pose greater difficulty. Decisions on the degree of hyperphenylalaninemia that commands treatment vary from clinic to clinic, but many referral centers use a blood phenylalanine level of 10 mg/dL (605 µmol/L) or greater. Experience has shown that dietary control should be continued into adulthood. Monitoring and control are especially important for females who wish to have children, since high levels of phenylalanine cross the placenta and are teratogenic. Thus, a restricted diet must be followed prior to conception and throughout pregnancy. Restriction should also include the artificial sweetener aspartame, a dipeptide of phenylalanine and aspartic acid.

In contrast to classic PKU, patients with cofactor variants are clinically unresponsive to phenylalanine restriction. These "malignant" forms of hyperphenylalaninemia require additional treatment, notably BH_4 replacement or supplementation with L-dopa, hydroxytryptophan, and folinic acid.

Notes on PKU Screening

Ferric Chloride Test. With a block in the conversion of phenylalanine to tyrosine, minor pathways of phenylalanine metabolism are activated, leading to increased production of phenylpyruvate (the phenylketone for which the disease is named) as well as other metabolites such as phenyllactate, phenylacetate, and o-hydroxyphenylacetate. The ferric chloride test is used to detect phenylpyruvate in urine but does not become positive until blood phenylalanine levels are >15 mg/dL (>908 μmol/L). By then, some degree of brain damage may have occurred. For this reason, the ferric chloride test has been abandoned as a screening test for PKU in newborns. Nevertheless, it remains useful in the diagnostic workup of older children with mental retardation or developmental problems.

Guthrie Test. The bacterial inhibition assay of Guthrie is a reliable, inexpensive method for detecting blood phenylalanine in a large number of samples. False negative and false positive results occur only rarely. Most false negatives occur in babies who have not experienced an adequate dietary protein challenge: breast-fed babies, babies discharged early from the hospital, and babies retained in intensive care units. Failure to test at birth and analytical errors are rare causes. Most false positive results occur in infants with liver immaturity or in those who are born prematurely.

References

1.   Scriver, C., Kaufman, S., and Woo, S.: The hyperphenylalaninemias. *In:* The Metabolic Basis of Inherited Disease. C.R. Scriver, A.L. Beaudet, W.S. Sly, and D. Valle, Eds. New York, McGraw-Hill, 1989.

2.   Guttler, F., and Lou, H.: Phenylketonuria and hyperphenylalaninemia. *In:* Inborn Metabolic Diseases: Diagnosis and Treatment. J. Fernandes, J.M. Saundubray, and K. Tada, Eds. Berlin, Springer-Verlag, 1990.

3.   Nyhan, W., and Sakiti, N.: Diagnostic Recognition of Genetic Disease. Philadelphia, Lea and Febiger, 1987, pp. 100-106.

4.   Silverman, L., Christenson, R., and Grant, B.: Amino acids and proteins. *In:* Textbook of Clinical Chemistry. N.W. Tietz, Ed. Philadelphia, W.B. Saunders Co., 1986.

5.   Mabry, C.: Phenylketonuria: Contemporary screening and diagnosis. Ann. Clin. Lab. Sci., *20:* 392-397, 1990.

WOMAN WITH MALAISE AND BLEEDING

Ewa Marciniak, Contributor

A 62-year-old woman was admitted to the hospital because of fever and general malaise. The patient had been well until two weeks before admission, when she had experienced fatigue and dyspnea on exertion and had developed a low grade fever. She took several aspirin tablets without resolution of symptoms. Two days before admission she suffered extensive epistaxis and noticed that large bruises had appeared on her arms.

The patient had been employed for 32 years as a clerk in a telephone company. She retired from this job at the age of 60. There was no history of hypertension, diabetes mellitus, cardiac or pulmonary disease, bleeding disorders, recent trauma, or weight change. She used no alcohol, tobacco, or prescription medications.

On admission her temperature was 100.8 °F (38.2 °C). On physical examination the patient appeared pale. Both upper extremities were covered with extensive ecchymotic lesions. Oozing of blood from a venipuncture site was noted. The chest and abdomen were normal. No lymphadenopathy was found.

Laboratory results showed the following:

Analyte	Value, conventional units	Reference range, conventional units	Value, SI units	Reference range, SI units
Hematocrit (B)	30 %	37-47	0.30	0.37-0.47
MCV (B)	83 fL	81-99	Same	
MCH (B)	27.5 pg	27-31	Same	
MCHC (BErcs)	33 g Hb/dL	33-37	20 mmol Hb/L	20-23
Leukocyte count (B)	$3.7 \times 10^3/\mu L$	4.8-10.8	$3.7 \times 10^9/L$	4.8-10.8
Differential count (B)				
Neutrophils	27 %	41-71	0.27	0.41-0.71
Immature myeloid cells with large promyelocytic granules	9 %	None		
Lymphocytes	47 %	24-44	0.47	0.24-0.44
Monocytes	17 %	3-7	0.17	0.03-0.07
Platelet count (B)	$32 \times 10^3/\mu L$	150-450	$32 \times 10^9/L$	150-450
Bleeding time (B)	15 min	<10	Same	
Prothrombin time (PT) (P)	15.7 s	11-13	Same	
Partial thromboplastin time (PTT) (P)	35 s	25-31	Same	
Thrombin time (TT) (P)	19 s	11	Same	
Fibrinogen (P)	63 mg/dL	150-450	0.63 g/L	1.5-4.5
Fibrin degradation products (FDP) (S)	>40 μg/mL	<10	>40 ng/L	<10

Because immature cells of myelocytic lineage were found in the peripheral blood, bone marrow examination was performed. It revealed a myeloblastic infiltrate; 90% of nonerythroid cells were hypergranular promyelocytes with kidney-shaped nuclei and cytoplasm packed with azurophilic granules. Multiple Auer rods were present in several of these cells; the cells stained intensely with myeloperoxidase. Cytogenetic studies revealed a translocation between chromosomes 15 and 17.

Discussion of Hematological Abnormalities and Diagnosis

This woman, previously well, developed over a short period of time progressive weakness, fever, and a hemorrhagic diathesis. She was found to have anemia, thrombocytopenia, and granulocytopenia with proliferation of marrow cells showing features characteristic of acute myelogenous leukemia (AML), such as the presence of Auer rods and specific histochemical staining with myeloperoxidase.

The predominant proliferation of abnormal hypergranular promyelocytes led to the diagnosis of acute promyelocytic leukemia (APL or M3, according to the French-American-British classification). APL is a morphological variant of AML. The form of APL found in this patient and the less frequent microgranular variant account for about 10% of cases of AML. The 15:17 translocations between chromosomes are typical for this type of leukemia. Anemia due to decreased production of red cells is a constant feature. Thrombocytopenia is nearly always present at the time of diagnosis. The absolute neutrophil count is most often reduced. In contrast to other forms of AML, APL is frequently associated with a coagulopathy characterized by a decreased fibrinogen level and moderately prolonged PT, PTT, and TT. Hemorrhagic manifestations are prominent. The manifestations appear not only in skin and mucous membranes but also as gastrointestinal, pulmonary, and intracranial bleeding.

A standard chemotherapy regimen including an anthracycline antibiotic and cytosine arabinoside was initiated and was continued for seven days, together with intravenous infusion of heparin at a low dosage. The patient also received daily infusions of platelets and fresh-frozen plasma. Five days after treatment was begun, the hemorrhagic skin lesions resolved and results of coagulation assays returned to normal. Changes in the patient's coagulation parameters in response to initial therapy are shown in Figure 1. About one month after treatment, the bone marrow examination showed remission of the leukemia; leukemic promyelocytes had decreased to less than 5% of nucleated cells. The platelet count at that time was 180,000/μL (180 x 10^9/L).

Discussion of Hemostatic Abnormalities

The bleeding phenomena in APL are generally accepted to be primarily the consequence of disseminated intravascular coagulation (DIC). DIC is a consumptive thrombohemorrhagic syndrome that appears in a variety of clinical disorders. All cases of DIC result from the activation of the coagulation cascade by a pathogen. The two major mechanisms by which DIC is triggered are endothelial cell injury and tissue injury. Endothelial injury appears mostly in infections. The endothelial surface altered by inflammatory mediators provides for the activation of factor XII, which initiates the intrinsic pathway of blood coagulation. Tissue injury occurs predominantly in malignancy. Procoagulant material released from tumor cells activates factor VII, initiating the extrinsic pathway of coagulation. Virtually all changes that develop in DIC reflect the uncontrolled action of two enzymes: thrombin and plasmin.

In APL, the subcellular structures of abnormal promyelocytes contain thromboplastic material. Release of this material into the vascular system leads to the production of thrombin and culminates in deposition of fibrin. Several coagulation factors including fibrinogen, prothrombin, and factors V, VIII, and XIII are consumed in the process of intravascular clotting. This is reflected in the prolongation of the PT and PTT.

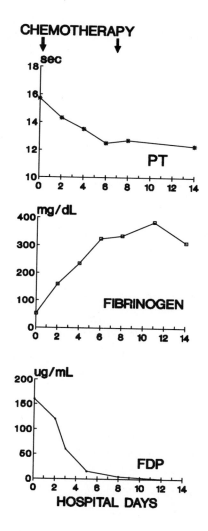

Figure 1. Changes in prothrombin time (PT), fibrinogen, and fibrin degradation products (FDP) levels induced by initial therapy. Arrows indicate the beginning and end of chemotherapy.

Microvascular deposits of fibrin obstruct the blood flow and cause ischemia with secondary release from the endothelium of tissue-type and urokinase-type plasminogen activators (t-PA and u-PA). These enzymes convert plasminogen to plasmin. Plasmin in the microcirculation contributes to the breakdown of fibrin with formation of FDP. In the systemic circulation, plasmin degrades fibrinogen and produces fragments that inhibit polymerization of fibrin monomers, thereby delaying hemostatic clot formation and aggravating bleeding.

Elaboration of thrombin in vivo also causes decreased survival of platelets. Thrombin binds to platelets at low concentration, thus inducing their aggregation, degranulation, and secretion. Platelet destruction intensifies the severity of thrombocytopenia initially caused by the malignant marrow infiltration. Platelets that survive contact with thrombin remain mostly agranular with decreased hemostatic activity. Therefore, the bleeding tendency in APL is usually greater than expected on the basis of existing platelet count.

Laboratory diagnosis of DIC is suggested when both the platelet count and fibrinogen level are markedly decreased; consumption of factors II, V, and X is usually less severe. PT and PTT are prolonged to a variable degree. Bleeding time may be markedly prolonged even when the platelet count remains above 50,000/μL (50 x 10^9/L) because of the presence of dysfunctional platelets. The diagnosis is supported by detection of high levels of FDP in serum. A prolonged thrombin time in the absence of heparin administration indicates that polymerization of fibrin is inhibited by fragments of lysed fibrinogen. The presence of so-called D dimer in plasma signifies lysis of intravascular thrombi. D dimer is a unique product of fibrin crosslinked by activated factor XIII. It is composed of two identical fragments cleaved from adjacent fibrin monomers covalently bound by crosslinks between their γ-chain remnants. Presence in the peripheral blood smear of fragmented red cells, schistocytes, and helmet cells is a less specific finding, since they occur often in other clinical conditions such as mitral valve stenosis and collagen vascular disorders.

Treatment

To control DIC, the triggering pathogenic mechanism must be eliminated. In APL, this is achieved by successful chemotherapy. During induction of chemotherapy, however, rapid lysis of tumor cells may transiently exacerbate the thrombohemorrhagic process. Concomitant treatment with heparin has been applied on the assumption that accelerated neutralization of thrombin by antithrombin III will limit DIC and lessen the risk of hemorrhage. However, heparin itself may cause bleeding. If used, the therapy should be closely monitored by coagulation tests and should be limited to doses that do not significantly prolong the PTT.

The efficacy of heparin as an agent that may limit or abolish the DIC process is questionable because antithrombin III does not neutralize factor VIIa, either in the presence of or in the absence of heparin; therefore heparin has little control over blood coagulation activated through the extrinsic pathway. Several studies have shown no apparent benefit from heparin therapy in DIC associated with a variety of underlying clinical disorders. In APL, however, heparin may lengthen the survival of infused platelets by preventing excessive destruction of platelets by thrombin. Replacement of consumed blood components with infusion of platelets, cryoprecipitate, or fresh-frozen plasma is a very important part of the initial therapy regimen in APL. During successful chemotherapy in combination with administration of hemostatic components alone, bleeding manifestations often disappear while levels of fibrinogen and other coagulation proteins gradually return to normal, signifying cessation of the consumptive process. The platelet count returns to normal only after marrow function is fully restored.

Additional Reading

Colman, R.W., and Rubin, R.N.: Disseminated intravascular coagulation due to malignancy. Semin. Oncol., *17:*172-186, 1990.

Feinstein, D.I.: Diagnosis and management of disseminated intravascular coagulation: The role of heparin therapy. Blood, *60:*284-287, 1982.

Lichtman, M.A., and Henderson, E.S.: Acute myelogenous leukemia. *In:* Hematology. W.J. Williams, Ed. New York, McGraw-Hill, 1990.

A YOUNG GIRL WITH DEEP VEIN THROMBOSIS
AND ABNORMAL COAGULATION TESTS

Ewa Marciniak, Contributor

A 16-year-old girl was admitted to the hospital because of the sudden onset of severe pain and swelling of the right thigh approximately 12 hours before admission. The patient was well until four months earlier when she experienced recurrent episodes of pain in the knees, ankles, and wrists, low grade fever, and anorexia with a gradual weight loss of about 20 lb (9 kg). During the last month before admission she had noticed the development of a nonpruritic rash on her face that flared up after even a short exposure to sunlight.

The patient was a high-school student. At the age of eight years she underwent uncomplicated appendectomy. There was no history of infections, bleeding, or allergies. She took no medications. On physical examination the temperature was 99.9 °F (37.7 °C). The patient appeared thin. A typical butterfly rash of the nasal and adjacent malar area was noted. There were a few palpable cervical nodes. The right calf and thigh were swollen and tender; otherwise the physical examination was noncontributory.

Laboratory tests gave the following results:

Analyte	Value, conventional units	Reference range, conventional units	Value, SI units	Reference range, SI units
Urinalysis (U)	Numerous erythrocytes; otherwise within normal limits			
Hematocrit (B)	31 %	37-47	0.31	0.37-0.47
Leukocyte count (B)	3.9 x 10^3/μL	4.5-13.0	3.9 x 10^9/L	4.5-13.0
Differential count (B)				
Neutrophils	33 %	41-71	0.33	0.41-0.71
Lymphocytes	59 %	21-51	0.59	0.21-0.51
Monocytes	8 %	2-9	0.08	0.02-0.09
Eosinophils	2 %	1-3	0.02	0.01-0.03
Platelet count (B)	115 x 10^3/μL	150-450	115 x 10^9/L	150-450
Erythrocyte sedimentation rate (ESR) (B)	39 mm/h	0-20	Same	
Bleeding time (bedside)	5 min	<10	Same	
Lupus anticoagulant test (B)	Distinctly positive	Negative		
Antithrombin III (P)	0.97 u/mL	0.80-1.15	Same	
Protein C (P)	1.14 u/mL	0.69-1.40	Same	
Prothrombin time (PT) (P) *	14.7 s	11.7 (control)	Same	
Partial thromboplastin time (PTT) (P) *	47 s	26 (control)	Same	
Anticardiolipin test (S)	Distinctly positive	Negative		
Urea nitrogen (S)	Within normal limits			
Creatinine (S)	Within normal limits			

* Both PT and PTT remained prolonged in a mixture of the patient's plasma with normal plasma.

Analyte	Value, conventional units	Reference range, conventional units	Value, SI units	Reference range, SI units
C3 complement (S)	50 mg/dL	80-175	0.5 g/L	0.80-1.75
Antinuclear antibodies (ANA) (S)	Strongly positive	Negative		
Anti-DNA antibodies (S)	Strongly positive	Negative		
VDRL (Venereal Disease Research Laboratory) test for syphilis (S)	Positive	Negative		

Phlebography and ultrasonography disclosed thrombotic occlusion of the right femoral vein. Several clinical symptoms in this young female, such as arthralgia, fever, anorexia, skin eruptions, and adenopathy, are consistent with the diagnosis of systemic lupus erythematosus (SLE).

Definition of the Disease

Systemic lupus erythematosus (SLE) is an autoimmune disorder of unknown etiology that develops predominantly in women, frequently at a young age. The picture is that of a chronic multisystemic inflammatory disease. It results from immunological dysregulation that leads to production of autoantibodies against host antigens. The most frequently targeted antigen is native DNA. Autoimmune reactions are responsible for tissue injury in many organ systems. Initial symptoms commonly include low grade fever, arthritis, and skin lesions often manifested as a typical butterfly rash. Hair loss, deterioration of renal function, neurological disorders, cardiac and pulmonary involvement, anemia, leukopenia, and thrombocytopenia vary greatly in the intensity and frequency of their appearance among individual patients. The course of the disease is unpredictable. It ranges from a benign, long-lasting disorder to a rapidly progressing fatal illness with simultaneous involvement of many organs. Remissions of variable duration are followed by exacerbations. No cure is available, but immunosuppressive and cytotoxic therapy have proved useful in controlling SLE manifestations. Patients without life-threatening symptoms may be managed conservatively with rest and nonsteroidal anti-inflammatory agents.

Discussion

Laboratory findings in SLE are, in general, either indicative of damage to an organ system or a reflection of the presence of pathological antibodies. The serum of patients with SLE may contain a variety of antibodies; most common are the antibodies to various epitopes of cell nuclei, present in over 90% of cases. Other diseases, however, may also cause a positive test for ANA. Anti-DNA antibodies, particularly those directed against native double-stranded DNA, are more specific. Reduced serum complement levels are the result of consumption of complement during immune complex formation and tissue damage.

Deep vein thrombosis (DVT), with which the patient presented, is not a specific symptom of SLE and is a rather uncommon manifestation in a juvenile subject. Normal levels of antithrombin III and protein C allow exclusion of a hereditary hypercoagulable disorder. However, the fact that significant prolongations in clotting assays were not corrected by normal plasma, together with positive tests for lupus anticoagulant and anticardiolipin, indicated the presence of antiphospholipid antibodies in blood. Development of these antibodies is known to be associated with a high risk of thrombosis.

On the basis of clinical and laboratory findings in this patient the following diagnoses were established: systemic lupus erythematosus; right femoral vein thrombosis; and hyper-coagulable state secondary to the presence of antiphospholipid antibodies.

Antiphospholipid Antibodies

Circulating antibodies, reacting specifically with negatively charged phospholipid, are heterogeneous immunoglobulins that may appear in a variety of clinical disorders including a significant number of cases with SLE. They may even occasionally appear in a subject without apparent disease. By binding to miscellaneous phospholipid reagents, these anti-bodies usually cause a distinct prolongation in all phospholipid-dependent clotting tests, especially the PTT (see Figure 1), and give positive results in one or more of the following laboratory tests: lupus anticoagulant test, anticardiolipin test, and VDRL test for syphilis.

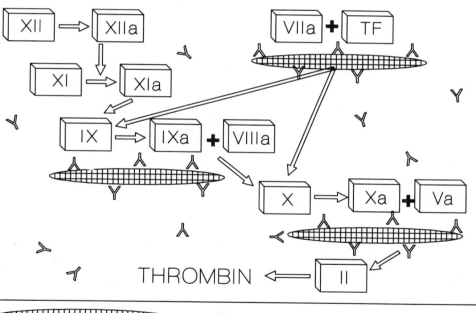

Figure 1. Scheme of the coagulation cascade. Antiphospholipid antibodies disturb binding of vitamin K-dependent clotting factors II, VII, IX, and X to the phospholipid surface, thereby delaying clotting in tests such as PT and PTT.

Historically, acquired antibodies with distinct anticoagulant properties were first reported in patients with SLE, thus leading to the term lupus anticoagulant. The lupus anticoagulant test is based on clotting assays specifically designed to utilize low concentrations of phospholipid and it is, therefore, most sensitive to the presence of these abnormal immunoglobulins.

Patients who develop lupus anticoagulant usually remain free of bleeding tendency. Only in rare cases complicated by immune hypoprothrombinemia or severe thrombocytopenia does bleeding occur. Lupus anticoagulant is closely related, if not identical, to the antibodies to cardiolipin, and the presence of either or both of these pathological immunoglobulins in blood leads to increased risk of thrombosis. In pregnant women these antibodies have been reported to contribute to fetal loss, probably due to placental thrombosis and infarction.

The relationship between antiphospholipid antibodies and thrombosis remains unclear. One possibility is that the antibodies may affect adversely the endothelial cell membrane, compromising its antithrombotic properties such as production of prostacyclin and activation of protein C. Protein C circulates in the form of an inactive enzyme precursor. To function as a coagulation inhibitor the precursor must be converted to the enzyme form, protein Ca. The conversion takes place on the vascular surface of the endothelium where only thrombin complexed with the endothelial membrane receptor, thrombomodulin, can rapidly activate protein C. If the expression of thrombomodulin on the cell membrane is suppressed, activation of protein C will diminish, and a thrombotic tendency may develop.

The apparent interference of lupus anticoagulant with binding of vitamin K-dependent proteins to a surface suggests yet another possibility, namely, that these antibodies may interfere with the catalytic function of already activated protein C. Protein Ca functions as a coagulation inhibitor primarily by destroying factor Va, which has been activated by thrombin. Factor Va plays a key role in blood coagulation since it functions as a nonenzymic cofactor in the activation of prothrombin by factor Xa. Proteolysis of factor Va by protein Ca terminates prothrombin activation and prevents increased production of thrombin. However, rapid proteolysis of factor Va by protein Ca takes place only when the enzyme, in the presence of calcium ions, binds through its vitamin K-dependent γ-carboxyglutamic acid residues to a surface provided by either isolated phospholipid or by platelets and endothelial cell membranes. Since antiphospholipid antibodies interfere with this binding, they may create conditions under which protein Ca will no longer function effectively; undegraded factor Va will remain in the circulation and lead to local accumulation of thrombin and thrombosis.

These associations need further studies to identify the precise mechanism by which antiphospholipid antibodies contribute to thrombosis. The risk of thrombosis is similar in all patients who have these antibodies, regardless of the underlying diagnosis. The antibodies usually persist for years and rarely disappear even after prolonged therapy with corticosteroids. Once an episode of venous thromboembolism has occurred, long-term anticoagulant therapy is mandatory.

Treatment

The patient was treated with intravenous infusion of heparin and with large daily doses of enteric-coated aspirin. On the fifth hospital day therapy with warfarin (Coumadin) was initiated, and the swelling and tenderness of the lower right extremity subsided. Heparin therapy was discontinued when the prothrombin time increased to 19.7 seconds. The patient became afebrile, and the skin rash disappeared. She was released from the hospital and treated with Coumadin and aspirin at home.

Additional Reading

Gastineau, D.A., Kazmier, F.J., Nichols, W.L., and Bowie, E.J.W.: Lupus anticoagulant: An analysis of the clinical and laboratory features of 219 cases. Am. J. Hematol., *19:* 265-275, 1985.

Shapiro, S.S., Thiagarajan, P., and DeMarco, L.: Mechanism of action of lupus anticoagulant. Ann. N.Y. Acad. Sci., *370:* 359-363, 1981.

Triplett, D.A., and Brandt, J.: Laboratory identification of the lupus anticoagulant. Br. J. Haematol., *73:* 139-142, 1989.

MEDICAL STUDENT WITH MILD BLEEDING DISORDER

Ewa Marciniak, Contributor
Richard A. Mc Pherson, Reviewer

A 21-year-old college student was struck in the knee by a baseball. Two hours later he started to experience increasing pain and swelling at the site of the injury and the development of an extensive hematoma in the tibial area of the right leg. He presented at the local health center where the diagnosis of right knee hemarthrosis was made. The knee was immobilized in splints, and the patient received an analgesic after which the pain rapidly diminished. He denied any previous bleeding episodes and was sent home without laboratory testing. After a few days the swelling subsided, and the mobility of the knee joint was restored. Six months thereafter this young man underwent dental extraction complicated by significant bleeding lasting three days. Two years later while working as a sophomore medical student on a summer project in the community blood bank, he was testing factor VIII stability in frozen plasma and cryoprecipitate. Out of curiosity he tested his own factor VIII activity and found that it was only 10% of the normal concentration. He suspected that he had hemophilia and sought medical advice from a hematologist at the University Hospital. The student had one sister, two brothers, and several maternal male relatives; there was no history of a bleeding disorder in the family. On physical examination no abnormalities were found.

Laboratory findings at this time were as follows:

Analyte	Value, conventional units	Reference range, conventional units	Value, SI units	Reference range, SI units
Platelet count (B)	375 x 10^3/µL	150-450	375 x 10^9/L	150-450
Bleeding time (bedside)	5 min	<10	Same	
Partial thromboplastin time (PTT) (P)	35.7 s	23-33	Same	
Prothrombin time (PT) (P)	11.7 s	11.5-13.5	Same	
Fibrinogen (P)	370 mg/dL	150-450	3.7 g/L	1.5-4.5
Factor VIII (FVIII) activity (P)	12 %	50-200	0.12	0.50-2.00
Factor IX (FIX) activity (P)	97 %	50-140	0.97	0.50-1.40
von Willebrand factor (P)	137 %	>60	1.37	>0.60

On the basis of clinical symptoms and laboratory results, the diagnosis of a mild form of hemophilia A was established. There were no further bleeding episodes. Recently, at the age of 27 years, the young man underwent extraction of his wisdom teeth. Before the surgery he was infused with DDAVP (1-desamino-8-D-arginine vasopressin), a synthetic analogue of vasopressin. The DDAVP induced a significant increase in plasma factor VIII activity as illustrated in Figure 1. For four days after the surgery an antifibrinolytic agent was administered; no bleeding complications occurred.

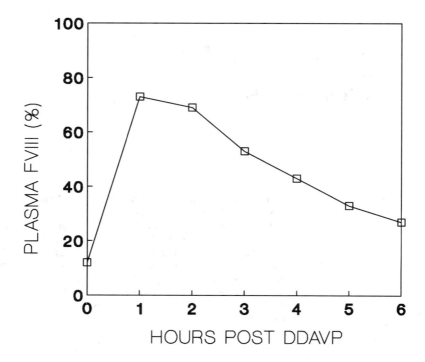

Figure 1. Change in the concentration of plasma factor VIII in response to intravenous infusion of DDAVP.

Genetics and Clinical Aspects of the Disease

Hemophilia is a sex-linked bleeding disorder that affects one in 5000 males world-wide. The disorder is transmitted by a gene on the X chromosome. There are two forms of hemophilia: hemophilia A (classic hemophilia) associated with the deficiency of factor VIII, and hemophilia B (Christmas disease) associated with the deficiency of factor IX. Hemophilia A is about four times more frequent than hemophilia B. Deficiency of factor XI, a non-sex-linked disorder, is sometimes termed hemophilia C.

The sons of a hemophilic man do not inherit hemophilia because they receive a paternal Y, not X, chromosome; their maternal X chromosome bears normal genes. All daughters of a hemophilic father receive his X chromosome and are therefore obligatory carriers of hemophilia. Since their second, maternal, chromosome is normal, they will transmit hemophilia to only 50% of their sons; 50% of their daughters will be carriers. In the plasma of a hemophilia carrier, factor VIII or factor IX activity is on the average 50% less than in genetically normal women. In individual carriers, however, the factor level ranges from that found in affected males to a high normal concentration. This distribution is in agreement with the Lyon hypothesis of random inactivation of one of the two X chromosomes in somatic female cells.

About 30% of hemophiliacs have "sporadic" hemophilia, i.e., no family history of the disorder. These cases reveal the introduction of a new genetic mutation into the population. The mutation may take place in the ovum from which the hemophiliac developed. More often, however, the mother of a sporadic hemophiliac is a carrier who has the mutated gene already in both somatic and germ cells. Due to the diversity in genetic mutations, there is a wide range of clinical severity in both types of the hemophilia. Severity relates directly to the level of factor VIII or factor IX in the blood (see Table 1). The phenotypic expression of hemophilia is constant throughout the life of an individual and is similar in all affected members of a given family.

Table 1. CLINICAL FORMS OF HEMOPHILIA

Severity	Factor, % of normal	PTT, s	Clinical manifestations
Severe	<1	>65	Severe bleeding into skin, joints, muscles, often with a delayed onset, may occur even after unrecognized trauma. The disorder is usually evident in the first year of life. Frequent and intense replacement therapy is required to prevent and arrest hemorrhage.
Moderate	1-5	50-65	Extensive bleeding occurs after trauma, but spontaneous bleeding and hemarthroses are less common. The need for replacement varies from sporadic to relatively frequent.
Mild	6-30	35-45	Absence of spontaneous bleeding. Excessive bleeding occurs only after major trauma or surgery. The patient may remain undiagnosed for several years.

The difference between the clinical pictures of severe and mild hemophilia is remarkable. A severely affected hemophiliac shows hemorrhagic diathesis early in life and is usually diagnosed in infancy. In about 50% of such patients the first bleeding episode occurs at the time of circumcision. In contrast, a mildly affected hemophiliac may remain free of serious bleeding for a long period of time and is often not diagnosed until late in life. The patient presented here is thus a typical case of sporadic mild hemophilia. Characteristic for all forms of hemophilia is the lack of excessive bleeding from superficial cuts, due to the normal primary hemostasis achieved by platelets.

About 5% of patients with severe hemophilia A, and 2% of patients with severe hemophilia B, who have been treated with blood products develop neutralizing alloantibodies to factor VIII or factor IX. In moderately severe or mild hemophilia these antibodies appear rarely. Although presence of antibody does not increase the frequency of hemorrhage, it makes the management of bleeding episodes exceedingly difficult. Not only is the infused clotting factor rapidly neutralized, but each exposure to the antigen is followed by a rise in the antibody titer. When the replacement therapy is withheld, the inhibitory activity gradually decreases or even disappears but will reappear with the next infusion.

Laboratory Diagnosis

Both factor IX and factor VIII participate in the process of blood coagulation as an enzyme-cofactor complex (FIXa-FVIIIa) essential for the activation of factor X. Selective deficiency of either factor IX or factor VIII contributes to a more or less extensive prolongation of PTT while other screening clotting assays remain normal. Measurement of these factors is based on the ability of plasma to correct PTT in plasma known to be deficient in the specific factor. A quantitative measure of the degree of deficiency is provided by presenting a test result as a percentage of normal corrective response. A variety of methods utilizing immunoassay techniques and chromogenic substrates have been developed, but these methods have not yet achieved a widespread acceptance. When a decreased factor VIII activity is detected, as in the case of the medical student, further testing for von Willebrand factor (also known as ristocetin cofactor) is necessary in order to distinguish hemophilia A from von

Willebrand's disease. The von Willebrand factor is a multimeric plasma protein with two important functions in hemostasis: it mediates platelet adhesion to the vessel wall at the site of injury and transports and stabilizes factor VIII in the circulation. Consequently, an apparent deficiency of factor VIII may be secondary to deficiency of von WIllebrand factor. In the case presented, the concentration of von Willebrand factor was normal. We may therefore assume that the reduction in factor VIII was primary and thus consistent with the diagnosis of hemophilia A.

For detection of the inhibitor, a simple screening test can be used. If the inhibitor is present, patient plasma will lengthen the PTT of normal plasma to a pronounced degree. Quantitative inhibitor assays are based on measurements of the amount of factor VIII or factor IX inactivated under specific conditions. One unit of the inhibitor (Bethesda unit) is defined as the reciprocal of the dilution of patient plasma that destroys 50% of factor VIII or factor IX activity present in 1 mL of normal plasma.

Treatment

Replacement therapy in hemophilia is usually given to combat hemorrhage or to prevent excessive bleeding in surgical procedures. Infusion of fresh-frozen plasma, cryoprecipitate, or factor VIII concentrate is given in hemophilia A, of plasma or factor IX concentrate in hemophilia B. Current methods for fractionating blood products and preparing factor concentrates reduce the risk for transmission of infectious agents such as hepatitis and AIDS viruses. Production of specific blood proteins by recombinant DNA technique eliminates this risk completely; factor VIII product of this origin is now in clinical trials.

The therapeutic dose of factors VIII and IX is expressed in units, 1 unit corresponding to the activity of the specific protein present in 1 mL of normal human plasma. When calculating dosage, 1 unit of factor VIII per kilogram body weight is expected to increase the recipient's factor level by 2%; 1 unit of factor IX per kilogram is expected to increase the factor level by 1%. The half-life of factor VIII is 11 hours, that of factor IX is 22 hours; thus in order to support similar levels of hemostasis, factor VIII must be administered twice as frequently as factor IX.

The minimal hemostatic level for treatment of mild bleeding is a factor level of 30%. In case of more extensive lesions, factor level should be maintained above 50%. Hemophiliacs undergoing major surgical operations require a factor level of 80%, or higher, in order to remain free of hemorrhage.

DDAVP, 1-desamino-8-D-arginine vasopressin, is helpful for treatment of patients with mild hemophilia A who are candidates for dental and surgical procedures. DDAVP stimulates release of factor VIII and von Willebrand factor from endothelial stores into the circulation. DDAVP infusion causes factor VIII level to peak at 3 to 8 times the baseline concentration, thus providing a level adequate to prevent bleeding.   Antifibrinolytic agents such as ε-aminocaproic acid and tranexamic acid inhibit clot lysis by blocking the binding of plasmin to its substrate, fibrin. These drugs are useful adjuvants to replacement therapy or DDAVP treatment.

Additional Reading

Brettler, D.B., and Levine, P.H.: Factor concentrates for treatment of hemophilia: Which one to choose? Blood, *73:* 2067-2073, 1989.

White, G.C., and Shoemaker, C.B.: Factor VIII gene and hemophilia. Blood, *73:* 1-12, 1989.

HIGH ANION-GAP ACIDOSIS WITH HIGH OSMOLAL GAP

Robert V. Blanke, Contributor

Case One*

A 51-year-old, 165-lb (75-kg) man with no history of ethanol abuse was brought to the emergency room 2.5 h after ingesting about 600 mL of an unknown liquid, apparently in a suicide attempt. His blood pressure was 158/96 mm Hg, pulse 128 BPM, and respirations 24/min. He was ataxic, dysarthric, and lethargic. Laboratory results were as follows:

Analyte	Value, conventional units	Reference range, conventional units	Value, SI units	Reference range, SI units
Sodium (S)	153 mmol/L	136-145	Same	
Potassium (S)	4.0 mmol/L	3.8-5.1	Same	
Chloride (S)	101 mmol/L	98-107	Same	
CO_2, total (S)	10 mmol/L	23-29	Same	
Urea nitrogen (S)	16 mg/dL	7-18	5.7 mmol urea/L	2.5-6.4
Calcium (S)	9.2 mg/dL	8.4-10.2	2.30 mmol/L	2.10-2.55
Osmolality (S)	422 mOsm/kg	275-295	422 mmol/kg	275-295
Osmolality, calculated (S)	312 mOsm/kg	275-295	312 mmol/kg	275-295
pH (aB)	7.18	7.35-7.45	Same	
pCO_2 (aB)	14 mm Hg	35-48	1.9 kPa	4.7-6.4
pO_2 (aB)	91 mm Hg	83-108	12.1 kPa	11.1-14.4

Because of the high osmolal and anion gaps (110 mOsm/kg and 42 mmol/L, respectively), alcohol or ethylene glycol intoxication was suspected, and a test for these two agents was ordered. The ethanol level was negative; the ethylene glycol concentration was 650 mg/dL (104 mmol/L). Emergency treatment was begun with intravenous sodium bicarbonate. Gastric lavage was performed, and activated charcoal was administered. The patient was then transferred to a larger medical center where, six hours after the ingestion, the physical examination showed no change. At this time, ethylene glycol was 325 mg/dL (52 mmol/L), and the blood ethanol was 10 mg/dL (2.2 mmol/L) despite two hours of intravenous administration of 5% ethanol. A loading dose of 114 mL of 50% ethanol was given by nasogastric tube. Since the patient had received activated charcoal upon admission, a second loading dose was required to obtain therapeutic blood ethanol concentrations. During hemodialysis therapy, blood ethanol concentrations were maintained at between 100 and 140 mg/dL (22-30 mmol/L). After six hours of dialysis, the ethylene glycol level was 60 mg/dL (10 mmol/L), dropping after further dialysis to undetectable concentrations 80 hours after ingestion. Serum creatinine rose to 3.0 mg/dL (265 μmol/L) on the fourth hospital day and dropped to 1.2 mg/dL (106 μmol/L) by the time of discharge. The kinetics of ethylene glycol elimination during therapy of this patient and the effectiveness of hemodialysis are illustrated in Figure 1.

---

*Adapted from Peterson, C.D., Collins, A.J., Himes, J.M., et al.[1]

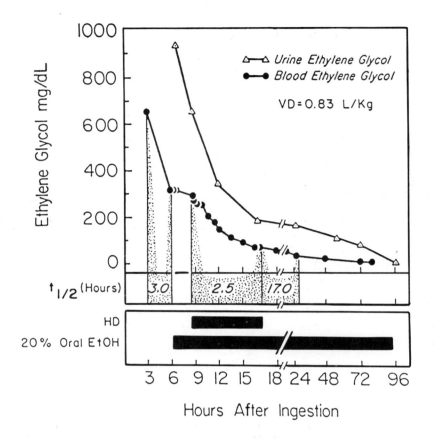

Figure 1. Blood and urine levels of ethylene glycol during hemodialysis (HD) and therapy with oral ethanol (EtOH). (Reprinted, by permission of the New England Journal of Medicine, from: Peterson, C.D., Collins, A.J., Himes, J.M., et al.: N. Engl. J. Med., *304:* 21-23, 1981.)

The half-life ($t_{1/2}$) of ethylene glycol was 3 h when no effective therapy was given. Note that during therapy with 20% oral EtOH alone, the $t_{1/2}$ of ethylene glycol was prolonged to 17 hours; hemodialysis effectively removed ethylene glycol ($t_{1/2}$ of 2.5 h). VD denotes volume of distribution. To convert ethylene glycol values to mmol/L, multiply mg/dL by 0.161.

Case Two*

A previously healthy 42-year-old male was brought to the emergency room after having ingested a large quantity of antifreeze 4.5 h earlier. Vomiting and polyuria soon developed. Upon admission to the emergency room, the patient appeared intoxicated and was becoming increasingly lethargic and drowsy. His plasma bicarbonate concentration was 13 mmol/L, with an anion gap of 27.5 mmol/L (reference range, 7-16 mmol/L) and a serum creatinine of 0.93 mg/dL (82 μmol/L). Initial emergency treatment consisted of gastric aspiration, oral administration of activated charcoal, and an intravenous infusion of 500 mmol of sodium bicarbonate.

*Adapted from Baud, F.J., Galliot, M., Astier, A., et al.[2]

After admission into the intensive care unit, eight hours after the ingestion, the patient was drowsy and hyperpneic.   Blood pressure was 130/90 mm Hg, pulse rate 140 BPM with numerous premature atrial beats.   Arterial blood analysis showed: pH, 7.31; pCO_2, 33 mm Hg (4.4 kPa); plasma HCO_3^-, 16 mmol/L; lactate, 25 mg/dL (2.8 mmol/L); anion gap, 21 mmol/L. The serum creatinine was 0.69 mg/dL (61 µmol/L), and plasma osmolality was 350 mOsm/kg. Gastric lavage was performed with 12 L of fluid followed by another dose of activated charcoal. Five percent dextrose was infused for the first two days after admission. Early recognition of the possibility of ethylene glycol poisoning resulted in the administration of 45 g of ethanol intravenously as a loading dose shortly after admission. Plasma ethylene glycol was 320 mg/dL (52 mmol/L) and blood ethanol only 12 mg/dL (2.6 mmol/L). No additional ethanol was administered, and hemodialysis was not performed. Instead, therapy using 4-methylpyrazole was initiated (based on earlier, favorable experimental trials).[2] The first dose of 4-methylpyrazole was administered nine hours after the ingestion and then given twice daily until plasma ethylene glycol concentration was minimal. Recovery was complete and uneventful. Acidosis did not recur, and the patient's serum creatinine remained normal throughout the hospitalization. This case suggests that 4-methylpyrazole is more effective than is ethanol in inhibiting the metabolism of ethylene glycol and therefore enhances urinary clearance and minimizes the risk of oxaluria.[3] The clinical course of the patient, as reflected by laboratory tests, is summarized in Figure 2.

Severe High Anion Gap, Metabolic Acidosis

The production of severe metabolic acidosis by toxic substances is infrequent. Methods for the confirmation of a specific causative agent may not be readily available, resulting in delays in the diagnosis. This delay is unfortunate since prompt, specific treatment is important to minimize renal failure, central nervous system injury, respiratory depression, and cardiovascular collapse. Frequently, patients suffering from ethylene glycol poisoning present with an alcohol-like intoxication. They may be in coma with a severe metabolic acidosis, a large anion gap, and an increased osmolal gap, i.e., difference between measured and calculated osmolality is above normal.*

Normally, the osmolal gap is <10 mOsmol/L, and the anion gap is in the ranges indicated below.† If these parameters are increased above these values, a variety of causes must be considered, such as chronic renal failure, diabetic ketoacidosis, administration of mannitol, or the presence of other osmotically active substances such as alcohols, acetone, or glycols. Thus, blood glucose, creatinine, and urea nitrogen should be measured, in addition to evaluating electrolytes. The presence of salicylates in urine can be tested easily by simple color tests on urine. If the result is positive, the possibility of salicylate overdose must be evaluated by a quantitative measurement of salicylates in serum. Similarly, the possibility of diabetic ketoacidosis can be ruled in or out by determining ketone bodies and serum glucose. If a toxic dose of ethylene glycol has been ingested, a qualitative test for oxalate in the urine will be positive. However, other toxic glycols cannot be ruled out by this test.

---

* Osmolality (Calc.) $= 2 \left[Na^+ (mmol/L) + \dfrac{glucose\ (mg/dL)}{18} + \dfrac{BUN\ (mg/dL)}{2.8} \right]$

Osmolal Gap $=$ Osmolality (Measured) $-$ Osmolality (Calculated)

† Anion Gap $= Na^+ - (Cl^- + HCO_3^-) =$ 7 to 16 mmol/L or
$= (Na^+ + K^+) - (Cl^- + HCO_3^-) =$ 10 to 20 mmol/L

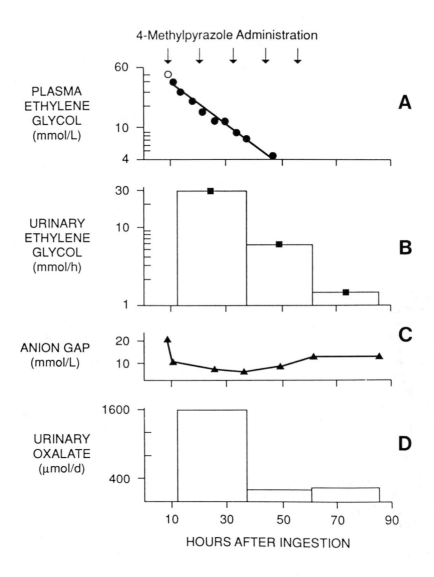

Figure 2. Assessments of levels of ethylene glycol and its metabolites in plasma and urine at various times after the ingestion of ethylene glycol. (Reprinted, by permission of the New England Journal of Medicine, from: Baud, F.J., Galliot, M., Astier, A., et al.: N. Engl. J. Med., *319:* 97-100, 1988.)

The times at which 4-methylpyrazole was administered are indicated by arrows. Panel A shows the plasma levels of ethylene glycol in mmol/L; the open circle denotes the ethylene glycol level on admission; the solid circles indicate the subsequent concentrations during treatment with 4-methylpyrazole. Panel B shows the rate of urinary excretion of ethylene glycol in mmol/h; solid squares denote the midpoint collection periods. Panel C shows the anion gap (in mmol/L), which was used as an estimation of plasma glycolate levels. Panel D shows the urinary excretion of oxalate in μmol/d.

Toxic solvents can be identified or ruled out best by examining serum with gas chromatography (GC)[4] or high-performance liquid chromatography (HPLC).[5] Either direct injection of serum diluted with an internal standard or head-space injection can demonstrate the presence or absence of methanol, ethanol, 2-propanol, and acetone. GLC or HPLC should be performed since toxic solvents may consist of mixtures of a variety of substances; alcoholics, when deprived of ethanol, may ingest any available liquid that is thought to contain alcohol. Specific analysis for ethylene glycol requires a different preparation of the specimen and modified chromatographic conditions. In both of the case reports described, ethylene glycol was identified as the causative agent by gas chromatography.

Ethylene Glycol Toxicity

Ethylene glycol is a colorless, slightly viscous, water-soluble liquid. It is said to have a somewhat sweet, not unpleasant taste. Together with other glycols, ethylene glycol is a common ingredient of antifreeze solutions, hydraulic fluids, and solvents with many industrial applications. Much like ethanol, it depresses the central nervous system, which, together with its ready availability and acceptable flavor, may be partly responsible for its choice as a suicide agent or as a cheap substitute for ethanol. Although its early effects are similar to those of ethanol, it is more toxic. Approximately 100 mL may be lethal in an adult. The toxicity of ethylene glycol is due to the accumulation of its major metabolites, which are:

$$
\begin{array}{ccccccccc}
\text{CH}_2\text{OH} & & \text{CH}_2\text{OH} & & \text{CH}_2\text{OH} & & \text{CHO} & & \text{COOH} \\
| & \xrightarrow{ADH} & | & \xrightarrow{ALD\ OX} & | & \xrightarrow{LDH\,/\,GLY\ AC\ OX} & | & \xrightarrow{LDH\,/\,ALD\ OX} & | \\
\text{CH}_2\text{OH} & & \text{CHO} & & \text{COOH} & & \text{COOH} & & \text{COOH} \\
\\
\text{Ethylene} & & \text{Glyoxal} & & \text{Glycolic} & & \text{Glyoxylic} & & \text{Oxalic} \\
\text{glycol} & & & & \text{acid} & & \text{acid} & & \text{acid}
\end{array}
$$

(*ADH* : alcohol dehydrogenase; *ALD OX*: aldehyde oxidase ; *LDH* : lactate dehydrogenase; *GLY AC OX*: glycolic acid oxidase.)

The above equations represent a postulated pathway for the metabolism of ethylene glycol. It is evident that the same enzyme that metabolizes ethanol, alcohol dehydrogenase, can also utilize ethylene glycol as a substrate. This can lead to the formation of glycolic acid, which contributes to severe anion-gap metabolic acidosis and leads to the formation of glyoxylic and oxalic acids. The profound metabolic acidosis leads to diminished renal blood flow. In addition, calcium oxalate crystals are deposited in the tubular epithelial cells, as well as in the lumina of the tubules, and diminish filtrate flow. If the condition remains untreated, renal failure results.[3]

Treatment of Ethylene Glycol Poisoning

The metabolic pathway outlined above for ethylene glycol also suggests the rationale for treatment of this type of poisoning. Ethanol is the preferred substrate for alcohol dehydrogenase. If administered in a controlled manner, it will displace ethylene glycol and thus will minimize the conversion of ethylene glycol to its toxic metabolites until all of the ethylene glycol is excreted. However, alternate pathways may operate when alcohol dehydrogenase is inhibited, permitting some oxalic acid to be formed. For this reason, an early hemodialysis followed by a forced diuresis, often with urinary alkalinization, is an important additional step to hasten the excretion of ethylene glycol.

Another recently introduced approach to the treatment of this condition has been used. It involves the use of 4-methylpyrazole, which is an inhibitor of the enzyme alcohol dehydrogenase. In animal studies, 4-methylpyrazole has been shown to reduce or eliminate the toxic effects of ethylene glycol and methanol. 4-Methylpyrazole has been used successfully in several clinical cases of ethylene glycol poisoning. Unfortunately, 4-methylpyrazole is only now undergoing Phase 1 clinical studies under the auspices of the Food and Drug Orphan Products Development Act. These initial studies suggest that this drug may soon be approved by the FDA for human use in the United States.

References

1. Peterson, C.D., Collins, A.J., Himes, J.M., et al.: Ethylene glycol poisoning: Pharmaco-kinetics during therapy with ethanol and hemodialysis. N. Engl. J. Med., *304:* 21-23, 1981.

2. Baud, F.J., Galliot, M., Astier, A., et al.: Treatment of ethylene glycol poisoning with intravenous 4-methylpyrazole. N. Engl. J. Med., *319:* 97-100, 1988.

3. Porter, G.A.: The treatment of ethylene glycol poisoning simplified (editorial). N. Engl. J. Med., *319:* 109-110, 1988.

4. Smith, N.B.: Determination of serum ethylene glycol by capillary gas chromatography. Clin. Chim. Acta, *14:* 269-272, 1984.

5. Gupta, R.N., Eng, F., and Gupta, M.L.: Liquid-chromatographic determination of ethyl-ene glycol in plasma. Clin. Chem., *28:* 32-33, 1982.

Additional Reading

Gosselin, R.E., Smith, R.P., and Hodge, H.C., Eds.: Clinical Toxicology of Commercial Products, 5th ed. Baltimore, Williams and Wilkins, 1984.

AN ANEMIC CHILD FROM AN UPPER MIDDLE-CLASS FAMILY

Robert V. Blanke, Contributor

A four-year-old Asian male was brought to the Pediatric Clinic by his concerned parents. The patient was pale and listless, and the parents related a history suggesting some type of gastrointestinal disorder. Abdominal pain was described that at times became severe and "colicky." Periods of constipation were followed by diarrhea, and the patient had experienced a 4 lb 14 oz (2.2 kg) weight loss during the preceding three months.

Subsequent to the physical examination, specimens were collected under fasting conditions. The following test results were obtained:

Analyte	Value, conventional units	Reference range, conventional units	Value, SI units	Reference range, SI units
Electrolytes (S)	Within normal limits			
Glucose (S)	75 mg/dL	60-100	4.2 mmol/L	3.3-5.6
Urea nitrogen (S)	8.2 mg/dL	5-18	2.9 mmol urea/L	1.8-6.4
Phosphorus, inorganic (S)	4.6 mg/dL	4.5-5.5	1.49 mmol/L	1.45-1.78
Creatinine (S)	0.19 mg/dL	0.3-0.7	16.8 µmol/L	27-62
Urate (S)	5.5 mg/dL	4.5-8.0	327 µmol/L	268-476
Calcium, total (S)	8.8 mg/dL	8.8-10.8	2.20 mmol/L	2.20-2.70
Iron, total (S)	180 µg/dL	50-120	32.2 µmol/L	9.0-21.5
Bilirubin, total (S)	1.2 mg/dL	<0.2-1.1	21 µmol/L	<3-19
ALP (S)	155 U/L	45-255	2.58 µkat/L	0.75-4.25
AST (S)	55 U/L	15-40	0.92 µkat/L	0.25-0.67
ALT (S)	94 U/L	10-40	1.57 µkat/L	0.17-0.67
Hematocrit (B)	28 %	31-43	0.28	0.31-0.43
Hemoglobin (B)	8.0 g/dL	11-16	4.96 mmol/L	6.83-9.93
Leukocyte count (B)	7.9 x 10³/µL	5.5-15.5	7.9 x 10⁹/L	5.5-15.5
MCH (B)	20 pg	27-31	Same	
MCV (B)	65 fL	73-85	Same	
Erythrocytes (B)	Showed basophilic stippling			

Alerted by the basophilic stippling and the increase in reticulocytes, the pediatrician ordered the following additional laboratory tests:

Analyte	Value, conventional units	Reference range, conventional units	Value, SI units	Reference range, SI units
Free erythrocyte proto-porphyrin (FEP) (B)	68 µg/dL	<35	1.2 µmol/L	<0.62
Lead (B)	45 µg/dL	<25	2.17 µmol/L	<1.21
δ-Aminolevulinic acid (U)	20 mg/d	1.3-7.0	153 µmol/d	10-53
Coproporphyrin (U)	720 µg/d	34-230	1100 nmol/d	52-351

Differential Diagnosis

This child had a severe microcytic hypochromic anemia that required precise diagnosis in order to select appropriate treatment. Three conditions that must be considered in the differential diagnosis are iron deficiency, thalassemia, and lead poisoning. Iron deficiency would not be accompanied by hemolysis or basophilic stippling of the erythrocytes. However, it does produce an increase in free erythrocyte protoporphyrin, as does lead poisoning. Iron deficiency is easily ruled out by measuring the serum iron and iron-binding capacity and/or serum ferritin.

The **thalassemias** result from diminished synthesis of hemoglobin due to gene deletion or to a deficiency or qualitative defect of messenger RNA leading to decreased production of a globin chain. Erythrocytes exhibit many morphological changes, including microcytic hypochromic anemia that must be differentiated from iron deficiency or plumbism in the laboratory.

β-Thalassemia is due to deficiency of the β-globin chain of hemoglobin and may be minor (one defective allele) or major (two defective alleles). α-Thalassemia shows a wider variation of findings because the α-globin chain is duplicated with four copies normally present. A single defective gene is silent (no clinical abnormality), whereas two defective genes on separate chromosomes cause moderate microcytic hypochromic anemia that occurs primarily in blacks. The presence of two defective genes linked on the same chromosome (found almost exclusively in patients of Asian ancestry) causes a more severe anemia with basophilic stippling. Three abnormal α-chain genes produce an even more severe condition, hemoglobin H disease (unstable β-chain tetramers), and the presence of four defective genes causes death *in utero* due to *hydrops fetalis*.

Diagnosis of thalassemia is guided by hemoglobin electrophoresis. β-Thalassemia is marked by increased hemoglobin A_2. Severe α-thalassemia shows hemoglobin H, but mild α-thalassemia may show no electrophoretic abnormality. In mild cases, diagnosis of α-thalassemia is frequently one of exclusion unless confirmed by measurement of α-/β-chain synthetic ratios in reticulocytes or by molecular biological definition of the gene abnormality.

Lead poisoning is a difficult diagnosis to make unless the physician suspects it in a context of occupational hazard. The diagnosis is particularly difficult in children, since no sign or symptom is pathognomonic. Early signs in children are progressive anorexia, drowsiness, stupor, and easy fatigue. Gastrointestinal effects may be noted; vomiting may occur, as well as complaints of abdominal pain. If plumbism is not recognized and treated early, encephalopathy may ensue; children under two years of age are especially susceptible to very rapid development of this condition.[1]

Increased numbers of reticulocytes, along with basophilic stippling observed in this patient's blood smear, were the clues that suggested lead poisoning. Although nonspecific, basophilic stippling of erythrocytes has long been associated with heavy metal poisoning. The patient's anemia was microcytic and hypochromic, similar to that seen in iron deficiency and also in lead poisoning. The pediatrician was quick to order blood lead and free erythrocyte protoporphyrin (FEP) and to ensure that the tests were performed on the same specimen. An elevation of the blood lead result may be due to contamination of specimen. If it is not, and the elevation is due to poisoning, then FEP should also be elevated. Zinc protoporphyrin (ZPP) assay serves the same purpose as the FEP assay.

Elevations of urinary δ-aminolevulinic acid (DALA) and coproporphyrin are also common findings in lead poisoning. Lead interferes at many sites in the biosynthetic path of the porphyrins (Figure 1). One enzyme particularly sensitive to inhibition is δ-aminolevulinic acid dehydratase (ALA-D). As blood lead levels increase linearly, activity of this enzyme decreases exponentially, and DALA accumulates. Coproporphyrinogen oxidase (COPRO-O) is also inhibited by lead, and coproporphyrinogen accumulates. The accumulations are reflected in increased urinary excretion of both DALA and coproporphyrin.[2]

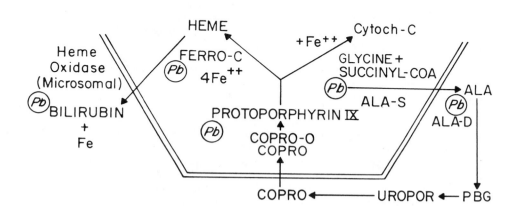

Figure 1. Scheme of heme synthesis showing sites where lead has an effect. *COA*, coenzyme A; *ALA-S*, δ-aminolevulinic acid synthetase; *ALA*, δ-aminolevulinic acid; *ALA-D*, δ-aminolevulinic acid dehydratase; *PBG*, porphobilinogen; *UROPOR*, uroporphyrinogen; *COPRO*, coproporphyrinogen; *COPRO-O*, coproporphyrinogen oxidase; *FERRO-C*, ferrochelatase; *CYTOCH-C*, cytochrome c ; (*Pb*), site for lead effect. (Reprinted with permission from: Amdur, M.O., Doull, J., and Klaassen, C.D., Eds.: Casarett and Doull's Toxicology: The Basic Science of Poisons, 4th ed. New York, Pergamon Press, Inc., 1991.)

Once the diagnosis of plumbism is made, interpretation of the other laboratory results of this patient becomes more obvious. Chronic lead poisoning may cause renal toxicity, although in this case serum urea nitrogen and urate appear normal. Lead tends to deposit in bone as a complex with calcium and phosphate, and in children the deposit can cause radiopaque lines in the epiphyses of long bones. An obsolete treatment for adults was once to encourage bone deposition by administration of calcium and phosphate compounds. The child in this case history displayed serum calcium and phosphorus concentrations near the lower limits of the reference ranges, 8.8-10.8 mg/dL (2.20-2.70 mmol/L) and 4.5-5.5 mg/dL (1.45-1.78 mmol/L) respectively, perhaps a suggestion that lead deposition in bone may have begun.

Insertion of iron into the protoporphyrin structure to form the product, hemoglobin, is also impaired in lead poisoning (Figure 1). Failure to incorporate iron properly may explain elevation of serum iron in this patient.

The elevation of ALP is not easy to explain. Perhaps it is a reflection of bone metabolism. Similarly, the increase in serum ALT and AST enzymes seems to suggest liver disease, although lead is not generally considered to be toxic to the liver.

Discussion

The greatest hazard of plumbism in developing children is irreversible damage to the central nervous system. High blood lead concentrations may lead to acute lead encephalopathy. Survivors of the severe convulsions may have permanent sequelae such as mental retardation, seizures, or both. Recent epidemiological studies have shown that relatively low blood lead concentrations can be associated with diminished IQ, hyperactivity, and behavioral disorders. Currently the Centers for Disease Control define lead toxicity in children as a blood lead concentration >25 µg/dL (>1.21 µmol/L). The critical level so defined has dropped steadily over past years as collection methods have improved, the sensitivity and quality of assay technology have increased, and clinical data have accumulated. The critical level may indeed change to 15 or even 10 µg/dL (0.48 µmol/L); one consequence of such a change would be a severe challenge for analytical methods currently in use.[3]

Recent studies have critically evaluated amounts of lead in drinking water. The Environmental Protection Agency has lowered the permissible lead content in drinking water from 50 parts per billion (ppb, µg/L) to 5 ppb. The mandate will have far-reaching effects on public water suppliers.[4]

Lead poisoning in children is usually associated with urban ghettos where children living unsupervised in old and substandard housing ingest peeling paint and putty that contain lead. But all children in any setting are at risk since lead is ubiquitous and can be encountered in many ways. Playing in outdoor areas where there are heavy concentrations of automobile exhaust or vapors from a nearby battery plant has been implicated; the dirt was found to be heavily contaminated with lead. Repeated use of cups or bowls of unglazed pottery, brought home from other countries as souvenirs, has been a cause of lead poisoning in children of wealthy families. Lead-based pigments leach from the container into the fluids subsequently ingested.

This case was an instance of poisoning occurring in an upper middle-class family. There seemed to be no obvious source of the lead. Nevertheless, every effort was made (and always *should* be made) to identify the source and to remove it permanently. Prolonged investigation, in this case, focused on a thickening agent used in cooking. The agent was imported from the Orient and contained a relatively high lead content. Other members of the family also had elevated blood lead concentrations that were, however, not sufficiently high to cause signs and symptoms of plumbism.

Treatment

The patient described in this case report was given one course of CaNa$_2$EDTA treatment, followed by oral D-penicillamine. His blood lead concentration fell to 23 µg/dL (1.11 µmol/L) immediately following these procedures and, after one year, had fallen to 16 µg/dL (0.77 µmol/L).

Treatment of lead poisoning falls into two categories. One is removal of unabsorbed lead from the gastrointestinal tract and of lead from the tissues. The second is alleviation of any acute signs and symptoms of encephalopathy, such as protracted vomiting and convulsions. The first stage of treatment may include gastric lavage with magnesium sulfate and use of the same agent as cathartic. Chelation therapy must be begun without delay.

Chelation therapy involves the intramuscular administration of a chemical that combines with lead and permits its excretion by the kidneys. The most thoroughly studied chelating agent is the calcium disodium salt of ethylenediaminetetraacetic acid or edetate calcium disodium (CaNa$_2$EDTA). Another, which penetrates cells more effectively than CaNa$_2$EDTA but has a weaker interaction with lead, is dimercaprol, or BAL (British anti-Lewisite). Subsequent to the CaNa$_2$EDTA administration, another chelating agent, D-penicillamine, may be given orally, if necessary. The selection of the type of agent depends on the degree of poisoning. After obtaining satisfactory blood lead measurements and determining that the renal function of the patient is satisfactory, de-leading the patient may proceed. Chronic chelation therapy promotes the excretion of essential metals in addition to lead and risks their depletion. During rest periods between therapy, dietary supplements of zinc and other essential metals are advisable.[5]

Convulsions are treated with diazepam or, in severe cases, with phenytoin. Abdominal pain should be treated with antispasmodics but may require morphine. Cerebral edema may be treated with intravenous mannitol or dexamethasone. Cerebral decompression, if necessary, must be done cautiously.

References

1. Waldron, H.A., and Stofen, D.: Sub-Clinical Lead Poisoning. New York, Academic Press, 1974.

2. Goyer, R.A.: Toxic effects of metals. *In:* Casarett and Doull's Toxicology: The Basic Science of Poisons, 4th ed. M.O. Amdur, J. Doull, and C.D. Klaassen, Eds. New York, Pergamon Press, 1991.

3. Boeckx, R.L.: Lead poisoning in children. Ther. Drug Monitoring - Tox., Am. Assoc. Clin. Chem., vol. 8, September 1986.

4. No author: Chem. Eng. News, May 13, 1991, page 17.

5. Gosselin, R.E., Smith, R.P., and Hodge, H.C.: Clinical Toxicology of Commercial Products, 5th ed. Baltimore, Williams and Wilkins, 1984.

SUICIDE ATTEMPT BY DRUG OVERDOSE

William H. Porter, Contributor

A 23-year-old woman was seen in the Emergency Department. She stated that she had ingested approximately 25 acetaminophen (Tylenol) tablets (500 mg each) six hours earlier, in a suicide attempt following an argument with her boyfriend. Subsequently she became frightened and sought medical help. She had not ingested other medications or alcohol.

On physical examination the woman appeared anxious. She was diaphoretic and complained of abdominal distress and nausea. Her blood pressure was 126/67 mm Hg; pulse, 98 BPM; respirations, 22/min; and temperature, 98.6 °F (37 °C). Otherwise the examination, including routine laboratory studies, was unremarkable. The patient was given syrup of ipecac to induce emesis. Activated charcoal was not administered.

On admission the patient's acetaminophen concentration, reported within the hour, was 263 µg/mL (1741 µmol/L). The Rumack-Matthew nomogram (see Figure 1) placed the patient at risk for developing hepatic necrosis. Treatment with *N*-acetylcysteine (NAC) was begun.

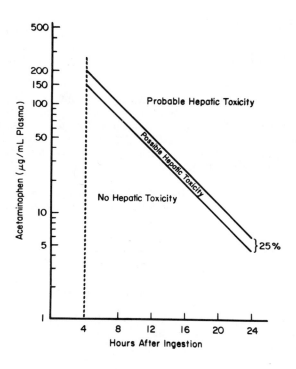

Figure 1. Rumack-Matthew nomogram for predicting acetaminophen toxicity. (Reprinted with permission of Pediatrics from: Rumack, B.H., and Matthew, H.: Pediatrics, *55:* 871-876. Copyright 1975.)

Three hours later, serum acetaminophen concentration was 170 µg/mL (1125 µmol/L). Based on the two acetaminophen values, the elimination half-life was estimated to be five hours, thus confirming the probable risk for hepatotoxicity.

The following liver function studies were performed:

Analyte	Day 1 (admission)	Day 2	Day 3	Day 5	Day 7
AST (S), U/L (µkat/L)	17 (0.28)	112 (1.87)	292 (4.87)	141 (2.35)	38 (0.63)
ALT (S), U/L (µkat/L)	22 (0.37)	123 (2.05)	324 (5.40)	139 (2.32)	33 (0.55)
Bilirubin (S), mg/dL (µmol/L)	0.9 (15)	1.0 (17)	1.7 (29)	1.3 (22)	0.8 (14)
Prothrombin time (P)					
patient, s	11.9	12.5	15.2	12.5	12.1
control, s	12.2	12.0	11.7	11.9	12.2

Based on the serum acetaminophen concentration, this patient ingested and absorbed sufficient acetaminophen to place her at risk for developing hepatic necrosis. Appropriate general and specific antidotal therapy was administered in a timely manner. The patient developed only mild indications of hepatic necrosis and was discharged on day 7 after psychiatric evaluation.

Clinical Manifestations of Acetaminophen Toxicity

The clinical course of acetaminophen intoxication occurs in three phases.[1] In the first phase, the patient is in no acute distress but may manifest nausea, vomiting, gastrointestinal irritability, diaphoresis, and pallor. Some patients may be completely asymptomatic during this initial period. The first phase generally begins shortly after acetaminophen ingestion and may last for 12 to 24 hours.

Before hepatotoxicity develops, there is typically a latent period of 24-72 hours (Phase 2). During this time, Phase 1 symptoms improve or disappear, and the patient appears to improve clinically. However, right-upper-quadrant abdominal tenderness may develop during this second phase, and liver enzymes (AST, ALT) may begin to rise. Many cases do not progress further, and there is a gradual return of normal liver function tests, especially if appropriate treatment is administered.

If substantial hepatic necrosis develops, progression to the third phase may occur typically three to five days after ingestion. Sequelae of hepatic necrosis may become prominent: nausea, vomiting, jaundice, marked increase in AST and ALT, increased pro-thrombin time, and hypoglycemia. Recovery is generally evident within seven to eight days. In severe cases, hepatic encephalopathy, hepatorenal syndrome, bleeding diatheses, cardiac abnormalities (rarely), or death due to hepatic failure may occur.

Mechanism of Acetaminophen-Induced Hepatotoxicity

Acetaminophen is readily absorbed from the gastrointestinal tract, with the peak serum concentration reached within 1-2 hours after ingestion. However, in instances of acetaminophen overdose, absorption may be delayed for up to four hours.

Acetaminophen is extensively metabolized in the liver, predominantly to glucuronide (55-60%) and sulfate (~30%) conjugates (see Figure 2). A lesser amount (~10%) is metabolized by the cytochrome P-450 mixed-function oxidase system.[2] Metabolism by this latter pathway is believed to involve a highly electrophilic intermediate (acetamidoquinone)

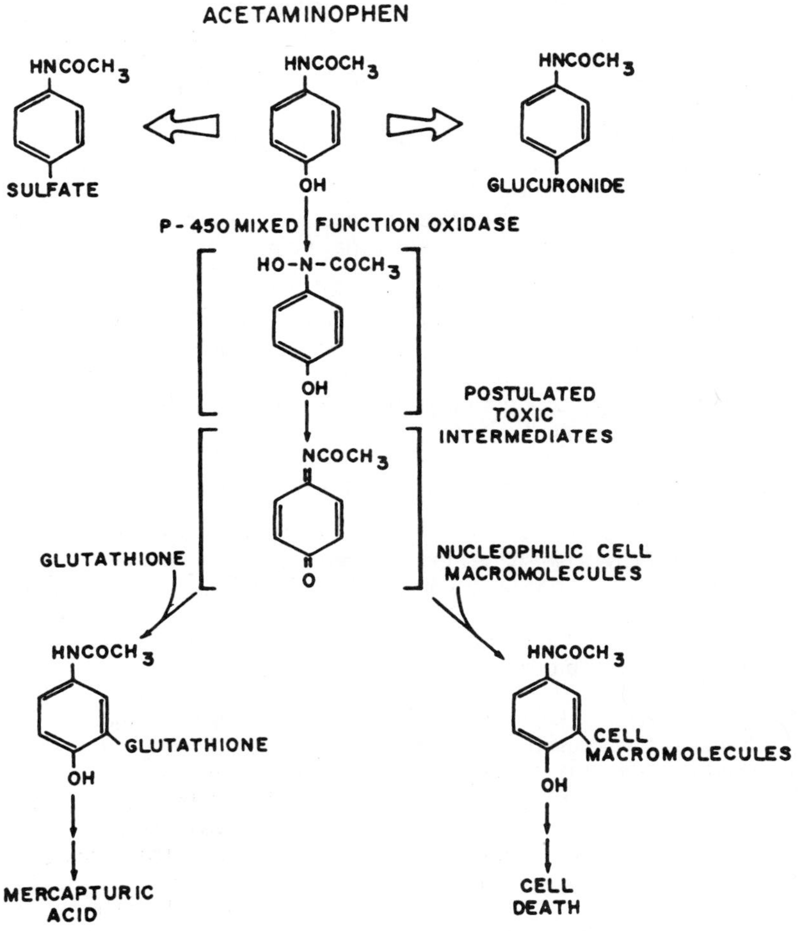

Figure 2. Metabolism of acetaminophen. (Reprinted with permission from: Mitchell, J.R., Thorgeirsson, S.S., Potter, W.Z., et al.: Clin. Pharmacol. Ther., *16:* 676-684, 1974.)

that normally reacts with glutathione.[3] The glutathione conjugate subsequently undergoes metabolic transformation to mercapturic acid and cysteine conjugates of acetaminophen.

With acetaminophen overdose, the sulfation pathway becomes saturated, perhaps because of limiting tissue levels of inorganic sulfate.[2] Concomitantly with or subsequent to this event, a larger proportion of acetaminophen is metabolized via the P-450 mixed-function oxidase pathway. Hepatotoxicity occurs when the available pool of glutathione is depleted by about 70%. The toxicity, characterized by diffuse centrilobular necrosis, is thought to be caused by arylation of cellular macromolecules by the reactive acetamidoquinone intermediate.[3]

Treatment of Acetaminophen Overdose

Specific antidote therapy to avoid or lessen the severity of acetaminophen-induced hepatic necrosis is oral administration of N-acetylcysteine (Mucomyst).[3] N-acetylcysteine (NAC) probably serves as a glutathione-surrogate,[4] although it may also act as a precursor for replenishment of hepatic glutathione stores[5] or to enhance sulfate conjugation[6] or both. Other sulfhydryl compounds such as cysteamine and methionine are also effective; glutathione has low efficacy due to poor uptake by hepatocytes.

The time of administration of NAC following an acetaminophen overdose is critical. The greatest efficacy is observed when NAC is administered within eight hours of acetaminophen ingestion. Efficacy declines sharply between 18 and 24 hours after ingestion.[7] Some investigators suggest the antidote is ineffective if administered more than 16 hours following ingestion, whereas others believe some benefit may be gained even with administration as late as 24 hours.

Initial administration of a loading dose (140 mg/kg) of NAC should be followed by 17 maintenance doses (70 mg/kg) given every four hours. Activated charcoal or cathartics should not be given because they interfere with the absorption of NAC. If the patient has ingested a mixed drug overdose, activated charcoal should be given and then removed by lavage before oral administration of NAC.

Assessment of Severity of Acetaminophen Intoxication

Histories of drug ingestion are often unreliable. Moreover, spontaneous or induced vomiting may significantly diminish the amount of drug actually absorbed. Because onset of clinical symptoms is delayed after acetaminophen overdose and because antidote therapy is ineffective after hepatotoxicity develops, early determination of the severity of the overdose is of paramount importance. Serum concentration of acetaminophen is measured to assess magnitude of overdose and probability of hepatic necrosis.

If the time of ingestion is known within two hours and at least four hours have passed, a single serum level can be used to predict the risk of hepatotoxicity, using the Rumack-Matthew nomogram (Figure 1). If acetaminophen concentration and time factor locate above the lower line, treatment with NAC should begin and be maintained for the full course. If results of the serum acetaminophen assay are not locally available within eight hours of ingestion, antidote therapy should begin and continue; therapy can always be discontinued if belated assay results indicate that it is superfluous.

When the time of acetaminophen ingestion is not accurately known, two or more blood specimens obtained at 2-3 hour intervals may be used to estimate the acetaminophen elimination half-life. Hepatotoxicity is more probable when the acetaminophen half-life is >4 hours, and hepatic coma is likely when the half-life is >12 hours. If the initial assay result indicates risk of hepatotoxicity, antidote therapy should not be delayed until the completion of the determination of half-life. Therapy can be discontinued later if not warranted by the analytical data. Some investigators believe the half-life determination to be a better predictor of hepatic necrosis than is interpretation based on a single acetaminophen serum concentration.[8]

Children under the age of nine years rarely develop significant hepatic necrosis, even when the serum acetaminophen concentration is well into the toxic range for adults.[1]

Prediction of risk of hepatotoxicity is based on the measurement of the potentially toxic parent drug and not the nontoxic sulfate, glucuronide, or mercapturic acid conjugates. Therefore, it is essential that the laboratory method measure only unconjugated acetaminophen.[9]

References

1. Rumack, B.H., and Augenstein, W.L.: Acetaminophen. *In:* Clinical Management of Poisoning and Drug Overdose. L.M. Haddad and J.F. Winchester, Eds. Philadelphia, W.B. Saunders Co., 1990.

2. Forrest, J.A.H., Clements, J.A., and Prescott, L.F.: Clinical pharmacokinetics of paracetamol. Clin. Pharmacokinet., *7:* 93-107, 1982.

3. Mitchell, J.R., Thorgeirsson, S.S., Potter, W.Z., et al.: Acetaminophen-induced hepatic injury: Protective role of glutathione in man and rationale for therapy. Clin. Pharmacol. Ther., *16:* 676-684, 1974.

4. Buckpitt, A.R., Rollins, D.E., and Mitchell, J.R.: Varying effects of sulfhydryl nucleophiles on acetaminophen oxidation and sulfhydryl adduct formation. Biochem. Pharmacol., *28:* 2941-2946, 1979.

5. Corcoran, G.B., Todd, E.L., Racz, W.J., et al.: Effects of N-acetylcysteine on the disposition and metabolism of acetaminophen in mice. J. Pharmacol. Exp. Ther., *232:* 857-863, 1985.

6. Lin, J.H., and Levy, G.: Sulfate depletion after acetaminophen administration and replenishment by infusion of sodium sulfate or N-acetylcysteine in rats. Biochem. Pharmacol., *30:* 2723-2725, 1981.

7. Smilkstein, M.J., Knapp, G.L., Kulig, K.W., and Rumack, B.H.: Efficacy of oral N-acetylcysteine in the treatment of acetaminophen overdose: Analysis of the national multicenter study (1976-1985). N. Engl. J. Med., *319:* 1557-1562, 1988.

8. Prescott, L.F., Roscoe, P., Wright, N., and Brown, S.S.: Plasma-paracetamol half-life and hepatic necrosis in patients with paracetamol overdose. Lancet, *1:* 519-522, 1971.

9. Porter, W.H., Stewart, M.J., Chambers, A.M., and Watson, I.D.: In acetaminophen assay, only unconjugated drug should be measured. Clin. Chem., *30:* 1884-1885, 1984.

CHILD WITH LETHARGY AND COMA

Dean A. Arvan, Contributor
William E. Neeley, Reviewer

A previously healthy nine-year-old white female was brought to the Emergency Department because of lethargy and unresponsiveness of about 12 hours' duration. Six days previously she had developed symptoms of an acute febrile respiratory illness that was treated with acetaminophen (Tylenol) and aspirin with some improvement. Approximately 36 hours prior to admission, the patient began vomiting, with 10-12 episodes occurring in the next few hours. There was vague abdominal discomfort but no crampy abdominal pain or diarrhea. On the day of admission, the patient became intermittently lethargic, exhibited inappropriate combative behavior and disorientation, and lapsed into sleep from which she could be aroused only with difficulty. After a quick evaluation by her family physician, she was referred to the hospital Emergency Department.

Questioning of her parents provided no clues about possible exposure to toxic substances. The child had no history or external evidence of trauma. Her past medical history was not contributory. She had had the usual childhood immunizations and except for intercurrent illnesses no previous similar episodes or hospitalizations. Two older siblings were healthy. There were no known inherited diseases in the family. Gestational diabetes had been diagnosed during her mother's last two pregnancies.

The blood pressure was 132/70 mm Hg, temperature 99.7 °F (37.6 °C), pulse 100 BPM, and respiratory rate 32/min. Breathing was deep but not labored. The skin was warm and dry, and her face was flushed. Pupils were equal but reacted sluggishly to light. Funduscopic examination showed no papilledema. Other than mild swelling of nasal passages, the ears, nose, and throat were normal. No significant adenopathy was found. The lungs were clear, and heart size and sounds were normal. The liver was enlarged to 2-3 cm below the costal margin, but the spleen was not palpable. The patient reacted with some combativeness when deep palpation in the right upper quadrant was attempted. There were no abdominal masses. The genitalia were those of a normal female child. Neurological examination revealed no deficits or lateralizing signs, and there were no signs of meningeal irritation. Reflexes were 2+ bilaterally.

The patient was assessed as being in Stage II coma and dehydrated. After obtaining appropriate specimens for laboratory tests, intravenous hydration therapy was begun, and the patient was transferred to the Pediatric Intensive Care Unit (PICU).

The following laboratory results were obtained in the Emergency Department:

Analyte	Value, conventional units	Reference range, conventional units	Value, SI units	Reference range, SI units
Sodium (S)	147 mmol/L	135-145	Same	
Potassium (S)	4.7 mmol/L	3.6-5.3	Same	
Chloride (S)	113 mmol/L	98-108	Same	
CO_2, total (S)	20 mmol/L	22-31	Same	
pH (aB)	7.36	7.34-7.46	Same	
pCO_2 (aB)	30 mm Hg	36-46	4.0 kPa	4.8-6.1

Analyte	Value, conventional units	Reference range, conventional units	Value, SI units	Reference range, SI units
pO₂ (aB)	95 mm Hg	95-100	12.7 kPa	12.7-13.3
Base excess	-6 mmol/L	(-3)-(+1)	Same	
Osmolality (S)	308 mOsm/kg	278-297	Same	
Glucose (S)	76 mg/dL	65-100	4.2 mmol/L	3.6-5.6
Urea nitrogen (S)	23 mg/dL	8-21	8.2 mmol urea/L	2.9-7.5
Creatinine (S)	0.9 mg/dL	0.5-1.0	80 µmol/L	44-88
Protein, total (S)	6.8 g/dL	5.8-7.8	68 g/L	58-78
Albumin (S)	4.8 g/dL	3.5-4.6	48 g/L	35-46
Bilirubin, total (S)	0.5 mg/dL	0.2-1.4	8.5 µmol/L	3-24
AST (S)	830 U/L	10-36	13.84 µkat/L	0.17-0.60
ALT (S)	624 U/L	9-41	10.40 µkat/L	0.15-0.68
GGT (S)	58 U/L	4-25	0.97 µkat/L	0.07-0.42
LDH (S)	582 U/L	100-190	9.70 µkat/L	1.67-3.17
ALP (S)	190 U/L	120-460	3.2 µkat/L	2.0-7.7
Ammonia (P)	272 µg/dL	10-63	160 µmol/L	6-37
Prothrombin time (P)	13.8 s	9.5-12.5	Same	
Hemoglobin (B)	14.2 g/dL	11.5-15.5	8.81 mmol/L	7.14-9.62
Leukocyte count (B)	8.6 x 10³/µL	4.8-14.5	8.6 x 10⁹/L	4.8-14.5

A differential blood count and urinalysis were within normal limits. A chest X-ray showed a streaky infiltrate in the left lower lobe. A spinal tap yielded normal opening pressure and clear, colorless fluid. Laboratory tests performed on various types of specimens gave the following results:

Analyte	Value, conventional units	Reference range, conventional units	Value, SI units	Reference range, SI units
Mononuclear cells (CSF)	2/µL	0-5	2 x 10⁶/L	0-5
Gram stain (CSF)	Negative	Negative		
Glucose (CSF)	58 mg/dL	40-70	3.2 mmol/L	2.2-3.9
Protein (CSF)	11 mg/dL	15-45	1.10 g/L	1.50-4.50
Viral culture				
CSF	Negative	Negative		
Nasopharyngeal swab	Negative	Negative		
Blood	Negative	Negative		
Cold agglutinin titer (S)	<1:8	<1:32		
Acetaminophen (S)	Negative	Negative		
Salicylate (S)	Negative	Negative		
Drug screen (U)	Positive for acetaminophen and salicylate	Negative		

Quantitative plasma and urine amino acid and organic acid analyses showed diffuse increases in several amino acids, including arginine, citrulline, and lysine. The pattern was not diagnostic of a specific disorder of amino acid metabolism, and the urinary amino acid pattern was essentially normal. The urine organic acid profile determined by capillary gas chromatography/mass spectrometry showed moderate lactic aciduria. The pattern was interpreted as being consistent with lactic acidosis. Urine orotic acid was normal.

The patient improved with intravenous fluids (10% dextrose in half-normal saline with 20 mmol KCl/L) and antibiotics. Plasma ammonia and serum levels of hepatic enzymes decreased rapidly in the next 48 hours, and she was discharged on the fourth day with no detectable residual neurological or other symptoms.

Differential Diagnosis

In formulating a differential diagnosis in this case, the clinical history is revealing and far more helpful than the physical findings. The following elements should be considered in formulating a list of diagnostic possibilities:

> Patient age at onset of the disease
> Lack of significant family or prior history of similar episodes
> The antecedent febrile, presumably viral, illness treated with antipyretics
> Relatively sudden and rapid progression through stages characterized by
>   vomiting, delirium, combative behavior, and semicoma
> Paucity of physical findings

The initial impression was that the patient had an infectious process, a mixed acid-base disorder, and was dehydrated. In addition, hyperammonemia, probably of hepatic origin, was thought to be a contributing factor to the patient's semicomatose state. Other causes, however, required exclusion. The differential diagnosis included the following:

> Mycoplasma pneumonia with possible encephalitis
> Reye's syndrome
> Inborn error of metabolism
> Acetaminophen or salicylate toxicity

The clinical history and absence of laboratory confirmation for an intracranial infection, exposure to toxins, or an inherited disorder in amino acid or organic acid metabolism led to the diagnosis of *Reye's syndrome.*

Definition of the Disease

Reye's syndrome is an acute, generally self-limited but potentially fatal, noninflammatory hepatic encephalopathy occurring principally in children over two years of age.[1] Characteristically, the syndrome follows an antecedent viral illness (e.g., influenza, varicella, adenovirus, or other infections), from which the patient appears at first to be recovering, only to develop within a week or less symptoms heralding encephalopathy. Patients may progress rapidly (i.e., within hours) through various stages of coma. Fatality rates are much lower now (10-15%) than 10-15 years ago (40-50%). Resolution of the encephalopathy generally leaves no permanent neurological deficits or liver function abnormalities. Cerebral edema is present, but the most prominent histological change is diffuse microvesicular infiltration of fat primarily in the liver but also in kidney, brain, heart, and pancreas. Characteristically, little or no infiltration of inflammatory cells or necrosis is seen. The most consistent ultrastructural abnormality is in liver mitochondria, which show swelling, variation in size and shape, and fragmentation of cristae and outer membrane. Among the biochemical consequences of these lesions are decreases in several mitochondrial enzymes including those of the pyruvate dehydrogenase complex. The changes are reversible, are generally attributed to the hyperammonemia, and may account for the serious derangements of glucose and fatty acid metabolism and resulting clinical symptoms. Other consistent changes are glycogen depletion and increased numbers of peroxisomes.

The precise etiology of Reye's syndrome is unknown. Strong epidemiological evidence points to a close linkage between the development of Reye's and use of salicylates to treat intercurrent viral illnesses in children.[2] Although a genetic susceptibility has been postulated, direct evidence for it is lacking. In the past, some patients with inborn errors of metabolism, particularly defects in urea cycle enzymes, were probably diagnosed incorrectly as having Reye's syndrome, but appropriate testing showed them to have hyperammonemic encephalopathy resulting from such defects.[3,4] Accurate diagnosis as well as a public campaign to avoid use of aspirin to treat children with acute respiratory or other viral illnesses accounts for the recent marked drop in both incidence and fatality rates. Rarely, Reye's syndrome has been reported in infants or adults. The reason for its predilection for children, especially white children, is unclear.

Clinical Features. Signs and symptoms of Reye's syndrome are typically those of any hepatic encephalopathy. Thus, clinical presentation is frequently identical to that of any disorder associated with hyperammonemia (see *Case 55*). Absence of a history of prior episodes of hyperammonemia or protein intolerance and the rapid development of vomiting, irritability, combative behavior, lethargy, dehydration, seizures, and coma that occur in a child immediately after an apparently resolving viral illness strongly suggest a presumptive diagnosis of Reye's syndrome. Use of aspirin in the course of the antecedent viral illness should further raise the suspicion. Severity and duration of symptoms and depth of coma vary widely and unpredictably. Progression to deep coma and death may occur within hours. Although this patient's history and clinical presentation are typical, atypical cases are common. Differentiation of Reye's syndrome from cases of encephalitis or of hyperammonemic coma such as those caused by a deficiency of one of the urea cycle enzymes (e.g., ornithine transcarbamylase [OTC], particularly of the late onset type) or of medium-chain acyl-CoA dehydrogenase, is essential.[5] The diagnosis of Reye's syndrome is, therefore, made only after other possibilities are excluded by history and appropriate diagnostic testing.

Laboratory Diagnosis

Routine laboratory measurements confirmed the clinical impression of dehydration in this patient. The markers were elevated serum sodium, chloride, osmolality, and urea nitrogen, the last associated with a normal creatinine. Whereas arterial blood pH was at the lower end of the reference range, the negative "base excess" is consistent with a metabolic acidosis, compensated by hyperventilation, and explains the low pCO_2. Such findings, of course, are not diagnostic of Reye's syndrome and could be consistent with a number of other possibilities, particularly salicylate toxicity. Subsequent serum and urine analyses established the presence of lactic acidosis and ruled out salicylate and acetaminophen toxicity. The normal serum glucose is helpful, because it tends to rule out inborn errors of metabolism resulting from disorders in fatty acid oxidation (e.g., carnitine deficiency, propionic acidemia) that are also associated with hyperammonemia. Hypoglycemia is rare in Reye's syndrome and is seen primarily in infants and children less than two years old, the group in which inborn errors of metabolism are most frequently confused with Reye's syndrome. In these young children, liver biopsy to locate the typical microvesicular fatty infiltration of Reye's syndrome may be required to differentiate it from other disorders. The generally negative neurological examination and lack of abnormalities in the cerebrospinal fluid virtually rule out an intracerebral infectious process as a cause of this patient's coma.

Plasma ammonia was moderately increased in this case, and the level was consistent with the patient's level of coma at the time of admission. Hyperammonemia is present in all patients with Reye's syndrome at the time of presentation; indeed, diagnosis is virtually impossible in its absence, although ammonia elevations may be transient. There is a close relationship between plasma ammonia levels and depth of coma. Ammonia concentrations > 350 µg/dL (>206 µmol/L) are associated with poor prognosis.[1]

Hyperammonemia as well as lactic acidemia and elevations of free fatty acids are frequently observed and are thought to be the result of mitochondrial damage. Transient reduction in tissue levels of mitochondrial enzymes, particularly those of the urea cycle, have been documented and may explain the hyperammonemia. The fatty acidemia can be explained by a block in mitochondrial β-oxidation compounded by release of fatty acids from peripheral tissues due to anorexia and vomiting.

Liver function test abnormalities in this case are entirely consistent with, but not diagnostic of, Reye's syndrome. As in other cases, increase in serum aminotransferases (AST, ALT), γ-glutamyltransferase (GGT), and lactate dehydrogenase (LDH) are in the range usually seen in patients with moderate to severe acute hepatocellular damage even though routine histological examination reveals only minimal necrosis or inflammation. Aminotransferases frequently reach serum levels observed in patients with viral hepatitis. The absence of jaundice and the rapid rate of increase in serum enzymes are more characteristic of toxic or hypoxic rather than viral hepatocellular damage. Mitochondrial enzymes (e.g., glutamate dehydrogenase, OTC) are released from liver cells, and marked increases may be found in serum, a finding consistent with mitochondrial damage observed by electron microscopy.[6] Typically, bilirubin levels are normal or only minimally elevated, probably because of the rapid onset of liver cell damage; the finding helps differentiate this type of liver damage from that usually associated with viral hepatitis. Prothrombin time, although usually prolonged, is generally unresponsive to vitamin K administration. Excessive spontaneous bleeding, however, is rare. The similarity in the array of liver function test abnormalities between Reye's syndrome and other types of hyperammonemic coma is obvious (see *Case 55*).

Differentiating among causes of hyperammonemic coma is primarily based on history, but the results of amino acid and organic acid analyses may be helpful. Such measurements, as well as liver biopsy to identify microvesicular fatty infiltration or to assay specific urea cycle enzymes, are usually reserved for difficult cases, particularly for those patients under two years of age. In this case, the absence of specific elevation of urinary orotic acid and the diffuse increase in several plasma amino acids, notably lysine, tend to rule out the more common urea cycle enzyme defects in which plasma citrulline and arginine are low and urinary orotate is high. Absence of elevated urinary organic acids also rules out enzyme defects in the metabolic paths of fatty acids, namely those leading to carnitine deficiency or to propionic or methylmalonic acidemias that are associated with hypoglycemia and unexplained metabolic acidosis.[1,7]

Treatment

Generally, patients with a presumptive diagnosis of Reye's syndrome are treated in intensive care units because they must be closely monitored. Treatment is entirely supportive and depends primarily on the patient's coma stage. Glucose infusion (with hypertonic dextrose with added insulin) and correction of electrolyte and acid-base abnormalities are essential. Insertion of arterial and central venous pressure lines, a nasogastric tube, Foley catheter, or endotracheal intubation with mechanical ventilation may be required. Neomycin is administered via nasogastric tube to eliminate ammonia-producing bacteria from the gut and thus reduce ammonia absorption and lower plasma ammonia levels. Severe coagulation abnormalities may require correction by infusion of fresh-frozen plasma or plasma exchange. Finally, intraventricular pressure monitoring in patients in advanced stages of coma and intravenous infusion of mannitol may be needed to reduce intracranial pressure.

References

1. Trauner, D.A.: Reye's syndrome. Curr. Probl. Pediatr., *12:* 1-31, 1982.

2. Hurwitz, E.S., Barrett, M.J., Bregman, D., et al.: Public Health Service study on Reye's syndrome and medications: Report of the main study. JAMA, *257:* 1905-1911, 1987.

3. Greene, C.L., Blitzer, M.G., and Shapira, E.: Inborn errors of metabolism and Reye's syndrome: Differential diagnosis. J. Pediatr., *113:* 156-159, 1988.

4. Gauthier, M., Guay, J., Lacroix, J., et al.: Reye's syndrome: A reappraisal of diagnosis of 49 presumptive cases. Am. J. Dis. Child., *143:* 1181-1185, 1989.

5. Rowe, P.C., Newman, S.L., and Brusilow, S.W.: Natural history of symptomatic partial ornithine transcarbamylase deficiency. N. Engl. J. Med., *314:* 541-547, 1986.

6. Holt, J.T., Arvan, D.A., and Mayer, T.K.: Masking by enzyme inhibitor of raised serum glutamate dehydrogenase activity in Reye's syndrome. Lancet, *2:* 4-7, 1983.

7. Romshe, C.A., Hifty, M.D., McClung, H.J., et al.: Amino acid pattern in Reye's syndrome: Comparison with clinically significant entities. J. Pediatr., *98:* 788-790, 1981.

LOW BACK PAIN

A. Ralph Henderson, Contributor

A 64-year-old general practitioner, otherwise in good health, had a three-month history of low back pain (that did not radiate or worsen with movement) and a family history of carcinoma of the prostate (father and uncle). There were no urinary symptoms such as incontinence, poor flow, or difficulty of micturition. The differential diagnosis of low back pain includes a very wide range of conditions (Table 1). His partner in the practice took blood samples and performed a general health review. Because of the history, the absence of other symptoms, and the patient's age, the general practitioner suspected a neoplastic cause.

Table 1. CAUSES OF BACK PAIN

Traumatic, mechanical, or degenerative (e.g., low back strain,
    degenerative disease of the spine)
Metabolic (e.g., osteomalacia, osteoporosis)
Infection of bone (e.g., osteomyelitis, tuberculosis)
Cardiac and vascular (e.g., spinal hemorrhage, dissecting aneurysm)
Gastrointestinal (e.g., peptic ulcers, pancreatitis)
Renal diseases
Drugs
Unknown causes (e.g., ankylosing spondylitis, ulcerative colitis)
Neoplastic (e.g., metastatic carcinoma, multiple myeloma)
Psychogenic

Blood pressure and pulse were normal. No abnormalities were detected on physical examination except that a firm prostatic nodule was palpated on rectal examination. The blood count, erythrocyte sedimentation rate (ESR), electrolytes, urea nitrogen, and creatinine were normal. Significant laboratory findings included the following:

Analyte	Value, conventional units	Reference range, conventional units	Value, SI units	Reference range, SI units
Calcium (S)	9.2 mg/dL	8.5-10.5	2.29 mmol/L	2.12-2.62
Protein, total (S)	7.4 g/dL	6.0-8.0	74 g/L	60-80
Albumin (S)	4.2 g/dL	3.5-4.9	42 g/L	35-49
Protein electrophoresis (S)	Within normal limits			
ALP (S)	96 U/L	18-113	1.6 μkat/L	0.3-1.9
Isoenzyme pattern (S)	Within normal limits			
Acid phosphatase, prostatic (Immunoassay) (S)	2.5 μg/L	<3.0	Same	
Prostate-specific antigen (PSA) (S)	95 μg/L	<4.0	Same	

Serum calcium was measured because metastases were suspected, and hypercalcemia is often a feature of secondary neoplastic spread to the bone. Evaluation of serum protein levels and electrophoretic pattern was appropriate because there is a correlation between serum calcium and albumin levels, and symptoms of bone pain may indicate multiple myeloma. Alkaline phosphatase isoenzyme pattern was important in the context of bone metastases.

On the basis of the physical examination and the very high PSA level, the patient was seen by a urological surgeon who confirmed the presence of a firm nodule in the prostate, thus establishing a probable diagnosis of carcinoma of the prostate. The nodule was biopsied, but findings were negative. A urinary infection arose as a result of the biopsy. Later, a transrectal ultrasonographic scan identified a "dark" area. Three biopsies were taken from it, and malignancy (carcinoma of the prostate) was confirmed. A nuclear magnetic resonance (NMR) study for secondary deposits was undertaken because the high PSA level suggested metastasis; however, none was detected.

A total prostatectomy was ruled out because the high PSA level suggested metastases. The patient was started on cyproterone acetate (a potent antiandrogen), 100 mg twice daily, and was referred to the Division of Oncology for radiotherapy. The radiotherapy staff first identified the exact location of the prostate by computed tomography (CT) before commencing radiotherapy. After discontinuing the cyproterone tablets, the patient received five daily radiotherapy treatments each week for six weeks. A sterile cystitis, with frequency, urgency, and strangury (painful excretion of urine due to spasmodic contraction of the urethra and bladder), occurred as a result of radiotherapy. Later, proctitis developed and produced diarrhea, flatulence, and tenesmus (painful defecation caused by spasm of the sphincter ani muscles).

The nodule was no longer palpable four months after radiotherapy, and PSA was undetectable. Follow-up was therefore arranged at three-month intervals; PSA remained undetectable during the following year.

Epidemiology of Prostatic Cancer

Prostatic cancer is now the most common cancer among males in the United States. Its incidence increases with age. Annually, nearly 400 cases are diagnosed per 100,000 men. Thus, in the United States over 100,000 new cases are identified yearly. Adenocarcinoma of the prostate is responsible for about 11% of cancer deaths in men (nearly 30,000 yearly), making it the third leading cause of such deaths after lung and colon cancer.[1]

One of every 12 white males and one of every 11 black males will develop prostatic cancer. Afro-Americans have the highest rates in the world for cancer of the prostate. However, the risk of dying from this cancer is only one out of 40 for Caucasian males and one out of 25 for Afro-American males; only one-third of all men diagnosed with prostatic cancer will actually die of it. There is a distinct racial and geographical prevalence of prostatic cancer. For example, it is rare in indigenous Asians, but the prevalence increases in those Asians who have migrated to the United States.

Pathology of Prostatic Cancer

Prostatic cancer[2] commonly arises in the peripheral posterior zone of the gland, allowing it to be palpated during rectal examination. Most lesions (90%) are adenocarcinomas that show well-defined gland patterns. Most are well differentiated, but some are not; these tend to grow in cords, nests, or sheets. Malignancy is indicated by the usual cytological features and by invasion of the perineurial spaces or the capsule with its lymphatic and vascular channels.

Spread occurs both by direct invasion and through the blood stream. Direct invasion may involve the neck of the bladder, causing urinary obstruction. Hematogenous spread is largely to bone structures such as the lumbar spine, femur, pelvis, and thoracic spine. These metastases may be osteolytic; but osteoblastic lesions also occur, and when these are detected, they strongly suggest the presence of prostatic cancer.

Regrettably, over 75% of all prostatic tumors that present clinically are past the early (A and B) stages. Typical symptoms at presentation include difficulty with micturition, dysuria, frequency, or hematuria. Some patients present with back pain due to vertebral metastases.

It is generally accepted that the majority of Stage A_1 tumors show latency; asymptomatic tumors are discovered at autopsy or following removal of hyperplastic tissue. It is estimated that a third of all males over age 50 carry a Stage A tumor. This incidence increases with age, approaching two-thirds of all males by age 80. Many of these latent tumors fail to progress to clinical disease over a 10-year period.

Grading and Staging

Like other tumors, prostatic cancer is graded and staged. Several grading schemes have been proposed. One such scheme is shown in Table 2. However, as techniques of investigation become more sensitive, such schemes require modification to incorporate these newer modalities. For example, the development of small probes for transrectal magnetic resonance imaging (MRI) has improved detectability of prostatic tumors. The results of routine use of PSA analysis, with its increased power of diagnostic resolution, have to be incorporated into current grading schemes. Finally, multiple biopsies can be obtained without anesthesia by using a biopsy gun. This gun replaces the more conventional large-bore core biopsy and fine-needle aspiration smear techniques. Its use appears to have increased the detection rate for such tumors.

Once prostatic cancer is diagnosed, the tumor must be staged in order to plan treatment. The process of staging requires a radionuclide bone scan. If the scan is negative, then CT or MRI or both are necessary to evaluate the pelvic lymph nodes. The extent of local disease may also be assessed by ultrasonography. Pelvic lymphadenectomy may also be required as a preliminary to radical prostatectomy.

Prostatic Acid Phosphatase

Although there are many acid phosphatase enzymes in human tissues, the acid phosphatase found in both the normal and malignant prostate has several unique characteristics that allow its specific quantitation. Enzyme activity methods capitalize on a selective substrate (the Roy method) or inhibition by tartrate ion to increase assay specificity; immunoassay methods determine enzyme mass rather than activity.[3] Until very recently, serum prostatic acid phosphatase was the most commonly used marker for adenocarcinoma of the prostate. Clinicians have, however, lost confidence in its reliability as more and more cases with advanced stages of cancer were found to have activities or levels within reference ranges. The discovery of prostate-specific antigen (PSA), a more sensitive marker for prostate cancer, tends to relegate determination of acid phosphatase to a lesser role, even though both are still often ordered together.

Table 2. CLINICAL STAGING OF PROSTATIC CANCER[1,3,4]

Clinical Stage	Description and Result of Digital Rectal Examination	Frequency of Prostatic Acid Phosphatase Elevation	Frequency of PSA Elevation	Bone Scan	Frequency of Lymph Node Metastases (%)
A_1	Microscopic, not clinically palpable, with focus in <5% of tissue examined	11%	67%	N	5
A_2	Microscopic, not clinically palpable, with multiple areas of >5%				25
B_1	Palpable, macroscopic tumor ≤1.5 cm in diameter, only in one lobe	22%	73%	N	8-21
B_2	Palpable, macroscopic tumor >1.5 cm in diameter, or several nodules in both lobes				14-45
C_1	Tumor with extracapsular extension but still clinically localized, palpably extending into seminal vesicle but not fixed to pelvic wall	39%	80%	N	40-80
C_2	Tumor with extracapsular extension still clinically localized, palpably extending into seminal vesicle but fixed to pelvic wall				
D_1	Demonstrated metastatic tumor with metastases, limited to 3 pelvic nodes or fewer	58%	88%	N	100
D_2	Demonstrated metastatic tumor with extensive nodal or extrapelvic (e.g., to bone) metastases			+	

Prostate-Specific Antigen

PSA is a serine protease uniquely synthesized in the cells of the prostatic epithelium.[4] It occurs in no other normal or cancerous tissue. It has been estimated that prostatic cancer produces at least 10 times more PSA than does normal prostatic tissue. Prostatic tissue injury or infection (prostatitis) may cause a transient elevation of serum PSA. Major trauma, such as multiple prostatic biopsies or total prostatectomy, may elevate the serum PSA levels 50-fold for up to two weeks. The serum half-life of PSA is about three days.

Nodular hyperplasia, by definition, increases the mass of the prostate and thus causes increased serum PSA levels; on the other hand, 30% of localized prostatic tumors have normal serum PSA levels. Indeed, only about 40% of Stage A or B tumors (see Table 2) have been found to be associated with PSA levels exceeding 10 µg/L (reference range, <4 µg/L). PSA has a role as a sensitive marker to follow treatment. Following successful radical prostatectomy for a Grade A or B tumor, the serum PSA falls to undetectable levels within a few days of the operation. A measurable level of PSA after the operation indicates that residual prostatic cancer cells remain. When radiotherapy is used, as in the present case of proven or suspected Grade C or D tumor, serial monitoring of serum PSA after therapy is valuable. Levels decline more slowly with radiotherapy than after surgery. Rising levels indicate failure of local treatment or the occurrence of systemic metastases.

Diagnosis of Prostatic Cancer

The need for multiple tests is underscored by a recent study[5] in which 12 of 37 men with prostatic cancer had normal findings on rectal examination. Five of the 12 had elevated PSA levels, and seven of them had abnormal ultrasonographic results. Serum PSA is not sufficiently sensitive to be used alone as a screening test for prostatic cancer. For example, of 61 men with prostatic cancer, 21% had serum PSA values <4.0 µg/L.[5] Patients with nodular prostatic hyperplasia may also have elevated PSA values, and such patients would be prime candidates for such screening. Accordingly, current opinion suggests the complementary use of a number of tests — rectal examination, PSA and prostatic acid phosphatase levels, and an ultrasonographic examination.[5]

Several diagnostic modalities have been described, but most of them still need to be assessed for effectiveness. The current approach is by receiver operating characteristic (ROC) curve analysis. In this process the tests to be compared are performed, preferably in a blinded fashion, on all patients and then their respective sensitivity and specificity are calculated for a range of decision thresholds (or cutoff points). An example of this process, for the diagnosis of carcinoma of the prostate, is referenced.[6]

Creatine kinase isoenzyme 1 (CK-BB) has often been found to be elevated in prostatic cancer and has been suggested as a tumor marker. However, this marker has not been subjected to the rigorous assessment necessary to establish its diagnostic utility.[6]

Benign Enlargement of the Prostate

Nodular prostatic hyperplasia (also incorrectly called benign prostatic hyperplasia or BPH) is extremely common in males over the age of 50. Autopsy findings suggest a prevalence of 70% by age 60 and 90% by the eighth decade.[2] Nodular hyperplasia is characterized by the formation of large nodules in the periurethral region of the prostate. Such nodules may be large enough to cause obstruction of the urethra.

Clinical presentation of nodular hyperplasia relates to compression of the urethra that causes difficulty in urination and retention of urine in the bladder. Retention may lead to distention and hypertrophy of the bladder, urinary infection, cystitis, and renal infections. Nodular hypertrophy is not a premalignant lesion, but cancer may be found in a hypertrophied prostate purely as a result of the age-related incidence of both conditions.

Discussion

The case described here is all too typical a presentation — carcinoma of the prostate detected when too advanced for surgical treatment. Annual rectal examination has been suggested for all asymptomatic males over the age of 40.[5] Presently some 12,000 cases are estimated to be detected per year by rectal examination. In view of the shortcomings noted above for rectal examination, multiple tests seem more effective for screening for the disease. However, more studies are needed to determine the cost/benefit ratio of multiple tests used in extensive screening. For patients with symptoms of prostatic hypertrophy or prostatitis that may mask cancer, transrectal ultrasonography and PSA assay should be included in a workup.

Treatment

Treatment of carcinoma of the prostate depends on the grade and stage of the tumor. If the tumor is localized within the capsule of the prostate and there is no evidence of metastases, radical prostatectomy is curative. The 15-year disease-specific survival rate is about 90% for such cases. If there are metastases and the tumor has spread beyond the prostatic capsule, then antitestosterone therapy or radiotherapy is considered as alternative or complementary treatment.

References

1.   Gites, R.F.: Carcinoma of the prostate. N. Engl. J. Med., *302:* 236-245, 1991.

2.   Cotran, R.S., Kumar, V., and Robbins, S.L.: Robbins Pathologic Basis of Disease, 4th ed. Philadelphia, W.B. Saunders Co., 1989.

3.   Moss, D.W., Henderson, A.R., and Kachmar, J.F.: Enzymes. *In:* Textbook of Clinical Chemistry. N.W. Tietz, Ed. Philadelphia, W.B. Saunders Co., 1986.

4.   Oesterling, J.E.: Prostate specific antigen: A critical assessment of the most useful tumor marker for adenocarcinoma of the prostate. J. Urol., *145:* 907-923, 1991.

5.   Catalona, W.J., Smith, D.S., Ratliff, T.L., et al.: Measurement of prostate-specific antigen in serum as a screening test for prostate cancer. N. Engl. J. Med., *324:* 1156-1161, 1991.

6.   Chybowski, F.M., Keller, J.J.L., Bergstralh, E.J., et al.: Predicting radionuclide bone scan findings in patients with newly diagnosed, untreated prostate cancer: Prostate-specific antigen is superior to all other clinical parameters. J. Urol., *145:* 313-318, 1991.

HEART FAILURE IN A MIDDLE-AGED WOMAN

Jonathan F. Plehn, Contributor
Gibbons G. Cornwell, III, Contributor

A 58-year-old white female presented with a complaint of a decline in exercise tolerance that had progressed to severe limitation in performing her routine housework. She had been active and vigorous until eight months prior to presentation. Her symptoms had started with a nonproductive cough and shortness of breath. She had gradually given up her regular walks and had noticed fatigue and weakness in her upper arms upon minimal exertion. Since her symptoms had worsened over the next six months, she had been evaluated by a pulmonary specialist who had performed pulmonary function tests and a bronchoscopy. The findings were normal, but the electrocardiogram (ECG) showed poor R-wave progression. Her physician was concerned about a silent infarct.

The patient was admitted to the hospital with further progression of her fatigue and shortness of breath. At that time, she gave a history of a 16-lb (7.3-kg) weight loss, numbness in her feet of more than one year's duration, chronic diarrhea, easy satiety, dry eyes, dry mouth, and occasional difficulty in focusing her vision. Past medical history included arthritis of hips, elbows, and shoulders for many years, and a bilateral carpal tunnel release one year previously for nocturnal hand numbness. In addition, she had a three-year history of hypertension that had spontaneously resolved over the last year. The family history was significant for hypertension, coronary artery disease, and malignancy. The patient denied the use of alcohol or tobacco. Her medications included furosemide, potassium chloride, nitroglycerin, and diphenoxylate.

On physical examination, the patient had a blood pressure of 95/60 mm Hg in the supine position with a regular pulse of 100 BPM. Examination of the neck demonstrated jugular venous distinction to 8-10 cm above the sternomanubrial notch in the 45-degree recumbent position. Cardiac examination revealed a hyperdynamic, nondisplaced apex with normal first and second heart sounds and no evidence of third or fourth sounds, murmurs, or rubs. There were bibasilar inspiratory rales on lung examination. On neurological testing there was some decreased sensation to light touch and pin-prick below the knees. Examination of the extremities failed to demonstrate edema, but small Heberden's nodes were evident.

The patient had a normal hemoglobin, leukocyte count, and platelet count. Serum electrolytes, urea nitrogen, creatinine, glucose, bilirubin, and alkaline phosphatase (ALP) were normal. The aspartate aminotransferase (AST) and alanine aminotransferase (ALT) were twice normal levels. Serum protein electrophoresis was normal, and a 24-h urine collection contained no protein. A chest X-ray showed bilateral Kerley B lines and an alveolar fluid pattern consistent with pulmonary edema secondary to diffuse failure. An ECG showed normal sinus rhythm with low voltage, right axis deviation, and poor R-wave progression across the precordium.

The patient died of progressive right- and left-sided heart failure less than one year later.

Differential Diagnosis

This patient's main complaints were fatigue and weakness, weight loss, dyspnea on exertion, and diarrhea. Less severe symptoms included numbness of the feet, dry eyes, dry mouth, and occasional difficulty with visual focusing. With the exception of the diarrhea, the major complaints could all be related to a problem with the cardiopulmonary system. Although there are many causes of diarrhea, a combination of diarrhea, difficulty in accommodation (focusing), decreased lacrimation and salivation, and paresthesias suggest autonomic and sensory peripheral neuropathy. In addition, there is considerable clinical evidence that this patient had biventricular heart failure. Right-sided failure is documented by jugular venous distention indicating an elevation in right atrial and right ventricular diastolic pressure. Left-sided heart failure is demonstrated by the presence of inspiratory rales or crackles with chest film findings of pulmonary alveolar fluid and lymphatic distention (Kerley B lines) caused by elevated left atrial and left ventricular diastolic pressure. The patient's symptoms of fatigue, exercise intolerance, and exertional dyspnea are all consistent with left-sided heart failure as well.

Determination of the cause of heart failure is greatly aided by the patient's history. Most important, the spontaneous disappearance of hypertension is an ominous finding suggestive of either autonomic neuropathy and uncontrolled vasodilation or a reduction in cardiac output. The ECG finding of diffuse low voltage is found in a number of conditions including obesity, chronic lung disease, hypothyroidism, multiple myocardial infarctions, and cardiomyopathy.

The constellation of findings — heart failure, spontaneous resolution of hypertension, and reduction of ECG voltage — suggests that this patient had developed a cardiomyopathy (disease of the heart muscle). There are three major classifications of cardiomyopathy: dilated, hypertrophic, and restrictive. *Dilated cardiomyopathy* most often either is caused by multiple myocardial infarctions or is idiopathic and possibly related to a viral infection. In patients with a dilated cardiomyopathy, there is a reduction in ventricular systolic function and, consequently, stroke volume. Physical examination reveals a displaced cardiac apex, consistent with ventricular dilation and, often, a third heart sound caused by ventricular volume overload. In *hypertrophic cardiomyopathy* the ventricular walls are thickened (as a result of congenital abnormality or hypertension) and the ventricular cavity is small or normal in size. There may be obstruction of the left ventricular outflow tract that causes a systolic, ejection-type murmur. The apex is not displaced, and left ventricular hypertrophy is often apparent on the ECG. A fourth heart sound is frequently audible on auscultation and indicates a stiff ventricle. The chest film is usually unrevealing.

Restrictive cardiomyopathy can be caused by endomyocardial fibrosis or fibroelastosis, but in the Western world it is most frequently caused by primary (AL) amyloidosis. (See Table 1 for nomenclature and classification of amyloidoses and amyloid proteins.) In this condition the ventricular walls are infiltrated by the amyloid protein and the ventricular chambers become small and noncompliant. Ventricular ejection fraction is usually maintained at normal or mildly reduced levels until the late stage of the disease. Heart failure results from diastolic abnormalities of ventricular filling (restriction) caused by myocardial or endocardial infiltration, leading to elevated pressures in all four cardiac chambers. Atrial infiltration is almost always found at autopsy and may account for the reduced contribution of the atrial kick to ventricular filling. On physical examination, signs of right-sided heart failure are usually more impressive than are signs of left-sided heart failure. There is often peripheral edema and jugular venous distention. Patients are often hypotensive for the reasons mentioned above. The cardiac apex is rarely displaced. The ECG demonstrates low voltage in advanced stages of the disease, and atrial fibrillation or premature ventricular contractions may be present.

Table 1. **NOMENCLATURE AND CLASSIFICATION OF AMYLOIDOSES AND AMYLOID PROTEINS** [1]

Clinical Condition	Protein Precursor	Amyloid Protein
Systemic Amyloidosis		
Primary (idiopathic) Myeloma- or macroglobulinemia-associated	IgL (κ or λ)	AL
Secondary (reactive)	Apo SAA	AA
Senile	Transthyretin	ATTR
Familial		
Neuropathic		
Portuguese, Japanese, Swedish	Transthyretin variant	ATTR
Finnish	Gelsolin	AGel
Cardiomyopathic	Transthyretin variant	ATTR
Nephropathic		
Familial Mediterranean fever	Apo SAA	AA
Familial amyloidotic nephropathy	Apo SAA	AA
Vascular		
Icelandic	Cystatin C variant	ACys
Dutch	β protein variant	Aβ
Associated with chronic dialysis	β_2-Microglobulin	Aβ_2M
*Localized Amyloids**		
Alzheimer's disease Down syndrome Hereditary cerebral hemorrhage	β protein	Aβ
Spongioform encephalopathies (Creutzfeldt-Jakob disease, kuru, etc.)	Scrapie proteins	AScr
Medullary carcinoma of thyroid	(Pro)calcitonin	ACal
Isolated atrial amyloid	Atrial natriuretic factor	AANF
Diabetes type II Insulinoma	Islet amyloid polypeptide	AIAPP

---

*There are many other forms of localized amyloid (e.g., aortic, adrenal, heart valve, joint, seminal vesicle, skin) for which specific amyloid proteins have not been identified.

The history and physical examination are extremely important in differentiating these three types of cardiomyopathy; however, the best test for making an objective diagnosis is echocardiography. In this patient the echocardiogram showed normal ventricular chamber size with thick ventricular walls that demonstrated a scintillation or sparkling pattern. There was normal systolic function of both ventricles and biatrial enlargement. On Doppler examination there was mild mitral regurgitation with mitral valve thickening seen on two-dimensional echocardiogram. Absence of the atrial kick was also found on Doppler examination. These findings, in combination, are virtually pathognomonic of cardiac amyloidosis.

The echocardiogram findings of normal ventricular size and function exclude the possibility of a dilated cardiomyopathy. The thick ventricular walls can be seen in hypertrophic or amyloid-restrictive cardiomyopathy. However, the myocardial sparkle, the depression in atrial systolic function, and the associated low voltage on ECG all point to the diagnosis of amyloid cardiomyopathy.

Cardiac catheterization was performed on this patient. It showed normal coronary arteries and mildly elevated pressures in all four chambers but not the equilibration of chamber pressures found in about 50% of restrictive cardiomyopathy cases.

Definitive diagnosis of amyloid cardiomyopathy was made by percutaneous endomyocardial biopsy of the right ventricular septum. This procedure is performed under fluoroscopic or echocardiographic visualization at the time of catheterization and uses a catheter-mounted bioptome. Congo red staining showed green birefringent positivity in polarized light (characteristic of amyloid deposits) in the vessel walls and interstitium.

Discussion

Amyloidosis is a family of diseases of systemic (multiple organ involvement) or localized (single organ involvement) type. All amyloid deposits are predominantly extracellular and consist of long, thin, nonbranching fibrils. The systemic amyloids are derived from various circulating protein precursors, whereas the localized amyloids are formed from proteins synthesized in the organ of deposit. The most common forms of systemic amyloidosis are primary (AL) amyloidosis, secondary (AA) amyloidosis, and senile systemic amyloidosis. On the basis of clinical presentation, this patient is most likely to have AL amyloidosis, since AA amyloidosis is usually associated with a chronic underlying infectious or inflammatory disease (such as rheumatoid arthritis) and senile systemic amyloid generally occurs in patients over the age of 80 years. The amyloid fibril protein associated with AL amyloid is immunoglobulin light (L) chain, and approximately 80% of patients with this type of amyloid have a monoclonal immunoglobulin or immunoglobulin light chain (so-called Bence Jones protein) in their serum or urine or both. Although such a protein was not found initially in this patient, subsequent protein electrophoresis of concentrated urine and of serum showed monoclonal proteins in the γ-region of both specimens. Immunofixation was carried out in an effort to identify the nature of these proteins. Immunofixation is performed by saturating individual cellulose acetate strips with anti-IgG, anti-IgA, anti-IgM, anti-free κ-chain, and anti-free λ-chain. The strips are laid side-by-side on an agarose gel following completion of the serum protein electrophoresis separation. The antibodies pass into the gel and form insoluble antigen-antibody complexes (precipitates). Free antigen and antibodies are washed away, and the remaining proteins are fixed and stained. The monoclonal proteins in this patient reacted exclusively with anti-free λ antibody. Moreover, a bone marrow examination showed an increased percentage of mature plasma cells that stained for cytoplasmic IgG-λ immunoglobulin. It is not known why certain circulating light chains cause amyloid fibril formation while others do not.

AL amyloidosis tends to involve the heart, gastrointestinal tract, liver, kidney, and peripheral nerves. AA amyloidosis rarely involves the heart, and when it does, resultant clinical deterioration is unusual. However, there is tremendous variability from patient to patient. In this patient, the heart and nerves were the dominant tissues involved. The mildly elevated hepatocellular enzymes are consistent with right-sided heart failure or amyloid infiltration of the liver. The diarrhea may result from either autonomic dysmotility or malabsorption secondary to small bowel amyloidosis. The carpal tunnel syndrome (median nerve entrapment) may be an early sign of amyloidosis.

Although all amyloid deposits show characteristic birefringent staining with Congo red dye under polarized light, other methods may be necessary to determine the specific amyloid fibril protein. AA amyloidosis can be distinguished from AL amyloidosis and other systemic types by the capacity of potassium permanganate to diminish Congo red staining of AA amyloid deposits. However, antibodies to specific amyloid fibril proteins provide the most reliable means of distinguishing one type of amyloidosis from another. The amyloid fibril protein of AL amyloid is generally composed of the variable region of the immunoglobulin light chain. Since commercial antibodies to complete κ and λ light chains react most avidly with the constant region, such antibodies may not detect AL amyloid. Thus, antibodies raised to isolated amyloid fibrils or fibril proteins have been used in some laboratories.

Antibody typing of amyloid utilizes immunohistochemistry. A tissue section is treated with a primary antiserum directed against the amyloid protein. A secondary antiserum, such as rabbit-anti-human IgG, is then added to react with the primary antiserum. The location of the amyloid deposit can then be detected microscopically by an enzyme complex bound to the secondary antiserum. This enzyme (e.g., peroxidase or alkaline phosphatase) converts an added substrate to a colored end-product.

The most definitive approach to making the diagnosis of amyloidosis is to biopsy the specific organ, such as heart, kidney, or liver, that is clearly associated with the patient's symptoms. However, a diagnosis can frequently be made with less risk by doing a biopsy under direct vision of the rectum (80% positive) or by aspiration of subcutaneous fat (80% positive).

Treatment

Since the cause of AL amyloidosis is unknown and there are no known specific means to eliminate amyloid deposits, therapy is directed toward alleviating symptoms. Since some patients with nephrosis appear to improve with melphalan (an antiproliferative agent), this drug can be tried. Patients with heart failure may be helped with diuretics, but digitalis may be contraindicated, since it predisposes patients to arrhythmias resulting from concentration of the drug in the amyloid tissue. Arrhythmias caused by the amyloid are often refractory to antiarrhythmic therapy. Some manifestations of autonomic neuropathy can be alleviated. Postural hypotension may be improved in a small percentage of patients by mineralocorticoid therapy and wearing a lower body stocking. Antidiarrheal agents can be helpful, and major efforts should be made to avoid dehydration and electrolyte depletion. If the patient has gastric atony secondary to autonomic dysfunction, maintenance of fluids, electrolytes, and calories will be difficult, and a nasogastric or gastrostomy tube may be required. A catheter may be required in patients with bladder atony.

Reference

1.   Natvig, J.B., Forre, O., Husby, G., et al., Eds.: Amyloid and Amyloidosis. Dordrecht, The Netherlands, Kluwer Academic Publishers, 1991, pp. 7-11.

Additional Reading

Buja, L.M., Khoi, N.B., and Roberts, W.C.: Clinically significant cardiac amyloidosis. Am. J. Cardiol., *26:* 394-405, 1970.

Carroll, J.D., Gaasch, W.H., and McAdam, K.P.W.J.: Amyloid cardiomyopathy: Characterization by a distinctive voltage/mass relation. Am. J. Cardiol., *49:* 9-13, 1982.

Falk, R.H., Plehn, J.F., Deering, T., et al.: Sensitivity and specificity of the echocardiographic features of cardiac amyloidosis. Am. J. Cardiol., *59:* 418-422, 1987.

Gertz, M.A., Kyle, R.A., and Greipp, P.R.: Response rates and survival in primary systemic amyloidosis. Blood, *77:* 257-262, 1991.

Glenner, G.G.: Amyloid deposits and amyloidosis. N. Engl. J. Med., *302:* 1283-1292, 1333-1343, 1980.

Kyle, R.A., and Bayrd, E.D.: Amyloidosis: Review of 236 cases. Medicine, *54:* 271-293, 1975.

A MAN WITH FEVER AND ACUTE POLYARTHRITIS

William Eugene Davis, Contributor

A 51-year-old Caucasian male was hospitalized in a local hospital after presenting to the emergency room with a two-day history of pain in the hands and shoulders and upper extremity weakness. He was febrile and reported a sore throat. Creatine kinase (CK) level and electromyography (EMG) were normal. Antinuclear antibodies and rheumatoid factor were absent. A throat culture grew group A streptococcus, and penicillin was given. On the third hospital day he developed difficulty walking due to pain in the knees and left ankle, and he was then transferred to the University Hospital with fever and polyarthritis.

The patient gave a history of occasional sore throats that were rarely treated with antibiotics and a history of intermittent knee pain for several years. He complained of dysuria of one-week duration. He had no regular sexual partner and reported a new sexual contact one month previously. Social history revealed a seventh grade education and employment as a parking lot attendant. His father died of cirrhosis and his mother of suicide. He did not smoke but drank approximately ten beers per week.

The temperature was 101.4 °F (38.6 °C), and other vital signs were normal. On physical examination he was mildly obese. The pharynx was not inflamed. A nonradiating systolic murmur was noted at the left sternal border. The physical examination was otherwise normal except for the musculoskeletal findings. Swelling, tenderness, and warmth were noted in the left second distal and third proximal interphalangeal joints, both wrists, the left elbow, both knees, and the left ankle, and the shoulders were tender. Joint pain precluded assessment of motor strength.

Upon admission, blood, urine, and throat cultures were obtained. Admission laboratory data included the following:

Analyte	Value, conventional units	Reference range, conventional units	Value, SI units	Reference range, SI units
Leukocyte count (B)	$10.8 \times 10^3/\mu L$	4.8-10.8	$10.8 \times 10^9/L$	4.8-10.8
Differential count (B)				
Neutrophils	55 %	40-76	0.55	0.40-0.76
Bands	9 %	0-10	0.09	0.00-0.10
Lymphocytes	23 %	20-52	0.23	0.20-0.52
Monocytes	12 %	1-10	0.12	0.01-0.10
Hemoglobin (B)	14 g/dL	12-16	8.69 mmol/L	7.45-9.93
Erythrocyte sedimentation rate (ESR) (B)	125 mm/h	0-15	Same	
Electrolytes (S)	Within normal limits			
Urea nitrogen (S)	12 mg/dL	7-18	4.3 mmol urea/L	2.5-6.4
Creatinine (S)	1.2 mg/dL	0.5-1.4	106 µmol/L	44-124
Glucose (S)	111 mg/dL	75-105	6.2 mmol/L	4.2-5.8
AST (S)	112 U/L	10-30	1.87 µkat/L	0.17-0.50
ALT (S)	139 U/L	8-30	2.32 µkat/L	0.13-0.50
LDH (S)	282 U/L	110-260	4.70 µkat/L	1.83-4.33
ALP (S)	161 U/L	100-310	2.7 µkat/L	1.7-5.2

Analyte	Value, conventional units	Reference range, conventional units	Value, SI units	Reference range, SI units
Bilirubin, total (S)	0.9 mg/dL	0.1-1.0	15 µmol/L	2-17
Urate (S)	6.4 mg/dL	2.4-7.5	381 µmol/L	143-446

Aspiration of synovial fluid from the right knee and left ankle revealed the following findings:

Analyte	Right knee	Left ankle	Reference range
Appearance	Straw-colored	Cloudy	Clear, straw
Leukocytes	8750/µL (8750×10^6/L)	62,200/µL ($62,200 \times 10^6$/L)	63/µL (63×10^6/L)
Polymorphonuclear cells	85% (0.85)	91% (0.91)	≤25% (≤0.25)

Both specimens were negative for gram-negative bacteria. Compensated polarized light microscopy disclosed intracellular, negatively birefringent crystals characteristic of monosodium urate.

All cultures were negative. Antistreptolysin O (ASO) and streptozyme titers were within normal limits. Hepatitis B surface antigen (HBsAg) was negative, and the C-reactive protein level was 20 mg/dL (200 mg/L), with a reference range of 0-1.4 (0-14).

The patient was treated with indomethacin and bed rest, and his symptoms resolved completely over the next five days. X-rays of his feet, prior to discharge, showed erosions at the right first metatarsal head. Upon discharge, he was continued on indomethacin.

One month later, his serum urate level was 10.0 mg/dL (595 µmol/L), and urine uric acid excretion was 1037 mg/d (6.12 mmol/d), reference range, 250-600 (1.48-3.54). He was subsequently treated with colchicine and allopurinol, and the serum urate level decreased to 6 mg/dL (357 µmol/L).

Differential Diagnosis

The differential diagnosis of fever and polyarthritis can be complex, including infectious disease, collagen vascular disorders, and a variety of miscellaneous conditions. In this patient, infectious causes had to be considered and excluded. Disseminated gonococcal infection was sought with appropriate cultures and acute rheumatic fever with throat cultures and serological tests. Empiric antibiotics were considered until synovial fluid analysis led to his diagnosis.

Collagen vascular disease is difficult to exclude in the acute setting. Some period of clinical observation is generally required. The absence of rheumatoid factor or antinuclear antibodies does not rule out rheumatoid arthritis or systemic vasculitis. Additional studies that may help include complement levels, tests for cryoglobulin, and antineutrophil cytoplasmic antibody.

Crystal-mediated arthropathies include pseudogout and gout. In pseudogout, acute arthritis is limited to one or two joints, chondrocalcinosis is evident on radiographs, and crystals characteristic of calcium pyrophosphate dihydrate (CPPD) are seen in synovial fluid.

This patient's diagnosis of gout was established when synovial fluid analysis revealed intracellular crystals characteristic of monosodium urate, in the absence of bacterial infection.

Definition and Classification

Gout represents a group of diseases in which prolonged hyperuricemia leads to deposition of urate salts in and around joints and in the kidneys. At physiological pH, most uric acid exists as monosodium urate. Saturation of serum occurs at a urate concentration of about 7 mg/dL (416 μmol/L). Above this value the potential for precipitation of monosodium urate crystals exists, although stable supersaturated solutions may allow the serum urate value to rise considerably higher.

The epidemiological definition of normouricemia (mean serum urate value plus or minus two standard deviations in a healthy population) varies depending on the analytic method. The uricase differential spectrophotometric method is more specific and gives an upper limit of 7.0 mg/dL (416 μmol/L) in men and 6.0 mg/dL (357 μmol/L) in women in most population studies. Less specific phosphotungstic acid methods are more widely used and overestimate the true urate level by up to 1 mg/dL (60 μmol/L), leading to a higher reference range.

Hyperuricemia leads to gout in a minority of instances. The majority of patients with asymptomatic hyperuricemia remain gout-free, but the greater the degree or duration of hyperuricemia, the more likely gout will develop.

When gout is present, hyperuricemia is classified as *primary*, if an inborn disorder of purine metabolism is present, or *secondary*, if another disease causes either overproduction or underexcretion of uric acid.

Overproduction of uric acid can be shown in 10-20% of patients with *primary hyperuricemia*. In these patients renal excretion of uric acid is >600 mg/dL (36 mmol/L) on a purine-restricted diet. Although the metabolic basis of overproduction is unidentified in most patients, two enzymatic defects have been defined — overactivity of 5-phosphoribosyl-1-pyrophosphate (PRPP) synthetase and partial deficiency of hypoxanthine guanine phosphoribosyltransferase (HPRT).

In humans, uric acid is the degradation end-product of purine metabolism. Inosinic acid, the parent purine compound, is synthesized *de novo* by a series of reactions including the condensation of PRPP and L-glutamine in the presence of the enzyme amidophosphoribosyltransferase. High concentrations of PRPP accelerate this reaction and increase purine synthesis.

Purine nucleotides are degraded to hypoxanthine and xanthine and ultimately oxidized to uric acid in reactions catalyzed by the enzyme xanthine oxidase. Normally a salvage pathway allows conversion of hypoxanthine to inosine monophosphate (IMP) in the presence of PRPP and HPRT. Deficiency of HPRT leads to increased degradation of hypoxanthine and to underutilization of PRPP (which fuels *de novo* purine synthesis), resulting in increased uric acid formation.

Both HPRT deficiency and PRPP synthetase overactivity are X-linked disorders. Affected males develop gout at an early age (15-30 years) and may be mentally retarded. The patient in this case was found to have normal HPRT and PRPP synthetase activity.

In the majority of patients with primary gout, hyperuricemia results from reduced renal uric acid clearance. Urinary uric acid levels are normal or low in the presence of increased serum levels. Specific renal defects have not been described.

Secondary hyperuricemia occurs when another primary disorder leads to either over-production of uric acid or underexcretion. In myeloproliferative disorders, increased nucleic acid turnover raises uric acid production. Renal failure, diuretic therapy, and lead intoxication reduce uric acid excretion.

Clinical Features

Persistent hyperuricemia may lead to deposition of monosodium urate crystals in and around articular tissues. Clinical attacks of gout occur when crystals incite an acute in-flammatory response in the synovial tissues. Physical trauma or rapid changes in the serum urate concentration may trigger attacks. The first attack is usually monoarticular and involves a lower extremity. Inflammation of the joint and periarticular tissues occurs rapidly, and joint effusions are large. Synovial fluid leukocyte counts are elevated (15,000-100,000/µL), and neutrophils predominate.

Acute attacks are self-limited and separated by asymptomatic, intercritical periods. Although the initial attack may be polyarticular, polyarthritis usually occurs later in the disease course. Fever may accompany acute attacks, along with elevations of the erythrocyte sedimentation rate (ESR) and acute phase reactants such as the C-reactive protein. Even-tually, uric acid deposition leads to grossly evident tophi around the joints or in subcutaneous tissue. Erosions may be visible on radiographs of the involved joints. Tophaceous gout is marked by chronic joint inflammation and deforming arthritis.

Diagnosis

The diagnosis of gout is made when intracellular crystals, typical of monosodium urate, are identified in the synovial fluid of an inflamed joint. Such crystals are needle shaped and strongly negatively birefringent when examined by compensated polarized light microscopy. They appear yellow when oriented parallel to the axis of the compensator and blue when oriented perpendicular to it. The CPPD crystals of pseudogout are rhomboidal and weakly positively birefringent. They appear blue when oriented parallel to the axis of the compen-sator and yellow when perpendicular. CPPD disease and gout may coexist. "False negative" results on synovial fluid may be due to an inadequate specimen or to inadequate microscopic examination. Demonstration of uric acid crystals in material aspirated from a suspected tophus also confirms the diagnosis of gout.

Although hyperuricemia is a prerequisite for uric acid deposition, the serum urate level during an acute attack of gout may be normal. Baseline serum and urine levels should, therefore, be obtained during intercritical periods.

Treatment

Therapy of gout includes treatment of the acute gouty arthritis and treatment of the underlying hyperuricemia. Acute attacks of gout are treated with nonsteroidal anti-inflamma-tory drugs (NSAID's), colchicine, or corticosteroids. When attacks become recurrent and frequent, colchicine or NSAID's may be given as prophylactic therapy. Although NSAID's may be preferred for acute therapy because of the gastrointestinal toxicity of large doses of colchicine, they may be less favored for chronic prophylaxis owing to the risk of NSAID-in-duced gastropathy. Small doses of colchicine as given for prophylaxis are usually tolerated very well.

Definitive hypouricemic therapy is indicated in recurrent gout or tophaceous gout. Probenecid increases urinary uric acid excretion and can be used in patients who are not "overproducers." Allopurinol, a xanthine oxidase inhibitor, inhibits uric acid formation. Either drug can be used to lower the serum urate level below 7 mg/dL (416 µmol/L) and allow dissolution of tissue deposits of monosodium urate. Although initiation of hypouricemic drugs may trigger an acute attack of gout, appropriate long-term use of these agents can prevent chronic tophaceous gouty arthritis.

Additional Reading

Holmes, E.W.: Clinical gout and the pathogenesis of hyperuricemia. *In:* Arthritis and Allied Conditions, a Textbook of Rheumatology. D.J. McCarty, Ed. Philadelphia, Lea and Febiger, 1985.

Lowry, G.V., Fan, P.T., and Bluestone, R.: Polyarticular versus monoarticular gout: A prospective, comparative analysis of clinical features. Medicine, *67:* 335-343, 1988.

Palella, T.D., and Fox, I.H.: Hyperuricemia and gout. *In:* The Metabolic Basis of Inherited Disease, 6th ed. C.R. Scriver, A.L. Beaudet, W.S. Sly, and D. Valle, Eds. New York, McGraw-Hill, 1989.

Rubenstein, J., and Pritzker, K.P.H.: Crystal associated arthropathies. Am. J. Roentgenol., *152:* 685-695, 1989.

Wyngaarden, J.B., and Kelley, W.N.: Gout and Hyperuricemia. New York, Grune and Stratton, 1976.

SUDDEN DEATH OF A COCAINE ADDICT
IN POLICE CUSTODY

John C. Hunsaker, III, Contributor

A 25-year-old unemployed male cocaine abuser suddenly exhibited bizarre behavior at his home in the presence of his girlfriend and another man. According to these witnesses, he became agitated and began to bang his head against the wall, while complaining of severe head and chest pain. Loudly accusing the other two of being after him and trying to kill him, he physically assaulted them. He shouted that bugs were crawling all over his body and started thrashing around inside the house and breaking furniture. Sweating profusely, he then stripped himself naked, used his arms to crash through a glass door, and ran into the street shouting that no one could harm him. In frenzied agitation he next started throwing rocks against the house.

Two police officers initially called to the scene found him writhing prone on the lawn. On their approach he vigorously struck out at the officers as they attempted to subdue and handcuff him. In the ensuing short struggle, one policeman first attempted a headlock without success. This officer then succeeded in applying a neck hold, and while the subject was briefly calm, several other officers hogtied him by tying rope around his wrists and ankles. Lying on his side on the flat sidewalk, he continued to struggle and curse for over 10 minutes. Rescue squad members, at the scene within 20 minutes of the officers' arrival, found him cyanotic, apneic, and pulseless with fixed and dilated pupils. Electrocardiographic monitoring showed no electrical activity. Cardiopulmonary resuscitation was carried out briefly without restoration of vital signs. He was declared dead within 25 minutes of the onset of his panic reaction.

Additional interrogation of the witnesses revealed that the decedent had received two intravenous injections of cocaine over a period of 30 minutes. The first was self-administered, the second given by his girlfriend less than one hour before the onset of delirious behavior. There was no history of significant medical or psychiatric problems.

Medicolegal/Forensic Investigation

Local news media soon reported that the decedent's death was due to a physical attack by police officers, as reported by witnesses. In addition, the local prosecutor started an investigation into probable negligent homicide in view of the girlfriend's admitted injection of cocaine into the decedent shortly before his death.

The coroner-authorized autopsy performed by the medical examiner began within six hours of death. Liver temperature then was 102.2 °F (39 °C). The external examination revealed two recent salmon-colored needle punctures with focal subcutaneous hemorrhage in the left antecubital fossa. There were no scars on the extremities, but both hands and forearms exhibited patchy superficial cuts deemed secondary to glass breakage. Recent abraded contusions corresponding to the rope ligatures encircled the wrists and ankles. Patchy conjunctival and mucosal petechiae of the lips were present. Nares were normal. There was no external cervical injury.

Internal findings at autopsy included focal, small bruises of the central bellies of both sternocleidomastoid muscles and the strap musculature (sternohyoid and cricothyroid). The cervical cartilages, soft tissues, vertebrae, and spinal cord were otherwise intact. Laryngeal petechiae were present. No external or internal craniocerebral trauma was detected. The only other internal finding of note involved the heart, which was slightly enlarged (weight 420 g) and showed moderate concentric left ventricular myocardial hypertrophy. The proximal left anterior descending coronary artery exhibited thrombotic occlusion in a region of eccentric thickening of the wall. Microscopical examination disclosed an acute intraluminal thrombus in a region of critical (>85%) stenosis by intimal hyperplasia. Rare foci of subendocardial contraction band necrosis of the hypertrophic myocytes were also observed.

At necropsy, the pathologist collecting the biological specimens for toxicological analysis initiated the legal chain of custody (see later). Toxicological analysis of the heart blood (preserved in sodium fluoride) yielded the following results: cocaine, 1.23 mg/L (4059 nmol/L); serum benzoylecgonine (a metabolite of cocaine), 2.07 mg/L (6831 nmol/L). Neither ethanol nor any other drugs were detected. Urine was not available.

Medicolegal Issues

Approach to Establishing the Cause and Manner of Death. This complex case history with lethal outcome constituted an event of paramount public interest. It therefore fell under the purview of laws requiring official medicolegal death investigation by the coroner or medical examiner of the relevant jurisdiction.

The purpose of official death investigation is to determine the cause of death (COD or why death occurred) and the manner of death (MOD or how death occurred) of humans under circumstances specified by pertinent law.[1] Such an investigation typically draws upon various specialists and investigators in the forensic sciences, among whom are forensic pathologists and toxicologists. In order to arrive at sound conclusions about COD and MOD, it is imperative to gather all relevant data surrounding the death. A minimal comprehensive investigation addresses the following: (1) background information, such as medical history and meticulous reconstruction of the terminal sequence of events; (2) structural evidence of disease or injury as seen by systematic external and internal examination of the body at autopsy; and (3) laboratory results.

The COD denotes the injury or disease, or combination of both disturbances, brief or prolonged, that produced the fatal outcome. The interpretive intellectual procedure to determine COD in forensic investigation involves two steps: first, recognition of structural or biochemical abnormalities or drug or poison levels incompatible with vital function; and, second, correlation of such abnormalities with pathophysiological mechanisms causing the lethal process. Correlation of apposite pathophysiological mechanisms (i.e., the biochemical or physiological derangements) produced by COD is mandatory in this process. Appropriate collection and disposition of all types of evidence, including samples taken for laboratory analysis, are legal prerequisites in forensic investigation. This ensures admissibility of expert testimony about relevant laboratory results that materially pertain to the COD and MOD in criminal or civil litigation.

The MOD represents an extrajudicial or administrative opinion as to how death came about. In most instances, the MOD is circumstance-dependent — derived from all sources of information at the end of the investigation — and not autopsy-dependent. In forensic investigation the principal reason to certify MOD is for statistical purposes as noted on the death certificate; the common certifiable manners of death are either natural (death solely from natural disease processes) or unnatural (death completely or in part due to some injurious agency). The latter category is further subdivided as follows: homicide, suicide, accident, or undetermined.   As an opinion, MOD is subject to interpretation: there are no universally accepted criteria among death investigators. Moreover, official certification of the MOD should not significantly affect decisions of other agencies (e.g., the prosecutor considering criminal action) or institutions (e.g., insurance companies), whose interests differ from those of forensic investigators. For example, a designation of "homicide" (on the death certificate) does not necessarily imply criminal culpability, a conclusion appropriately left to legal proceedings.

Establishing Legal Chain of Custody. All personnel handling or possessing physical evidence (e.g., pathologists or other physicians, toxicologists, laboratorians, and police) have a legal duty to maintain the evidentiary chain of custody. Preservation of the integrity of physical evidence undergoing subsequent analysis affords admissibility of test results at trial. The results may then be entered as proof of an issue in question by establishing credibility in the minds of the court and jury.

This axiom applies particularly to specimens of biological or chemical evidence, which as a class may be consumed in analysis and are susceptible to contamination or spoilage. The law requires written documentation reflecting positive identification and the absence of significant alterations or tampering of chemical specimens from the time of collection through analysis. Such documentation comprises not only the laboratorian's reports and work sheets but also written notes or forms documenting an uninterrupted chain of custody.

In this case study the pathologist collecting the specimens initiated the legal chain of custody. Upon collection he first labeled the containers with data identifying the deceased, case number, time and date of collection, body site of collection, and character or description of sample, and then affixed his name or initials. The same data were simultaneously entered on a specially designed standard form consisting of a master sheet and duplicates. He next preserved the specimen in appropriate locked storage or refrigeration with limited access in preparation for transfer of custody to the next official in the chain for final delivery to the analyst. Every person involved in the evidentiary escort of the physical evidence records similar data on the form upon taking possession. This may involve few or many custodians. Finally, the receiving analyst at the end of the chain records all data as to time and type of analysis and also notes whether and how any retained sample is stored. This paper trail of documentation may then be properly referred to at trial by any official witness in the chain as a means of establishing the integrity of the specimen.

Differential Diagnosis of Investigative and Medical Findings

In this case reasonable arguments could be raised to justify any of the listed manners of death, dependent upon determination of COD. The forensic pathologist at the outset must consider not only natural causes (organic heart disease) but also unnatural (injurious) causes to justify certification, such as homicide because of lethal injection of illicit drugs by the girlfriend or, alternatively, asphyxia due to cervical constriction by police; suicide because of deliberate high-risk self-administration of an illicit drug with established lethal potential; accident because of untoward reaction to drug during recreational use; or, if none of these preponderate, undetermined.

Homicide. All deaths of persons occurring while they are held in official custody are controversial, requiring comprehensive and meticulous forensic investigation.[2] Moreover, police attempts to restrain deranged, violent subjects lead to accusations of police brutality and excessive use of force. Police departments are charged to formulate appropriate procedures for restraint and apprehension of suspects. The law permits these officials to employ reasonable force under the circumstances to safely restrain violent subjects. The fundamental procedural goals are to prevent injury to the psychotic individual and others, including the police officials, and to arrange for prompt medical attention. Some methods of apprehension involving a rapidly moving, uncooperative subject are potentially lethal even with appropriate by-the-book application. Various types of choke holds (i.e., either the carotid sleeper or the bar arm control) to subdue thrashing subjects with inordinate strength not only may cause loss of consciousness but also may trigger asphyxial or reflex neural mechanisms that produce sudden death.[3] The technique of hogtying, moreover, may cause death by positional asphyxia by hampering motion of the thorax for effective respiration. The autopsy findings of internal cervical hemorrhage and petechiae are compatible with the story of forcible external neck compression. Mechanical or positional asphyxia was not considered to cause death, however, because the subject continued to remain conscious for minutes after the restraint maneuvers, and the upper airway was patent and normally configured.

There was no evidence that his girlfriend intended his death, although she deliberately and unlawfully injected the illicit drug into the decedent. State laws on this issue are variable. Some jurisdictions permit prosecution under the felony murder rule (unintended death during commission of a felony), whereas others invoke laws pertinent to involuntary manslaughter or reckless homicide.

Suicide. By consensus, suicide as an MOD is applicable when the preponderance of all evidence conduces to establish that the decedent by his own act intended to kill himself and simultaneously understood the probable consequences of the act. The subject deliberately self-administered cocaine intravenously — an act arguably reducing his chances of survival to a minimum because of the unpredictable physiological effects of the drug, even at low levels. Most forensic investigators, however, require considerably more social, medical, and psychiatric background information than developed here before concluding that the death was intentionally self-inflicted.

Natural Cause. In this case history there are nontraumatic anatomical findings sufficient to account for sudden death. Specifically, occlusion of a single major epicardial coronary artery by any disease process greatly predisposes one to sudden and frequently unexpected death during arousal or sleep. A grossly observable myocardial infarct may occasionally be apparent, but the more common physiological mechanism is an ischemia-induced lethal cardiac dysrhythmia, such as ventricular fibrillation. In view of current research into the physiological and psychological effects of cocaine on the human organism under the above-described circumstances of death, the coronary artery pathology in this case was not deemed to be the underlying cause of death. At most, the lesion may be listed as a contributory cause so that an MOD other than natural is more appropriate.

Accident. Accidental deaths result from inadvertent or negligent action by the victim or another (i.e., no intent to do harm) in the setting of a hazardous internal or external environment. Deaths from acute toxicity or overdose of a licit medication, ethyl alcohol, or an illicit drug in the absence of intent to kill, even for individuals who regularly abuse the substances, are generally regarded as accidents. On the basis of all investigative and medical considerations, including the discussion of cocaine-induced sudden death outlined below, the medical examiner certified the COD as acute cocaine intoxication and the MOD as accidental.

Patterns and Etiology of Cocaine-Induced Sudden Death

Cocaine, initially isolated as an alkaloid from *Erythroxylum coca* in the l9th century, has since been condemned as the "third scourge of the mankind."[4] First used as an anesthetic and briefly later as a therapeutic elixir (once an ingredient of Coca-Cola), its physiological and adverse side effects were quickly elucidated so that, by the early 1900's, reports of toxicity and death associated with its use or abuse occasionally appeared. Outlawing of cocaine by federal law early in this century appeared to curtail this trend until the 1970's, after which there was a dramatic resurgence of cocaine-related morbidity and mortality attributable to its abundance and cheap street price.

For many years cocaine was formulated in crystalline powder (cocaine HCl), which was suitable for administration by nasal insufflation ("snorting"), parenterally and mainly intravenously because of its water solubility, or less commonly by oral ingestion. More recently, alkaloidal cocaine has been prepared by adding ammonia and baking soda to an aqueous solution of cocaine HCl. The precipitate thus formed is mixed with ether. This product, cocaine free base, vaporizes with moderate heating to facilitate self-administration by smoking through a water pipe ("base pipe"). Since the mid-1980's "crack," as a nearly pure form of cocaine, has been manufactured by a similar process but without adding ether; this product is a dry crystalline precipitate sold or used as "rock." Crushed rock, or crack, is sprinkled on marijuana or tobacco and then smoked either as a cigarette or in an ordinary pipe. This form of ingestion has supplanted snorting as the most common method for "recreational" use. The resultant craving developed from free basing or crack use rapidly leads to addiction.

Pharmacologically, cocaine acts as a local anesthetic and is a powerful sympathomimetic agent that produces marked central nervous system stimulation. The effects of central and adrenergic stimulation are due to excess of neurotransmitters, i.e., the catecholamines epinephrine, norepinephrine, and dopamine, as well as serotonin. Potentiation of these neurotransmitters is caused by increased postsynaptic concentration at the receiving nerve cell, which results from blockage of the "pump" (i.e., plasma membrane neurotransmitter transporters) for presynaptic reuptake.[4] (See Figure 1.)

Major stimulant effects include tachycardia and hypertension. The desired immediate psychological effect of this psychoactive drug is intense euphoria, which characteristically degenerates into a dysphoric "crash" that quickly engenders repetitive use and addiction.

Individuals display great pharmacokinetic variability in their reaction to cocaine and its metabolites.[4] Acted upon by plasma and hepatocytic cholinesterases, 90% of cocaine is rapidly metabolized at one or both of the ester linkages. Its major metabolite, benzoylecgonine, is thought to be produced in vivo not by esterases, but instead by nonenzymatic hydrolysis. The plasma $t_{1/2}$ of the parent drug is about one hour. Small amounts of cocaine are eliminated in the urine primarily as unchanged drug, benzoylecgonine, or other metabolites. Dependent upon duration of use, the major metabolite may be detected in urine any time from two days up to three weeks. Degradation by esterases in blood continues after death. Prompt storage on ice and preservation by sodium fluoride are required for stabilization and accurate detection of levels at the time of death.

Risks of use are high because undesirable biological or toxic reactions are not necessarily dose-related. A plethora of well-documented adverse reactions — in the form of strong temporal associations and probable causal relationships — may cause sudden death. Various potentially fatal complications may occur simultaneously. Grand mal seizures, hyperpyrexia, and acute psychotic reactions are not infrequent. Untoward cardiovascular reactions include either life-threatening cardiac dysrhythmias or coronary artery spasm with development of angina pectoris and acute myocardial infarct. Accumulating reports also describe cocaine-induced myocarditis that, if survived, may lead to a crippling dilated cardiomyopathy. Acute hypertensive crises occur as well and are occasionally complicated by aortic dissection, rupture of intracranial saccular aneurysms with subarachnoid hemorrhage, or intracerebral hemorrhage (stroke).

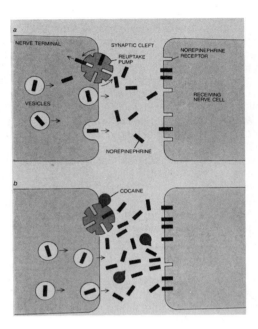

Figure 1. Schematic depiction of (*a*) normal and (*b*) cocaine-altered synaptic activity of biogenic amines such as norepinephrine. (*a*) shows that, after its release and action at the respective nerve terminals, norepinephrine is taken up at the presynaptic site by the plasma membrane transporter (i.e., the reuptake "pump"), which terminates neurotransmission. (*b*) depicts the action of a psychomotor stimulant such as cocaine, which creates its sympathomimetic effects by direct binding on the pump so as to inhibit reuptake of norepinephrine. The resultant increased concentration of the amine at the receiving nerve cell terminal thereby potentiates the stimulative effects. (Reprinted with permission from: "Cocaine" by Craig van Dyke and Robert Byck. Copyright © March, 1982 by Scientific American, Inc. All rights reserved.)

The principal cerebro- and cardiovascular complications of cocaine use and abuse are related to systemic catecholamine excess, which causes vasoconstriction by affecting vascular smooth muscle both directly through changes in calcium flux and indirectly by preventing neurotransmitter reuptake at sympathetic nerve terminals.[5,6] Thus, with anatomically normal arteries, prolonged vasospasm is hypothesized to compromise regional blood flow and produce ischemic sequelae in the affected system. Cocaine is also deemed under certain circumstances to alter and stenose the vasculature (spasm-produced endothelial injury) so as to either accelerate the process of atherosclerosis or induce nonatherosclerotic intimal hyperplasia. In this context, catecholamine excess not only leads to a mismatch of myocardial oxygen demand and supply but also predisposes the cocaine user to thrombotic occlusion due to enhanced thrombogenicity by platelet aggregation. In addition to these acute vascular complications, other changes secondary to postulated direct toxic effects on the myocardium include catecholamine-induced cardiomyopathy, expressed variably as myocarditis, myocardial contraction band necrosis, and chronic heart failure with dilated cardiomyopathy.

Cocaine-induced psychiatric syndromes, characteristically a function of dose and duration of use, include dysphoria, acute psychoses, particularly paranoid schizophreniform psychosis without disorientation, and delirium.[7] Usually, elimination of cocaine alleviates the psychiatric symptoms, but there are accumulating reports of sudden death attributable to cocaine-induced psychosis or "excited delirium" seen in recreational users and in the body packer syndrome.[8] Deaths associated with this uniquely dramatic syndrome involve a "body packer" or, in street jargon, "mule," a person who swallows packets of contraband cocaine out of the country and, after clearing customs, excretes them from the bowel. Poorly designed or ruptured packets in the gut may cause severe cocaine intoxication.

Dysphoria presents as a profound change of mood, agitation, paranoid thinking, irritability, and impulsiveness. The attendant distortion of thought processes with impairment of judgment and attention can increase the probability of homicidal or suicidal acts or lead to injury-related accidents. Delirium itself is an organic mental disorder in which the primary symptoms are perceptual and attentional deficits, disordered thought processes, disorientation, delusions, and hallucinations. Cocaine-induced excited delirium represents a panic reaction and is a medical emergency that is typically characterized by the acute development of paranoia, violent and bizarre behavior, herculean feats of strength, hyperpyrexia, and ongoing struggle in the face of attempted restraint. Visual misperceptions such as flashing lights ("snow lights") and tactile hallucinations (formication or, more commonly, "coke bugs") are frequent features as well.

Because of the idiosyncratic human response to cocaine intake, many of these syndromes tend to overlap. However, there is a developing consensus that differentiates those sudden deaths due to cocaine overdose from those due to intoxication.[9] In general, deaths attributable to overdose are sudden, and generalized convulsions precede acute respiratory arrest. The average postmortem blood levels in overdose deaths are around 6 mg/L (19,800 nmol/L), whereas mean concentrations of 0.6 mg/L (1980 nmol/L) are reported in fatalities of cocaine psychosis attributable to acute intoxication. For comparison, the serum concentration in surgical patients treated with cocaine or its derivatives for local anesthe- sia is only 0.31 mg/L (1023 nmol/L), and the average "recreational" level is 0.4 mg/L (1320 nmol/L). As suggested, however, the range of concentrations reported in cocaine- related fatalities is wide; values vary from minimal to over 60 mg/L (198 μmol/L).

The reason for such confounding patterns is due at least in part to the method of intake and formulation of the drug. Clearly, sudden death may occur by any form of intake, and toxic or fatal reactions are not inevitably dose-dependent. Moreover, many fatalities involve combinations of cocaine and other substances, such as ethyl alcohol and drugs, any of which may potentiate the deleterious effects by direct cardiotoxic and other mechanisms.

Treatment of Cocaine-Induced Psychiatric Syndromes

As noted, many psychiatric symptoms are resolved by elimination of cocaine from the body. No *specific* treatment for overdose exists. In cases of medical emergency with a psychiatric presentation of delirium, however, the differential diagnosis includes cocaine toxicity. After the patient is safely under control and medically stabilized, therapeutic efforts are directed to control those life-threatening features. The following measures may be indicated: rapid cooling for hyperthermia; ventilatory support for potential respiratory arrest; and administration of antiseizure medication such as diazepam or phenobarbital for convulsions, agitation, and anxiety. More powerful tranquilizers such as haloperidol may be required to control paranoia. To overcome the sympathomimetic effects of cocaine, antiarrhythmic or antihypertensive agents such as propranolol, sodium nitroprusside, or lidocaine (the last cautiously) may be administered. Continuous monitoring should be in force until the acute phase resolves.

Comment

This multifaceted case of cocaine-related fatality underscores the complex law enforcement and medical complications of cocaine use or abuse reaching epidemic proportion in the United States. The case also highlights the difficult issues confronting medical and police officials having the responsibility to control and treat the vast range of human behaviors related to such use or abuse.

References

1. Kircher, T., and Anderson, R.: Cause of death: Proper completion of the death certificate. JAMA, *258:* 349-352, 1988.

2. Copeland, A.R.: Deaths in custody revisited. Am. J. Forensic Med. Pathol., *5:* 121-124, 1984.

3. Reay, D.T., and Eisele, U.W.: Deaths from law enforcement neck holds. Am. J. Forensic Med. Pathol., *3:* 253-258, 1982.

4. Ellenhorn, M.J., and Barceloux, D.G.: Cocaine. *In:* Medical Toxicology Diagnosis and Treatment of Human Poisoning. New York, Elsevier Publishing Co., 1988.

5. Levine, S.R., Brust, J.C.M., Futrell, N., et al.: Cerebrovascular complications of the use of the "crack" form of alkaloidal cocaine. N. Engl. J. Med., *323:* 699-704, 1990.

6. Karch, S., and Billingham, M.E.: The pathology and etiology of cocaine-induced heart disease. Arch. Pathol. Lab. Med., *112:* 225-230, 1988.

7. Post, R.M.: Cocaine psychosis: A continuum model. Am. J. Psychiatry, *132:* 225-231, 1975.

8. Wetli, C.V., and Fishbain, D.A.: Cocaine-induced psychosis and sudden death in recreational cocaine users. J. Forensic Sci., *30:* 873-880, 1985.

9. Escobedo, L.G., Ruttenber, A.J., Agocs, M.M., et al.: Emerging patterns of cocaine use and the epidemic of cocaine overdose deaths in Dade County, Florida. Arch. Pathol. Lab. Med., *115:* 900-905, 1991.

Additional Reading

DiMaio, D.J., and DiMaio, V.J.M.: Forensic Pathology. New York, Elsevier Publishing Co., 1989.

Spitz, W.V., and Fisher, R.S., Eds.: Medicolegal Investigation of Death, 2nd ed. Springfield, IL, Charles C Thomas, 1980.

Wetli, C.V., Mittleman, R.E., and Rao, V.J.: Practical Forensic Pathology. New York/Tokyo, Igaku-Shoin Medical Publishers, Inc., 1988.

CHILD WITH NAUSEA AND VOMITING
EIGHT DAYS POST-CRANIOTOMY

Susan A. Fuhrman, Contributor
Ronald J. Whitley, Reviewer

A six-year-old female was admitted to the University Hospital with a history of nausea and vomiting over the past 24 hours. She had been discharged the previous day, eight days post-craniotomy for removal of a craniopharyngioma. Her previous admission had been characterized by an episode of central diabetes insipidus, and she had been sent home with 1-desamino-8-D-arginine vasopressin (DDAVP), an antidiuretic hormone analogue, to be given if required. Her parents had taken her to a local hospital when she developed nausea and vomiting at home; laboratory studies there revealed a very low serum sodium of 114 mmol/L. She was then referred to the University Hospital, where she was admitted to the neurosurgical service.

Physical examination revealed an alert six-year-old who denied any lightheadedness, although she was nauseated. Blood pressure was 110/60 mm Hg without postural changes, pulse 85 BPM. Skin turgor was normal; no edema was identified. The remainder of the physical examination was normal.

The following laboratory results were obtained:

Analyte	Value, conventional units	Reference range, conventional units	Value, SI units	Reference range, SI units
Sodium (S)	115 mmol/L	135-145	Same	
Chloride (S)	73 mmol/L	95-105	Same	
Potassium (S)	4.4 mmol/L	3.5-5.5	Same	
CO_2, total (S)	28 mmol/L	22-29	Same	
Urea nitrogen (S)	8 mg/dL	9-23	2.9 mmol urea/L	3.2-8.2
Creatinine (S)	0.5 mg/dL	0.3-1.0	44 µmol/L	27-88
Glucose (S)	102 mg/dL	72-106	5.7 mmol/L	4.0-5.9
Calcium (S)	9.6 mg/dL	8.8-10.6	2.40 mmol/L	2.20-2.64
Magnesium (S)	1.6 mg/dL	1.6-2.4	0.66 mmol/L	0.66-0.99
Phosphorus (S)	5.6 mg/dL	3.8-6.5	1.81 mmol/L	1.23-2.10
Osmolality (S)	237 mOsm/kg	279-301	237 mmol/kg	279-301
Osmolality (U)	418 mOsm/kg	250-900	418 mmol/kg	250-900
Sodium, random (U)	37 mmol/L			

The initial clinical assessment was severe hyponatremia probably due to water intoxication. She was clinically euvolemic, i.e., without evidence of volume depletion or volume overload. Differential diagnosis included the syndrome of inappropriate antidiuretic hormone secretion (SIADH) and the possibility of overdose with DDAVP or other drugs associated with water retention and adrenal insufficiency. Criteria for a diagnosis of SIADH are shown in Table 1.

Table 1. CRITERIA FOR THE DIAGNOSIS OF SIADH

Hyponatremia (sodium <136 mmol/L) with hyposmolal plasma
    (osmolality <275 mOsmol/kg H_2O)
Urine less than maximally dilute (osmolality >100 mOsmol/kg H_2O);
    urine osmolality high relative to plasma osmolality
Inappropriate increase in urine sodium (>20 mmol/L)
No clinical evidence of volume depletion or overload
Absence of other possible causes of euvolemic hyposmolality, e.g., hypo-
    thyroidism, hypocortisolism, renal impairment, recent diuretic therapy
Absence of medication with drugs known to stimulate ADH release,
    e.g., amitriptyline, chlorpropamide, clofibrate, cyclophosphamide,
    morphine, vincristine

This patient met all the criteria listed in Table 1, except for rigorous exclusion of other causes of euvolemic hyponatremia, particularly hypothyroidism, adrenal insufficiency, and renal impairment. Renal impairment was, however, unlikely since the patient had a normal serum urea nitrogen and creatinine and demonstrated ability to concentrate urine (urine osmolality, 418 mOsmol/kg H_2O). Adrenal insufficiency, although capable of causing hyponatremia without evidence of water depletion, was considered unlikely because of the marked hyponatremia in this patient. Hypothyroid patients who develop hyponatremia usually have other clinical symptoms of thyroid disease; nonetheless a thorough workup of a hyponatremic patient should include screening studies for thyroid disease. Such studies were not done in this case. The child's mother denied giving her DDAVP or any other drug that could cause water retention (Table 2). In view of the recent surgery on the pituitary and the high incidence of manifestation of SIADH in such cases, the attending physicians concluded the most probable diagnosis was SIADH. The child was treated conventionally by restricting fluid intake. Sodium and plasma osmolality values returned to normal within two days.

Table 2. DISORDERS AND DRUG THERAPIES ASSOCIATED WITH SIADH

Central nervous system disorders
    Cerebral tumor
    Infection (encephalitis, meningitis, abscess)
    Acute psychosis
    Neuropathy
    Acute intermittent porphyria
    Guillain-Barré syndrome
    Cerebral vascular thrombosis or hemorrhage

Carcinoma
    Lung (small-cell undifferentiated, oat cell)
    Duodenum
    Pancreas
    Thymus
    Ureter

Pulmonary disorders
    Pneumonia
    Abscess
    Asthma
    Tuberculosis
    Pneumothorax

Drugs
    Cyclophosphamide
    Carbamazepine
    Vincristine
    Haloperidol
    Amitriptyline
    Monoamine oxidase inhibitors
    Thioridazine
    Bromocriptine

Definition of the Disease

SIADH has been associated with a variety of primary disease processes as well as drugs and has been shown to be the most common cause of hyponatremia in hospitalized patients.[1] Table 2 shows diseases and therapies that may precipitate hyponatremia.

Pituitary surgery was the proximate cause of this patient's SIADH. Most patients who develop diabetes insipidus (DI) following pituitary surgery experience an acute onset of polyuria that resolves within 3-5 days. Another group of patients develop permanent DI. The least common response is the triphasic type, illustrated by this case and presenting as a significant therapeutic challenge. In the first phase, classic DI due to decreased secretion of ADH occurs in the first 24 postoperative hours. The second or antidiuretic phase varies in severity but may take on the characteristics of full-fledged SIADH. This patient presented in the second phase. The third phase is always DI, reflecting progressive death of magno-cellular neurons by retrograde axonal degradation. The result is permanent DI.[2]

Clinical Features. There are no specific signs or symptoms of SIADH *per se.* Patients present with symptoms reflecting low serum sodium levels. In less severe cases, the symptoms may be only those of mild water intoxication, namely, weakness and apathy. In more severe cases, signs of disturbance of the central nervous system are seen; the level of consciousness is decreased, and confusion and coma occur. Those patients most severely affected may develop *grand mal* seizures.

Diagnosis

The traditional criteria for SIADH are shown on Table 1. SIADH remains primarily a diagnosis of exclusion. Supportive evidence for the diagnosis of SIADH includes (1) failure of correction of hyponatremia following sodium administration; (2) improvement of hyponatre-mia following water restriction; (3) an abnormal water load test; and (4) plasma vasopressin (ADH) level that is inappropriately increased relative to low plasma osmolality in the absence of known stimuli for ADH release.

Antidiuretic hormone (ADH) is synthesized in the supraoptic and ventricular nuclei located in the hypothalamus. It is transported down the axons to be stored in the pituitary. ADH is normally released from the posterior pituitary as the result of specific physiological stimuli. *Inappropriate* ADH secretion is characterized as such because autonomous ADH release occurs in the absence of known stimuli that are normally mediated through osmo-receptors located in the hypothalamus and through baroreceptors located in the right atrium and carotid sinus. These stimuli include increased plasma osmolality and decreased effective blood volume and blood pressure. The baroreceptor-mediated response takes precedence over osmoregulation; therefore, decreased effective blood volume will stimulate ADH release even in the presence of decreased osmolality. Consequently, volume-depleted patients have *appropriate* ADH release mediated by the baroreceptor mechanism, as do patients in cardiac failure and those with edema. Such patients release ADH and retain water even in the presence of profound hyponatremia and hyposmolality, but ADH secretion is still appropriate.

Patients with SIADH develop hyponatremia because of increased reabsorption of water by the renal tubules in response to stimulation by high ADH levels. The result is decreased urine volume and increased urine sodium and osmolality. The increase in intravascular volume brought about by increased tubular reabsorption of water causes hemodilution accompanied by hyponatremia, hyposmolality, and reduced serum urea nitrogen. The increase in intravascular volume also decreases renal sodium reabsorption and thus further increases the urine sodium concentration. Since the urine sodium level and the urine and serum osmolality are such important factors in the mechanisms that control sodium balance, laboratory determinations are very useful in evaluating patients and identifying the cause of the hyponatremia (see Figure 1).

Although the urinary sodium level is useful as a criterion for diagnosis of SIADH, it can be misleading. Other disorders besides SIADH can cause increased sodium excretion in the face of hyponatremia. These include renal loss of sodium, adrenal insufficiency, and use of diuretics (Figure 1). These patients usually appear somewhat volume-depleted. Furthermore, patients with SIADH may have low sodium excretion if they become hypovolemic, a condition that may occur following sodium and water restriction.

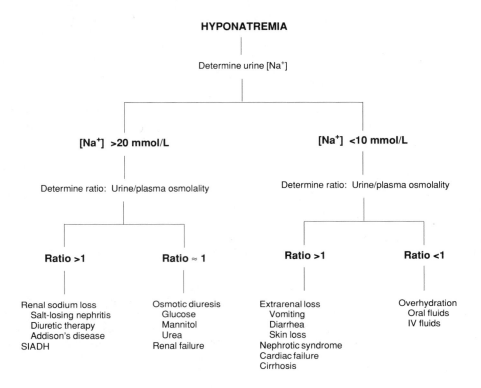

Figure 1. Determination of etiology of hyponatremia. (Adapted from Walmsley, R.N., and White, G.H., Eds.: A Guide to Diagnostic Clinical Chemistry. Boston, Blackwell Scientific Publications, 1983, p. 35.)

Plasma ADH assay has not been included in traditional criteria for diagnosis of SIADH because the assay has not been widely available. ADH levels may be useful in some cases but are not generally necessary to make the diagnosis. Values in patients with SIADH are usually within the physiological reference range but are inappropriately elevated relative to plasma hyposmolality. Interpretation is further complicated because ADH levels are undetectable in 10-20% of patients with SIADH. As assays with better sensitivity become available and low normal values can be distinguished from truly suppressed values, the assay of ADH may become more valuable in the diagnosis of SIADH. Since elevated ADH levels cannot be documented in all cases, the name SID (syndrome of inappropriate diuresis) rather than SIADH (syndrome of inappropriate antidiuretic hormone) has been suggested.[3,4]

The water load test is rarely necessary to make a diagnosis of SIADH; it may even be dangerous in patients with severe hyponatremia. Water loading can be of value in patients with only mild hyponatremia when the etiology is still in question. Normal response is defined as urinary excretion, within four hours, of >90% of the administered water, with concomitant suppression of urine osmolality to <100 mOsmol/kg H_2O.[3] Patients with SIADH have impaired excretion of the water load; they often excrete <40% in five hours and fail to dilute the urine.

As important as laboratory tests for the diagnosis of SIADH is exclusion of other known causes of euvolemic hyponatremia: adrenal insufficiency, hypothyroidism, renal disease, and recent diuretic therapy. These disorders can present with similar laboratory results, including elevated levels of ADH, which do not represent *inappropriate* ADH secretion. SIADH has traditionally been associated with a variety of clinical conditions (Table 2). It was previously thought to be a rare condition, commonly associated with specific tumors of the pancreas or small-cell, undifferentiated (oat cell) carcinoma of the lung, as well as with pulmonary disease and a variety of central nervous system disorders. We now know that it occurs relatively frequently, especially in hospitalized patients and particularly postoperatively.[1] The etiological mechanism of these idiopathic cases is now being sought. An association between stress and sympathetic nervous system response has been considered, particularly among patients who have recently undergone surgery. In these patients, SIADH appears to occur in a context of increased plasma epinephrine and norepinephrine levels. Whether SIADH in these cases represents activation of baroreceptor-mediated nonosmotic stimulation of ADH secretion remains to be proved, but the theory is currently tenable.

Treatment

Standard treatment for patients with SIADH is restriction of free water intake. The treatment is effective because the cause of SIADH is water excess, not sodium deficiency. Therapy by saline infusion will not be helpful since the patients respond by excreting the administered sodium so that hyponatremia is not corrected. In fact, saline infusion has been suggested as a diagnostic ploy, and its failure to correct hyponatremia is used as a marker for SIADH.

This patient's free water intake was restricted. Her sodium and plasma osmolality returned to normal within two days. Studies have shown that water restriction for patients particularly susceptible to development of SIADH prevents the hyponatremia commonly seen. When patients are on drugs with a risk factor for SIADH, water restriction as well as careful monitoring of intake and of plasma sodium and osmolality is important. Demeclocycline, an ADH antagonist, may be useful when water restriction alone is ineffective in reversing hyponatremia. The drug is not, however, useful in the acute phase because onset of action is delayed for a week or more after therapy is initiated.[5]

References

1. Anderson, R.J., Chung, H., Kluge, R., and Schrier, R.W.: Hyponatremia: A prospective analysis of its epidemiology and the pathogenic role of vasopressin. Ann. Intern. Med., *102:* 164-168, 1985.

2. Ober, K.P.: Diabetes insipidus. Crit. Care Clin., *7:* 109-123, 1991.

3. Verbalis, J.G.: Hyponatraemia. Bailliere's Clin. Endocrinol. Metab., *3:* 499-529, 1989.

4. Robertson, G.L.: Diseases of the posterior pituitary. *In:* Endocrinology and Metabolism. P. Felig, J.D. Baxter, A.E. Broadus, and L.A. Frohman, Eds. New York, McGraw-Hill, 1987.

5. Department of Medicine, Washington University School of Medicine: Hyponatremia. *In:* Manual of Medical Therapeutics, 26th ed. W.C. Dunagan and M.L. Ridner, Eds. Boston, Little, Brown and Co., 1989.

AN ELDERLY WOMAN WITH BILATERAL HIP PAIN

Eric L. Hume, Contributor
William H. Porter, Reviewer

A petite, white 72-year-old woman was referred to an orthopedic surgeon with a complaint of progressive hip pain over several months prior to the office visit. She gave no history of trauma and had otherwise been in her usual state of good health. She complained of bilateral pain in the inguinal ligament areas that radiated into the anterior and medial thighs. The pain resolved with rest, grew worse with activity, and was most severe upon rising from a chair, getting out of bed, or climbing stairs.

Upon physical examination, the patient had a healthy appearance, was of slight build with small muscle mass, and had no remarkable signs or symptoms aside from the pain in her hips and thighs. Gentle rotation of her hips caused no significant pain, but forced range of motion reproduced the pain in the groin region. There was local tenderness over the inguinal ligaments and over the inferior gluteal folds bilaterally. Heel percussion also reproduced the pain.

The following laboratory results were obtained:

Analyte	Value, conventional units	Reference range, conventional units	Value, SI units	Reference range, SI units
Hemoglobin (B)	12.8 g/dL	12-16	7.94 mmol/L	7.45-9.93
Sedimentation rate (B)	12 mm/h	0-20	Same	
Leukocyte count (B)	8.3 x 10³/µL	4.8-10.8	8.3 x 10⁹/L	4.8-10.8
Protein, total (S)	6.8 g/dL	6.2-7.6	68 g/L	62-76
Albumin (S)	4.2 g/dL	3.2-4.6	42 g/L	32-46
Calcium (S)	8.8 mg/dL	8.8-10.0	2.20 mmol/L	2.20-2.50
Phosphorus (S)	2.3 mg/dL	2.3-3.7	0.74 mmol/L	0.74-1.19
Urea nitrogen (S)	26 mg/dL	8-21	9.3 mmol urea/L	2.9-7.5
Creatinine (S)	1.2 mg/dL	0.7-1.2	106 µmol/L	62-106
ALP (S)	95 U/L	53-141	1.6 µkat/L	0.9-2.4
Protein (U)	Negative	Negative		

X-ray evaluation showed incompletely healed bilateral fractures of the pubis and ischial rami and severe osteopenia (decrease in bone mass). Additional testing was ordered as follows:

Analyte	Value, conventional units	Reference range, conventional units	Value, SI units	Reference range, SI units
PTH, intact (S)	65 pg/mL	15-60	7.0 pmol/L	1.6-6.4
25(OH)D* (S)	50 ng/mL	9-52	125 nmol/L	22-130
1,25(OH)₂D† (S)	12 pg/mL	15-60	29 pmol/L	36-144
Creatinine clearance	60 mL/min	60-102	0.58 mL/s per m²	0.58-0.98

*25-Hydroxyvitamin D.
†1,25-Dihydroxyvitamin D.

Based on the patient's age, X-ray evaluation, and fracture site, a working diagnosis of senile osteoporosis was recorded. She was treated with calcitriol and calcium supplements every other day and instructed to exercise, initially with an assisting device (a walker) until full healing of the fracture occurred. Laboratory values improved within two weeks, and after two years of treatment the patient felt well, had no recurrent fractures, and maintained serum calcium and parathyroid hormone (PTH; parathormone) levels in the reference ranges. Fracture healing was documented with follow-up radiographs.

Definition of the Disease

Osteoporosis is a common disorder, especially among the elderly. Its prevalence in the United States is about 50 million. The disease is characterized by reduction of bone mass, sufficient to render the skeleton fragile and vulnerable to fractures. Bone loss is above that seen during the normal aging process, and it occurs in both sexes but more in females than in males; it is more pronounced in Caucasians than in Afro-Americans. Osteoporosis is said to exist when bone loss is associated with pain and increased susceptibility to fractures. There are two forms of the disease, postmenopausal and senile osteoporosis.

Postmenopausal osteoporosis was the most likely alternative diagnosis to senile osteoporosis in this particular case. It is important to recognize, however, that not all elderly Caucasian women with atraumatic fractures are automatic candidates for a diagnosis of postmenopausal osteoporosis. A woman with postmenopausal osteoporosis is typically 15-20 years past the loss of ovarian function, whether the loss occurs by natural menopause in the fourth or fifth decade or from surgical oophorectomy. The atraumatic fractures, when they occur, are characteristically of the spine or wrists; secondary sites are cancellous bone regions of the skeleton (i.e., the ends of long bones). These patients may have slightly decreased levels of serum $1,25(OH)_2D$, but most laboratory results are normal. Speculation as to the etiological factors focuses on increased activity of osteoclasts subsequent to estrogen withdrawal. Acceleration of bone resorption and increase in ionized calcium could then depress PTH levels and thus cause inhibition of $1-\alpha$-hydroxylation of 25(OH)D.

Senile osteoporosis is also associated with decreased bone density and increased incidence of bone fractures. In senile osteoporosis, however, fractures occur predominantly in the hip and the age of patients is generally >72 years. The disease occurs in women and men at a ratio of $\approx 2:1$. Speculation as to the etiological mechanism of senile osteoporosis has included the proposition that the mild degree of hyperparathyroidism sometimes seen in elders contributes to the accelerated bone loss of senile osteoporosis. Studies demonstrating a slight decline in the serum concentrations of $1,25(OH)_2D$ with advancing age have led to speculation that the decline stems from the general decline in renal function that occurs with aging. Some observers think the decline implicates an effect of aging to decrease the efficiency of renal activation of 25(OH)D by $1-\alpha$-hydroxylation. The slight increase in serum PTH observed with increasing age has been postulated to be secondary to decreased levels of $1,25(OH)_2D$, or perhaps a consequence of decreased renal clearance of the hormone. However, not all patients with senile osteoporosis and hip fracture display alterations in serum levels of PTH or $1,25(OH)_2D$ or both. Moreover, therapy with vitamin D metabolites has not been demonstrated consistently to prevent or reverse the bone loss of osteoporosis. Nevertheless, vitamin D therapy is often instituted if a deficiency of its intake or production is demonstrated or suspected. Although this agent has been found effective by some investigators, it has not yet been approved for this purpose by the Food and Drug Administration (FDA).

Differential Diagnosis

Diagnosis of osteoporosis is problematic since laboratory findings are not distinctively abnormal in either pattern or direction, and the physical signs of bone loss are not unique to any given disease. This patient had laboratory values that suggest slight secondary hyperparathyroidism, namely, increased PTH and low normal calcium and phosphorus values; normal levels of 25(OH)D were present together with levels of 1,25(OH)$_2$D that were inappropriately low relative to the increased PTH concentration.

The laboratory findings were compatible with secondary hyperparathyroidism and focused on the possibility of vitamin D deficiency, early renal disease, or intestinal malabsorption. PTH in this patient was only slightly increased; the concentration of 25(OH)D was normal, and that of 1,25(OH)$_2$D was low. The normal level of 25(OH)D implied normal intake and absorption and adequate exposure to sunlight. Sufficient substrate was therefore available for the synthesis of the 1,25(OH)$_2$D metabolite by renal tubular cells. The increase of PTH, which drives 1-α-hydroxylation, should have led to normal or increased levels of 1,25(OH)$_2$D. Low levels found in this patient cast some doubt on the efficiency of renal hydroxylation of vitamin D; however, values obtained for creatinine clearance and serum urea nitrogen appear to rule out frank renal disease as a cause.

Other possible causes of this patient's osteopenia included neoplasia metastatic to bone, multiple myeloma, primary hyperparathyroidism, hyperthyroidism, and hypercortisolism. **Neoplasia** and **multiple myeloma** could be excluded because history and physical and X-ray examinations revealed no signs and symptoms of chronic disease or primary tumor sites. Laboratory data did not indicate anemia or hypercalcemia; increased sedimentation rate and abnormal serum or urine proteins were not found.

Primary hyperparathyroidism was not considered because the patient was normocalcemic despite a slight elevation in PTH, and she had none of the abdominal complaints, renal calculi, or psychiatric dysfunction usual in affected patients. Cases of primary hyperparathyroidism are ordinarily detected by routine screening of asymptomatic patients for hypercalcemia.

The patient was also free of symptoms of **hyperthyroidism**, namely, nervousness, anxiety, weight loss, thin hair and skin, increased pulse, and hyperreflexia. Furthermore, the patient had no history of treatment with thyroid medication; iatrogenic hyperthyroidism is an important cause of bone loss. Had hyperthyroidism been a real consideration, evaluation of serum T$_4$ and TSH would have been appropriate to rule out or confirm the diagnosis.

Hypercortisolism in this age group is frequently caused by overmedication with steroids for asthma, rheumatoid arthritis, or inflammatory bowel disease, but the patient had no history of these diseases or therapies and no signs and symptoms of primary adrenocortical or pituitary disorders. History is a critical discriminator in detecting primary hypercortisolism. Physical examination detecting characteristic signs of dowager's hump, moon face, or change in skin pigmentation or texture should lead to investigation of serum or urine corticosteroids and metabolites.

One concern the clinician faces in reaching a confident diagnosis of either type of osteoporosis is how far to go in a workup in order to exclude treatable causes of osteopenia. In general, in the primary evaluation of a person with an initial fracture and an age likely for postmenopausal or senile osteoporosis, the clinician should order simple screening tests that index on hyperparathyroidism, hyperthyroidism, and hypercortisolism. History and physical examination indicating chronic disease symptoms (weight loss, change in appetite, malaise, fever, other constitutional symptoms), regardless of laboratory findings, should heighten the clinical level of suspicion for a disease entity other than osteoporosis and trigger aggressive workup for primary tumors. Examination of undecalcified sections of bone biopsy material can be helpful in looking for neoplastic disease or for evaluating bone change characteristic of menopause.

Evaluation of Osteoporosis

Although a variety of methods for measuring mineral density and turnover rates of bone are available and may be applied to quantitate the progress of osteoporosis,[1] the measurements are more applicable to research of the etiological and pathophysiological factors and to trials of preventive and therapeutic modalities than to routine follow-up and treatment of the patient with evident bone loss.

Treatment

Prevention of osteoporosis is greatly preferred over treatment. Some patients have diets that are, relative to their physiological needs, deficient in calcium and vitamin D; these patients benefit from supplementation. Lack of exercise or physical activity contributes to bone loss, and forms and degrees of exercise appropriate for almost any kind of patient can be designed and prescribed to prevent or reduce the rate of progression of bone loss. Recent evidence indicates that estrogen replacement therapy for women has a beneficial effect on the rate of fractures in patients with both senile and postmenopausal osteoporosis and on the risk for cardiovascular disease. Nevertheless, increased risk of breast cancer prevents universal use of estrogen therapy.

Considerable controversy remains regarding other treatments for postmenopausal osteoporosis. *Sodium fluoride*, because it has been shown to increase bone mineral density as evidenced by radiographic examination, was used in the early 1980's. However, a recent study[2] suggested that the fracture rate of the spine was not decreased and that the fracture rate of long bones might even be slightly increased. The study of sodium fluoride treatment with modified dosages continues.

An FDA-approved drug for treating osteoporosis is *calcitonin*, which acts by interfering with osteoclastic activity. Measurements of bone mineral density demonstrate decreased loss in osteoporotic patients treated with calcitonin, especially in high-turnover osteoporosis.[3]

A recent development is the potential for use of *bisphosphonates*. A prospective randomized study[4,5] has shown a decrease in the rate of spinal fractures in patients treated with diphosphonates. More extensive experience with this class of drugs will be required before specific agents can be recommended for widespread use.

Combination of various agents may be important in the future. Drugs used in sequence promise greater effectiveness than when used separately and independently and in a nonsequential pattern.

References

1. Johnston, C.C., Melton, L.J., Lindsay, R., and Eddy, D.M.: Clinical indications for bone mass measurements. J. Bone Miner. Res., *4(Suppl. 2):* 1-28, 1989.

2. Riggs, B.L., Hodgson, S.F., and O'Fallon, W.M.: Effect of fluoride treatment on the fracture rate in postmenopausal women with osteoporosis. N. Engl. J. Med., *322:* 802-809, 1990.

3. Chesnut, C.H., III: Synthetic salmon calcitonin, diphosphates, and anabolic steroids in the treatment of postmenopausal osteoporosis. *In:* Osteoporosis, vol. 2. C. Christiansen, Ed. Proceedings of the Copenhagen International Symposium on Osteoporosis, June 3-8, 1984.

4. Storm, T., Thamsborg, G., Steiniche, T., et al.: Effect of intermittent cyclical etidronate therapy on bone mass and fracture rate in women with postmenopausal osteoporosis. N. Engl. J. Med., *322:* 1265-1271, 1990.

5. Watts, N.B., Harris, S.T., Genant, H.K, et al.: Intermittent cyclical etidronate treatment of postmenopausal osteoporosis. N. Engl. J. Med., *323:* 73-79, 1990.

Additional Reading

Barth, R.W., and Lane, J.M.: Osteoporosis. Orthop. Clin. North Am., *19:* 845-858, 1988.

Compston, J.E.: Osteoporosis. Clin. Endocrinol., *33:* 653-682, 1990.

Cooper, C., McLaren, M., Wood, P.J., et al.: Indices of calcium metabolism in women with hip fractures. Bone Miner., *5:* 193-200, 1989.

Hordon, L.D., and Peacock, M.: Osteomalacia and osteoporosis in femoral neck fracture. Bone Miner., *11:* 247-259, 1990.

Philllips, S., Fox, N., Jacobs, J., and Wright, W.E.: The direct medical costs of osteoporosis for American women aged 45 and older, 1986. Bone, *9:* 271-279, 1988.

Raisz, L.G.: Local and systemic factors in the pathogenesis of osteoporosis. N. Engl. J. Med., *318:* 818-828, 1988.

Raisz, L.G., and Smith, J.: Pathogenesis, prevention, and treatment of osteoporosis. Ann. Rev. Med., *40:* 251-267, 1989.

Rapin, C.H., Lagier, R., Boivin, G., et al.: Biochemical findings in blood of aged patients with femoral neck fractures: A contribution to the detection of occult osteomalacia. Calcif. Tissue Int., *34:* 465-469, 1982.

Silverberg, S.J., Shane, E., de la Cruz, L., et al.: Abnormalities in parathyroid hormone secretion and 1,25-dihydroxyvitamin D_3 formation in women with osteoporosis. N. Engl. J. Med., *320:* 277-281, 1989.

GAIT DISTURBANCE AFTER EXTENSIVE BOWEL RESECTION

Zilla Huma, Contributor
Joseph M. Gertner, Contributor

A four-year-old girl first presented at age five months with an abdominal mass that was found to be a retroperitoneal teratoma. This was successfully resected, but postoperatively she developed bowel ischemia and necrosis. Large necrotic areas of small bowel including the terminal ileum were resected, leaving only 30 cm of small bowel intact and leading to development of short-gut syndrome. The child had multiple other postoperative complications including superior vena cava obstruction and resultant hydrocephalus.

For the next two years she was fed through a gastrostomy tube and deep line for total parenteral nutrition (TPN). Gradually she was weaned off TPN and maintained on Peptamen Formula (hydrolysate formula, lactose-free, and containing medium-chain triglyceride oil) through the gastrostomy tube. The formula was supplemented with a meager oral diet and multivitamin supplementation that included the fat-soluble vitamins A, D, E, and K.

When the child was four years of age, her physician noted elevation of the serum aminotransferase levels. Further inquiry revealed accidental overdosage of vitamin A. Hypervitaminosis A was confirmed by a liver biopsy and by an elevated vitamin A serum concentration of 128 μg/dL (4.47 μmol/L); reference range, 30-95 μg/dL (1.05-3.32 μmol/L).

Shortly thereafter her physician noted an abnormal gait for which he suspected a metabolic cause. Accordingly she was referred to the metabolism service for further investigations. On physical examination she measured 37 inches (94.1 cm; 5th percentile) in height and 31 lb (14 kg; 25th percentile) in weight. The enlargement of her head, already greater than the 95th percentile, had remained unchanged over the last year. Apart from a distinct muscular weakness, she appeared to be in good general health and was not in any distress. There was no evidence of jaundice or anemia. The patient exhibited marked bowing of the legs with a waddling toed-in gait. No obvious thickening at the wrist or rachitic rosary (enlargement of the costochondral junctions) was seen. There was marked abdominal protuberance with hepatomegaly measuring 4 cm below the right rib margin. A gastrostomy tube was sited 5 cm below the left rib margin in the anterior clavicular line. All other systems were normal on examination. Chvostek's sign for hypocalcemia could not be elicited. Despite a history of supplementation with calcium glubionate, vitamin D₂ (ergocalciferol), and multivitamins, the radiographic studies were suggestive of rickets.[1] In particular the epiphyseal plates were irregularly widened, with a frayed and cupped appearance seen most prominently at the wrists, knees, and ankles. The child was therefore investigated for possible malabsorption of calcium and vitamin D. The following laboratory data were obtained:

Analyte	Value, conventional units	Reference range, conventional units	Value, SI units	Reference range, SI units
Calcium (S)	9.4 mg/dL	8.5-10.5	2.35 mmol/L	2.12-2.62
Phosphorus (S)	2.0 mg/dL	3.6-6.2	0.65 mmol/L	1.16-2.00
Magnesium (S)	2.1 mg/dL	1.5-1.9	0.86 mmol/L	0.62-0.78
ALP (S)	1674 U/L	100-330	27.9 μkat/L	1.67-5.50
1,25(OH)₂D (S)	92.6 pg/mL	20-40	222 pmol/L	48-96

Analyte	Value, conventional units	Reference range, conventional units	Value, SI units	Reference range, SI units
25(OH)D (S)	7.1 ng/mL	15-45	18 nmol/L	37-112
PTH (S)	123 pg/mL	<65	13.2 pmol/L	<7.0
Vitamin B$_{12}$ (S)	382 pg/mL	160-970	282 pmol/L	118-716
Folic acid (S)	18.8 ng/mL	2-17	43 nmol/L	5-39

Calcium Absorption Test *	Prechallenge	Postchallenge
Calcium (S)	9.2 mg/dL (2.30 mmol/L)	10.1 mg/dL (2.52 mmol/L)
Calcium (U)	8.3 mg/dL (2.07 mmol/L)	6.8 mg/dL (1.70 mmol/L)
Creatinine (S)	0.4 mg/dL (35 μmol/L)	0.4 mg/dL (35 μmol/L)
Creatinine (U)	54.5 mg/dL (4.8 mmol/L)	14.4 mg/dL (1.3 mmol/L)

Explanation of Test. The calcium absorption test is an indirect approach to the assessment of intestinal calcium absorption. The end points are the postload increases, if any, in serum calcium, i.e., the calcemic effect, and the urinary calcium excretion corrected for renal function (in $Ca_{U(corr)}$), i.e., the calciuric effect. The following equation is used to calculate $Ca_{U(corr)}$:

$$Ca_{U(corr)} = (Ca_U \times Cr_S)/Cr_U$$

where Ca_U and Cr_U are the urinary calcium and creatinine concentrations, respectively, and Cr_S is the serum creatinine.

In the present case the calcemic effect of the load was 0.9 mg/dL, and the calciuric effect was 0.28-0.06 = 0.22 mg/dL. The calcemic effect was normal while the calciuric effect was high for an adult or child. These were unexpected findings in nutritional rickets when, *a priori*, one would expect to find poor indices of intestinal calcium absorption.

25(OH)D Absorption Test †	Patient value	Mean reference value
Baseline 25(OH)D (P)	6.7 ng/mL (17 nmol/L)	20 ng/mL (50 nmol/L)
Postchallenge (P)		
2 h	5.2 ng/mL (13 nmol/L)	62 ng/mL (155 nmol/L)
4 h	6.5 ng/mL (16 nmol/L)	110 ng/mL (275 nmol/L)
6 h	8.5 ng/mL (21 nmol/L)	114 ng/mL (285 nmol/L)
8 h	8.8 ng/mL (22 nmol/L)	118 ng/mL (295 nmol/L)
18 h	9.7 ng/mL (24 nmol/L)	100 ng/mL (250 nmol/L)
24 h	9.1 ng/mL (23 nmol/L)	86 ng/mL (215 nmol/L)

---

* **Calcium Absorption Test:**[2] Have patient void urine upon waking and discard urine. Collect next two hours of urine passed (prechallenge specimen). At the end of this period, collect baseline blood specimens for serum creatinine, calcium, phosphorus, magnesium, PTH, and vitamin D metabolites. Then administer the oral challenge of whole milk, 4 mL/kg body weight, plus calcium glubionate (Neo-Calglucon), 0.5 mL/kg body weight. Collect urine over the next two hours and discard it. Collect the urine over the *next* two hours and label it postchallenge specimen. Halfway through this collection period (three hours after challenge) collect blood specimens for serum calcium and creatinine.

† **25(OH)D Absorption Test:**[3] Obtain baseline blood specimen. Administer 25(OH)-cholecalciferol (25-hydroxyvitamin D; 25[OH]D) orally (10 μg/kg body weight) and obtain blood specimens at 0, 2, 4, 6, 8, 18, and 24 hours postchallenge. Analyze blood specimens for plasma 25(OH)D.

Explanation of Test. Figure 1 demonstrates poor absorption of the fat-soluble 25(OH)D. These results support the view that the child's vitamin D deficiency, as manifested by a subnormal basal 25(OH)D level, was due to gastrointestinal factors.

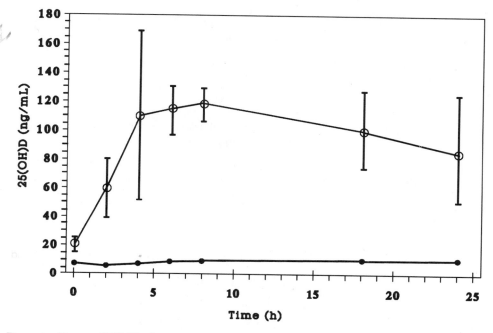

Figure 1. Plasma 25(OH)D after an oral dose of 10 μg of the vitamin. Patient values: ● ;   mean reference values: ○ .

Definition of the Disease

The term *rickets* describes a constellation of physical, histopathological, radiological, and biochemical findings. On histological examination, epiphyseal growth plate cartilage is hypertrophic with the mineralization process delayed and irregular. Since adults do not possess cartilaginous growth plates, rickets is, of necessity, a disease of children. Rickets, however, is always accompanied by poor mineralization and hyperosteoidosis of trabecular bone, the characteristics of osteomalacia in all age groups. Physically, children with rickets have bony deformities, especially of weight-bearing bones. Additionally, bossing or prominence of the frontal part of the skull and hypertrophy of the costochondral junctions may be seen when the onset of rickets occurs before two years of age.

Bone pain and proximal muscular weakness are often features of nutritional rickets. Both can contribute to the disturbance in gait that was the primary presenting feature in this case. The bone pain is probably due to an abnormal response to mechanical stress in pathologically soft bones. The muscle weakness is not well understood. It may be due to a direct effect of a vitamin D metabolite on muscle power, to an effect of hypophosphatemia, or to some combination of both.

Since rickets is essentially the end result of inadequate bony mineralization in a growing child, it follows that it may be a consequence of any disorder that interferes with such mineralization. These causes have recently been reviewed[4,5] and can be simply classified as follows:

Inadequate intake or absorption of vitamin D
Interference with the metabolic activation of vitamin D
End-organ resistance to 1,25-dihydroxyvitamin D (1,25[OH]$_2$D)
Phosphate deficiency, usually due to renal tubular dysfunction
Chronic acidosis, especially distal type renal tubular acidosis
Calcium deficiency due to very unusual diets

In developed countries rickets due to nutritional calcium or phosphorus deficiency, or both, is almost entirely confined to rapidly growing premature infants.[6]

The biochemical aberrations associated with rickets depend on the cause. Alkaline phosphatase (ALP) is always elevated since this enzyme is directly released from cells of the hypertrophic osteoid. Levels of other circulating factors, together with some causes of rickets associated with them, are shown in Table 1.

Table 1. LABORATORY VALUES IN RICKETS DUE TO VARIOUS CAUSES

Cause	Calcium	Phosphorus	ALP	1,25(OH)$_2$D	25(OH)D	PTH
Nutritional D deficiency	Low	Low to High	High	Low to High	Low	High
1,25(OH)$_2$D synthesis defect	Low	Low	High	Low	Normal	High
Resistance to 1,25(OH)$_2$D	Low	Low	High	High	Normal	High
Renal tubular phosphorus wasting	Normal	Low	High	Normal to Low	Normal	Normal

Discussion

Despite vitamin D and calcium supplementation after extensive bowel resection, this patient developed vitamin D deficiency rickets. The biochemical findings suggested a relatively mild deficiency with normal serum calcium but with hypophosphatemia attributable to secondary hyperparathyroidism. The elevated ALP, however, indicated defective bone mineralization, whereas the radiological findings confirmed the presence of rickets. The calcium absorption test demonstrated a detectable rise in serum calcium and low basal urinary calcium excretion, with a considerable increase in postload urinary calcium excretion. The low basal calcium excretion could be due to vitamin D deficiency, to steatorrhea *per se*, or to a combination of these factors. The postload increase in urinary calcium excretion was hard to explain but did suggest that some calcium was absorbed under the special conditions of the test. It is noteworthy that this patient had a high 1,25(OH)$_2$D level despite clinical and biochemical evidence (low 25[OH]D) of vitamin D deficiency. We have observed this phenomenon quite often in vitamin D deficient children, and it has been reported in the literature.[7] Normally, the concentration of 1,25(OH)$_2$D in the plasma is about 1/1000 of that of its precursor. Parathyroid hormone (PTH; parathormone) is trophic for the renal conversion of 25(OH)D to 1,25(OH)$_2$D, and we assume that under the conditions of hyperparathyroidism prevalent in patients with nutritional rickets that a substantial amount of substrate is converted to the active metabolite. We have not routinely performed calcium absorption tests in children with nutritional rickets, but as noted before, poor calcium absorption and low urinary calcium excretion have generally been considered pathognomonic of this deficiency disease.

The 25(OH)D absorption test produced no significant rise in the serum values of the metabolite. Typical "nutritional" vitamin D deficiency is due to dietary deficiency of vitamin D coupled with inadequate exposure to sunlight. Affected patients would have a normal absorption curve for oral 25(OH)D. In the present case, however, the lack of vitamin D is due to a failure to absorb vitamin D rather than to dietary deficiency.[8]

Treatment

Native vitamin D exists in two closely related chemical forms, cholecalciferol (vitamin D_3) and ergocalciferol (vitamin D_2). The form produced in mammalian (including human) skin is cholecalciferol; the manufactured form, used most commonly for the production of medications and the fortification of food, is ergocalciferol. Each form has a corresponding 25-hydroxylated and 1,25-dihydroxylated form, but these forms are probably physiologically equivalent in humans.

The recommended daily allowance for vitamin D is 400 IU. For treatment of rickets due to dietary or sunlight deprivation, 2000 IU/d should be adequate. Here, however, intestinal dysfunction mandated parenteral treatment. The child was treated with intramuscular vitamin D_2 (500,000 IU); serum calcium and phosphate levels increased, serum ALP decreased, and plasma 25(OH)D levels, the best measure of an individual's vitamin D nutritional status, rose into the normal range after treatment (see Figure 2).

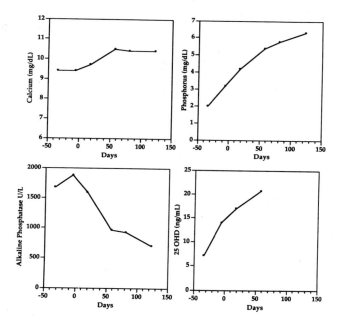

Figure 2. Serum biochemistry values before and after therapy with a single intramuscular injection of ergocalciferol (vitamin D_2). X-axis numbers indicate days relative to the injection.

In the months following the intramuscular injection, marked improvement occurred in her gait and in muscle strength. Because intestinal malabsorption persists, further treatment with parenteral vitamin D will probably be necessary in the future.

References

1. Harrison, H.E., and Harrison, H.C.: Rickets and osteomalacia. *In:* Disorders of Calcium and Phosphate Metabolism in Childhood and Adolescence. Philadelphia, W.B. Saunders Co., 1979.

2. Broadus, A.E., Horst, R.L., Littledike, E.T., et al.: Primary hyperparathyroidism with intermittent hypercalcaemia: Serial observations and simple diagnosis by means of an oral calcium tolerance test. Clin. Endocrinol., *12:* 225-235, 1980.

3. Stamp, T.C.: Intestinal absorption of 25-hydroxycholecalciferol. Lancet, *2:* 2121-2123, 1974.

4. Glorieux, F.H.: Rickets, the continuing challenge. N. Engl. J. Med., *325:* 1875-1877, 1991.

5. Jacobsen, S.T, Hull, C.K., and Crawford, A.H.: Nutritional rickets. J. Pediatr. Orthop., *6:* 713-716, 1986.

6. Gertner, J.M., and Globerman, H.: Mineral metabolism and skeletal disorders in the newborn. *In:* Principles and Practice of Pediatrics. F.A. Oski, C.D. DeAngelis, R. Feigin, and J.B. Warshaw, Eds. Philadelphia, J.B. Lippincott Co., 1989.

7. Garabedian, M., Valnsel, M., Mallet, E., et al.: Circulating vitamin D metabolite concentrations in children with nutritional rickets. J. Pediatr., *103:* 381-386, 1983.

8. Gertner, J.M., Lilburn, M., and Domenech, M.: 25-Hydroxycholecalciferol absorption in steatorrhoea and postgastrectomy osteomalacia. Br. Med. J., *1:* 1310-1312, 1977.

PERSISTENT COUGH AND DYSPNEA

Robert C. Noble, Contributor

A 20-year-old white, single engineering student complained of shortness of breath and cough over a three-week period.

The patient had been in good health all of his life. He was born in Merced, California, and visited his parents there last summer. He described himself as a "health nut" in that he worked out in the gym regularly and ran five miles daily. For the past three months, he had noticed enlarged lymph nodes, particularly in his neck. Despite a good appetite, he had lost approximately 15 lb (6.8 kg). He had to stop running three weeks ago because of lack of energy, shortness of breath, and a dry, hacking cough. For the past several days, he had noticed that he was sweating at night and had to get up at least once to change his pajamas. For the past two days, he had become short of breath with almost any physical activity.

The physical examination revealed a well-developed, well-nourished young man who was sweating and breathing rapidly. His height was 70 inches (1.78 m) and his weight 154 lb (70 kg). The vital signs were temperature, 100.4 °F (38 °C); pulse, 115 BPM; respirations, 48/min; blood pressure, 115/65 mm Hg. Abnormal physical findings included shotty axillary, inguinal, and anterior cervical nodes and scattered rales on auscultation of the chest.

Laboratory tests included the following:

Analyte	Value, conventional units	Reference range, conventional units	Value, SI units	Reference range, SI units
Sodium (S)	135 mmol/L	136-145	Same	
Potassium (S)	4.1 mmol/L	3.8-5.1	Same	
Chloride (S)	100 mmol/L	96-104	Same	
CO$_2$, total (S)	25 mmol/L	23-29	Same	
Urea nitrogen (S)	7 mg/dL	7-18	2.5 mmol urea/L	2.5-6.4
Creatinine (S)	0.8 mg/dL	0.7-1.3	71 µmol/L	62-115
Glucose (S)	100 mg/dL	65-95	5.6 mmol/L	3.6-5.3
Protein, total (S)	7.3 g/dL	6.0-7.8	73 g/L	60-78
Albumin (S)	2.4 g/dL	3.5-5.0	24 g/L	35-50
Urate (S)	5.0 mg/dL	4.5-8.0	297 µmol/L	268-476
Cholesterol (S)	95 mg/dL	140-225	2.46 mmol/L	3.63-5.83
Bilirubin, total (S)	1.1 mg/dL	<0.2-1.0	19 µmol/L	<3-17
AST (S)	20 U/L	15-40	0.33 µkat/L	0.25-0.67
ALT (S)	15 U/L	13-40	0.25 µkat/L	0.22-0.67
LDH (S)	301 U/L	100-190	5.02 µkat/L	1.67-3.17
ALP (S)	151 U/L	49-120	2.5 µkat/L	0.8-2.0
pH (aB)	7.44	7.35-7.45	Same	
pCO$_2$ (aB)	33 mm Hg	35-48	4.4 kPa	4.7-6.4
pO$_2$ (aB)	79 mm Hg	83-108	10.5 kPa	11.1-14.4
Hemoglobin (B)	13.2 g/dL	14-18	8.19 mmol/L	8.69-11.17
Hematocrit (B)	37.9 %	40-54	0.38	0.40-0.54
Leukocyte count (B)	6.6 x 10^3/µL	4.8-10.8	6.6 x 10^9/L	4.8-10.8

Analyte	Value, conventional units	Reference range, conventional units	Value, SI units	Reference range, SI units
Platelet count (B)	156 x 10³/μL	150-450	156 x 10⁹/L	150-450
Differential count (B)				
Segmented neutrophils	79 %	41-71	0.79	0.41-0.71
Band forms	6 %	5-10	0.06	0.05-0.10
Lymphocytes	9 %	24-44	0.09	0.24-0.44
Monocytes	6 %	3-7	0.06	0.03-0.07
Urinalysis (U)	Within normal limits			
Occult blood (F)	Negative	Negative		

A chest X-ray showed diffuse bilateral densities consistent with pneumonia. The lower lobes were more involved than the upper lobes. The cardiac size and silhouette were normal.

On further questioning, the patient stated that he was homosexual and had been sexually active since age 15. He thought that he had AIDS and that he had been infected with the human immunodeficiency virus (HIV) when he worked as a waiter one summer in San Francisco. He had not sought medical attention because he was afraid that his fellow students in the College of Engineering would learn of his homosexuality. His current lover had not been tested for the HIV antibody.

Because of this new information, the following laboratory tests were ordered: HIV antibody to detect infection with human immunodeficiency virus; tuberculin skin test to test for current or prior infection with *Mycobacterium tuberculosis*; syphilis serology to test for infection with *Treponema pallidum*; and a hepatitis serological panel consisting of HBsAg, anti-HBc, and anti-HBs. Both hepatitis B virus infection and syphilis are common among homosexual men. Serological testing for HIV involves two steps: an enzyme-linked immunosorbent assay (ELISA) test and a Western blot test.[1] The ELISA test is a screening test that detects antibodies to whole virus extracts or recombinant proteins of HIV-1. A Western blot test is performed on sera that exhibit a positive ELISA result initially and upon repeat testing. The Western blot assay detects antibodies to HIV-1 and also identifies individual viral components to which the antibodies are reactive. A positive Western blot test is currently the most common method for definitively diagnosing HIV infection. The patient's ELISA and Western blot tests were both positive.

In consideration of the presence of pneumonia with a nonproductive cough, a bronchoscopy was performed to collect sputum for analysis and culture. The most common cause of pneumonia in HIV-positive patients is the parasite *Pneumocystis carinii*. The bacterium *Mycobacterium avium-intracellulare* is the second most common cause of pneumonia. The bronchoscopy specimen was positive for cysts of *Pneumocystis carinii*. The patient was treated with intravenous trimethoprim-sulfamethoxazole and oral prednisone. The latter drug is used to suppress inflammation and to improve oxygenation of the lung.

One final test was performed on the patient, a CD4+ lymphocyte count. This test enumerates the lymphocytes that are specifically infected by the human immunodeficiency virus, HIV-1. HIV is a small RNA virus that is cytolytic for CD4+ or T "helper" lymphocytes. HIV becomes part of the host DNA, and infection with the virus is lifelong.[2,3] As the HIV infection progresses over months and years, the CD4+ count drops. The CD4+ count is not diagnostic of HIV infection, and the measurement is only helpful in directing therapy. When the number of CD4+ lymphocytes reaches 500/μL, the patient is started on zidovudine (Retrovir), an antiviral agent. When the CD4+ count reaches 200/μL, the patient is also placed on trimethoprim-sulfamethoxazole as prophylaxis to prevent *Pneumocystis carinii* pneumonia. Since the patient already had *Pneumocystis* pneumonia, it was likely that his CD4+ count was less than 200/μL, and he would require continual prophylaxis for *Pneumocystis* in any case. His CD4+ count was found to be 16/μL.

The patient's *Pneumocystis* pneumonia responded to three weeks of antibiotic therapy. There was no evidence of prior infection with *Mycobacterium tuberculosis* as his TB skin test was negative; his syphilis and hepatitis B serological tests were negative as well. He was placed on zidovudine and trimethoprim-sulfamethoxazole prophylaxis and followed in the outpatient clinic.

Differential Diagnosis

Fever, cough, and abnormal chest film were suggestive of pneumonia. The patient's history, however, was not typical for a community-acquired bacterial pneumonia. His dyspnea and cough had been present for at least three weeks. Bacterial pneumonias are usually associated with elevated blood neutrophil counts, but the patient's neutrophil count was normal. Pulmonary tuberculosis might cause this X-ray finding, but there was no sputum production, and the infiltrates seen on the roentgenogram were not found in the apices of the lungs. Mycoplasma can also cause pneumonia in a young person, but mycoplasma pneumonia is usually a more acute illness with prostration, headache, and an unremitting, dry cough. Since the patient came from the San Joaquin Valley in California, coccidioidomycosis, caused by the fungus *Coccidioides immitis*, required consideration. The patient's weight loss was ominous and suggested a chronic illness.

Tests included in the laboratory screening panel were relatively normal with a few exceptions. The blood studies revealed low serum albumin, low cholesterol, and elevated LDH and ALP   A low cholesterol is often seen in patients with malnutrition, severe liver cell damage, hyperthyroidism, and chronic anemia. Low albumin levels are seen in malnutrition, liver disease, and hypothyroidism. Elevated serum LDH levels are seen in patients with hepatitis, acute myocardial infarction, pernicious anemia, pulmonary embolism, and pulmonary infarction. The serum ALP may be elevated in certain bone and liver diseases.

Consideration of laboratory results raises the possibility of malnutrition, liver disease, pulmonary disease, a chronic infectious disease, or a combination of such conditions. However, in view of the patient's symptoms and the presence of a normal AST and ALT, primary liver disease was unlikely. Thus, malnutrition and pulmonary disease could account for the abnormal values. A chronic infectious disease of the lungs was consistent with the patient's weight loss and pulmonary symptoms.

Late HIV Infection

After the initial infection with HIV, the patient may experience a flu-like illness. Seroconversion to HIV antibody is usually complete at 2-3 months but may take up to 36 months.[4] Subsequently, there may be a period lasting 10-12 years in which the patient feels well.[5] The earliest symptoms of progressive disease may be the presence of lymphadenopathy and low grade fever. Commonly, patients also complain of a sore mouth due to infection with *Candida albicans*. A clue to the diagnosis is a history of homosexuality, intravenous drug abuse, a blood transfusion between 1978 and 1985, or a history of intercourse with an HIV-infected sexual partner. Since the virus attacks the cellular immune system, the patient becomes susceptible to many infectious diseases or so-called "indicator" diseases.[6] These include

Candidiasis of esophagus, trachea, bronchi, or lungs
Extrapulmonary cryptococcosis
Cryptosporidiosis with diarrhea persisting for more than one month

Cytomegalovirus disease of an organ other than liver, spleen, or lymph
nodes in a patient more than one month of age
Herpes simplex virus infection causing a mucocutaneous ulcer that persists
longer than one month
Bronchitis, pneumonitis, or esophagitis of any duration affecting a patient
more than one month of age
Kaposi's sarcoma affecting a patient less than 60 years of age
Lymphoma of the brain (primary) affecting a patient less than 60 years
of age
Lymphoid interstitial pneumonia and/or pulmonary lymphoid hyperplasia
affecting a child less than 13 years of age
Mycobacterium avium complex or *M. kansasii* disease disseminated at a
site other than, or in addition to, lungs, skin, or cervical or hilar
lymph nodes
Pneumocystis carinii pneumonia
Progressive multifocal leukoencephalopathy
Toxoplasmosis of the brain affecting a patient more than one month of age

References

1. Davey, R.T., and Lane, H.C.: Laboratory methods in the diagnosis and prognostic staging of infection with human immunodeficiency virus type I. Rev. Infect. Dis., *12:* 912-930, 1990.

2. Green, W.C.: The molecular biology of human immunodeficiency virus type I infection. N. Engl. J. Med., *324:* 308-317, 1991.

3. Merigan, T.C., and Katzenstein, D.A.: Relation of the pathogenesis of human immunodeficiency virus infection to various strategies for its control. Rev. Infect. Dis., *13:* 292-302, 1991.

4. Imagawa, D.T., Lee, M.H., Wolinsky, S.M., et al.: Human immunodeficiency virus Type I infection in homosexual men who remain seronegative for prolonged periods. N. Engl. J. Med., *320:* 1458-1462, 1989.

5. Lifson, A.R., Rutherford, G.W., and Jaffe, H.W.: The natural history of human immunodeficiency virus infection. J. Infect. Dis., *158:* 1360-1366, 1988.

6. Centers for Disease Control: Revision of the CDC surveillance case definition for acquired immunodeficiency syndrome. MMWR, *36(Suppl.):* 1S-15S, 1987.

Index

Note: Page numbers in *italics* refer to illustrations; page numbers followed by t indicate tables.

Abdomen, acute, differential diagnosis of, 100
Abdominal pain, in acute hepatic porphyria, 89
 in acute pancreatitis, 99
 in cholelithiasis, 85
 in diabetic ketoacidosis, 111, 112
 in pancreatitis, 303
ABO incompatibility, fetomaternal, 232. See also *Erythroblastosis fetalis.*
Abscess, in acute pancreatitis, 104
Accident, in cocaine-related fatality, 380
Acetaminophen metabolism, 348–349, *349*
Acetaminophen poisoning, case study of, 347–350
 clinical manifestations of, 348
 hepatotoxicity following, mechanism of, 348–349
 liver function studies in, 348
 Rumack-Matthew nomogram in, 347, *347*, 350
 severity of, assessment of, 350
 treatment of, 350
N-Acetylcysteine, for acetaminophen poisoning, 350
Acid phosphatase, in prostatic carcinoma, 361
Acidosis, metabolic. See *Metabolic acidosis.*
 renal tubular, 30–32
 uremic, 30
ACTH stimulation test, in Addison's disease, 178
ACTH-producing tumor, ectopic, case study of, 171–174
 clinical features of, 172–173
 Cushing syndrome due to, 172. See also *Cushing syndrome.*
 dexamethasone screening test for, 173
 diagnosis of, 173–174
 laboratory findings in, 164
 metyrapone and, 173–174
 petrosal sinus sampling in, 174
 serum corticol levels in, 173
 treatment of, 174
Acute hepatic porphyria, case study of, 89–96
 δ-aminolevulinate in, 91, 92–95, 94t
 diagnosis of, 95–96
 laboratory findings in, 94t
 Hoesch test for, 90, 95

Acute hepatic porphyria *(Continued)*
 management of, 96
 porphobilinogen in, 91, 92–95, 94t
 porphyrins in, 91, 92
Acute intermittent porphyria, 92
 laboratory findings in, 94t
Acute myelogenous leukemia, definition of disease, 267
Acute progranulocytic leukemia, Auer bodies in, 267
 bone marrow aspiration and biopsy in, 266, 267
 case study of, 265–268
 definition of disease, 267
 diagnosis of, 266–267
 discussion of, 266
 treatment of, 268
Acute promyelocytic leukemia, Auer rods in, 322
 bleeding phenomena in, 322. See also *Disseminated intravascular coagulopathy (DIC).*
Acute renal failure. See *Renal failure, acute.*
Acute tubular necrosis, renal failure secondary to, 35, 38
Addison's disease, ACTH stimulation test for, 178
 case study of, 177–180
 causes of, 179–180
 diagnosis of, 179
 differential diagnosis of, 178–179
 hyperpigmentation in, 179
 hypopituitarism vs., 179
 plasma cortisol in, 179
 treatment of, 180
ADH (antidiuretic hormone), inappropriate secretion of, 387. See also *Syndrome of inappropriate antidiuretic hormone secretion (SIADH).*
Adrenal cortical carcinoma. See also *Cushing syndrome.*
 case study of, 167–169
 differential diagnosis of, 168–169
 discussion of, 169
 treatment of, 169
 urinary 17-ketosteroids in, 168

Adrenal failure (insufficiency), primary. See *Addison's disease.*
  secondary. See *Hypopituitarism.*
Adrenal hyperplasia, congenital. See *Congenital adrenal hyperplasia.*
Adrenal tumor, laboratory findings in, 164
Adrenergic blockers, preoperative management of pheochromocytoma with, 205
Adrenoleukodystrophy, 180
Adrenomyelodystrophy, 180
Alcohol, tissue damage caused by, 79–80
Alcoholic liver disease, anemia in, 81
  ascites in, 80–81
  case study of, 77–82
  cirrhosis in, 80–81
  coagulation tests in, 82
  definition of, 79
  drug sensitivity in, 82
  encephalopathy in, 82
  esophageal varices in, 81
  feminization in, 82
  hepatitis in, 80
  hypersplenism in, 81
  hypoalbuminemia in, 82
  liver function tests in, 81–82
  Mallory bodies in, 80
  stages of, 79
  treatment of, 82
Alkaline phosphatase activity, in gallbladder disease, 87
Alkalosis, metabolic, in pyloric stenosis, 135
Allograft rejection, following renal transplantation, 29–30
Alpha-fetoprotein (AFP), in genetic hemochromatosis, 66
  in hepatocellular carcinoma, 62, 63–64
  maternal serum, in neural tube defects, 286–287
    screening for, 288, *289*, 290
      results of, 286
Alpha-thalassemia, vs. lead poisoning, 342
Amino acid assays, in ornithine transcarbamylase (OTC) deficiency, 310
δ-Aminolevulinic acid, elevation of, in lead poisoning, 342–343, *343*
  in acute hepatic porphyria, 91, 92–95, 94t
Ampulla of Vater, carcinoma of, case study of, 107–110
  differential diagnosis of, 109–110
Amyloid proteins, antibody typing of, 369
  nomenclature and classification of, 367t
Amyloidosis, amyloid deposits in, 369
  Bence Jones protein in, 368
  cardiac, 367
  carpal tunnel syndrome in, 368
  case study of, 365–369
  differential diagnosis of, 363–368
  discussion of, 368–369
  nomenclature and classification of, 367t
  primary, 368
  secondary, 368

Amyloidosis *(Continued)*
  senile systemic, 368
  treatment of, 369
Androgen(s), excess of, in Cushing disease, 162, 163
Anemia, hemolytic, in Wilson's disease, 74
  in alcoholic liver disease, 81
  in chronic renal disease, 250–251
  in cystic fibrosis, 15–16
  in lead poisoning, 342
  in malabsorption, 124
  in sickle cell disease, 253–254
  pernicious. See *Pernicious anemia.*
Anencephaly. See also *Neural tube defect (NTD).*
  definition of disease, 287
Angina pectoris, definition of, 12
  stable, 12
  unstable, 13
Anion gap, in ethylene glycol poisoning, 335, 336, *338*
Antibiotics, for chorioamnionitis, 222
  contraindications to, 222t
Antidiuretic hormone (ADH), inappropriate secretion of, 387. See also *Syndrome of inappropriate antidiuretic hormone secretion (SIADH).*
Anti-DNA antibodies, in systemic lupus erythematosus, 326
Antiphospholipid antibodies, in systemic lupus erythematosus, *327*, 327–328
Anti-Rho (D), in erythroblastosis fetalis, 229, 232, 233
Aplastic crisis, in sickle cell disease, 256
Apolipoprotein B, elevated, in familial hypercholesterolemia, 298, 299, 300
Apolipoprotein C11, genetic defect in, 305. See also *Hypertriglyceridemia, familial.*
Ascites, in alcoholic cirrhosis, 80–81
  evaluation of, 81
    treatment of, 81
  in ovarian cancer, 242–243
  new onset, associated with liver disease, 66
    evaluation of, 67
Atherosclerosis, associated with familial hypercholesterolemia, 299
  reversal of, 300
Atresia, biliary. See *Biliary atresia.*
Auer bodies, in acute promyelocytic leukemia, 322
  in leukemia, 267
Australia antigen. See *Hepatitis B surface antigen (HBsAg).*
Azotemia, prerenal, differential diagnosis of, 37
  urea nitrogen/creatinine ratio in, 14

Babinski's sign, in multiple sclerosis, 291, 294
Back pain, causes of, 359t
  in prostatic carcinoma, 359, 361

Bacterial peritonitis, spontaneous, diagnosis of, 67

Bence Jones protein, in amyloidosis, 368
in multiple myeloma, 281, 282

Beta-thalassemia, vs. lead poisoning, 342

BH_4-deficient hyperphenylalaninemia, spectrum of, 316t

Bicarbonate, fractional clearance of, calculation of, 31
reduced renal threshold for, 31

Bile acid sequestrants, for familial hypercholesterolemia, 301

Biliary atresia, extrahepatic, case study of, 127–131
diagnosis of, 130
discussion of, 128–131
hepatic biopsy in, 131
neonatal cholestasis associated with, 128
surgical treatment of, 131
vs. neonatal hepatitis, 130–131

Biliary colic, in cholelithiasis, 86

Biliary system, carcinoma of, case study of, 107–110
differential diagnosis of, 109–110

Bilirubin, in gallbladder disease, 87
in stone formation, 86
in Wilson's disease, 72

Biphosphates, for osteoporosis, 394

Bleeding phenomena, in acute promyelocytic leukemia, 266, 267, 322

Blood glucose, self monitoring of, 116

B-ly7 antibody, in hairy-cell phenotype, 278

Body packer syndrome, 383

Bone Gla protein, in high-turnover renal osteodystrophy, 198–199

Bone marrow biopsy, in acute promyelocytic leukemia, 266, 267
in chronic myelogenous leukemia, 270

Bone marrow myeloid cell analysis, in chronic myelogenous leukemia, 270

Bone marrow transplantation, for chronic myelogenous leukemia, 273

Bone pain, in rickets, 399

Bone pathology, in renal osteodystrophy, 197–198

Bowman's space, erythrocytes in, 41

Breast cancer, case study of, 235–238
discussion of, 236–238
prognosis of, cathepsin D in, 237–238
DNA cell content in, 237
epidermal growth factors in, 238
estrogen/progesterone receptors in, 236–237
histopathological features in, 236
neu oncogene in, 238
risk factors for, 236
screening for, 236
treatment of, multiple modalities in, 238

Breast cancer–ovarian cancer syndrome, 241

Breath, shortness of, comments on, 24
with cough, 21

Bronchitis, chronic, comments on, 24
discussion of, 23

Calcitonin, for osteoporosis, 394
in familial MEN 3, 184, 184
in medullary thyroid carcinoma, 147, 186

Calcium absorption test, 398
explanation of, 398

Calcium assay, for hyperparathyroidism, 192

Calcium oxalate stones, in malabsorption, 124

Calcium pyrophosphate dihydrate (CPPD) crystals, in pseudogout, 372, 374

Calculi, calcium oxalate, 124
in gallbladder. See Cholelithiasis.

CALLA (common acute lymphoblastic leukemia-associated antigen), definition of, 270

$CaNa_2EDTA$ (edetate calcium disodium), for lead poisoning, 344–345

Cancer. See Carcinoma; Neoplasia; specific neoplasm or anatomic site.

Cancer antigen 125 (CA 125) assay, in ovarian cancer, 240, 242

Carcinoembryonic antigen (CEA) assay, in ovarian cancer, 240

Carcinoid tumors, case study of, 213–216
definition of, 214–215
diagnosis of, 215–216
diagnostic laboratory tests for, 215–216
facial flushing in, 213, 216
foregut, 215
hindgut, 215
histochemical tests for, 215
histologic tests for, 215
imaging techniques in, 213, 216
midgut, 215
serotonin and 5-HIAA levels in, 214, 216
and response to antineoplastic therapy, 214t
treatment of, 214, 214t, 216

Carcinoma, adrenal cortical. See Adrenal cortical carcinoma.
hepatocellular. See Hepatocellular carcinoma.
medullary thyroid. See Thyroid carcinoma, medullary.
of biliary system, case study of, 107–110
differential diagnosis of, 109–110
prostatic. See Prostatic carcinoma.

Cardic shunt-related pulmonary vascular dynamics, congenital, 9

Cardiomyopathy, amyloid, diagnosis of, 368. See also Amyloidosis.
dilated, 366
echocardiogram in, 367
hypertrophic, 366
restrictive, 366

Carpal tunnel syndrome, in amyloidosis, 368

Catecholamines, in MEN-associated pheochromocytoma, 287

Catecholamines *(Continued)*
  in pheochromocytoma, 203–205, *204*
Cathepsin D, as prognostic predictor, in breast
    cancer, 237
Cause of death (COD), in cocaine-related
    fatality, 378
CD4+ lymphocyte count, in HIV-positive
    patient, 404–405
CD10, definition of, 270
Celiac disease. See *Gluten-sensitive
    enteropathy.*
Central nervous system, damage to, lead
    poisoning and, 344
  involvement of, in hyperparathyroidism, 191–
    192
Cerebral necrosis, causes of, 10
  in congenital heart disease, 10
Cerebrospinal fluid (CSF), in multiple sclerosis,
    analysis of, 292
  electrophoresis of, 293, *293*
    measurement of IgG synthesis rates of, 293
Ceruloplasmin assay, in Wilson's disease, 74
Chelation therapy, for lead poisoning, 344–345
Chenodeoxycholic acid, for gallstones, 88
Chest pain, in myocardial infarction, 11, 12, 297
Chest X-ray, in congenital heart disease, 8
  in emphysema, 22
  in myocardial infarction, 12
  in tumor metastasis, 61
Chloride/phosphorus ratio, in
    hyperparathyroidism, 192
2-Chlorodeoxyadenosine (2-CDA), for hairy-cell
    leukemia, 279
Cholecystectomy, for gallstones, 88
Cholecystitis, definition of, 86
Cholecystogram, in gallbladder disease, 87
Cholelithiasis, case study of, 85–88
  cholescintigram in, 87
  clinical features of, 86
  definition of, 86
  development of stones in, 86
  diagnosis of, 86–87
  laboratory tests for, 87
  oral cholecystogram in, 87
  serum enzyme activity in, 87
  treatment of, 87–88
  ultrasonogram in, 86
Cholescintigram, in gallbladder disease, 87
Cholesterol, in stone formation, 86
Cholesterol desmolase deficiency, clinical and
    laboratory findings in, 153t
Chorioamnionitis, 220
  definition of, 220
  discussion of, 220–221
  treatment of, 222, 222t
Choriocarcinoma, case study of, 225–227
  clinical features of, 227
  extraembryonic differentiation in, 246
  hCG levels in, 225
    following treatment, 226
  treatment of, 226, 227

Christmas disease (hemophilia B), factor IX
    deficiency causing, 332
Chronic myelogenous leukemia, aggressive
    phase of, 272
  blast phase of, 272
  bone marrow aspiration and biopsy in, 270
  case study of, 269–273
  diagnosis of, 271
  differential diagnosis of, 271
  discussion of, 272
  hydroxyurea for, 270
  immunophenotype of blast cells in, 270
  myeloid cell analysis in, 270
  Philadelphia chromosome in, 270, 271, 272
  splenomegaly in, 269, 271
  treatment of, discussion of, 272
Cirrhosis, alcohol-induced, 79, 80–81
  ascites associated with, 80–81
    new onset, 67
  associated with Wilson's disease, 73
  genetic hemochromatosis causing, 66
CK-BB (creatine kinase isoenzyme 1), in
    prostatic carcinoma, 363
Clinical staging, of prostatic carcinoma, 361,
    362t
Clubbing, in hypoxemic states, 10
Coagulation cascade, scheme of, *327*
Coagulation tests, in alcoholic liver disease, 82
Cobalamin deficiency, in pernicious anemia,
    258, 259–260, 261, 261t
Cocaine, administration of, 381
  as sympathomimetic agent, 381, *382*
  "crack," 381
  reaction to, pharmacokinetic variability in, 381
  use and abuse of, 380–381
    cerebral and cardiovascular complications
      of, 382–383
Cocaine-related fatality, accident in, 380
  case study of, 377–384
  comment on, 384
  differential diagnosis of, 379–380
  establishing cause of death in, 378
  establishing legal chain of custody in, 379
  establishing manner of death in, 378–379
  homicide in, 379–380
  medicolegal issues in, 378–379
  medicolegal/forensic investigation into, 377–
    378
  natural cause of death in, 380
  patterns and etiology of, 380–383
  postmortem blood levels and, 383
  suicide in, 380
COD (cause of death), in cocaine-related
    fatality, 378
Colic, biliary, in cholelithiasis, 86
Collagen vascular disease, differential diagnosis
    of, 372
Coma, hyperammonemic, 310
  in Reye's syndrome, 353, 357

Common acute lymphoblastic leukemia-associated antigen (CALLA), definition of, 270

Congenital adrenal hyperplasia, clinical and laboratory findings in, 153t
    definition of disease, 150
    due to 21-hydroxylase deficiency, 150. See also *21-Hydroxylase deficiency.*
    rapid growth and precocious sexual maturity in, 149–150

Congenital erythropoietic porphyria, 95

Congenital heart disease, case study of, 7–10
    cerebral necrosis in, 10
    chest X-ray in, 8
    cyanotic, complications of, 9–10
    discussion of, 9
    Eisenmenger physiology in, 8, 9, 10
    electrocardiogram in, 8
    erythroid hyperplasia in, 10
    heart murmur in, 7
    heart sounds in, 7
    hypoxemia in, 9–10
    morphological vascular changes in, 9
    oxygen saturation in, 8

Conjugated hyperbilirubinemia, definition of, 128

Convulsions, treatment of, 345

Copper, absorption, utilization, and excretion of, in Wilson disease, 72, 73
    hepatic, in Wilson's disease, 74

Copper diet, low, for Wilson's disease, 72, 74

Copper incorporation test, for Wilson's disease, 75

Coproporphyria, hereditary, 92
    laboratory findings in, 94t
    photosensitivity in, 95

Cor pulmonale, comments on, 24
    discussion of, 23
    ECG in, 22

Corneal arcus, in familial hypercholesterolemia, 299
    in familial hypertriglyceridemia, 305

Coronary artery occlusion, CK and CK-MB values in, 13

Corticosteroids, for minimal change nephrotic syndrome, 51

Corticosterone methyl oxidase deficiency, clinical and laboratory findings in, 153t

Corticotropin-releasing factor (CRF) syndrome, ectopic, 157, 160. See also *Cushing syndrome.*

Cough, and sputum production, 21
    comments on, 24
    in human immunodeficiency virus (HIV) infection, 403

C-peptide test, for insulin reserve, 115

"Crack" cocaine, 381

C-reactive protein, in multiple myeloma, 282, 283

Creatine kinase isoenzyme 1 (CK-BB), in prostatic carcinoma, 363

Creatinine, urinary, diabetes mellitus and, 114

Creatinine clearance, calculation of, 31

Cretinism (congenital hypothyroidism), 143

CSF. See *Cerebrospinal fluid (CSF).*

Cushing disease, androgen excess in, 162, 163
    case study of, 161–165
    definition of disease, 162–163
    diagnosis of, 163–164
    laboratory findings in, 164
    pituitary microadenoma in, 164
    treatment of, 165

Cushing syndrome, adrenal cortical carcinoma in, 169. See also *Adrenal cortical carcinoma.*
    adrenocortical-pituitary axis tests in, 157
    clinical features of, 158, 163
    definition of, 157
    definition of disease, 162–163
    definition of syndrome, 172–173
    diabetes insipidus in, 156, 158–159
    diagnosis of, 158–160, 163–164
    differential diagnosis of, 163
    ectopic ACTH-producing tumor in, 172. See also *ACTH-producing tumor.*
    endocrinological studies in, 156
    hypercortisolism in, 157–158, 171
    metabolic features of, 157–158
    metastatic carcinoma in, 157, 158, 160
    panhypopituitarism in, 156, 159
    pathophysiology of, 162–163
    pituitary microadenoma in, 164. See also *Cushing disease.*
    suspected, 159
    treatment of, 160, 165
    tumors associated with, laboratory findings in, 164

Custody, legal chain of, in cocaine-related fatality, 379

Cyanosis, in congenital heart disease, 9

Cyclosporine, as immunosuppressant, effects of, 29
    toxicity of, 29
    for minimal change nephrotic syndrome, 51

CYP21 gene, in 21-hydroxylase deficiency, 150
    mutations in, 150

Cyproterone acetate, for metastatic prostatic carcinoma, 360

Cystic fibrosis, case study of, 15–19
    clinical features of, 18
    definition of, 16–17
    diagnosis of, 17
    fertility in, 18
    gene for, 17
    incidence of, 17
    life expectancy with, 19
    malabsorption in, 18
    postural drainage of chest in, 18
    sweat chloride test for, 16, 17
    transmembrane regulatory protein in, 16–17
    treatment of, 18

DCF (deoxycoformycin), for hairy-cell leukemia, 279
DDAVP (1-desamino-8-D-arginine vasopressin), for hemophilia A, 331, 332, 334
Death, cause of, in cocaine-related fatality, 378
  natural, 380
  manner of, in cocaine-related fatality, 378–379
  sudden, cocaine-induced, patterns and etiology of, 380–383
Deep venous thrombosis, associated with systemic lupus erythematosus, 326
Delirium, excited, cocaine-induced, 383
Deoxycoformycin (DCF), for hairy-cell leukemia, 279
Deoxyribonucleic acid (DNA), cell content of, in breast cancer prognosis, 237
1-Desamino-8-D-arginine vasopressin (DDAVP), for hemophilia A, 331, 332, 334
Dexamethasone suppression test, in ectopic ACTH-producing tumors, 173
Diabetes insipidus, in Cushing syndrome, 156, 158–159
Diabetes mellitus, case study of, 111–117
  clinical features of, 113–114
  complications of, 113–114
  control of, monitoring, 116–117
  diagnostic criteria for, 114–115
  differential diagnosis of, 112–113
  glucose tolerance test for, 114–115
  incidence of, 113
  microalbuminuria in, 114
  screening tests for, 115
  treatment of, 115
  Type I (insulin-dependent), 113
  Type II (noninsulin-dependent), 113
  urinary protein and creatinine concentrations in, 114
Diabetic ketoacidosis, diagnosis of, 112
  metabolic acidosis in, 112–113
Diarrhea, in gluten-sensitive enteropathy, 119
  in malabsorption, 123
  in Zollinger-Ellison syndrome, 207, 208, 210
DIC. See Disseminated intravascular coagulopathy (DIC).
Diet, for phenylketonuria, 319
  in cystic fibrosis, 18
  low fat, for familial hypercholesterolemia, 300–301
  for familial hypertriglyceridemia, 306
1,25–Dihydroxyvitamin D, reduced, in renal osteodystrophy, 196–197
Dipstick protein test, in minimal change nephrotic syndrome, 49
Disseminated intravascular coagulopathy (DIC), acute promyelocytic leukemia associated with, diagnosis of, 322
  treatment of, 322, 323
  case study of, 321–324
  hematological abnormalities in, discussion of, 322, 323

Disseminated intravascular coagulopathy (DIC) (Continued)
  hemostatic abnormalities in, discussion of, 322–324
  laboratory diagnosis of, 324
  treatment of, 324
DNA (deoxyribonucleic acid), cell content of, in breast cancer prognosis, 237
Down syndrome, definition of disease, 287
  risk of, calculation of, 286
  screening for, 288
    AFP levels in, 288
    hCG levels in, 288
    recommended AFP profile in, 288, 289
    results of, 286
    sensitivity of AFP profile in, 290
    unconjugated estradiol levels in, 288
Drinking water, lead in, permissible levels of, 344
Drug overdose. See Acetaminophen poisoning.
Drug sensitivity, in alcoholic liver disease, 82
Drug therapy. See also named drug.
  for familial hypercholesterolemia, 301
Duodenal ulcer, 209
Dysgerminoma, 245
  discussion of, 246
Dysphoria, cocaine-induced, 383
Dyspnea, 24. See also Shortness of breath.
  in human immunodeficiency virus (HIV) infection, 403

Ecchymoses, in acute promyelocytic leukemia, 265, 266
Echocardiogram, in cardiomyopathy, 367
  in myocardial infarction, 12
Edema, associated with minimal change nephrotic syndrome, 45, 47
  associated with pulmonary disease, 24
Edetate calcium disodium (CaNa$_2$EDTA), for lead poisoning, 344–345
EGFR (epidermal growth factor receptors), in breast cancer, 238
Eisenmenger physiology, 8, 9, 10
Electrocardiogram, in congenital heart disease, 8
  in cor pulmonale, 22
  in myocardial infarction, 11, 12
Electrophoresis, of cerebrospinal fluid, in multiple sclerosis patient, 293
ELISA (enzyme-linked immunosorbent assay), for human immunodeficiency virus, 404
Embryonal carcinoma, embryonic differentiation in, 246
Emphysema, chest X-ray for, 22
  comments on, 24
  discussion of, 23
Encephalopathy, in alcoholic liver disease, 82
  in Reye's syndrome, 355, 356

Endodermal sinus tumor, extraembryonic differentiation in, 246
End-stage renal disease. See *Renal disease, end-stage.*
Enteropathy, gluten-sensitive. See *Gluten-sensitive enteropathy.*
Enzyme-linked immunosorbent assay (ELISA), for human immunodeficiency virus, 404
Epidermal growth factor receptors (EGFR), in breast cancer, 238
Erythroblastosis fetalis, alternative considerations in, 233–234
    amniocentesis in, 229, *230–231*
    case study of, 229–234
    discussion of, 233
    exchange transfusion in, 230–231
    intrauterine transfusion of Rh-negative erythrocytes in, 233
    pathogenesis of, 232
    prevention of, 234
    Rh antibody titers in, 229, 233
    simple transfusion in, 233
Erythrocyte indices, in glomerulonephritis, 41
Erythrocytic protoporphyria, laboratory findings in, 94t
    photosensitivity of, 95
Erythroid hyperplasia, in congenital heart disease, 10
Esophageal varices, in alcoholic liver disease, 81
Estriol, unconjugated, in Down syndrome, screening for, 288
    results of, 286
Estrogen/progesterone receptors, in breast cancer prognosis, 236–237
Ethanol, tissue damage caused by, 79–80
Ethylene glycol, plasma and urinary levels of, *338*
    toxicity of, 339
Ethylene glycol poisoning, anion gap in, 335, 337, *338*
    case studies of, 335–340
    high osmolal gap in, 335, 337
    metabolic acidosis in, 337
    treatment of, 335, 336–337, 339–340
    urinary oxalate in, 337, *338*
Excited delirium, cocaine-induced, 383

Facial flushing, carcinoid tumors and, 213, 216
Factor Va, in blood coagulation, 328
Factor VIII, change in concentration of, DDAVP infusion and, 331, *332*
    deficiency of, 332. See also *Hemophilia A.*
    half-life of, 334
Factor IX, deficiency of, 332
Factor XI, deficiency of, 332
Failure to thrive, in cystic fibrosis, 15
Familial hypercholesterolemia. See *Hypercholesterolemia, familial.*

Familial hyperchylomicronemia, 305
Familial hypertriglyceridemia. See *Hypertriglyceridemia, familial.*
Fatty acids, omega-3, for familial hypertriglyceridemia, 306
Feminization, male, in alcoholic liver disease, 82
Ferric chloride test, in PKU screening, 319–320
Ferritin, measurement of, in genetic hemochromatosis, 68
Fertility, in cystic fibrosis, 18
Fetal lung immaturity, discussion of, 221–222
    lecithin/sphingomyelin ratio in, 221
    shake test (foam stability index) in, 221–222
    surfactant/albumin ratio in, 222
    treatment of, 223
Fever, 33
FEV_1/FVC ratio, in airway obstruction, 23
Fibric acid agents, for familial hypertriglyceridemia, 306
Fine-needle aspiration biopsy, of thyroid nodule, 138, 145, 183, 185
Finger clubbing, in hypoxemic states, 10
Flank pain, associated with adrenal cortical carcinoma, 167
Fludrocortisone, for Addison's disease, 180
Foam stability index, in fetal lung maturity, 221–222
Folate deficiency, in pernicious anemia, 260, 261, 261t
Fractional clearance, of bicarbonate, calculation of, 31
Fractional excretion, of compound, 31
    of sodium, determination of, 37
Free thyroxine index, calculation of, 142
    definition of, 137, 141
Fructosamine assay, for glycemia, 117
Fucosylation index, in hepatocellular carcinoma, 463

Gait, abnormal, in rickets, 397
Gallstone(s). See also *Cholelithiasis.*
    development of, 86
    diagnosis of, 86–87
    treatment of, 87–88
Gallstone ileus, definition of, 86
Gastric ulcer, 209
Gastrinoma, in Zollinger-Ellison syndrome, 209
Gene, CYP21, in 21-hydroxylase deficiency, 150
    mutations in, 150
    for cystic fibrosis, 17
    for ornithine transcarbamylase deficiency, 310
Genetic hemochromatosis. See *Hemochromatosis, genetic.*
Genital ambiguity, female, in 21-hydroxylase deficiency, 151
    surgery for, 154
Germ cell tumors, case study of, 245–247
    classification of, 246

Germ cell tumors *(Continued)*
  discussion of, 246–247
  hCG levels in, 247
  metastatic, 245
  oncofetal antigens in, 246
  summary of, 247
  treatment of, 247
  tumor markers in, 246
Gestational diabetes. See also *Diabetes mellitus.*
  diagnostic criteria for, 115
Gestational trophoblastic neoplasia, 226
  clinical features of, 226–227
  treatment of, 227
Gibson-Cooke pilocarpine iontophoresis, 17
Glomerular filtration rate, reduction of, uremic acidosis associated with, 30
Glomerulonephritis, Bowman's space in, erythrocytes in, 41
  case study of, 39–43
  creatinine values in, 40
  discussion of, 41–43
  erythrocyte indices in, 41
  immune-complex, 49
  membranoproliferative, 49
  rapidly progressive, 42
Glucose tolerance, impaired, diagnosis of, 114
Glucose tolerance test, for diabetes mellitus, 114–115
Glucose-6-phosphate dehydrogenase (G6PD) deficiency, vs. sickle cell disease, 254
γ-Glutamyltransferase, in gallbladder disease, 87
Gluten-sensitive enteropathy, antigliadin and antiendomysial antibodies in, 121
  case study of, 119–122
  definition of disease, 120–121
  differential diagnosis of, 121
  genetic markers in, 122
  malabsorption in, 120, 121
  pathogenesis of, 122
  recurrent diarrhea in, 119
  treatment of, 122
Glycemia, control of, fructosamine assay in, 117
  glycosylated hemoglobin measurement in, 116–117
Goiter, in Hashimoto's thyroiditis, 143
Goodpasture's syndrome, diagnosis of, 42
Gout, case study of, 371–375
  clinical features of, 374
  definition and classification of, 373–374
  diagnosis of, 374
  differential diagnosis of, 372–373
  HPRT deficiency and PRPP overactivity in, 373
  hyperuricemia in, classification of, 373–374
  treatment of, 374–375
Graves' disease, and thyroid cancer, 140
  case study of, 137–140
  differential diagnosis of, 138
  ^{123}I uptake and scan in, 138

Graves' disease *(Continued)*
  laboratory results in, 139–140
  treatment of, 140
Growth, rapid, in 21-hydroxylase deficiency, 149–150
Guthrie test, in PKU screening, 320

Haemophilus influenzae, bronchitis caused by, 23
Hairy-cell leukemia, case study of, 275–279
  clinical findings in, 276–277
  definition of disease, 276
  diagnosis of, 277–279
  differential diagnosis of, 277
  laboratory features of, 278–279
  morphological features of, 277
  natural history of, 277
  serum concentration of sIL-2R in, 278–279
  Southern blot analysis in, 278
  tartrate-resistant acid phosphatase activity in, 278
  treatment of, 279
  variants of, 278
Hashimoto's thyroiditis, causing primary hypothyroidism, 142, 143
  goiter in, 143
HAV (hepatitis A virus), 55
HBcAg (hepatitis B core antigen), 55
HBeAg (hepatitis B e antigen), 55
HBsAg (hepatitis B surface antigen), 55
HBV (hepatitis B virus), 55–57, *56*
  associated with hepatocellular carcinoma, 63
  vertical transmission of, 62
hCG. See *Human chorionic gonadotropin (hCG).*
HCV (hepatitis C virus), 58
HDV (hepatitis D virus), *57*, 57–58
Headache, in pheochromocytoma, 202
Heart disease, congenital. See *Congenital heart disease.*
Heart failure, left-sided, Kerley B lines in, 365, 366
Heart murmur, in congenital heart disease, 7
  in myocardial infarction, 13
Heart-lung transplantation, for cystic fibrosis, 18
Heme pathway, porphyrias and, *92, 93*
Hemiparesis, in multiple sclerosis, 291
Hemochromatosis, 252
  genetic, case study of, 65–69
    diagnosis of, 67–68
    iron index in, 66
    iron-loading in, 68
    pathophysiology of, 67–68
    screening for, 68–69
Hemodialysis therapy, for ethylene glycol poisoning, 335, *336*
Hemoglobin A (Hb A), glycosylation of, in diabetes mellitus, 116

Hemoglobin A$_{1c}$ (Hb A$_{1c}$), concentration of, determination of, 116–117
Hemoglobin S (Hb S), in sickle cell disease, 255
Hemolytic anemia, of Wilson's disease, 74
Hemophilia A, case study of, 331–334
  clinical aspects of, 332–333, 333t
  factor VIII deficiency causing, 332
  genetics of, 332–333
  laboratory diagnosis of, 333–334
  neutralizing alloantibodies in, development of, 333
  "sporadic," 332
  treatment of, 334
  vs. von Willebrand's disease, 333–334
Hemophilia B (Christmas disease), factor IX deficiency causing, 332
Hemophilia C, factor XI deficiency causing, 332
Hemoptysis, 40
Hemorrhage, in Zollinger-Ellison syndrome, 207, 208
Hemosiderosis, due to transfusion, 255
Heparin therapy, for disseminated intravascular coagulopathy, 324
Hepatic copper, in Wilson's disease, 74
Hepatic porphyria, acute. See *Acute hepatic porphyria.*
Hepatic underperfusion, in myocardial infarction, 14
Hepatitis, alcoholic, 77
  diagnosis of, 80
    enzyme levels in, 81–82
  associated with Wilson's disease, 73–74
  case study of, 53–59
  causes of, 55
  discussion of, 58–59
  neonatal, vs. extrahepatic biliary atresia, 130–131
  serological test results for, 54
  treatment of, 59
  types of, 55–58, *56, 57*
Hepatitis A virus (HAV), 55
Hepatitis B core antigen (HBcAg), 55
Hepatitis B e antigen (HBeAg), 55
Hepatitis B surface antigen (HBsAg), 55
Hepatitis B virus (HBV), 55–57, *56*
  associated with hepatocellular carcinoma, 63
  vertical transmission of, 62
Hepatitis C virus (HCV), 58
Hepatitis D virus (HDV), *57,* 57–58
Hepatitis E virus (HEV), 58
Hepatocellular carcinoma, alpha-fetoprotein levels in, 62, 63–64
  case study of, 62–64
  comments on, 63–64
  hepatitis B virus associated with, 63
  metastasis from, 61–62
  screening test for, 64
  treatment of, 64
Hepatolenticular degeneration. See *Wilson's disease.*

Hepatoportoenterostomy-Kasai operation, for extrahepatic biliary atresia, 131
Hepatorenal syndrome, 81
Hepatotoxicity, acetaminophen-induced, 348–349
Hereditary coproporphyria, 92
  laboratory findings in, 94t
  photosensitivity of, 95
HEV (hepatitis E virus), 58
5-HIAA (5-hydroxyindoleacetic acid), in carcinoid tumors, 214, 216
  and response to antineoplastic therapy, 214t
Hip pain, in osteoporosis, 391
Hirsutism, in Cushing disease, 162, 163
HIV infection. See *Human immunodeficiency virus (HIV) infection.*
HLA. See *Human leukocyte antigen (HLA).*
Hoesch test, for acute hepatic porphyria, 90, 95
Homicide, in cocaine-related fatality, 379–380
Howell-Jolly bodies, in sickle cell disease, 254
HPRT (hypoxanthine guanine phospho-ribosyltransferase), deficiency of, 373
Human chorionic gonadotropin (hCG), α-subunit of, 225
  β-subunit of, 225, 226, 227
  definition of, 225
  in choriocarcinoma, 225
    following treatment, 226
  in Down syndrome, screening for, 288
    results of, 286
  in germ cell tumors, 247
Human immunodeficiency virus (HIV) infection, case study of, 403–406
  CD4+ lymphocyte count in, 404–405
  cough and dyspnea in, 403
  differential diagnosis of, 405
  ELISA test for, 404
  "indicator" diseases in, 405–406
  late, 405–406
  Pneumocystis carinii pneumonia in, 404, 405
  tuberculin skin test for, 404
  Western blot test for, 404
Human leukocyte antigen (HLA), in genetic hemochromatosis, 66
  in renal transplantation, 28–29
Hyaline membrane disease, inadequate surfactant in, 221
Hydatidiform mole, clinical features of, 226–227
  treatment of, 227
Hydrops fetalis, 233
Hydroxycobalamin, for pernicious anemia, 258
5-Hydroxyindoleacetic acid (5-HIAA), in carcinoid tumors, 214, 216
  and response to antineoplastic therapy, 214t
11-Hydroxylase deficiency, clinical and laboratory findings in, 153t
17α-Hydroxylase deficiency, clinical and laboratory findings in, 153t

21-Hydroxylase deficiency, case study of, 149–154
  classic form of, 151–152
  clinical features of, 151–152
  CYP21 gene in, 150
  definition of disease, 150, *151*
  diagnosis of, 152
    clinical and laboratory findings in, 153t
  helpful diagnostic notes on, 154
  nonclassic form of, 150, 152
  treatment of, 152–154
21-Hydroxylase enzyme, genetic markers for, 150
3-Hydroxy-3-methylglutaryl-CoA reductase inhibitors, for familial hypercholesterolemia, 301
3β-Hydroxy-steroid dehydrogenase deficiency, clinical and laboratory findings in, 153t
Hydroxyurea, for chronic myelogenous leukemia, 270
Hyperactivity, in hyperphenylalaninemias, 315
Hyperammonemia. See also *Ornithine transcarbamylase (OTC) deficiency.*
  in females, 310
  in males, 310
  in Reye's syndrome, 356–357
  treatment of, 312
  vomiting in, 309, 310
Hyperamylasemia, causes of, 101t
Hyperbilirubinemia, classification of, 108
  conjugated, 109
    definition of, 128
  jaundice in, 108–109
Hypercalcemia, causes of, 190t
  hyperparathyroidism and, 189–190
  in renal osteodystrophy, 198
Hypercholesterolemia, familial, case study of, 297–302
  clinical features of, 299
  definition of disease, 299
  diagnosis of, 300
  elevated LDL-cholesterol and apolipoprotein B in, 298, 299, 300
  fasting state in, laboratory results of, 298
  heterozygous, 299
  homozygous, 299
  treatment of, 300–302
    dietary, 300–301
    drug, 301
Hyperchylomicronemia, familial, 305
Hypercortisolism. See also *Cushing syndrome.*
  in Cushing syndrome, 157–158, 171
  vs. osteoporosis, 393–394
Hyperlipidemia, in minimal change nephrotic syndrome, 50
Hyperoxaluria, enteric, 124
Hyperparathyroid bone disease, 197, 198
Hyperparathyroidism, case study of, 189–193
  chloride/phosphorus ratio in, 192
  clinical features of, 190–191
  CNS involvement in, 191–192

Hyperparathyroidism *(Continued)*
  definition of disease, 190–191
  diagnosis of, 191–192, *193*
  immunometric PTH assay for, 191–192
  ionized calcium assay for, 192
  parathyroid hormone-related peptide (PTHrP) assay for, 192
  primary, vs. osteoporosis, 393
  secondary, treatment of, 199
  tertiary, 198
  treatment of, 192
Hyperphenylalaninemia(s). See also *Phenylketonuria (PKU).*
  definition of disease, 316
  diagnosis of, 318–319
    prenatal, 319
  enzyme and genetic defects in, 316–317
  inherited, spectrum of, 316t
Hyperphosphatemia, treatment of, 199
Hyperpigmentation, in Addison's disease, 179
Hypersplenism, in alcoholic liver disease, 81
Hypertension, in pheochromocytoma, 201, 202
  in renal failure, 33
Hypertriglyceridemia, familial, case study of, 303–307
  clinical features of, 305–306
  definition of disease, 305
  diagnosis of, 306
  laboratory evaluations in, 304
  metabolic defects in, 305
    associated, 306
  treatment of, 306–307
Hyperuricemia, primary, 373
  secondary, 374
Hypervitaminosis A, confirmation of, 397
Hypoalbuminemia, alcoholic liver disease and, 82
  differential diagnosis of, 49
Hypochloremia, in pyloric stenosis, 134–135
Hyponatremia, in syndrome of inappropriate antidiuretic hormone secretion, *383*, 387
Hypopigmentation, in phenylketonuria, 318
Hypopituitarism, vs. Addison's disease, 179
Hypothyroidism, case study of, 141–144
  cause of, 142, 143
  congenital (cretinism), 143
  definition of disease, 143
  presentation of, 142–143
  treatment of, 143–144
Hypoventilation, and pulmonary vasoconstriction, 23
Hypoxanthine guanine phosphoribosyl-transferase (HPRT), deficiency of, 373
Hypoxemia, and pulmonary vasoconstriction, 23
  arterial O_2 and pCO_2 in, 23
  clubbing associated with, 10
  in congenital heart disease, 9–10

Immune-complex glomerulonephritis, 49

Immunoglobulin G (IgG) synthesis, CSF, during multiple sclerosis exacerbation, 293
Infarction, myocardial. See *Myocardial infarction*.
Insulin, for diabetes mellitus, 113, 115
Insulin reserve, C-peptide test for, 115
Insulin-dependent diabetes mellitus, 113. See also *Diabetes mellitus*.
Interferon, for hairy-cell leukemia, 279
Invasive mole, 226
  clinical features of, 227
^{123}Iodine uptake, in Graves' disease, 138
IQ values, in phenylketonuria, 318
Iron index, calculation of, 68
  in genetic hemochromatosis, 66
Iron therapy, for anemia, 252
Iron-loading, in genetic hemochromatosis, 68

Jaundice, in hyperbilirubinemia, 108–109, 127, 128
Juvenile diabetes mellitus, 113. See also *Diabetes mellitus*.

Kasai procedure, for extrahepatic biliary atresia, 131
Kayser-Fleischer rings, in Wilson's disease, 72, 74
Kerley B lines, in left-sided heart failure, 365, 366
17-Ketosteroids, in adrenal cortical carcinoma, 168
Kidney(s). See *Renal* entries.
Klimmelstiel-Wilson disease, 113

Labor, premature onset of, discussion of, 221
  treatment of, 223
Laboratory test(s), choice of, 1–2
  groups of, use of, 4
  optimizing use of, 4–5
  predictive value of, 3
  results of, interpretation of, 2–3, *3*
  sensitivity of, 2–3
  specificity of, 2–3
LDH-1/LDH-2 ratio, in myocardial infarction, 13
LDL-cholesterol, elevated, in familial hypercholesterolemia, 298, 299, 300
Lead, in drinking water, permissible levels of, 344
Lead poisoning, anemia in, 342
  δ-aminolevulinic acid levels in, 342–343, *343*
  case study of, 341–345
  CDC definition of, 344
  diagnosis of, 342–343
  differential diagnosis of, 342–343
  discussion of, 344

Lead poisoning *(Continued)*
  laboratory findings in, 94t
  treatment of, 344–345
  vs. porphyria, 93
Lecithin/sphingomyelin (L/S) ratio, in fetal lung maturity studies, 221
Legal chain of custody, in cocaine-related fatality, 379
Leukemia, acute, multiple myeloma and, 283
  acute myelogenous, definition of disease, 267
  acute progranulocytic. See *Acute progranulocytic leukemia*.
  acute promyelocytic, Auer rods in, 322
    bleeding phenomena in, 266, 267, 322
  chronic myelogenous. See *Chronic myelogenous leukemia*.
  hairy-cell. See *Hairy-cell leukemia*.
Lhermitte's phenomenon, in multiple sclerosis, 291, 294
Lipase assay, in acute pancreatitis, 102
Lipoprotein lipase disorder, defect causing, 305. See also *Hypertriglyceridemia, familial*.
Lithotripsy, for gallstones, 88
Liver, cirrhosis of, alcohol-induced, 79, 80–81
  ascites associated with, 80–81
    new-onset, 67
  associated with Wilson's disease, 73
  genetic hemochromatosis causing, 66
  inflammation of. See *Hepatitis*.
Liver biopsy, in alcoholic liver disease, 80
  in extrahepatic biliary atresia, 131
  in genetic hemochromatosis, 68
  in hepatocellular carcinoma, 62
  in Wilson's disease, 74
Liver cancer. See *Hepatocellular carcinoma*.
Liver disease, alcoholic. See *Alcoholic liver disease*.
  stigmata of, 65
Liver failure, fulminant, associated with hepatitis, 53
  due to Wilson's disease, 74
  evidence of, 58
Liver function tests, in alcoholic liver disease, 81
Liver transplantation, for Wilson's disease, 74
Lung. See also *Pulmonary* entries.
Lung immaturity, fetal. See *Fetal lung immaturity*.
Lung infection(s), in cystic fibrosis, 18
Lupus anticoagulant, 328
17,20-Lyase deficiency, clinical and laboratory findings in, 153t
Lynch Type II syndrome, 241

Magnetic resonance imaging, in multiple sclerosis, 294
Malabsorption syndrome, anemia in, 124
  case study of, 123–126
  chronic diarrhea in, 123
  differential diagnosis of, 121

Malabsorption syndrome *(Continued)*
    drastic anatomic alterations causing, 125
    enteric hyperoxaluria in, 124
    hepatic status in, 125
    in cystic fibrosis, 18
    in gluten-senstive enteropathy, 120, 121
    nutritional deficiencies in, 124–125
    steatorrhea in, 124, 125
    stone formation in, 124
Maldigestion, case study of, 123–126
    drastic anatomic alterations causing, 125
Mallory body(ies), in alcoholic liver disease, 80
Manner of death (MOD), in cocaine-related
        fatality, 378–379
Maternal serum alpha-fetoprotein, in neural tube
        defects, 286–287
    screening for, 288, *289*, 290
        results of, 286
Maturity-onset diabetes mellitus, 113. See also
    Diabetes mellitus.
MBP (myelin basic protein), elevated CSF levels
    of, in multiple sclerosis, 293
MCNS. See *Minimal change nephrotic
    syndrome (MCNS).*
Meconium ileus, in cystic fibrosis, 18
Medicolegal issues, in cocaine-related fatality,
        378–379
Medicolegal/forensic investigation, into cocaine-
    related fatality, 377–378
Medullary thyroid carcinoma. See *Thyroid
    carcinoma, medullary.*
Membranoproliferative glomerulonephritis, 49
MEN Type 1. See *Multiple endocrine neoplasia
    syndrome (MEN Type 1).*
MEN Type 2. See *Multiple endocrine neoplasia
    syndrome (MEN Type 2).*
MEN Type 3. See *Multiple endocrine neoplasia
    syndrome (MEN Type 3).*
Metabolic acidosis, hyperchloremic, 30
    in diabetic ketoacidosis, 112–113
    in ethylene glycol poisoning, 337
Metabolic alkalosis, in pyloric stenosis, 135
Metabolic defect(s), in familial
        hypertriglyceridemia, 305
    associated, 306
Metabolism, acetaminophen, 348–349, *349*
    triglyceride-rich lipoprotein, defect in, 305
Metastasis, from hepatocellular carcinoma, 61–
        62
    from prostatic carcinoma, 359, 361, 364
4-Methylpyrazole, for ethylene glycol poisoning,
        337, *338*, 339–340
Microalbuminuria, in nephropathy, 114
β_2-Microglobulin, in multiple myeloma, 282, 283
Mineralization, inadequate, in rickets,
    classification of, 400
Minimal change nephrotic syndrome (MCNS),
        case study of, 45–51
    clinical findings in, 47
    consequence of protein loss in, 51
    diagnosis of, 46

Minimal change nephrotic syndrome (MCNS)
        (Continued)
    differential diagnosis of, 49
    edema associated with, 45, 47
    etiology of, 49
    pathophysiology of, 47–49, *48*
    selection and interpretation of results in, 49–51
    treatment of, 51
    urine protein in, 49
MOD (manner of death), in cocaine-related
        fatality, 378–379
Molar pregnancy, clinical features of, 226–227
    treatment of, 227
MoM (multiples of median value), definition of,
    286
Muehrcke's lines, associated with minimal
        change nephrotic syndrome, 47
Multiple endocrine neoplasia syndrome (MEN
        Type 1), gastrinoma in, 209
    organ involvement in, 186t
Multiple endocrine neoplasia syndrome (MEN
        Type 2), medullary thyroid carcinoma in,
        146
    organ involvement in, 186t
Multiple endocrine neoplasia syndrome (MEN
        Type 3), familial, case study of, 183–187
    definition of disease, 185
    diagnosis of, 185–187, 186t
    genetics of, 185
        medullary thyroid carcinoma in, 183–184,
            185, 187
        pheochromocytoma in, 184, 186–187, 203
    treatment of, 187
    medullary thyroid carcinoma in, 146
    organ involvement in, 186t
Multiple myeloma, and acute leukemia, 283
    Bence Jones proteinuria in, 281, 282
    β_2-microglobulin in, 282, 283
    case study of, 281–283
    C-reactive protein in, 282, 283
    definition of disease, 282–283
    differential diagnosis of, 281
    plasma cell labeling index in, 282, 283
    presentation of, 283
    treatment of, 283
    vs. osteoporosis, 393
Multiple sclerosis, Babinski's sign in, 291, 294
    case study of, 291–294
    clinical features of, 292
    CSF analysis in, 292–293
    CSF electrophoresis in, 293, *293*
    CSF IgG synthesis rates in, 293
    definition of disease, 292
    diagnosis of, 292–294
    elevated CSF levels of MBP in, 293
    hemiparesis in, 291
    Lhermitte's phenomenon in, 291, 294
    magnetic resonance imaging in, 294
    sensory evoked potentials in, 294
    signs and symptoms of, 292
    treatment of, 294

Multiples of median value (MoM), definition of, 286

Murmur, heart. See *Heart murmur*.

Mutation, in cystic fibrosis, 17

Myelin basic protein (MBP), elevated CSF levels of, in multiple sclerosis, 293

Myeloma, multiple. See *Multiple myeloma*.

Myocardial infarction, case study of, 11–14
chest pain in, 11, 12, 297
discussion of, 12–14
ECG changes in, 11, 12, 13
hepatic underperfusion in, 14
LDH-1/LDH-2 ratio in, 11, 12, 13
serial enzyme studies in, 11, 12, 13
thrombolytic agents for, 13
ventricular wall rupture in, 14

Natural cause of death, in cocaine-related fatality, 380

Neonatal cholestasis, causes of, 128
disorders associated with, 128t–129t
workup for, 130t

Neonatal hepatitis, vs. extrahepatic biliary atresia, 130–131

Neoplasia, gestational trophoblastic, 226
clinical features of, 226–227
treatment of, 227
vs. osteoporosis, 393

Nephritic syndrome, 41

Nephritis, definition of, 47
vs. nephrosis, 47

Nephrosis, definition of, 47
diseases causing, 49
symptoms of, 48
vs. nephritis, 47

Nephrotic syndrome, minimal change. See *Minimal change nephrotic syndrome (MCNS)*.
primary, 49

Neu oncogene, in breast cancer, 238

Neural tube defect (NTD), case study of, 285–290
causes of, 290
definition of disease, 287
forms of, 287
screening for, 288
AFP profile in, 288
recommended protocol for, 288, 289
sensitivity of, 290
results of, 286

Neutrophil alkaline phosphatase, definition of, 270

Nicotinic acid, for familial hypercholesterolemia, 301
for familial hypertriglyceridemia, 307

Nodular prostatic hyperplasia, 363

Noninsulin-dependent diabetes mellitus, 113. See also *Diabetes mellitus*.

Non-phenylketonuria hyperphenylalaninemia, diagnosis of, 318
PAH activity in, 317
spectrum of, 316t

Normouricemia, epidemiological definition of, 373

NTD. See *Neural tube defect (NTD)*.

5′-Nucleotidase, in gallbladder disease, 87

25(OH)D absorption test, explanation of, 399, *399*
in assessment of vitamin D deficiency, 398

1,25(OH)D levels, in osteoporosis, 392, 393

Oliguria, 27

Omega-3 fatty acids, for familial hypertriglyceridemia, 306

Oncofetal antigen(s), in germ cell tumors, 246

Oncogene, *neu*, in breast cancer, 238

Ornithine transcarbamylase (OTC) deficiency, biochemical findings in, 312
case study of, 309–313
clinical features of, 310
diagnosis of, *311*, 311–312
definitive, 312
enzyme defect in, 310
genetic defect in, 310
helpful notes on, 312–313
hyperammonemia in, 310, 311
treatment of, 312
plasma amino acid and urinary organic acid assays in, 310
site of defect in, *311*
treatment of, 312

Osmolal gap, in ethylene glycol poisoning, 335, 336

Osteitis fibrosa, 197, 198

Osteocalcin, in high-turnover renal osteodystrophy, 198–199

Osteodystrophy, renal. See *Renal osteodystrophy*.

Osteomalacia, low-turnover, etiological factors in, 197–198

Osteoporosis, case study of, 391–394
1,25(OH)D and PTH levels in, 392, 393
differential diagnosis of, 393–394
evaluation of, 394
hip pain in, 391
postmenopausal, definition of disease, 392
senile, definition of disease, 392
diagnosis of, 392
treatment of, 394

Ovarian cancer, abdominal distention in, 239
case study of, 239–243
CEA and CA 125 assays in, 240, 242
clinical features of, 242–243
definition of disease, 241
diagnosis of, 242
differential diagnosis of, 241
incidence of, 241

Ovarian cancer *(Continued)*
  risk factors for, 241
  thoracocentesis in, 240–241
  transudative effusions in, 241
  transvaginal sonography for, 242
  treatment of, 243
Oxalate, urinary, in ethylene glycol poisoning, 337, *338*
Oxygen saturation, in congenital heart disease, 8
Oxygen therapy, for congenital heart disease, 8

P-450 enzyme, 21-hydroxylase deficiency and, 150, *151*
PAH. See *Phenylalanine hydroxylation (PAH)*.
Pain. See at specific anatomic site.
Pan-B cell antigens, in hairy-cell leukemia, 278
Pancreatic deficiency, in cystic fibrosis, treatment of, 18
Pancreatitis, abdominal pain in, 303
  acute, amylase activity in, 100, 101
    case study of, 99–104
    causes of, 102–103, 103t
    clinical manifestations of, 103
    complications of, 103–104
      multisystem, 102
    definition of, 100–101
    differential diagnosis of, 100
    discussion of, 100–102
    incidence of, 102
    index of disease severity in, 102
    laboratory findings in, 100, 101t
    lipase activity in, 102
    Ranson's criteria in, 103, 104t
    treatment of, 104
    unfavorable prognostic indices in, 104t
  diagnosis of, 304
Parathyroid hormone (PTH), in high-turnover renal osteodystrophy, 199
  in osteoporosis, 392, 393
Parathyroid hormone (PTH) assay, for hyperparathyroidism, 191–192
Parathyroid hormone-related peptide (PTHrP) assay, for hyperparathyroidism, 192
Partial thromboplastin time (PTT), in systemic lupus erythematosus, 325
  prolonged, alcoholic liver disease and, 82
D-Penicillamine, for Wilson's disease, 72, 75
Peptic ulcer, 208–209
  caused by Zollinger-Ellison syndrome, 209–210
Percussion, in cystic fibrosis, 18
Pericardial tamponade, 14
Perinatal pulmonary vascular dynamics, 9
Peritonitis, bacterial, spontaneous, diagnosis of, 67
Pernicious anemia, case study of, 257–262
  clinical features of, 260

Pernicious anemia *(Continued)*
  cobalamin deficiency in, 258, 259–260, 261, 261t
  definition of disease, 259–260
  diagnosis of, 260–262, 261t
  fatigue and pallor in, 257
  folate deficiency in, 260, 261, 261t
  IF-cobalamin complex in, 259
  Schilling test for, 258, 261–262
  serum cobalamin, serum folate, and erythrocyte folate levels in, 261, 261t
  signs and symptoms of, 260
  treatment of, 262
Petrosal sinus test, for ectopic ACTH-producing tumor, 174
Phenylalanine hydroxylation (PAH), and cofactor transformations, 316, *317*
  inherited defect in, 315–316. See also *Phenylketonuria (PKU)*.
Phenylketonuria (PKU), case study of, 315–320
  clinical symptoms of, 317–318
  definition of disease, 316
  diagnosis of, 318–319
    prenatal, 319
  enzyme and genetic defect in, 316–317
  ferric chloride test for, 319–320
  Guthrie test for, 320
  hepatic PAH activity in, 317
  hyperactivity and delayed speech in, 315
  prognosis of, 319
  screening for, 319–320
  spectrum of, 316t
  treatment of, 319
  vs. non-phenylketonuria hyperphenylalaninemia, 316t, 317, 318
Pheochromocytoma, bilateral, 185
  case study of, 201–201
  catecholamines in, 203–205, *204*
  clinical features of, 202–203
  definition of disease, 202
  diagnosis of, 203–205, *204*
  headache in, 202
  hypertension in, 201, 202
  localization of, 205
  MEN-associated, 146, 184, 186, 203
    catecholamine secretion in, 187
  treatment of, 205
  vanillylmandelic acid in, 203
Philadelphia chromosome, in chronic myelogenous leukemia, 270, 271, 272
Phlegmon, as complication of acute pancreatitis, 104
5-Phosphoribosyl-1-pyrophosphate (PRPP) synthase, overactivity of, 373
Photosensitivity, in porphyrias, 95
Pineal gland, germ cell tumors of, 246. See also *Germ cell tumors*.
Pituitary gland, adenoma of. See also *Cushing disease*.
  diagnosis of, 163–164

Pituitary gland *(Continued)*
   germ cell tumors of, 245. See also *Germ cell tumors.*
PKU. See *Phenylketonuria (PKU).*
Plasma cell labeling index, in multiple myeloma, 282, 283
Pleural effusion, in ovarian cancer, 242–243
Plumbism. See *Lead poisoning.*
Plummer's disease, 138
Pneumocystis carinii pneumonia, in HIV-positive patient, 404, 405
Pneumonia, in sickle cell disease, 253
   Pneumocystis carinii, in HIV-positive patient, 404, 405
   recurrent, in cystic fibrosis, 15
Poisoning, acetaminophen, case study of, 347–350
   ethylene glycol, case studies of, 335–340
   lead, case study of, 341–345
Polyarthritis, 371
   differential diagnosis of, 372
Polydipsia, in diabetic ketoacidosis, 111, 112
Polyuria, in diabetic ketoacidosis, 111, 112
Porphobilinogen, 92
   determination of, 91
   screening test for, 95
Porphyria(s), acute hepatic. See *Acute hepatic porphyria.*
   acute intermittent, 92
      laboratory findings in, 94t
   ALA synthase in, 94–95
   congenital erythropoietic, 95
   definition of, 92–95
   diagnosis of, laboratory findings in, 94t
   heme pathway and, 92, 93
   hereditary coproporphyria, 92
      laboratory findings in, 94t
   management of, 95
   photosensitivity in, 95
   variegate, 92
      laboratory findings in, 94t
   vs. lead poisoning, 93
Porphyria cutanea tarda, 95
   laboratory findings in, 94t
Porphyrins, 92
   determination of, 91
Portosystemic encephalopathy, 82
Postmenopausal osteoporosis, definition of disease, 392
Postural drainage, in cystic fibrosis, 18
Prednisone, for Addison's disease, 180
   for minimal change nephrotic syndrome, 51
Pregnancy, diabetes during, 115. See also *Diabetes mellitus.*
   molar, 226–227
   sickle cell disease and, 219. See also *Sickle cell disease.*
Premature onset of labor, discussion of, 221
   treatment of, 223
Prerenal azotemia. See *Azotemia, prerenal.*
Prolymphocytic variant of hairy-cell leukemia, 278

Prostate gland, benign enlargement of, 363
Prostate-specific antigen (PSA), 362–363
Prostatic carcinoma, acid phosphatase in, 361
   case study of, 359–364
   diagnosis of, 363
   discussion of, 363
   elevated prostate-specific antigen in, 362–363
   epidemiology of, 360
   grading and staging of, 361, 362t
   low back pain in, 359, 359t
   pathology of, 360–361
   treatment of, 364
Protein, Bence Jones, in amyloidosis, 368
   in multiple myeloma, 281, 282
   bone Gla, in high-turnover renal osteodystrophy, 198–199
   C-reactive, in multiple myeloma, 282, 283
   loss of, in nephrotic patient, 51
   thyroxine-binding, 51
   transmembrane regulatory, in cystic fibrosis, 16–17
   urinary, diabetes mellitus and, 114
      nephrotic syndrome and, 49
Protein Ca, as coagulation inhibitor, 328
Proteinuria, presence of, in minimal change nephrotic syndrome, 49
Prothrombin time (PT), in systemic lupus erythematosus, 325
   prolonged, alcoholic liver disease and, 82
Protoporphyria, erythrocytic, laboratory findings in, 94t
   photosensitivity of, 95
PRPP (5-phosphoribosyl-1-pyrophosphate) synthase, overactivity of, 373
PSA (prostate-specific antigen), 362–363
Pseudocyst, as complication of acute pancreatitis, 104
Pseudogout, 372
   CPPD crystals of, 372, 374
Pseudomonas aeruginosa, mucoid coating of, in cystic fibrosis, 18
Psychiatric manifestation(s), in Wilson's disease, 71, 74
Psychiatric syndromes, cocaine-induced, 382–383
   treatment of, 383
PT (prothrombin time), in systemic lupus erythematosus, 325
   prolonged, in alcoholic liver disease, 82
PTH (parathyroid hormone), in high-turnover renal osteodystrophy, 199
   in osteoporosis, 392, 393
PTT (partial thromboplastin time), in systemic lupus erythematosus, 325
   prolonged, in alcoholic liver disease, 82
Pulmonary function test(s), 22
Pulmonary vascular dynamics, cardiac shunt-related, congenital, 9
   perinatal, 9
Pulmonary vascular resistance, measurement of, 8
Pyloric stenosis, case study of, 133–135

Pyloric stenosis *(Continued)*
  discussion of, 134–135
  hypochloremia in, 134–135
  metabolic alkalosis in, 135
  palpation of "olive" in, 134
  treatment of, 135
  vomiting in, 133, 134

Ranson's criteria, in acute pancreatitis, 103, 104t
Rapidly progressive glomerulonephritis (RPGN), 42. See also *Glomerulonephritis.*
Receiver operator characteristic (ROC) curve analysis, in prostatic carcinoma, 363
Recombinant human erythropoietin (r-HuEPO), for anemia, 252
Renal allograft, rejection of, 28, 29–30
Renal biopsy, as indicator of allograft rejection, 29
  in glomerulonephritis, 40
Renal disease, chronic, anemia of, 250–251
  differential diagnosis of, 250–251
  recombinant human erythropoietin for, 252
  study of, 249–252
  treatment of, 251–252
  congenital, renal osteodystrophy secondary to, 196
  end-stage, case study of, 27–32
    transplantation for. See *Renal transplantation.*
  in diabetes mellitus, 113–114
Renal failure, acute, 37–38
  case study of, 33–38
  differential diagnosis of, 36–38
  secondary to acute tubular necrosis, 35, 38
  treatment of, 38
Renal function, decreased, in minimal change nephrotic syndrome, 50
Renal osteodystrophy, bone pathology in, 197–198
  case study of, 195–199
  etiology of, 196–197
  high-turnover, 197
  hypercalcemia in, 198
  laboratory evaluation of, 198–199
  low-turnover, 197
  reduced 1,25-dihydroxyvitamin D in, 196–197
  treatment of, 199
Renal transplantation, allograft rejection following, 29–30
  cyclosporine toxicity following, 29
  HLA matching in, 28–29
  renal tubular acidosis in, 30–31
  uremic acidosis in, 30
Renal tubular acidosis, 30–32
  bicarbonate in, reduced renal threshold for, 31
  proximal, 31–32

Respiratory distress syndrome, inadequate surfactant in, 221
Reticulocyte count, in Wilson's disease, 72
Retinoid therapy, for acute progranulocytic leukemia, 268
Reye's syndrome, case study of, 353–357
  clinical features of, 356
  coma in, 353, 357
  definition of disease, 355–356
  diagnosis of, 355
  differential diagnosis of, 355
  encephalopathy in, 355, 356
  hyperammonemia in, 356–357
  laboratory diagnosis of, 356–357
  liver function tests in, 357
  salicylates and, 356
  treatment of, 357
Rh antibody titers, in erythroblastosis fetalis, 229, 233
Rh hemolytic disease of newborn. See *Erythroblastosis fetalis.*
r-HuEPO (recombinant human erythropoietin), for anemia, 252
Rickets, biochemical aberrations associated with, 400, 400t
  bone pain in, 399
  calcium absorption test for, 398
    explanation of, 398
    results of, 398
  case study of, 397–402
  25(OH)D absorption test in, 398
    explanation of, 399, *399*
    results of, 398
  definition of disease, 399–400
  discussion of, 400–401
  gait disturbances in, 397
  inadequate mineralization in, classification of, 400
  laboratory values in, due to various causes, 400t
  results of, 398
  treatment of, *401*, 401–402
Ristocetin cofactor. See *Von Willebrand factor.*
RPGN (rapidly progressive glomerulonephritis), 42. See also *Glomerulonephritis.*
Rumack-Matthew nomogram, in acetaminophen poisoning, 347, *347*, 350

Salicylates, Reye's syndrome and, 356
"Salt-wasting" phenotype, in classic 21-hydroxylase deficiency, 151
Schilling test, for pernicious anemia, 258, 261–262
Seminoma, discussion of, 246
Senile osteoporosis, definition of disease, 392
Sensory evoked potentials, in multiple sclerosis, 294
Serotonin, in carcinoid tumors, 214, 216

Serotonin *(Continued)*
   and response to antineoplastic therapy, 214t
Serum albumin concentration, in minimal change nephrotic syndrome, 50
Serum amylase assay, in acute pancreatitis, 100, 101
Serum ceruloplasmin, in Wilson's disease, 72, 74
Serum glucose, in Wilson's disease, 72
Sexual maturation, precocious, in 21-hydroxylase deficiency, 149–150
Shake test, in fetal lung maturity, 221–222
Shortness of breath, comments on, 24
   with cough, 21
SIADH. See *Syndrome of inappropriate antidiuretic hormone secretion (SIADH).*
Sickle cell crisis, 219, 256
Sickle cell disease, acute sickle cell crisis in, 256
   anemia in, 253–254
   aplastic crisis in, 256
   case study of, 253–256
   definition of, 220
   differential diagnosis of, 253–255
   hemoglobin electrophoresis in, 254–255
   hemoglobin S in, 255
   Howell-Jolly bodies in, 254
   infection in, 255
   pneumonia in, 253
   pregnancy complicated by, 219
      amniocentesis in, 220
      case study of, 219–223
      chorioamnionitis in, 220
      discussion of, 220
      fetal lung maturity studies in, 221–222
      premature onset of labor in, 221
   reticulocyte count in, 254
   transfusion hemosiderosis in, 255
   treatment of, 255–256
   vaso-occlusive crisis in, 256
sIL-2R test, for hairy-cell leukemia, 278–279
SLE. See *Systemic lupus erythematosus (SLE).*
SLVL (splenic lymphoma with circulating villous lymphocytes), 278
Small bowel biopsy, in gluten-senstive enteropathy, 121
Sodium, fractional excretion of, determination of, 37
Sodium fluoride, for osteoporosis, 394
Southern blot analysis, in hairy-cell leukemia, 278
Speech, delayed, in hyperphenylalaninemias, 315
Spina bifida. See also *Neural tube defect (NTD).*
   definition of disease, 287
Splenic lymphoma with circulating villous lymphocytes (SLVL), 278
Splenomegaly, in chronic myelogenous leukemia, 269, 271

Spontaneous bacterial peritonitis, diagnosis of, 67
Sputum production, 21
   comments on, 24
Staging, of prostatic carcinoma, 361, 362t
Starling forces, 48
Steatorrhea, in malabsorption, 124, 125
Stenosis, pyloric. See *Pyloric stenosis.*
Steroidogenesis, pathways of, *151*
Steroids, following renal transplantation, 27–28
Stones, calcium oxalate, 124
   in gallbladder. See *Cholelithiasis.*
Suicide, in cocaine-related fatality, 380
Sulfosalicylic acid test, in minimal change nephrotic syndrome, 49
Surfactant, inadequate, in hyaline membrane disease, 221
Surfactant/albumin ratio, in fetal lung maturity studies, 222
Sweat chloride test, for cystic fibrosis, 16, 17
Syndrome of inappropriate antidiuretic hormone secretion (SIADH), case study of, 385–389
   clinical features of, 387
   definition of disease, 386–387
   diagnosis of, 387–389, *388*
      criteria for, 386t
   disorders associated with, 386t, 389
   drug therapies associated with, 386t
   hyponatremia in, *383*, 387
   treatment of, 389
   water load test for, 388
Systemic lupus erythematosus (SLE), anti-DNA antibodies in, 326
   antiphospholipid antibodies in, *327*, 327–328
   case study of, 325–328
   deep vein thrombosis in, 326
   definition of disease, 326
   discussion of, 326–327
   factor Va in, 328
   lupus anticoagulant in, 328
   protein C in, 328
   treatment of, 328
Systemic vascular resistance, calculation of, 8

T_4. See *Thyroxine* entries.
Tartrate-resistant acid phosphatase (TRAP) activity, in hairy-cell leukemia, 278
TdT (terminal deoxynucleotidyl transferase), definition of, 270
Teratoma, embryonic differentiation in, 246
Terminal deoxynucleotidyl transferase (TdT), definition of, 270
Test(s). See named test, e.g., *Guthrie test.*
Thalassemia, vs. lead poisoning, 342
   vs. sickle cell disease, 254
Thrombocytopenia, alcoholic liver disease and, 82
Thrombolytic agents, use of, in myocardial infarction, 13

Thrombosis, deep venous, associated with systemic lupus erythematosus, 326
Thrombotic thrombocytopenic purpura-hemolytic uremic syndrome (TTP-HUS), 35
differential diagnosis of, 36–37
Thyroid autoimmunity, pretibial myxedema and thyroid acropachy in, 139
Thyroid carcinoma, Graves' disease and, 140
medullary, calcitonin levels in, 147, 186
case study of, 145–147
definition of disease, 146
differential diagnosis of, 146–147
laboratory tests in, 145–146
of MEN 2, 146
of MEN 3, 146, 183–184, 185, 187
pheochromocytoma and, 146
treatment of, 147
papillary, ^{131}I whole-body scanning in, 138
treatment of, laboratory studies following, 138
Thyroid nodule, fine-needle aspiration of, 138, 145, 183, 185
treatment of, modes of, 138
Thyroidectomy, for medullary thyroid carcinoma, 147, 187
Thyroiditis, Hashimoto's, causing primary hypothyroidism, 142, 143
goiter in, 143
Thyrotoxicosis, definition of disease, 139–140
differential diagnosis of, 138
laboratory tests in, 138
presentation of, 139
Thyroxine (T_4), expression of, 142
Thyroxine (T_4) index, free, calculation of, 142
definition of, 137, 141, 145
Thyroxine-binding protein, 51
Thyroxine-binding ratio, definition of, 137, 141, 145
Toe clubbing, in hypoxemic states, 10
Toxicity, of cyclosporine, 29
of ethylene glycol, 339
Transferrin, in genetic hemochromatosis, 68
Transfusion, in erythroblastosis fetalis, 230–231, 233
problems associated with, 255
Transmembrane regulatory protein, in cystic fibrosis, 16–17
Transplantation, heart-lung, for cystic fibrosis, 18
liver, for Wilson's disease, 74
renal. See Renal transplantation.
Transvaginal sonography, in ovarian cancer screening, 242
Tremor, in Wilson's disease, 71, 74
Triglyceride-rich lipoprotein metabolism, defect in, 305. See also Hypertriglyceridemia, familial.
Trisomy 21. See Down syndrome.
Trypsin levels, in cystic fibrosis, 17
TTP-HUS (thrombotic thrombocytopenic purpura-hemolytic uremic syndrome), 35

TTP-HUS (Continued)
differential diagnosis of, 36–37
Tuberculin skin test, 404
Tubular acidosis, renal, 30–32
Tubular necrosis, acute, renal failure secondary to, 35, 38
Tumor(s). See specific type, e.g., Carcinoid tumors.

Ulceration, in Zollinger-Ellison syndrome, 209–210
peptic, 208–209
Ultrasound, in gallbladder disease, 86
transvaginal, in ovarian cancer screening, 242
Urea cycle enzymes, defect in, 310. See also Ornithine transcarbamylase (OTC) deficiency.
Urea nitrogen/creatinine ratio, in liver failure, 58
in prerenal azotemia, 14
Uremia, erythrocyte indices in, 41
Uremic acidosis, 30
Uremic syndrome, 42–43
Urinary creatinine, diabetes mellitus and, 114
Urinary organic acid assay, in ornithine transcarbamylase deficiency, 310
Urinary oxalate, in ethylene glycol poisoning, 337, 338
Urine, specific gravity of, in minimal change nephrotic syndrome, 50
Urine output, decreased, in minimal change nephrotic syndrome, 45
Urobilinogen, absence of, from stool, in gallbladder disease, 87
Ursodeoxycholic acid, for gallstones, 88

Vanillylmandelic acid, in pheochromocytoma, 203
Varices, esophageal, in alcoholic liver disease, 81
Variegate porphyria, 92
laboratory findings in, 94t
photosensitivity of, 95
Vascular resistance, pulmonary, measurement of, 8
systemic, calculation of, 8
Vaso-occlusive crisis, in sickle cell disease, 256
Vertebral metastasis, back pain in, 359, 361
Virilism, in classic 21-hydroxylase deficiency, 151
Virilization, in Cushing disease, 162, 163
Vitamin D, for rickets, 401, 401
Vitamin D-deficiency osteomalacia, vs. low-turnover osteomalacia, 197
Vitamin D-deficiency rickets. See also Rickets.
25(OH)D absorption test for, 401
discussion of, 400–401
treatment of, 401, 401–402

Vomiting, in hyperammonemia, 309, 310
  in pyloric stenosis, 133, 134
Von Willebrand factor, 333, 334
Von Willebrand's disease, vs. hemophilia A,
  333–334

Water load test, for syndrome of inappropriate
  antidiuretic hormone secretion, 388
Watson-Schwartz test, modified, for acute
  hepatic porphyria, 90, 95
Western blot test, for human immunodeficiency
  virus, 404
Wilson's disease, abnormal liver studies in,
  evaluation of, 72
  bilirubin in, 72
  case study of, 71–75
  copper incorporation test for, 75
  diagnosis of, 74–75
  hemolytic anemia of, 74
  hepatic copper in, 74
  hepatic involvement of, 73–74
  Kayser-Fleischer rings in, 72, 74
  manifestations of, 73–74

Wilson's disease (Continued)
  neurological and psychiatric presentations of,
    74
  pathophysiology of, 73
  reticulocyte count in, 72
  serum ceruloplasmin in, 72, 74
  treatment of, 72, 75
  tremor in, 71

Xanthelasma, in familial hypertriglyceridemia,
  305
Xanthomas, in familial hypercholesterolemia,
  299, 300
  in familial hypertriglyceridemia, 305
X-ray, chest. See Chest X-ray.

Zollinger-Ellison syndrome, case study of, 207–
  211
  diarrhea in, 207, 208, 210
  differential diagnosis of, 208
  discussion of, 210
  hemorrhage in, 207, 208
  peptic ulcers caused by, 209
  treatment of, 210–211